Oxford Handbook of
Children's and
Young People's
Nursing

PUBLISHED AND FORTHCOMING
OXFORD HANDBOOKS IN NURSING

Oxford Handbook of General and Adult Nursing
George Castledine and Ann Close

Oxford Handbook of Children's and Young People's Nursing
Edited by Alan Glasper, Gillian McEwing, and Jim Richardson

Oxford Handbook of Mental Health Nursing
Edited by Patrick Callaghan and Helen Waldock

Oxford Handbook of Midwifery
Janet Medforth, Susan Battersby, Maggie Evans, Beverley Marsh, and Angela Walker

Oxford Handbook of Nurse Prescribing
Sue Beckwith and Penny Franklin

Oxford Handbook of Cancer Nursing
Edited by Mike Tadman and Dave Roberts

Oxford Handbook of Primary Care Nursing
Edited by Vari Drennan and Claire Goodman

Oxford Handbook of Cardiac Nursing
Edited by Karen Rawlings-Anderson and Kate Johnson

Oxford Handbook of
Children's and Young People's Nursing

Edited by

Edward Alan Glasper

Professor of Child Health Nursing,
School of Nursing and Midwifery,
University of Southampton, UK

Gillian McEwing

Senior Lecturer, Faculty of Health and Social Care,
University of Plymouth, UK

Jim Richardson

Principal Lecturer, School of Health Care Sciences,
University of Glamorgan, Pontypridd, UK

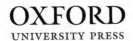

OXFORD
UNIVERSITY PRESS

OXFORD
UNIVERSITY PRESS

Great Clarendon Street, Oxford OX2 6DP

Oxford University Press is a department of the University of Oxford.
It furthers the University's objective of excellence in research, scholarship,
and education by publishing worldwide in

Oxford New York

Auckland Cape Town Dar es Salaam Hong Kong Karachi
Kuala Lumpur Madrid Melbourne Mexico City Nairobi
New Delhi Shanghai Taipei Toronto

With offices in

Argentina Austria Brazil Chile Czech Republic France Greece
Guatemala Hungary Italy Japan Poland Portugal Singapore
South Korea Switzerland Thailand Turkey Ukraine Vietnam

Oxford is a registered trade mark of Oxford University Press
in the UK and in certain other countries

Published in the United States
by Oxford University Press Inc., New York

British Library Cataloguing in Publication Data
Data available

Library of Congress Cataloging in Publication Data
Data available

Typeset by Newgen Imaging Systems (P) Ltd., Chennai, India
Printed in Italy
on acid-free paper by Legoprint S.p.A.

ISBN 0–19–856957–2 (flexicover.:alk.paper) 978–0–19–856957–2 (flexicover:alk paper)

10 9 8 7 6 5 4 3 2 1

Foreword

This handbook provides those inspired to and accepting of the challenges of nursing children with fundamental insight and essential knowledge to underpin their competent delivery of care.

Nursing children and young people is a privilege. In your care is a precious young life, deeply loved by many close family members and the very future of our society and world. If thus reflectively considered, the responsibility accepted by children's nurses to get care right is onerous. We must not only ensure the highest possible quality of age-specific physical care is given, but must also make sure that we protect and enhance the child's psychological, emotional, and social development.

The effects of our care will last a lifetime not only on the recipient child or young person, but potentially on all who care for or come into contact with them. Children's nursing not only includes the complexity of caring for our young at every stage of development, from neonate to young person, but also necessitates nursing skills involved in caring for the whole family. All this delivered within the tight confines of time available for healthcare delivery. This handbook is specifically designed for quick and easy access to essential elements of knowledge. It supports not only immediate safe delivery of care, but also prompts further in-depth exploration of a particular subject and provides a useful reminder of faded knowledge or expertise.

It is an essential handbook for the experienced and inexperienced within children's nursing.

Dr Judith Ellis MBE
Chair of Association of Chief Children's Nurses

Oxford University Press makes no representation, express or implied, that the drug dosages in this book are correct. Readers must therefore always check the product information and clinical procedures with the most up-to-date published product information and data sheets provided by the manufacturers and the most recent codes of conduct and safety regulations. The authors and the publishers do not accept responsibility or legal liability for any errors in the text or for the misuse or misapplication of material in this work.

Preface

As editors of this book, we are very conscious of how the world of children and young people's health care has changed in recent years. The health care of children, young people and their families is being delivered in new service formats and a range of settings. These demand nurses who are able to use high level skills in a versatile and transferable fashion. As a consequence these health care professionals must have accurate and up to the minute information that allows them to deliver the optimum standards of care expected by the families who put their trust in the National Health Service. Our aim is that this book will seamlessly bridge theory and practice in contemporary children's and young people's nursing. The prestigious Oxford University Press, in publishing this essential and timely book recognise that evidence-based practice must lie at the heart of children's and young people's health care .

In developing the Oxford Handbook of Children's and Young People's Nursing we decided at the outset to approach clinical and academic experts in this field of nursing to give our readers the utmost confidence in the provenance of the material embedded within the text. We therefore sourced many of our expert contributors through the membership of the Association of Chief Children's Nurses (ACCN) and we are confident that this Oxford Handbook represents the very best benchmarked practice from across the four countries of the United Kingdom. It has been a pleasure to have worked with the over three hundred children's and young people's nurses who contributed to this exciting new handbook with its imaginative design features. In launching this handbook we are conscious that our readers will want a quick and easy reference book which allows them to inform safe and effective practice in a range of clinical settings across the health care continuum. We have no doubts that this will be an indispensable book for any nurse working within the field of children's and young people's health care.

Alan Glasper, Gill Mcewing
and Jim Richardson
September 2006

Contents

Detailed contents

Key informants

Jane Coad
(also contributor) University of
West of England

Brenda Creaney
(also contributor) Royal Belfast
Hospital for Sick Children

Judith Ellis
Great Ormond Street
Hospital for Sick Children

Becky Healey
Cardiff & Vale NHS Trust

Angela Horsley
(also contributor) Royal Aberdeen
Children's Hospital

Nigel Lawrence
Royal Devon and Exeter NHS
Foundation Trust

Jan Newton
Southampton University Hospitals
NHS Trust

Lynne Robertson
Royal Hospital for Sick Children Glasgow

List of contributors

Penelope Aitken
Southampton University Hospitals
NHS Trust

Marion Aylott
University of Southampton

Jacqueline Baker
Maelor Hospital
Wrexham

Sarah Baker
Royal Devon and Exeter Hospital
NHS Foundation Trust

Zoe Baker
Royal Cornwall Hospital Trust

Lynne Barnes
Central Manchester and
Manchester Children's Hospitals
NHS Trust

Susie Barnes
Queen's University Belfast

John Bastin
University of Plymouth

Rebecca Battrell
Canterbury Christ Church
University

Nicola Birchley
Coventry University

Julie Black
Robert Gorden University,
Aberdeen

Neil Bloxham
Plymouth Hospitals NHS Trust

Eileen Brennan
Great Ormond Street Hospital
for Children NHS Trust

Nicola Brogan
Central Manchester and
Manchester Children's University
Hospitals NHS Trust

Gilly Bromilow
Royal Devon and Exeter NHS
Foundation Trust

Keith Bromwich
University of Coventry and
Warwickshire

Debra Broom
Royal Gwent Hospital Newport

Mark Broom
University of Glamorgan

Andrew J.S. Brown
Plymouth Hospitals NHS Trust

Pauline Carson
University of Wolverhampton

Rachel Carter
University of Plymouth

Anne Casey
Royal College of Nursing

Stefan Cash
University of Central England,
Birmungham

Margaret Chambers
University of Plymouth

Carol Chamley
Coventry University

Debbie Chant
South Devon Youth Offending
Team

Celia Charlton
Royal Devon and Exeter NHS
Foundation Trust

Alan Charters
Portsmouth Hospitals Trust

Janina Chell
Royal Cornwall Hospital Trust

Anna Chick
Royal Cornwall Hospital Trust

Sonya Clarke
Queen's University Belfast

Gerri Clay
University of Plymouth

Jane Coad
University of West of England

Annie Cole
Birmingham Children's Hospital
NHS Trust

Kerry Cook
Coventry University

Doris Corkin
Queen's University Belfast

Brenda Creaney
Royal Hospitals, Northern Ireland

Marc Crocker
Birmingham Children's Hospital
NHS Trust

Sue Danby
Royal Aberdeen Children's
Hospital

Pete Darley
Central Manchester and
Manchester Childrens University
Hospitals NHS Trust

Ruth Davies
Royal Devon and Exeter NHS
Foundation Trust

Sheila Davies
Contact a Family, London

Yvonne Davies
West Wales General Hospital
Carmarthen

Paula Dawson
Nottingham University Hospitals
NHS Trust

Nettie Dearmun
Oxford Brookes University

Jayne Deaves
South Devon Healthcare
NHS Trust

Fionnuala Diamond
Royal Belfast Hospital for Sick
Children

Maggie Doman
University of Plymouth

Pauline Donaldson
Royal Aberdeen Children's
Hospital

Mary Donnelly
University of Hertfordshire

Sarah Doyle
Royal Liverpool Children's
Hospital NHS Trust

Sue Earney
University of Glamorgan

Stephen Earnshaw
Royal Liverpool Children's Trust
(Alder Hey)

Julia Edge
South Devon Healthcare
NHS Trust

Marie Elen
Napier University
Edinburgh

Sarah Elworthy
Royal Devon and Exeter NHS
Foundation Trust

Andrea Fairclough
South Devon Youth Offending
Team

Rory Farrelly
Derby Hospitals NHS Foundation Trust

Claire Ferguson
Royal Liverpool Children's Hospital NHS Trust

Lynn Findlay
Royal Aberdeen Children's Hospital

Martin Firth
University of Nottingham

Paula Flint
Central Manchester and Manchester Children's University Hospitals NHS Trust

Anne Fothergill
University of Glamorgan

Jenny Freeman
Royal Devon and Exeter NHS Foundation Trust

Michelle Fuller
Southampton University Hospitals NHS Trust

Carmel Geoghegan
Central Manchester and Manchester Children's University Hospitals NHS Trust

Nicola J. Gibbons
Nottingham University Hospital NHS Trust

Andrea Gibson
Queen's University Belfast

Linda Gibson
Royal Devon and Exeter NHS Foundation Trust

Laura Gilbert
Canterbury Christ Church University

Alan Glasper
University of Southampton

James E. Glasper
Citizen's Advice Bureau Lymington Hampshire

Graham Gordon
Birmingham Children's Hospital NHS Trust

Liz Gormley-Fleming
University of Hertfordshire

Joanne Groves
Southampton University Hospitals NHS Trust

Carol Hall
University of Nottingham

Maureen Harrison
University of Southampton

Alison Hayes
Royal Devon and Exeter NHS Foundation Trust

Sarah Haywood
Royal Devon and Exeter NHS Trust

Pauline Heaton
Central Manchester and Manchester Children's University Hospitals NHS Trust

Alison Hegarty
Central Manchester and Manchester Children's University Hospitals NHS Trust

Janet Hetherington
Birmingham Children's Hospital, NHS Trust

Leyonie Higgins
Central Manchester and Manchester Children's University Hospitals NHS Trust

Sarah Hill
Royal Cornwall Hospital Trust

Louise Holliday
Royal Aberdeen Children's Hospital

Angela Horsley
NHS Grampian

Rachael Hufton
Central Manchester and
Manchester Children's University
Hospitals NHS Trust

Liz Hutchinson
Nottingham Children and
Young People's Rheumatology
Service

Melanie Hutton
Royal Hospital for Sick Children
Glasgow

Pam Iles
Southampton University Hospitals
NHS Trust

Jackie Imrie
Central Manchester and
Manchester Children's University
Hospitals NHS Trust

Kate Jackson
Napier University
Edinburgh

Pamela Joannidis
Hospital for Sick Children
Glasgow

Jackie Johnston
Napier University
Edinburgh

Denise Jonas
University of Salford & CMMC
NHS Trust

Christopher Jones
University of Nottingham

Kirsten Jones
Royal Devon and Exeter NHS
Foundation Trust

Julia Judd
Southampton University Hospitals
NHS Trust

Di Keeton
Southampton University Hospitals
NHS Trust

Melanie Kelly
Royal Cornwall Hospital Trust

Janet Kelsey
University of Plymouth

Marjorie Keys
Napier University
Edinburgh

Julie Kitchen
Royal Devon and Exeter NHS
Foundation Trust

Elizabeth Lane
Royal Devon and Exeter NHS
Foundation Trust

Gill Langmack
University of Nottingham

Helen Langton
University of Coventry

Angela Ledsham
University of Southampton

Gilli Lewis
Queen's University Belfast

Lorna Liggett
Queen's University Belfast

Tony Long
University of Salford

Geraldine Lyte
University of Manchester

Andrea Macarthur
Central Manchester and Manchester Children's University Hospitals
NHS Trust

Fiona MacDonald
Royal Aberdeen Children's
Hospital

Gill McEwing
University of Plymouth

Catherine Macfarlane
Royal Hospital for Sick Children
Edinburgh

Debbie McGirr
Napier University
Edinburgh

Brian McGowan
University of Ulster

Wendy M. McInally
Napier University and Royal
Hospital for Sick Children
Edinburgh

Lizanne McInnes
Royal Hospital For Sick
Children Glasgow

Lucelia Mackay
Robert Gordon University
Aberdeen

Irene McTaggart
University of Dundee

Nichola Maggs
Royal Gwent Hospital Newport

Elaine Mahoney
University of Glamorgan

Hazel Marriott
Nottingham University Hospitals
NHS Trust

Debbie Martin
Hertfordshire Partnership NHS
Trust

Kathryn Martin
Maelor Hospital
Wrexham

Sue Mason
Royal Devon and Exeter NHS
Foundation Trust

Pearl Mathews
Southampton University Hospitals
NHS Trust

Fiona Maxton
Napier University
Edinburgh

Lindy May
Great Ormond Street Hospital
for Children NHS Trust

Jean Mercer
Central Manchester and
Manchester Children's University
Hospitals NHS Trust

Ruth Mitchell
Napier University
Edinburgh

Sarah Mitchell
Royal Aberdeen
Children's Hospital

Hermione Montgomery
Birmingham Children's Hospital
NHS Trust

Fiona Moore
Action for Sick Children London

Dave Morgan
Central Manchester and
Manchester Children's University
Hospitals NHS Trust

Phil Morrow
Queen's University Belfast

Louise Mould
Royal Devon and Exeter NHS
Foundation Trust

Gary Mountain
University of Leeds

Pauline Musson
Southampton University Hospitals
NHS Trust

Jody Nevile
Royal Cornwall Hospital Trust

Frances Northeast
Nottingham University Hospitals
NHS Trust

Andrea O'Donnell
Royal Liverpool Children's Trust
(Alder Hey)

Anna Oddy
Central Manchester and
Manchester Children's University
Hospitals NHS Trust

Jan Orr
Royal Cornwall Hospital Trust

Lisa Owen
North East Wales NHS Trust
Wrexham

Fiona Smith
Royal Aberdeen Children's Hospital

Mary Smith
University of Glamorgan

Rosemary Smith
Robert Gordon University
Aberdeen

Barbara Southcombe
Royal Devon and Exeter NHS
Foundation Trust

Anne Spiers
Royal Hospital
for Sick Children Glasgow

Anne Squire
Central Manchester and
Manchester Children's University
Hospitals NHS Trust

Amanda Stoner
University of Leeds

Helen Strike
Southmead Hospital Bristol

Rhona Stuart
Royal Aberdeen Children's Hospital

Kathryn Summers
Canterbury Christ Church
University

Krystyna Sutkowski
North East Wates NHS Trust

Karen Swanson
Southampton University Hospitals
NHS Trust

Sue Swift
Royal Aberdeen Children's
Hospital

Alison Tait
University College London
Hospitals NHS Trust

Chris Taylor
Southampton University Hospitals
NHS Trust

John Thain
University of Wolverhampton

Catherine Thornton
Central Manchester and
Manchester Children's University
Hospitals NHS Trust

Donald Todd
Royal Aberdeen Children's
Hospital

Jayne Tomlinson
Birmingham Children's Hospital
NHS Trust

Denise Toplis
Royal Devon and Exeter NHS
Foundation Trust

Angie Tims
University Hospitals Coventry and
Warwickshire NHS Trust

Ruth Trengove
South Devon Healthcare NHS
Trust

Catherine Trower
Royal Hospital for Sick Children

Jacqueline Ulyatt
Nottingham University Hospitals
NHS Trust

Ruth Underhill
Southampton University Hospitals
NHS Trust

Peter Vickers
University of Hertfordshire

Louise Viljoen
Southampton University Hospitals
NHS Trust

Angela Waddell
Royal Hospital For Sick Children
Edinburgh

Jan Walmsley
Royal Cornwall Hospital Trust

Janice Watson
University of Southampton

Lesley Wayne
University of Plymouth

Fiona White
Central Manchester and
Manchester Children's University
Hospitals NHS Trust

Sarah Wiggins
Royal Devon and Exeter NHS
Foundation Trust

Veronica Wilbourn
University of Huddersfield

Lisa Marie Wilkie
Royal Devon and Exeter NHS
Foundation Trust

Leanna Will
Robert Gordon University
Aberdeen

Caroline Williams
West Wales General Hospital
Carmarthen

Jo Williams
Birmingham Children's Hospital
NHS Trust

Maureen Wiltshire
Southampton University Hospitals
NHS Trust

Sarah Jane Woolliscroft
Central Manchester and
Manchester Children's University
Hospitals NHS Trust

Elizabeth Wright
Southampton University
Hospital NHS Trust

Symbols and abbreviations

5-ASA	5-aminosalicyclic acid
ABC	airway, breathing, and circulation
ABCD	airway, breathing, circulation, disability
ABO	blood groups
ACE	angiotensin-converting enzme
ADHD	attention-deficit/hyperactivity disorder
AGN	acute glomerulonephritis
AIDS	acquired immunodeficiency syndrome
ALL	acute lymphoblastic leukaemia
AML	acute myeloid leukaemia
AOI	apnoea of infancy
AOP	apnoea of prematurity
APLE	apparent life-threatening event
ASC	action for Sick Children
ATLS	acute tumour lysis syndrome
ATP	adenosine triphosphate
AVPU	alert, responds to voice, pain, unresponsive
BIH	benign intracranial hypertension
BMI	body mass index
bpm	beats per minute
BSA	bovine serum albumin
CAB	Citizens Advice Bureau
CAMHS	Child and Adolescent Mental Health Services
CDGP	constitutional delay of growth and puberty
CF	cystic fibrosis
CFTR	cystic fibrosis transmembrane receptor
CJD	Creutzfeldt-Jakob disease
CO_2	carbon dioxide
COSHH	control of substances hazardous to health
CMV	cytomegalovirus
CNS	central nervous system
CPAP	continuous positive airway pressure
CPK	creatinine phosphokinase
CPM	continual passive movement
CPR	cardiopulmonary resuscitation
CRP	C-reactive protein
CRT	capillary refill time
CSF	cerebrospinal fluid

CT	computed tomography
CVAD	central venous access device
CVP	central venous pressure
DDH	developmental dysplasia of the hip
DfES	Department for Education and Skills
DIC	disseminated intravascular coagulation
DKA	diabetic ketoacidosis
DMARD	disease-modifying anti-rheumatic drug
DMD	Duchenne muscular dystrophy
DMSA	Dimescaptosuccinic acid (renal scan)
DNA	deoxyribonucleic acid
DOH	Department of Health
DTaP/dTaP	diphtheria, tetanus, and pertussis (vaccine)
ECG	electrocardiogram
EEG	electroencephalogram
EMLA	Eatectic Mixture of Lidocaine and Prilocaine
ENT	ear, nose, and throat
ET	endotracheal
EUA	examination under anaesthetic
FDA	Federal Drug Administration
FiO_2	Inspired fraction of oxygen
FLACC	Faces, Legs, Activity, Cry and Consolability
FOG	frequency of grammar
FS	febrile seizure
FSA	Food Standards Agency
FSH	follicle-stimulating hormone
FTU	finger-tip units
GABHS	group A beta-haemolytic streptococci
GAG	glycosaminoglycan
Gal-L-P	galactose-L-phosphate
Gal-L-PUT	galactose-L-phosphate uridyl transferase
GBS	group B streptococci
GCS	Glasgow coma scale
G-CSF	granulocyte-colony stimulating factor
GnRH	gonadotrophin-releasing hormone
GOR	gastro-oesophageal reflux
GP	general practitioner
HAART	highly active antiretroviral therapy
HAI	healthcare-associated infection
HAV	hepatitis A virus
HbA	haemoglobin A (Adult)
HbAlc	type of Haemoglobin checked to monitor diabetes control

HbS	haemoglobin S (sickle)
HBV	hepatitis B virus
HCV	hepatitis C virus
HbcAb	hepatitis B core antibody
HbeAb	hepatitis B e antibody
HbeAg	hepatitis B e antigen
HbsAb	hepatitis B surface antibody
HbsAg	hepatitis B surface antigen
HDU	high-dependency unit
HHV-6	human herpes virus 6
Hib	*Haemophilus influenzae b*
HIV	human immunodeficiency virus
HMA	Homeopathic Medical Association
HSV	herpes simplex virus
HUS	haemolytic uraemic syndrome
HVA	homovanillic acid
HVS	high vaginal swab
IBD	inflammatory bowel disease
IBS	irritable bowel syndrome
ICP	intracranial pressure
Ig	immunoglobulin
IPV	polio (vaccine)
IQ	intelligence quotient
ITP	idiopathic thrombocytopenic purpura
IUGR	intra-uterine growth retardation
IV	intravenous
IVF	*in vitro* fertilization
JCA	juvenile chronic arthritis
JIA	juvenile idiopathic arthritis
LAD	language-acquisition device
LH	luteinizing hormone
LP	lumbar puncture
LRD	living-related donor
LREC	local research ethics committee
LTB	laryngotracheobronchitis
MAS	meconium aspiration syndrome
M, C&S	Microscopy, culture, and sensitivity
MCU	micturating cystourethrogram
MCV	Molluscum contagiosum virus
MenC	meningitis C
MHRA	Medicines and Healthcare Products Regulations Authority
mIBG	meta-iodo-benzyl-guanidine

MMR	measles, mumps, and rubella (vaccine)
MODY	maturity-onset diabetes mellitus in the young
MPS	mucopolysaccharidoses
MREC	Medical Research Ethics Committee
MRI	magnetic resonance imaging
MRSA	methicillin-resistant *Staphylococcus aureus*
NAO	National Audit Office
NAWCH	National Association for the Welfare of Children in Hospital
NBM	nil by mouth
NES	NHS Education Scotland
NG	nasogastric
NHS	National Health Service
NICE	National Institute for Clinical Excellence
NMC	Nursing and Midwifery Council
NPA	Nasopharyngeal aspirate
NPIS	National Poisons Information Service
NASID	non-steroidal anti-inflammatory drugs
NSF	National Service Framework
PCA	patient-controlled analgesia
P_{CO_2}	partial pressure of CO_2
PCOS	polycystic overian syndrome
PCR	Polymerase chain reaction
PEEP	positive end-expiratory pressure
PFM	peak expiratory flowmeter
PIPP	Premature Infant Pain Profile
PICU	paediatric intensive care unit
PKU	phenylketonuria
PN	parenteral nutrition
PNET	primitive neuro-ectodermal tumour
P_{O_2}	partial pressure of oxygen
PPE	personal protective equipment
PPP	Paediatric Pain Profile
PREP	post-registration education and practice
PUV	posterior urethial valves
PVC	Polyvinyl choloride
RCN	Royal College of Nursing
RDS	respiratory distress syndrome
RhD	rhesus positive
RMS	rhabdomyosarcoma
RNA	ribonucleic acid
RPE	retinal pignant epithelium
rpm	respirations per minute

RSV	respiratory syncytial virus
SaO_2	arterial oxygen saturation
SCD	sickle cell disease
SCID	severe combined immunodeficiency
SDLD	surfactant-deficient lung disease
SICP	standard infection control precautions
SIDS	sudden infant death syndrome
SIMV	synchronized intermittent mechanical ventilation
SMBG	self-monitoring of blood glucose
SMOG	standard measure of gobbledegook
SpO_2	saturation pressure of oxygen
SRNS	steroid-resistant nephrotic syndrome
SSNS	steroid-sensitive nephrotic syndrome
SSRI	serotonin re-uptake inhibitor
STC	slow-transit constipation
STI	sexually transmitted infection
$t_{1/2}$	half-life
T_3	triiodothyronine
T_4	thyroxine
TBSA	total body surface area
TENS	transcutaneous electrical nerve stimulation
T_d	volume doubling time
TPR	Temperature, pulse, and respiration
TSH	thyroid-stimulating syndrome
TTN	transient tachypnoea of the newborn
O_2	oxygen
OI	oxygen index
OSA	obstructive sleep apnoea
PaO_2	partial pressure of oxygen
U&Es	urea and electrolytes
UKCCSG	UK Children's Cancer Group
UTI	urinary tract infection
UVB	ultraviolet B
VMA	vanillic mandelic acid
VNS	vagal nerve stimulation
VUR	vesico-ureteral reflux
VZV	Varicella zoster virus
WCC	white cell count
WHO	World Health Organization
XLA	X-linked gammaglobulinaemia
YAG	Yttrium aluminium garnet
ZIG	zoster immunoglobulin

Normal growth and development

Physical growth and its measurement

Pattern of growth

Growth proceeds in a continuous pattern but can be sporadic; the most rapid growth takes place *in utero*, during the first 2 years of life and in adolescence. However, the growth rate of an individual can accelerate or decelerate in response to illness, changes in nutrition, or environmental changes.

Length/height

- An infant's length increases by 12 cm during the first 6 months.
- By 1 year the infant's height has increased by almost 50% and by the age of 2 years the child is about half his/her adult height.
- After 2 years the increase in height is 5–7.5 cm/year.
- Adolescence then brings a 'growth spurt', following which height and weight are gained slowly until adult size is achieved.

Measurement

- Measure an infant's length on a measuring board (figure). Place the baby with his/her head against the top of the board and the heels of his/her feet at the foot board.
- Measure the height of a child when he/she is standing upright. Ask the child to remove his/her shoes and stand as tall and straight as possible with his/her head in the mid line and his/her line of vision in parallel to the floor. Most accuracy is gained by using a wall-mounted stadiometer (figure).

Weight

- On average an infant gains 600–800 g in weight per month.
- Birth weight doubles by 6 months.
- Weight triples by 1 year.
- From 2 years weight is gained at approximately 3 kg/year.

Measurement

- Infants should be weighed naked, and preferably at the same time of day if repeated measurements are needed.

Head circumference

- The head growth of an infant is rapid: in the first 6 months the circumference increases by between 8 and 9 cm.
- By the first year there is an increase of 33% in the overall size of the head.
- The size of the skull is closely related to the size of the brain.

Measurement

- Use a paper disposable tape-measure for this measurement as linen tape-measures stretch and produce inaccurate results.
- Measure the infant's head around the point of greatest circumference—this is usually slightly above the eyebrows and pinna of the ears and around the occipital prominence at the back of the skull (figure).

Gill McEwing University of Plymouth

Surface area

- This measurement is important for the prescription of some drugs.
- Once the child's height and weight are known you can calculate his surface area using the body surface area nomogram.

Further reading

Hockenberry, M.J., Wilson, D., Winkelstein, M.L., and Kline, N.E. (2003). *Wong's Nursing Care of infants and children*, 7th edn. Mosby, St Louis.

Measuring board

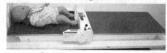

Stadiometer

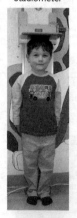

Circumferential measurements

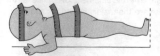

Figures reproduced by kind permission of Elsevier.

Physical development

Factors affecting growth and development

- Genetic/chromosomal
- Racial factors
- Endocrine system
- Drugs
- Illness: children grow more slowly during periods of illness, but after recovery there may be increased growth to catch up
- Nutrition: poorly nourished children grow more slowly and do not reach full potential size; malnutrition can have a permanent effect on some parts of the brain and nervous system
- Environment: the ability to practise skills, e.g. crawling, walking.

Measuring development

Development is measured using developmental scales. There are four major areas.
- *Physical:* growth, vision, hearing, locomotion, and coordination
- *Cognitive:* language and understanding
- *Psychosocial:* adapting to the society and culture to which the child belongs
- *Emotional:* control of feelings and emotions

The charts by Sheridan (1975) and Denver (1990) cited in Bee (1997) were developed to show what can be expected at key stages of development.

Differences in rate

There may be individual differences in the rate and timing of developmental progress.

Developmental assessment

The health visitor usually carries out these assessments, but they could be carried out by a general practitioner or paediatrician. They include the evaluation of:
- Locomotion or gross motor development, referring to large muscle skills
- Fine motor or manipulation skills: referring to small muscle skills
- Hearing and speech
- Vision
- Social development, e.g. feeding, dressing, and social behaviour

In order to assess deviations from the normal, it is first necessary to know about normal development. The development of a child birth to 18 months is very complex. These are the major milestones and their approximate age of appearance:

- smiles   1–2 months
- laughs   6 months
- sits
  - with support   6 months
  - without support   8–9 months

- crawls   8–9 months
- stands/walks   12 months
- pincer grip   12 months
- delicate pincer   18 months
- walks backwards   18 months

All aspects of development are interlinked, and skills are acquired sequentially. An example of this is the sequence of development of motor skills, which is often described as cephalocaudal, i.e. head (cephalo) to toe via the spine (caudal). Initially head control is developed before the baby is able to sit independently; this is followed by crawling and finally control of the lower limbs for standing and walking.

Further reading

Bee, H. (1997). *The developing child*, 6th edn. London, Harper Collins.

Hockenberry, M.J., Wilson, D., Winkelstein, M.L., Kline, N.E. (2003) *Wong's nursing care of infants and children*, 7th edn. St Louis, Mosby.

www.childdevelopmentinfo.com/development/

Developmental milestones

Newborn

In ventral suspension the head droops below the plane of the body. When the baby is pulled to sit there is marked head lag.

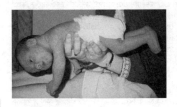

One month

Posture and large movement

- When the baby is pulled to it, the head lags until the body is vertical, when head is held momentarily erect before falling forward.
- When held sitting, the back is one complete curve.
- In ventral suspension, the head is in line with body and the hips are semi-extended.

 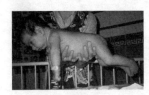

Vision and fine movement

- Pupils react to light.
- Shuts eyes tightly when light is shone in them.
- Fixes and follows.
- Watches mother's nearby face when she feeds or talks to him.

Hearing and speech

- Startled by sudden noise.
- Stops whimpering and (usually) turns towards sound of nearby soothing voice.
- Cries lustfully when hungry or uncomfortable.
- Guttural noises when content.

Social behaviour and play

- Sucks well.
- Sleeps most of the time when not being fed or handled.
- Expression still vague—more alert later, progressing to social smile and responsive vocalizations at 5–6 weeks.

Gill McEwing, University of Plymouth

Three months
Posture and large movement
- Supine, prefers to lie with head in midline, limb movements smoother.
- Pulled to sit little or no head lag.
- In ventral suspension, head held well above line of body.
- Prone lifts head and upper chest, uses fore arms for support, buttocks flat.

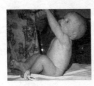
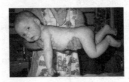

Vision and fine movement
- Visually alert, turns head deliberately to look around.
- Watches movements of own hands and demonstrates finger play.
- Recognizes feeding bottle and makes eager movements as it approaches.
- Defensive blink present.
- Holds rattle for a few seconds but does not look at it at the same time.
Hearing and speech
- Sudden loud noise still causes distress
- Definite quietening or smiling in response to mother's voice.
- Vocalizes happily when spoken to; can also vocalize when playing alone.
- Cries when uncomfortable or angry.
Social behaviour and play
- Intense gaze at mother's face when being fed.
- Reacts to familiar situations by showing excitement.
- Enjoys bathing.
- Responds with obvious pleasure when played with.

Six months
Posture and large movement
- Supine raises head to look at feet, lifts legs into vertical, and grasps feet.
- When hands are held, braces shoulders and pulls self to sit.
- Held sitting, head firmly erect, and back straight. Can sit momentarily alone.
- Held standing, bears weight on feet and bounces up and down.
- When placed prone, lifts head and chest well up, supporting him/herself on extended arms.

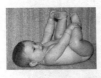

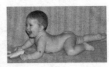

Figures in this topic reproduced by kind permission of Elsevier.

Vision and fine movement
- Visually insatiable, moves head and eyes eagerly.
- Immediate fixation on interesting small objects at 30 cm.
- Uses whole hand to palmar grasp and passes object from one hand to the other.
- When toys fall outside visual field, eyes do not follow them.

Hearing and speech
- Vocalizes tunefully to self and others.
- Using single or double syllables—adah, goo, aroo.
- Laughs and chuckles.
- Screams with annoyance.
- Demonstrates different responses to mother's tone of voice.

Social behaviour and play
- Reaches out and grasps small toys.
- Plays with feet and hands.
- Puts hands around bottle and pats it.
- Shakes rattle deliberately to make sound.
- Friendly with strangers but does show some anxiety if approached too quickly.

One year
Posture and large movement
- Crawls on hands and knees, shuffles on buttocks or bear walks.
- Usually able to stand alone, may walk.

Vision and fine movement
- Looks in correct place for toys dropped out of sight.
- Recognizes familiar people at 7 m distance.

Hearing and speech
- Turns immediately to own name.
- Comprehends simple instructions associated with gesture, e.g. 'come to mummy'.

Social behaviour and play
- Drinks from a cup.
- Waves 'bye-bye', plays 'pat-a-cake'.
- Helps with dressing, e.g. holding out arm for sleeve.

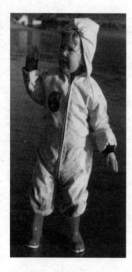

Further reading

Hockenberry, M.J., Wilson, D., Winkelstein, M.L., Kline, N.E. (2003). *Wong's nursing care of infants and children*. 7th Edition. Mosby, St Louis.
MacGregor, J. (2000). *Introduction to the anatomy and physiology of children*. Routledge, London.
www.childdevelopmentinfo.com

Cognitive development

The question of *how* children learn has been an area of development that has been debated at great length, but what we do know is that within the first few years of a child's life, including the time *in utero*, he/she will learn more than at any other period of existence. The concept of cognition is a vast subject covering memory, attention, language, social cognition, reasoning, and problem solving.

Cognition is the process by which the developing individual becomes acquainted with the world in which they live. Children ultimately have the ability to reason abstractly, to think logically, and to organize intellectual functions or performances into higher-order structures. Cognitive development consists of age-related changes that occur in mental activities.

Nature versus nurture debate

The nature (genetics) versus nurture (environment) debate is one of the most contested arguments in relation to age-related developmental changes. The debate wrestles with the question of 'What is the best possible explanation for how development takes place?' The ideal position is that all human activities are a product of both nature and nurture.

Influential learning theorists

Piaget's theory of cognitive development

Jean Piaget (1896–1980) developed the most comprehensive theory of cognitive development. Piaget viewed the child as an organism adapting to his/her environment, and cognition progressing through a series of hierarchical stages. These stages are described as *universal* across all cultures and *invariant*, meaning that all children pass through the same stages in the same sequence, unless there are underlying problems. In the process of learning, the child is viewed as an isolated individual who adapts the world around himself/herself through processes of:

- schemas
- assimilation
- accommodation
- equilibrium.

Piaget developed four stages of cognitive development	
Stage	**Approximate age**
Sensorimotor	Birth to 2 years
Pre-operational	2–7 years
Concrete operational	7–11 years
Formal operational	11 years plus

Carol Chamley, Coventry University

Vygotsky's theory of cognitive development

Lev Vygotsky (1896–1934) believed that the child is born into a complex cultural world of social relationships. Vygotsky proposed two aspects of development:

- natural line of organic growth and maturation
- cultural improvement of psychological function.

He proposed the *zone of proximal development,* which is the distance between the actual developmental level as determined by independent problem solving, and the *level of potential development* as determined through problem solving under adult guidance or in collaboration with a capable peer.

Bruner's theory

Bruner (1966) describes three modes of representing the world: *enactive, iconic,* and *symbolic.* He proposed the idea of *scaffolding,* which is a form of apprenticeship or guided participation, where children engage in cultural processes where adults guide, model, and scaffold between old and new practices.

Information-processing theories

The information-processing approach to cognitive development is based on an analogy between the computer and the human mind. This represents the view that the mind is like a system that manipulates symbols according to a set of rules.

Further reading

Bukatko, D., Daehler, M.W. (2004). *Child development: a thematic approach,* 5th edn. Houghton Mifflin, New York.

Gross, R. (2005). *Psychology: the science of the mind and behaviour,* 5th edn. Hodder Arnold, London.

Psi-Café. www.psy.pdx.edu/PsiCafe/Cognitive Development.

www.psy.pdx.edu/PsiCafe?Areas?Developmental/CogDev-Child#WhatIs

Language development

Many theories have attempted to explain language development It is known that children learning any language progress through similar periods of development. They begin by learning the elements of the sound of their own language, progressing through the stages of one-word and then two-word utterances to begin using words in combinations integrating appropriate grammatical forms. By the age of 3 years they are producing short sentences intelligible to most adults, and finally they progress to using sentences recognizable as matching adult forms. Theorists have argued that language is learned just like any other behaviour and that by repeating back infant vocalizations adults positively reinforce the development of speech. Some believe language to be an innate ability and that children are born with a genetic mechanism for the acquisition of language, called a 'language-acquisition device' (LAD). It has also been proposed that critical periods exist that determine the universality and invariant order for the process of language development. However, we cannot ignore the importance of social influences on language development; interactions between the parent and child establish the communicative function of vocalization, and throughout development adults both correct and reinforce speech through everyday communications and play.

Further reading

Cusson, R.M. (2003). Factors influencing language development in preterm infants. *Journal of Obstetric, Gynecologic, and Neonatal Nursing*, **32**, 402–9.

🖳 www.childdevelopmentinfo.com/development/language_development.shtml

Janet Kelsey, University of Plymouth

Language development

Age	Normal language development	Normal speech development	Intelligibility
Infant	Cooing	Non-cry vocalic sounds	
	Babbling	Consonant–vowel syllables with intonation patterns	
1 year	Appearance of first 2–3 words	Omits most final and some initial consonants	Usually no more than 25% intelligible to familiar listener
	Imitates sounds of animals	Substitutes consonants m, w, p, b, k, g, n, t, d, and h for more difficult sounds	
2 years	Uses 2–3-word phrases	Uses above consonants with vowels but inconsistently and with substitution	50–65% of spoken language can be understood
	Has a vocabulary of 250–300 words. Can put together simple 2–3-word phrases	Word usage and comprehension develops but comprehension lags behind expressive ability	
	Uses I, me, and you	Can understand much adult communication directed to them	
3 years	Says 4–5-word sentences, with a vocabulary of about 900 words. Uses who, what, and where. Uses plurals, pronouns, and prepositions	Says b, t, d, k, and g, but r and l may be unclear. W is either omitted or substituted. Often repeats self	75% of communications are intelligible
4–5 years	Vocabulary has increased to about 1500–2100 words. Sentences are complete and most grammar correct	Says f and v. May still have some distortion of r, l, s, z, sh, ch, y, and th	All speech can be understood, although some words may not be perfectly enunciated
5–6 years	Vocabulary of 3000 words	May still distort s, z, ch, sh, and j	

Social development

Human beings are social animals. In every society children must learn the rules, behaviours, and values in order to function within that group. This is called socialization; it is achieved by observational learning and direct teaching.

A society's rules and standards of behaviour are called social 'norms'; they are not usually written down, yet they govern our behaviour and our expectations of the behaviour of others. Children tend to learn them as facts. Social norms are developed and perpetuated because they give society stability.

The individual is required to:
• recognize self, develop self-concept, and personality
• enter relationships: parents, family, peers, and others
• go beyond people's behaviour to their intentions and perceived expectations.

The ultimate of aim of socialization is to give children the ability to discipline themselves, to compromise between what they want and what society demands of them. Socialization is a lifelong process; there is a need to learn new norms at each stage of the life span. Children will have to cope with learning new rules at playgroup, school, groups, university, and employment.

To understand social development, it must be remembered:
• it is closely connected to both psychological and cognitive development
• children are part of a large network of people and activities
• it is influenced by the relationship of the child to his/her mother, and to other important relationships that the child engages in from the beginning of life.

Theories of social development

A number of theories have been proposed to assist in our understanding of social development of children. Piaget (1932) argued that children's relationships with adults were structured along a *vertical dimension*, meaning that relationships were unequal or *asymmetrical*. By contrast, he viewed children's relationships with other children as more balanced or *symmetrical* and egalitarian, and structured upon a *horizontal plane*.

Identity

The differentiation of *self* begins in infancy and continues throughout childhood where there are changes in the development of the *self concept* and the relationship of self to others. As children move through childhood their self-descriptions become more complex, and by adolescence they forge a more coherent view of self which integrates various characteristics.

Carol Chamley, Coventry University

Theorists consider biological factors, social learning theory, cognitive–developmental factors, gender schemas, and social–cognitive theories important to the development of identity. Furthermore, there are several theories relating to the inherent processes of acquiring a sex role or sex-role identification.

Ethnicity

Ethnic identity can be considered as awareness of one's own ethnicity and it is closely linked to, and parallels, developing ethnicity in others. By the age of 4–5 years children seem to be able to identify fundamental differences, and by 8–9 years children understand that ethnicity is constant.

Relationships

Once the infant has formed a rudimentary concept of self and established particular habits, the next stage is the utilization of these skills to form relationships. Relationships are based on interactions, but require the integration of self with others. Types of relationships include parental relationships, family relationships, sibling relationships, peers/friendship relationships, acquaintance relationships, and love/sexual relationships.

Summary of social development (adapted from Keenan 2002).[1]

Age	Milestones
0–6 months	By 6 months of age, infants are aware of, and are interested in, other infants
6–12 months	Infants show an interest in their peers
12–24 months	Engage in parallel play, use language, development of self-understanding, first evidence of behaviours such as empathy, engagement in rules of social exchange, child operates according to desire
3 years	Engage in cooperative play, behaviours are based on desire, dominant hierarchies evolve in peer groups
4 years	Engage in associative play, emergence of socio-cognitive conflict
6 years	Desire to spent more time with peers, shared interests, coordinated successful play
7–9 years	The goal of friendship is peer acceptance
Early adolescence	Friendship is centred on self-disclosure and intimacy, peer group is organized around crowds and cliques, first appearance of adolescent egocentrism
Late adolescence	Friends increasingly provide emotional support, adolescent egocentrism declines

Further reading

Schaffer, R. (2003). *Social development*. Blackwell, London.
Taylor, J., Woods, M. (2005). *Early childhood studies: a holistic introduction*, 2nd edn. Hodder Arnold, London.
National Electronic Library for Child Health ▣ www.libraries.nelh.nhs.uk/childhealth

Psychological theories of attachment

Attachment theory overlaps with behavioural, biological, and interpersonal theories and cognitive development, and aims to:

- describe the character of the lasting relationships between a person and significant others (often the person's carers, in the case of the child)
- explain those relationships in terms of behaviours, emotions, and cognition.

Attachment styles

Secure attachment

These are seen in the way the child responds to their carer—with sensitivity, empathy, and affection. There is often a degree of perception, insightfulness, nurturing, and consideration for the other person, which can result in altruistic behaviours. If children see their carer as responsive, supporting, and available, they are cooperative, easily comforted, and eager to explore new situations.

Insecure attachments

These develop in response to inconsistencies, uncertainty, and abuse or neglect by the carer(s):

- *Anxious–ambivalent:* the child appears hostile and dependent when upset. As seen in separation anxiety: there are often reactions of protest, despair, and detachment when the parent leaves the child, and avoidance of the parent by the child when he or she returns.
- *Anxious–avoidant:* distrust and a lack of confidence in getting a response from his/her carers results in the child becoming distant, not seeking support if upset.
- *Disorganized–disorientated:* the child demonstrates a mixture of avoidance, anger, and behavioural issues.

John Bowlby (1969) proposed a model for early parent–child interactions that influence development of the infant's understanding of, and connections to, others. Genetically pre-programmed and instinctive, this development also depends on the degree of attention and care given by the significant carer, serving as a guide for the child's social expectations, perceptions, and behavioural interactions, not only in childhood but also in adolescence and adulthood.

A reciprocal complex relationship results. Fundamental to the child's psychological well-being, the strength and quality of the emotional attachment of the carers/parents to each other affects the emotional and behavioural ability of the child. Likewise, the behaviour of the child will also affect the parents.

Gill Langmack, University of Nottingham

Erikson's eight stages of development

Infant	Trust vs mistrust
	Needs maximum comfort with minimal uncertainty to trust him/herself, others, and the environment
Toddler	Autonomy vs shame and doubt
	Works to master physical environment while maintaining self-esteem
Pre-schooler	Initiative vs guilt
	Begins to initiate, not imitate, activities; develops conscience and sexual identity
School-age child	Industry vs inferiority
	Tries to develop a sense of self-worth by refining skills
Adolescent	Identity vs role confusion
	Tries integrating many roles (child, sibling, student, athlete, worker) into a self-image under role model and peer pressure
Young adult	Intimacy vs isolation
	Learns to make personal commitment to another as spouse, parent, or partner
Middle-age adult	Generativity vs stagnation
	Seeks satisfaction through productivity in career, family, and civic interests
Older adult	Integrity vs despair
	Reviews life accomplishments, deals with loss and preparation for death

Further reading

Grossmann, K.E., Grossmann, K. (2003). Universality of human social attachment as an adaptive process. In *Attachment and bonding: a new synthesis* (Dahlem Workshop Report 92), (ed. C.S. Carter, L. Ahnert, K.E. Grossmann *et al.*). MIT Press, Boston, MA. ▣ www.fu-berlin.de/dahlem/DWR%2092_Attachment/Chapter%2010.pdf

International Attachment Network (2002). *Questions and Answers* ▣ www.attachmentnetwork.org/questions.html

Sondin, D.J. (2005). Attachment theory and psychotherapy. *The Therapist*, Jan/Feb. ▣ www.daniel-sonkin.com/attachment_psychotherapy.htm

Promoting child health and health promotion models

It is difficult to put boundaries around health promotion, as much of nursing children, young people, and their families is about promoting their health in the widest and narrowest sense, e.g. influencing social policy or immunizing children.

- Health promotion = health education + healthy public policy
- Health promotion = empowering people to take control of their own health.
- Nursing children = empowering children and their families to achieve the best outcomes possible for their individual situations.
- National Service Framework (NSF) for Children and Young People (2004) suggests that the focus should be child centred.

Greater emphasis on public health is occurring because it is recognized that some daily activities have an enormous influence on health from, for example, the narrow confines of personal nutrition to the wider impact of social policy around nutrition. Public health medicine focuses on disease prevention, monitoring, and management.

Health promotion is about the protection and promotion of health. The models of health promotion demonstrate that public health and health promotion are inextricably linked.

Hall and Elliman (2003) is a review of child health in Britain. This report, plus other government policies, suggest that nutrition is a crucially important aspect of child health—the prevention of obesity being a prime target at present due to its increasing prevalence. Good nutrition will also maintain dental health, skin integrity, hydration, and pain-free elimination. A new problem related to diet is the development of type 2 diabetes mellitus in children in the UK.

Approaches used in health promotion

There are five main approaches to promoting health.

Approach	Objective
1. Medical or preventive	To prevent disease
2. Behaviour change	To facilitate individuals/groups to make healthy choices
3. Educational/information giving	To provide individuals/groups with information about how to be healthy
4. Empowerment/client centred	To enable individuals/groups to take control of their own health
5. Social change/radical/ political	To develop/adapt policies/environments that support healthy choices

Christine Rhodes and Veronica Wilbourn, University of Huddersfied

Models of health promotion

Various theoretical frameworks of health promotion have been developed, known as models. These models provide structure to help direct and manage practice.

There are a number of health promotion models. The Tannahill model has been selected to demonstrate different ways of promoting health in relation to preventing obesity in childhood. Historically, malnutrition has been the main focus of practice but today, in our comparatively affluent society, obesity is of great concern.

Tannahill's model of health promotion

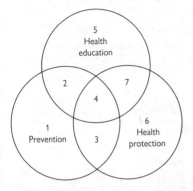

Reproduced from *Health promotion: Models and Values* (2nd ed), Figure 4.1 (p.59) by Downie, R.S., Tannahill, A (1996), by permission of Oxford University Press.

A Venn diagram demonstrates the different relationships between the various health promotion activities described by Tannahill's model. Domains 1, 5, and 6 are the main areas of activity, because health promotion is about prevention, education, and protection, as highlighted by Tones and Tilford's equation. Domain 4 is central to all activities concerned with promoting health.

Tannahill's seven domains

	Domain	Examples in practice	Obesity
1	Preventive services	Developmental surveillance, immunization	Monitor growth in children
2	Preventive health education	Educating to influence lifestyle	Education about physical activity, change eating patterns. e.g. promote family meal times
3	Preventive health protection	Fluoridation of water supplies; motor cycle helmet and seat belt legislation; making healthy choices easier	National school fruit scheme; 4–6-year-olds receive a free piece of fruit each day
4	Health education for preventive health protection	Central to all practice—involves *all* aspects of health promotion	All examples + 5-a-day campaign—recommends at least five portions of fruit and vegetables a day
5	Positive health education	Positive reinforcement of health promoting behaviour, e.g. exercise, to develop fitness, health-related life skills	National curriculum: personal health social education—information about healthy food, exercise
6	Positive health protection	Promotion of no smoking environments/provision of user-friendly leisure facilities	Healthier school meals—Jamie Oliver's campaign
7	Health education aimed at positive health protection	Raising awareness of health issues amongst general population and policy makers	Lobbying for healthier school tuck shops/educating parents

Further reading

Department of Health (2004). *National service framework for children, young people and maternity services*. DoH, London.

Hall, D.M.B., and Elliman, D. (2003). *Health for all Children*, 4th edn. Oxford University Press, Oxford.

Downie, R.S., Tannahill, C., Tannahill, A. (2004). *Health promotion: models and values*, 2nd edn. Oxford University Press, Oxford.

Immunization

To achieve herd immunity in a population it is vital to ensure that children are appropriately immunized against preventable diseases. Inaccurate press coverage related to the adverse effects of certain vaccines has frightened some parents, resulting in less than optimum uptake of immunizations. This not only puts individual children in jeopardy but potentially exposes larger groups of not yet immunized children to unnecessary risk. It is, therefore, an integral part of the admission process for a nurse to ascertain and record the immunization status of every child admitted. Remedial immunization must be available for children who have not adhered to the policy below.

When to immunize	What is given	How it is given
2, 3, and 4 months old	Diphtheria, tetanus, pertussis (whooping cough), polio, *Haemophilus* (DTaP/IPV/Hib)	One injection
	Meningitis C (MenC)	One injection
Around 13 months old	Measles, mumps, and rubella (MMR)	One injection
3 years and 4 months to 5 years old	Diphtheria, tetanus, pertussis (whooping cough), and polio (dTaP/IPV or DTaP/IPV)	One injection
	Measles, mumps, and rubella (MMR)	One injection
13–18 years old	Diphtheria, tetanus, and polio (Td/IPV)	One injection

2, 3, and 4 months old
- When the baby is 2 months old, parents are asked to attend for their first DTaP/IPV/Hib injection against diphtheria, tetanus, pertussis (whooping cough), polio (inactivated polio vaccine, IVP), and Hib.
- They will also be offered the meningitis C (MenC) vaccine, which can be given at the same time.
- They will then be asked to come back for another two doses of both DTaP/IPV/Hib and MenC when the baby is 3 and 4 months old.

Around 13 months old
- When the infant turns 1 year old, they will be offered their first dose of the triple MMR vaccine against measles, mumps, and rubella.
- This is given as a single injection.

3 years and 4 months to 5 years old
- Before the child starts school, they will be offered the dTaP/IPV or DTaP/IPV vaccines which protect against diphtheria, tetanus, pertussis (whooping cough), and polio.

Alan Glasper, University of Southampton

- This is given as a single injection.
- They will also be offered a booster dose of MMR against measles, mumps, and rubella, which is also given as a single injection.

13–18 years old

13–18-year-olds are offered Td/IPV at school. It is given as a single injection in the upper arm and protects against diphtheria, tetanus, and polio.

Further reading

Glasper, E.A. (2002). New evidence reaffirms the safety of the MMR vaccine. *British Journal of Nursing*, **11**(12), 794. ☐ www.immunisation.nhs.uk/

Care of the child/young person and family

Working with families

Introduction

Families contribute greatly to the care and wellbeing of the child, but to do so effectively must be considered part of the healthcare team. The nature of interaction between the family and professionals will impact upon team functioning. Developing positive relationships is a complex demanding task which, to be successful, requires respect for each other's knowledge, skills, and expertise.

Paternalism

- Professionals, with the best intentions, decide what is best and expect compliance.
- Power lies with professionals.
- Assumptions are made which may be incorrect.
- The family has a limited controlled contribution to care.
- The family may feel frustrated at their perceived lack of input.
- The family may be relieved that they do not have to make decisions.

Collaboration

- Partnership, where power is shared with child/family, increases family choices.
- Decision making meets a family's need to be included in care delivery and increases the prospect of compliance.
- There is a danger that the family may feel overwhelmed and abandoned by professionals.

Empowerment

- The family is educated and informed regarding condition, treatment, and care.
- They are encouraged to participate in care delivery.
- Support is provided in a non-judgemental way.
- The family feels prepared for their role in care delivery.
- Family wishes are taken into account when care is planned.

Important points

Team working:
- Role clarity is crucial.
- Be consistent, confusion/resentment arises when the family is part of the team one minute and then disregarded the next.
- The family should not be pressured into carrying out care they feel unprepared or unable to do.
- If truly collaborative, child/family decisions are accepted even if different to yours.

Communication

- Acknowledge that often the child/family know what is best for them.
- Be truthful at all times.
- Give the family time to assimilate information and make decisions.
- Speak to family members as individuals, as well as part of a group.
- Remember to respect confidentiality of all family members.

Irene McTaggart, University of Dundee

Further reading

Booth, K., Luker, K. (ed.) (1999). *A practical handbook for community health nurses: working with children and their parents*. Blackwell Science, Oxford.

Smith, L. (ed.) (2002). *Family centred care: concept, theory and practice*. Palgrave, Basingstoke.

Communication with the child and family

Definition
Communication is a two-way multifaceted process, consisting of verbal and non-verbal strategies. Communication takes place on an informal and formal basis, throughout which it is just as important to observe and listen as it is to talk.

General points
Purpose:
- to gain information
- to give information
- to establish a therapeutic relationship
- social.

Set scene
- Ensure privacy.
- Avoid interruptions, e.g. phones, staff.
- Organize furniture avoiding confrontational arrangement, e.g. chairs at an angle, not face to face.
- Allow for personal space, e.g. leg room.
- Do not position chairs in front of window, reduces non-verbal aspect of communication, while backlight may be discomforting for those facing it.

Plan
Consider:
- purpose
- developmental level of recipient(s)
- stage of child's illness/condition
- emotional state of child/family, and their readiness for communication.

Explain to child/family purpose of discussion; allow them preparation time if possible.

Implement
Verbal
- Adjust vocabulary/tone to gain maximum understanding.
- Speak clearly, express yourself unambiguously.
- Use layman's language, not technical jargon.
- Give small amounts of information at a time.
- Minimize barriers between you and the child/family.

Non-verbal
- Open, friendly, professional approach.
- Avoid judgemental facial expressions, body posture.
- Use appropriate responses, e.g. facial expression, touch.
- Encourage dialogue by eye contact, nodding, etc.

Irene McTaggart, University of Dundee

- Use diagrams and leaflets.
- Observe for signs of discomfort, change subject, and revisit later if possible/necessary.
- Respond to verbal and non-verbal cues; do not rush to fill silences.

Evaluate

- Summarize discussion or ask child/parents to do so; checks/reinforces understanding.
- Ensure child/family do not feel pressurized to give a *correct* answer.
- Give child/family an opportunity to ask questions, state concerns, etc.

Follow-up

- Arrange further discussion if necessary, e.g. Tuesday, not 2.30 pm Tuesday; avoids potential deterioration of relationship if emergency occurs.
- Encourage child/family to:
  - write down any concerns arising in interim
  - ask questions any time to avoid excess worry or delay.

Important point

It is just as important to know when not to ask a question as when to ask it.

Useful website

Organization for parents of babies requiring special care:
🖳 www.bliss.org.uk

Further reading

Arnold, E., Boggs, K.U. (2003). *Interpersonal relationships: professional communication skills for nurses*, 5th edn. W.B. Saunders, St Louis.
Hargie, O., Dickson, D. (2004). *Skilled interpersonal communication: research, theory and practice*, 4th edn. Routledge, London.

Family nursing

Conceptual clarification

Represents a paradigm shift from family-centred care to family nursing focus.

There is ongoing debate within the profession as to what constitutes 'family nursing' and a little understanding of nursing interventions that might begin to address family needs. The extent to which we have developed family nursing in paediatric practice is debatable.

Family nursing can be perceived as:
• a philosophy of care
• an ethos of care
• an approach to care.

The family

• Definitions are diverse and often unclear. It is a dynamic concept which is culturally influenced.
• Understanding of family systems is fundamental to understanding family nursing.

Family systems

• Parts of a family are related to each other.
• One part of the family cannot be understood in isolation from the rest of the system.
• Family functioning is more than just the sum of the parts.
• A family's structure and organization are important in determining the behaviour of family members.
• Changes (e.g. change in overall health status) in one family member create changes in other family members, which in turn create a new change in the original member.
• Family health has been reported to be a significant factor in the child's recovery from illness and/or adjustment to disability.

Family assessment

In order to practise family nursing, it is necessary first to conduct a comprehensive family assessment. Four intrinsic elements in family nursing assessments include:
• having a human caring presence
• acknowledging multiple perceptions
• respecting diversity
• valuing each person in the context of family.

Each of the above is consistent with family nursing systems, in that all members are involved in the assessment process.

Child health nurses need to critically appraise various family nursing assessment tools available for possible adoption in their practice context.

Gary Mountain, University of Leeds

Family nursing interventions

Family systems nursing targets the cognitive, behavioural, and affective domains of family functioning. Interventions that meet these three domains of family functioning may assist the family in finding new solutions to their problems arising from such changes in health status.

Typical interventions

- Behaviour modification
- Contracting
- Case managing/coordinating
- Collaborative strategies
- Empowering/participating
- Family advice
- Environmental modification
- Family crisis intervention
- Networks/self-help groups
- Information and technical expertise
- Role modelling
- Role supplementation
- Teaching strategies

The above list is by no means exhaustive and points to synonyms, related roles, and prerequisites for family nursing.

Further reading

Neabel, B., Fothergill-Bourbonnais, F., Dunning, J. (2000). Family assessment tools: a review of the literature from 1978–1997. *Heart and Lung*, **29**(3), 196–209.

Friedman, M.M., Bowden, R.V., Jones, E.G. (2003). *Family nursing: research, theory and practice*, 5th edn. Prentice Hall, Upper Saddle River, NJ.

Working with siblings

Siblings of all ages are affected by having an ill brother or sister, especially if this illness is chronic.

Young children

Parents report that they feel that babies, toddlers, and pre-school siblings miss out on the normal cuddles and prolonged contact that they would have from mum, as she is constantly caring for her ill child. One parent's solution to this was to ensure that another carer attended to her sick child for a full day once a week so she could give undivided attention to her other son on his special day. Other relatives or care team members may be available to give parents time to devote to siblings.

Older children

As children get older, parents report that they are often angry, frustrated, ashamed, attention seeking, and naughty.

Children under 10 years of age may not understand what is happening with their sibling. They may feel they are at risk of getting the disease or that they have caused the illness in some way. They may feel embarrassed and confused as they see their sibling is different to others. Parents need to acknowledge the feelings that their well child has, and discuss with the child how difficult it is to live with a poorly sibling, allowing them to feel free about discussing their feelings.

Adolescents

Adolescents may struggle with their own need for independence and may feel guilty about not wanting to be available for care giving. They need to be reassured that their life does not revolve around caring for their sibling and that they should be attentive to their own needs. Most children of any age like to feel useful, but the burden of care should not be on their shoulders.

Interventions

In a study looking at psychosocial support for siblings of children with cancer, Murray and John (2002) reported that the most helpful interventions were emotional and instrumental support, followed by informational and appraisal support. It was noted that the greatest difficulty siblings remembered was being left out and not being able to share their feelings.

Support

Respite, especially in children's hospices, is a valuable asset to allow siblings more access to family activities, as the care team takes over some of the parents' care roles.

Support groups, e.g. SIBS, are available to provide centres where children of all ages can meet, socialize, and discuss concerns. They provide short breaks and holidays, enabling siblings to meet others in their situation.

Jackie Imrie, Central Manchester and Manchester Children's University Hospitals NHS Trust

Further reading

Murray, L.T.C., John, S. (2002). A qualitative exploration of psychosocial support of children with cancer. *Journal of Pediatric Nursing*, **17**(5).

Post, C.E. (1991). When the youngest becomes the oldest. *Exceptional Parent*, March.

🖳 www.sibs.org.uk

Using nursing models in practice

Models of nursing

Models are representations of reality. Like a model of a building, a nursing model shows how parts fit together to make a whole. The universal *concept model* of nursing has four elements:

- person
- environment
- health
- nursing.

Definitions of these concepts and the relationships between them differ in the many models that exist to represent different approaches to nursing.

A *process model* widely used in nursing consists of the steps taken to plan individualized care:

- assessment
- planning
- intervention
- evaluation (the nursing process).

Choosing a model

Consider what the model is supposed to represent.

- Does it fit with your view of nursing? Is it culturally appropriate?
- What is it for, i.e. what aspects of nursing, person, health, and environment does it describe? Does that fit with what you want to use it for?
- Has the model been evaluated for use in your care setting?
- Is it understood by, and acceptable to, the child, young person, and family?

Models in use

A team of nurses used the Casey partnership model to decide on audit criteria. They evaluated the quality of the support provided for children and families and found that support needs were not assessed, supportive care was not planned systematically, nor was it evaluated.

Community nurses in East London used the model to argue for better translation services, making the case that they could not teach and support families in care without good translation.

When nurses in an acute ward were provided with a nursing model their records no longer described care in terms of medical diagnosis but reflected the model, including:

- continuity of usual care by parents
- support for family members
- impact of illness and hospitalization
- participation by parents in nursing and medical care.

Anne Casey, Royal College of Nursing

Evaluation

As with any aspect of practice, use of nursing models should be evaluated. Begin with your reasons for using a model and then assess whether the model is meeting your needs. Does the model help you to:
- think about, describe and improve your practice?
- teach students about practice?
- direct research and audit?
- argue for resources and facilities?

Further reading

Pearson, A. (2005). Nursing models for practice, 3rd edn. Butterworth Heinemann, Oxford.

Mason, G., Webb, C. (1997). Researching children's nurses' clinical judgments about assessment data. *Clinical Effectiveness in Nursing*, **1**, 47–55.

Partnership model of nursing

Principles

Partnership nursing is based on recognition of, and respect for, the child/young person and family's rights and preferences, as well as their knowledge about, and expertise in, (their own) care and treatment. It involves the following:

- ongoing provision of information, teaching, and support to enable them to be involved in decision making, care, and treatment to the extent that they wish to be.
- negotiation of choices and care responsibilities, balancing the child/young person and family's needs and preferences with available resources and professional views of what is needed.

Partnership is an approach to child- and family-centred care; it differs from family involvement in that there is no assumption that the child and family will be involved.

Practice

Assess

- Ask the child; ask the parents/carer.
- Invite the child/parent to observe and measure; observe and measure.
- Confirm your impressions and conclusions with the child and parents, especially their view of priorities.

Plan

- Agree goals with the child and parents.
- Discuss possible actions and assist them in making choices.
- Agree plan for what needs to be done, who will do it, when and how.
- Plan for regular shared review of the plan, care responsibilities, and teaching and support needs.

Implement

- Perform direct care as planned (child, parents, nurse).
- Facilitate learning and information sharing.
- Provide support and supervision.
- Monitor progress and re-assess as planned (child, parents, nurse).
- With consent, refer to other professionals and coordinate care.

Evaluate

- Invite the child and parents to observe and measure outcomes and report their experience of care.
- Review and reflect on the care process from the child and family perspective and from the professional nursing perspective.

Outcomes

Evaluation and audit of the partnership model for nursing children and young people address the following questions.

Anne Casey, Royal College of Nursing

- Did the child/young person and family feel that their views and preferences were heard and their knowledge and experience respected?
- Were they involved in decisions, care, and treatment to the extent they wished to be?
- Did they feel adequately informed and supported in making decisions and carrying out care/treatment?

Further reading

Casey, A. (2005). Assessing planning care in partnership. In *A Textbook of Children's Nursing*, (ed. E.A. Glasper and J. Richardson). Churchill Livingstone, London.

How to write a care plan

What is a care plan?

- A nursing care plan is a written structured plan of action for patient care based on a holistic assessment of patient requirements, the identification of specific problems, and the development of a plan of action for their resolution.
- Care plans are designed to provide the organizing frame for the planning, provision, and evaluation of nursing care, and they operate as a vehicle for communication and a record of care given.
- The Nursing and Midwifery Council (NMC) views record keeping as an essential aspect of nursing care and not a distraction from its provision. It is a professional requirement for nurses to construct and maintain accurate care plans.

The structure of a care plan

- The structure of a care plan is dependent on the nursing model on which it is based, and as there are many models, there is also a wide range of formats for a nursing care plan. Whichever nursing model the care plan is based on, it should involve all four elements of the nursing process, i.e. the assessment, planning, implementation, and evaluation of nursing care.
- The nursing care plan must be factual and accurate. It should be seen as a structured tool for documenting holistic care, including a balanced assessment of patient need.
- The care plan should contain sufficient detail for a nurse to care for the patient without further information.

How to write a care plan

- Following the nursing assessment, the nurse must identify the patient's needs and document accordingly.
- A plan must be written for each identified need, consisting of a nursing diagnosis (what the problem/need is), expected outcome(s) and/or goals, nursing interventions and rationales required to meet the outcome, and a time at which the plan should be reviewed.
- The intended goal may not be a return to full health but should be appropriate to the patient and the individual circumstances.
- There may be more than one goal for each diagnosis, and each goal should have a set of interventions/rationales required for its achievement.
- The nurse caring for the patient should follow each care plan, which should be assessed and evaluated following every intervention or change in the patient's condition.
- Care plans should remain contemporary—they must be reviewed regularly and rewritten or changed to accurately reflect the patient's current needs.

Paula Flint, Central Manchester and Manchester Children's University Hospitals NHS Trust

Date	Problem number	1

| 01.01.06 | **Nursing Diagnosis**: Sally Smith has pain related to removal of drain from abdomen |
| | **Patient Goal**: Sally will experience no pain or reduced level of pain acceptable to her |

Nursing interventions/*rationales*

1. Administer analgesics as prescribed *for pain*
2. Do not wait until pain is occurring *in order to prevent pain from occurring*
3. Avoid palpating area unless necessary to *minimize risk of pain*
4. Allow Sally to find own position of comfort unless contraindicated
5. Perform nursing procedures and activities (e.g. dressing changes) after analgesia to *minimize risk of pain occurring*
6. Monitor effectiveness of analgesics *to ensure Sally is receiving and has been prescribed adequate and appropriate pain relief*
7. Discuss all care and treatment with Sally and encourage her participation in care *to minimize her distress and anxiety and allow the opportunity for Sally to inform staff if she is experiencing any pain*

Nursing Evaluation

Date

Evaluation of nursing care following care plan 1

Sign & print name and designation

Further reading

Nursing and Midwifery Council (2005). *Guidelines for records and record keeping.* www.nmc-uk.org/nmc/main/publications/Guidelinesforrecords.pdf

Foster, E., Harrison, M. (2000). Setting up a collaborative care plan. *Nursing Standard*, **15**(8), 40–3.

Mason, C. (1999). Guide to practice or 'load of rubbish'? The influence of care plans on nursing practice in five clinical areas in Northern Ireland. *Journal of Advanced Nursing*, **29**(2), 380–7.

Evaluation of care

In order to measure the effectiveness of the care that is delivered, and to justify the contribution that we as nurses make to the patient experience, evaluation of that care is essential to identify whether the goals or outcomes of that care has been achieved.

Evaluation involves
- Comparison of the outcome with the original goal or outcome statement.
- If the goal or outcome is not achieved, then reassessment and re-formulation of the nursing outcomes or goals for the child.

The evaluation of care cannot take place if there is no statement or tool to measure it against. For example, how can you evaluate the effectiveness of analgesia that you administered to a child if you have no nursing outcome statement with which to compare it?

Evaluation skills are similar to assessment skills, and are intrinsically linked. By continually evaluating the care delivered to the child, predictions and effectiveness of interventions will become known to both the nurse and the child, thus affording the child choice in his/her future care.

Evaluation of care is an ongoing process and it is an essential component of the nursing process. This may be referred to as formative evaluation, with summative evaluation taking place once the nurse is no longer involved in the care of the child. In evaluating the care given and its effectiveness, the nurse must also critically examine the implementation of the care given, to identify if it was delivered by the most effective means and what it was like for the child and family. Any difficulties encountered in carrying out the plan of care should be documented, as should any changes to the plan of care. Nursing records serve to protect the patient and should contain an accurate account of the treatment given and the care planned and delivered.

Although it is the final part of the nursing process, it is a continual activity, and best practice should advocate the involvement of the child and family so that assumptions will not be made about the effects of care; thus making evaluation objective and empowering the child and parent.

Further reading
Aggleton, P, Chalmers, H. (2000). *Nursing models and nursing practice*, 2nd edn. Macmillan Press, Basingstoke.
Nursing and Midwifery Council (2005). *Guidelines for records and record keeping*. NMC, London.

Liz Gormley-Fleming, University of Hertfordshire

The importance of play

Play can be described as the engagement in activities for pleasure rather than for a serious or practical purpose. It is a source of enjoyment for both the player and the observer of play activity.

Play is the language of children, an essential tool through which they attain knowledge about themselves and the world around them. Play is a rich learning medium, and the ability to play develops earlier in children than the ability to communicate through language, making it a valuable communication tool for children of all ages.

For children there are no extrinsic goals in play activity. Nevertheless play makes an important contribution to normal growth and development. Play and playing are vital parts of children's lives, and through play children learn how to learn and how to do things.

The child uses play:
- for physical development (e.g. fine and gross motor skills, strength, and stamina)
- for social development (e.g. social skills and social behaviours, control of aggression)
- for moral development (e.g. learning to take turns, to win and lose, not to cheat, self-control, and consideration for others)
- for psychological development (e.g. the development of self-awareness and self-actualization)
- for cognitive development (Piaget linked play to cognitive development)
- for problem solving
- as a communication tool (e.g. to demonstrate misconceptions about information received)
- to normalize the environment
- to practise adult behaviours and skills
- for language development
- for distraction from anxiety-provoking situations
- to master/make sense of the environment (play helps children to understand the world in which they live and to differentiate between what is real and what is not)
- to have fun!

Play is an important outlet for anxiety, frustration, emotional tension, and fear, and it enables the child to make sense of anxiety-provoking situations such as invasive medical procedures. In this sense play becomes therapeutic and is emotionally enhancing for the child.

Margaret Chambers, University of Plymouth

Further reading

Piaget, J. (1963). *The origins of intelligence in children*. Norton, New York.
LeVieux-Anglin, L., Sawyer, E. (1993). Incorporating play interventions into nursing care. *Pediatric Nursing*, **19**(5), 459–63.
www.nncc.org/Curriculum/better.play.html

Diversionary/normal play

- In order to enable medical/nursing staff to examine a child in the way that is least traumatic for the child, time needs to be given to build a relationship of trust through play.
- Play can then be used for distraction, should unpleasant invasive procedures be required.
- Ensure that the activity is developmentally age appropriate, taking into account any special needs the child may have.
- The effect on parents is reduced stress. They are more relaxed, which improves communication.

Children need to be able to access play wherever they are. Play is their way of making sense of the world and coping with their feelings. Play areas provide a safe child-friendly environment in which they are surrounded by familiar things that provide them with a link to home. This creates an environment away from the clinical areas, which is conducive to building relationships and trust with play staff.

The play provided needs to be age and ability appropriate, taking into account special needs, and must also be appropriate for black and ethnic minority children. Staff need to take account of language and communication barriers as well as religious beliefs.

Taking time to build a relationship with parents and children can prove invaluable in gaining trust and identifying the most appropriate and effective activities.

It is important to gain as much information from parents as possible at admission with regard to the child's special toy and any special vocabulary they may have. In addition, it is important to take into account any previous bad experiences the child may have had in hospital and any knowledge of any abuse or neglect the child has experienced.

Include parents and siblings wherever possible. This also has the benefit of creating a home-from-home environment.

Where access to the play room/teenage room is available, children/young people can be provided with an opportunity to self-select activities of their choice. When children are unable to access play independently, the necessary support needs to be provided to enable them to access play. In the event that the child is unable to access the playroom, every effort should be made to identify the favoured activities and provide them at the bedside.

Suggested distraction tools
Infants:
- tactile soothing
- cuddling
- music tapes

Pam Iles, Southampton University Hospitals NHS Trust

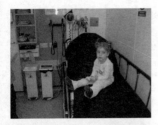

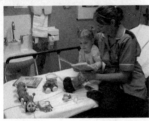

Toddlers:
- blowing bubbles/feathers
- pop-up toys and books
- songs or rhymes

Pre-school children:
- *Where's Wally?* books/posters
- songs and rhymes
- puppets

School-age children:
- joke books
- counting games
- songs and rhymes
- puppets
- kaleidoscopes (with/without glitter wand)
- guided imagery
- games consoles

Further reading

National Association of Hospital Play Specialists (2002). *Guidelines for professional practice: Distraction therapy*. National Association of Hospital Play Specialists.

Preparation and post-procedural play

Understanding what is happening is important to help children/young people and parents relax and accept treatment.

Parents do not always prepare their child for hospital, but all children should be prepared in a way that is appropriate to their cognitive ability, taking into account any special needs and/or cultural and/or religious beliefs.

Illness, accidents, or invasive medical investigations can all bring the emotional challenge of:
• the threat of physical harm
• separation from one's parents and other trusted people
• the threat of strange and unforeseeable experiences
• uncertainty about acceptable behaviour
• relative loss of control and personal autonomy.

Preparation play

A range of quality play helps in preparing children/young people for procedures. This can be achieved through attending a pre-admission club, which will introduce children to the environment and equipment. They will have an opportunity to become familiar with the surroundings, including the theatre waiting room and the recovery room for those children who are to undergo surgery. The familiarization of hospital equipment and routines reduces stress and anxiety, helping the child/young person to come to terms with his/her condition.

Play specialists, in conjunction with the healthcare team, can develop presentation programmes for children undergoing surgical, clinical, and diagnostic procedures, to develop their understanding of what is going to happen, thus reducing fear.

Role play is particularly useful when enabling children who do not have the necessary language and/or cognitive skills to develop an understanding of the procedure and familiarize them with the equipment.

Good-quality preparation play in the radiotherapy department, for example, enables children, who would otherwise need a general anaesthetic to keep still for treatment, to lie still without fear.

Post-procedural play

Post-procedural play is particularly important for children admitted as emergencies. Post-procedural play should be offered and should include:
• praise; certificates and/or stickers will reinforce this
• an evaluation of the coping strategies used
• an opportunity to express feelings following the procedure
• planning, if future admissions are necessary.

Pam Iles, Southampton University Hospitals NHS Trust

Further reading

Journal of the National Association of Hospital Play Staff, Spring/Summer 1994.

National Association of Hospital Play Specialists (2002). *Guidelines for professional practice*. National Association of Hospital Play Specialists.

Directed and hospital role play

P participation in play introduces normality into a strange setting
L lessens the impact of pain and anxiety
A allows the child/young person to work through feelings and fears, so that hospitalization can become a positive experience
Y yields results: recovery is faster and the in-patient stay is reduced

Being in hospital can be a frightening experience. Directed play enables the child to regain some control over what is happening by acting out his/her feelings and fears. Hospital role play involves playing with clinical equipment in order to gain familiarity and reduce fantasies about it. Gaining the child's/young person's confidence/trust enables medical/nursing staff to observe the patient's reactions and to pick up and deal with fears and misconceptions. In order to achieve this, an attractive and inviting child-friendly environment is required, where children can feel confident and safe to explore and investigate the equipment and activities provided. For example, dolls that children can use to insert a central line enable them to ask questions, develop their understanding of the procedure that they will undergo, and reduce fears. Role play creates a relaxed forum where children, parents, and siblings are free to take their time and ask questions and develop their understanding in a non-judgemental environment. This activity is best carried out whenever possible by a member of the play staff in a non-clinical area, where children are in surroundings that are familiar to them and with people whom they know are safe (not going to undertake any painful procedures).

The effect on the child of skilled directed role play is to reduce fears and anxiety. The child will then be more responsive to procedures and treatments, thus aiding the medical/nursing staff in carrying out what would otherwise be a very distressing procedure. This is particularly important where the child may have to undergo the treatment on more than one occasion. Any distress that is experienced by the child initially will be compounded with each episode experienced. This will make the work of those carrying out the procedure stressful and time consuming. The effect of not making time for role play results in the child potentially having a bad experience. It is extremely difficult to regain a child's trust once this has happened, and it will take substantially more time for the play specialist to develop the child's understanding and acceptance of the treatment/procedure that he/she is required to undergo.

Further reading

Sylvia, K. (1995). Play in hospital: When and why it is effective. *Current Paediatrics*, **3**, 247–9.
Barry, P. (2000). *A child's recollection of hospital*. National Association of Hospital Play Specialists.

Pam Iles, Southampton University Hospitals NHS Trust

Guided imagery

Guided imagery is a 'therapeutic technique that allows two people to communicate on a reality that one of them has chosen to describe through the process of imaging.

It can be used with children in hospital as a form of pain management.

Before the imagery can start, it is important to carry out an assessment of the child you hope to use this technique with. You need to look at:
- age/cognitive level of child
- what type of pain they may be experiencing, e.g. procedural, anxiety, chronic
- emotional state of the child
- expectations of the child (remember always to be realistic and do not make promises)
- any existing coping strategies the child may use
- environment
- staff to be involved are needed at least two people: one to carry out the procedure and the other to guide the imagery at an appropriate point
- organization of procedure

Guided imagery technique
- Building a rapport and gaining the child's trust.
- 'I know a way we could help to make this easier. Would you like to try?'
- Child to identify what they would like to imagine (should be something fun!).
- Start by getting the child to do some deep breathing and progressive muscle relaxation.
- Child begins to describe imagery.
- You begin to guide and be guided by child's imagery.
- Ask questions such as what can you see? What's happening now? Is anyone there with you? Tell me what it looks like.
- Always inform the child what is happening while they are in imagery, e.g. the tourniquet is going on now, we are going to remove the dressing now.
- Reinforce imagery when necessary.

Always round off imagery:
- Ask the child if he/she would like to finish his/her imagery.
- Encourage him/her to take a big deep breath in and out slowly.
- Think backwards from 4 to 1 (younger children count 1–4).
- Open his/her eyes slowly.
- Wiggle toes and fingers.

Ask the child how he/she feels and encourage him/her to sit still for a few moments, as he/she may feel a little 'funny'.

Joanne Groves, Southampton University Hospitals NHS Trust

Guided imagery response indicators

- Eyes closed (not always at first)
- Eye movements under closed lids
- Slowing of breathing
- Relaxed, absence of muscle tension
- Speech normal—calm
- Easy flowing description of imagery

Points to consider

- Guided imagery can be used with children from an age when they are able to use their imagination. It may not be suitable for children with special needs.
- Imagery can be guided by play specialists, nurses, doctors, and parents, as long as, when it is used during a procedure, there is at least one other person to carry out the procedure.
- Remember to review each case. It will not work for everybody. What was easy to focus on? What were the goals? How can I improve the outcome?

'Guided imagery, a form of relaxed focused concentration is a natural and powerful coping mechanism.'

Further reading

- www.guidedimageryinc.com
- www.phoenixchildrens.com

Education and the ill child

Children with medical conditions have an increased likelihood of experiencing, at some time, a constellation of factors that may directly or indirectly place their education at risk. The importance of school for children with chronic diseases cannot be underestimated.

If education is to be effective for children with medical conditions, education authorities, schools, and staff must make positive responses to these issues. Section 19 of the 1996 Education Act says that 'each local education authority shall make arrangements for the provision of suitable education at school or otherwise than at school for those children of compulsory school age who, by reason of illness ... may not for any period receive suitable education unless arrangements are made'. Because each case is unique, it is not possible to quantify this.

Most establishments are ill-prepared in terms of experience, professional development, knowledge, skills, and attitudes, to take up and sustain the challenge in an in-depth way.

When parents are considering their child's education, they are mindful not only of academic and performance-related matters, but also of care, medical, and quality-of-life issues. For a family whose life is totally affected and controlled by the child's illness, the quality of the child's school life assumes an enormous significance.

Some children go through their entire schooling suffering the effects of their condition and experiencing difficulties. Schools should not underestimate the difference they can make to the child's quality of life. With careful planning, appropriate activities, and sensitive teaching, the school can make a significant contribution. Teachers and support staff can be content in the knowledge that their input has the double benefit of being therapeutic and educational.

It is important that a holistic approach is adopted by all working with the family and its individual members. Sick children do not exist in isolation; they are members of a family group that functions as a unit. All members of the family are affected by the illness.

There are many other reasons why an ill and disabled child may not be able to attend school but still benefit from home tuition, such as a susceptibility to serious chest infections, difficulties over school transport, or supervision problems at school associated with distressing, unpredictable, and possibly life-threatening symptoms.

Home tuition for children with degenerative disorders, for example, is not an extension of school per se but rather is a unique service provision, a specially crafted resource to meet the needs of a child and family living under difficult, stressful, and peculiar circumstances.

Jackie Imrie, Central Manchester and Manchester Children's University Hospitals NHS Trust

Patient and parent information and education

The provision of adequate information is an essential prerequisite to the formation and development of a trusting relationship between practitioner, child, and family. It is, therefore, extremely important that all information provided should be clear, factual, and aimed at empowering and enabling the family in relation to their understanding, consent, and participation.

This may include the creative use of verbal communication, non-verbal communication, abstract communication, and aids such as leaflets, books, and posters, or interactive methods such as videos, CDs, DVDs, and computers with internet access.

All information provided needs to be good quality, based on up-to-date evidence, and adapted to take account of the age, development, and level of understanding of all involved.

This will require knowledge and skills on the part of the practitioner, not only in relation to their understanding of child development and inter-personal communication strategies, but also the ability to assess and evaluate information needs and understanding. Linked to this, it must never be assumed that parents lack knowledge in relation to their child or their child's condition. With the increasing influence of the internet, it follows that children and their parents now have improved access to information, which can, in many cases, lead to an expert knowledge and understanding on their part. It is important that practitioners do not perceive this as a threat to their own expertise. Rather, it should be viewed as a basis on which to develop communication strategies based on partnership, mutual trust, and respect. In this way further exploration and explanation of specific issues can be provided and appropriate skills acquired by all, with guidance given towards reliable sources of good-quality information.

Factors to note when providing information include the following.
- Information should be appropriate in its presentation and linked to the age, ability, and level of understanding of those involved.
- Verbal information should be clear and factual and spoken at a normal pace.
- Technical terms or jargon should be avoided and explanations should be simple and uncomplicated.
- Adequate time should be allocated; include time for questions and discussion.
- Not all information will be understood at first and back-up material, such as leaflets, videos, or books, should be provided for reinforcement and further explanation.

Elaine Mahoney, University of Glamorgan

Further reading

HMSO (2001). *Learning from Bristol: the report of the public inquiry into children's heart surgery at the Bristol Royal Infirmary 1984–1995*. CM5207(1). HMSO, London.

Matthews, J. (2006). Communicating with children and their families. In *A textbook of children's and young people's nursing*, (ed. A. Glasper and J. Richardson). Elsevier, London.

⊟ www.deafnessatbirth.org.uk

Dealing with parental aggression

In today's society, having the skills to manage anger, aggression, and violent behaviour successfully is very important for a children's nurse. However, prevention of the occurrence and escalation of these situations will be more satisfying and productive for all involved. Where prevention has not been possible and aggression or violence is a reality, nurses must have the ability to utilize high-level interpersonal skills in order to effectively relate to the individuals involved.

It is important that you can:
• define and differentiate between anger, aggression, and violence
• understand the possible causes of anger, aggression, and violence
• identify what signs to look for
• understand how to respond
• develop the skills required to prevent and deal with situations as they occur.

Factors that can lead to families becoming angry and aggressive can include:
• staff shortages and increased workload that lead to a reduction in the time you can spend with families
• unrealistic expectations of the family
• poor planning and prolonged waiting times
• poor communication
• lack of appropriate information
• inadequate resources
• inappropriate discharge planning.

In relation to this, an important aspect is the ability of the children's nurse to become self-aware. Self-awareness will enable you to learn about your own behaviour and reactions. This, in turn, will lead to an understanding of how your own behaviour is perceived by others and how, in certain circumstances, if responses are deemed to be inappropriate, this may contribute to increasing the frustration and anger experienced by the family. Along with the development of self-awareness, you must strive to incorporate some of the basic principles of communication. Communication involves content and context factors, and situations may escalate if one person misinterprets or misunderstands what the other person has said or done.

It is also essential that you learn to become tuned in and perceptive to the possible predisposing factors and emotions that can lead to a person becoming frustrated, angry, or aggressive. These may include:
• fear—for the welfare of the child or of the environment
• stress and anxiety
• feelings of loss of control
• blaming themselves and feelings of guilt for their child's illness
• perceived inappropriate waiting times
• insufficient information.

Elaine Mahoney, University of Glamorgan

By developing this understanding, the skills and strategies aimed at calming the situation and preventing escalation can be more successfully applied. These include:
- effective listening
- remaining calm and actively engaging with the family
- demonstrating empathy and understanding of the situation
- being responsive but remaining in control
- being aware of the environment and personal safety.

Arnold, E., Underman Boggs, K. (2003). *Interpersonal relationships: communication skills for nurses*, 4th edn. WB Saunders, St Louis.

Hollinworth, H., Clark, C., Harland, R., Johnson, L., Partington, G. (2005). Understanding the arousal of anger: a patient-centred approach. *Nursing Standard*, **19**(37), 41–7.

Writing a patient information leaflet

Written and other information resources play an increasingly important role in the care of families with sick children. A fundamental component of the NSF is the giving of information, which is complete and clearly communicated. All healthcare staff who treat children should receive training in communicating with young people and their parents.

Production of local information

Writing a patient information leaflet may appear superficially easy but the reality is that it cannot just be typed on a word processor one evening using a home computer.

- Readability formulae can help writers of patient information leaflets to assess how well their writing can be understood by the reader. The FOG and standard measure of gobbledegook (SMOG) indices are widely available for this. Remember that the average reading age of UK adults is at the level of the *Sun* newspaper.
- Keep sentences short, using simple explanations.
- Use familiar, but avoid unnecessary, words.
- Use action verbs and terms your reader can picture.
- Make sure the leaflet is comprehensible, usable, and easy to navigate.

Before rushing to your computer

- Know your purpose. What do you want to achieve?
- Know your target audience. Who are you writing for, a child or a carer?
- Know your subject. If you do not, get help.
- Know the setting under which your intended audience will read the leaflet.

Make sure your information leaflet contains:

- Awareness information.
- Information that allows the reader to optimize the purpose of the leaflet.
- Principles information which gives, for example, real concrete information on how certain drugs work.

The style of patient information leaflets

- Use informative headings.
- Personalize the leaflet by using personal pronouns such as 'I, we, or you'.
- Use decisive, clear, and unambiguous language.
- Describe actions positively ('give only after meals', or 'give only if wheezing').
- Only use familiar words and avoid professional jargon.
- Use short paragraphs with strong topic sentences.
- Use simple visual images and 12-point type.
- Leave lots of white space.

Alan Glasper, University of Southampton

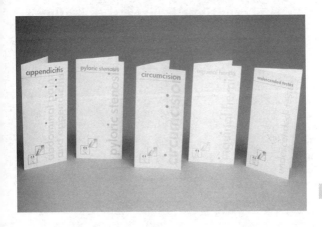

Remember to always:

- Base your leaflet on best evidence.
- Have it peer reviewed.
- Use families to pilot and develop the leaflet.
- State explicitly by using a date when the leaflet should be updated.

Further reading

Glasper, A., Burge, D. (1992). Developing family information leaflets. *Nursing Standard*, **25**, 24–7.

Glasper, E.A., McWilliams, R. (1998). Developing a centre for health information and promotion. In *Innovations in paediatric ambulatory care*, (ed. E.A. Glasper and S. Lowson). Macmillan, Basingstoke.

Care of the child/young person and family in hospital

Risk assessment

A *risk assessment* is a careful examination of what, in your work, could cause harm to people. Once a *hazard* has been identified, assess the precautions in place to reduce the *risk*.

It is a *legal requirement* to assess and minimize risk to anyone in a work-place.

You will have a Health and Safety Department with a Risk Manager. There should also be at least one trained Risk Assessor in a unit, but it is everyone's personal responsibility to raise awareness of potential hazards so they can be removed or the risk minimized.

The five steps to risk assessment:
- look for hazards
- decide who might be harmed and how
- evaluate the risks and decide if existing precautions are enough or if more should be done
- record your findings
- review and revise if necessary.

Common workplace injuries are from manual handling, slips, trips and falls, and contact with harmful substances. The cost of injuries can be huge, with sick leave, stress, bad publicity and reputation, and poor staff performance and morale.

Be aware that in nursing there can be constant change. Risks should be evaluated when there is:
- new equipment
- a new way of working
- awareness of policy changes
- MHRA Medical Devices alerts
- challenging behaviour of patients or relatives
- new chemicals in the workplace (COSHH)
- changes in your environment
- the increased risks for pregnant mothers, children, elderly, and adolescents.

Most simple hazards can be identified and acted upon, and risks reduced quickly, but potentially serious hazards require formal recording on a risk assessment form, which should be available with instructions in your Health and Safety Manual, and shown to your manager to act upon.

Recording of incidents/accidents or 'near misses' on a unit and prompt reporting to your Health and Safety Department to audit can quickly highlight problems in particular areas and reduce the risk of injury.

Additional control methods to reduce risks are:
- elimination
- substitution
- risk control at source
- safe procedures

Alison Hayes, Royal Devon and Exeter NHS Foundation Trust

- training
- instruction
- supervision
- personal protective equipment (PPE): clothing, gloves, etc.

Further reading

Medicines and Healthcare Products Regulations Authority. 🖳 www.medical-devices.gov.uk
NHS Plus Health at work. 🖳 www.nhsplus.nhs.uk/law&you/employers_riskassessment.asp

The effects of hospitalization

Children's and young people's nurses now adopt a range of initiatives to minimize the potentially harmful effects of hospital admission.

From Victorian times through to the 1960s and beyond, some hospitals only allowed parents to visit once a week or less often. Bed rest for children until the advent of antibiotics was long and continuous, and the screams and incessant crying bouts which accompanied each weekly visit convinced the nursing staff that parents were generally a hindrance rather than a help.

The recognition that psychological trauma might be perpetrated on children during their hospital stay owes much to the work of psychiatrist John Bowlby and his colleague James Robertson. Their work was to play a crucial role in improving the conditions under which children were cared for in hospital. Because of this Sir Harry Platt launched 'The Welfare of Children in Hospital' in 1959 which fundamentally changed practice.

However, much of the credit for changing the way children are cared for in hospital and the introduction of open and unrestricted visiting must be attributed to the National Association for the Welfare of Children in Hospital (NAWCH), now Action for Sick Children (ASC).

The important process of bonding and attachment is put at risk by any form of separation between mother and infant, leading Bowlby to pronounce: 'Motherlove in infancy and childhood is as important for mental health as are vitamins and proteins for physical health'.

Stages of maternal deprivation

Protest

This stage can last from a few hours to a few days. The child has a strong conscious need of his mother and the loud crying exhibited is based on the expectation built on previous experience that the mother will respond to his/her cries. During this stage of the maternal deprivation sequence, the child will cry noisily and look eagerly towards any sound that might be his/her mother.

Despair

This stage succeeds protest and can best be compared to clinical depression. It is a sign of increasing hopelessness and despondency. The child becomes less active and vocal, and in the past this was interpreted by the nursing staff as a sign that the child was settling into the ward.

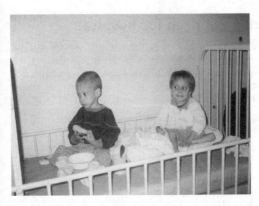

Children deprived of parental contact may fail to thrive.

Denial/detachment
In this final stage of maternal deprivation the child represses his/her longing for his mother and begins to loose his attachment. He/she appears, at least superficially, to have settled into the hospital routine and will respond positively, if shallowly, to kind adults who take an interest in him/her. Importantly, he/she will react badly to brief reappearances of mother, for example during the weekly visiting periods, giving rise to the fallacy that parents actually made matters worse. There is no wonder that generations of children's nurses dreaded 'Sunday afternoon visiting'.

Further reading
Glasper, E.A., Heggarty, R. (2005). The psychological preparation of children for hospitalisation. In *A textbook of children's and young people's nursing* (ed. E.A. Glasper and J. Richardson). Churchill Livingstone, Edinburgh.

Preparing children for hospital

Emotional factors may be an even greater source of concern than the child's physical condition during a hospital admission.

There are five key potential threats to a child on admission to hospital:
- fear of the unknown
- fear of physical harm and pain
- loss of control and identity
- uncertainty about what is expected of them
- separation from security and family routine.

The way in which children interact with the world and how they understand and interpret what they see and hear is influenced enormously by their age and stage of development. A number of different strategies have been developed to help children and their families cope with hospital admission.

Family preparation for day- and in-patient surgery may be important in reducing the psychological effects of hospitalization. This has led to the development of paediatric pre-admission programmes throughout the UK, which aim to protect children from the stresses of hospital admission.

Pre-admission preparation programmes (cited as good practice in the NSF) offer the child and family the opportunity to visit the hospital and be familiarized with the environment and personnel. At the same time, practical issues can be discussed and the child and family informed about anticipated specific events.

Invitations to programmes are often sent out in the mail with all the other information prior to admission. These programmes often consist of a PowerPoint or video/DVD presentation followed by a visit to the ward/unit to which the child will be admitted. Additionally the children may have the opportunity of visiting the anaesthetic room with their carers, where they can see first hand where they will receive their anaesthetic and, importantly, know that their parent will be allowed to go with them on the day.

The role of the skilled play specialist is another essential element of pre-admission preparation, but not to the exclusion of the skilled children's nurse. A major benefit of these programmes is that they facilitate interaction between hospital staff and parents, who are encouraged to ask programme workers about their child's admission.

Children learn through play, and time set aside for hospital-type play gives the child an ideal opportunity to find out about their hospital experience. In doing so their fears may be allayed and their abilities to cope enhanced.

Alan Glasper, University of Southampton

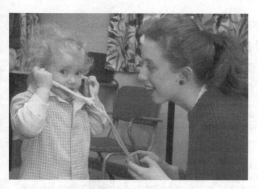

Preparing a child for hospital admission.

Further reading

Eiser, C. (1988). Do children benefit from psychological preparation for hospitalisation? *Psychology and Health*, **2**, 133–8.

Glasper, E.A., Thompson, M. (1993). Preparing children for hospital. In *Advances in child health nursing*, (ed. E.A. Glasper and A. Tucker), Scutari, London.

Making the environment child and young person orientated

Children and young people require age-appropriate care when experiencing hospitalization. Modernization of the National Health Service (NHS) promotes the right of paediatric patients to be treated as individuals.

A carefully designed hospital environment can help a child cope with the sense of loss experienced from the absence of home.

An environment that encourages and displays play will aid its beneficial process:
• equipment used for treatment will be covered with colourful sheeting to alleviate fears
• bright colours and pictures will project a friendly atmosphere where play is easily accessible
• messy play is used to relieve anxiety
• role-play is facilitated to act out experiences with the help of puppets, dolls, and dressing up
• visits from pets enable links with home
• brightly coloured materials are used to make tabards for uniforms
• posters and toys can be used to reflect and accommodate cultural diversity, including various languages and dolls of different ethnic mix.

Young people are a group quite distinct from children, and attention should be paid to their particular needs:
• hospital school provides a routine for the older child, and can also be delivered to the school-age bed-bound patient
• a teenage room can provide an escape from younger children
• a dedicated adolescent unit with specially trained staff would be the ideal
• patient's beds can be grouped according to age, as resources and patient condition allow.

Children's nurses work in the family, delivering the ethos of family-centred care with an environment that:
• encourages normal family routine
• recognizes the parent as the expert in their child
• provides resident parenting.

Play is an integral part of family-centred care. Collaborate with the hospital play specialist or play leader to maintain a child-focused environment.

A dedicated child's and young person's environment can be achieved with practical measures, supported by a philosophy of care to strengthen its delivery.

Nicola Birchley, Coventry University

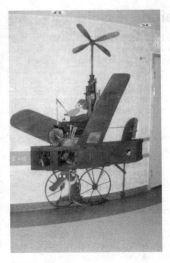

Child-friendly environment.

Further reading

Smith, F.(1995). *Children's nursing in practice the Nottingham model*. Blackwell Science, Oxford.

Admission to hospital

The aim of the contemporary NHS is to deliver hospital services to meet the needs of children, young people, and their parents in a suitable, child-friendly, and child-centred environment by appropriately trained and skilled staff.

Admission to hospital may be an anxiety-provoking experience for both the child and the parents alike. The role of parents in the care of their child in hospital cannot be overstated and has been advocated in many policy documents.

Admission to hospital may be planned, as in the case of a child attending for investigations or for elective surgery. This can be undertaken through pre-admission programmes, the provision of written information, and visits to the ward/unit and pre-operative assessment clinics. However, many infants, children, and young people will have unplanned attendance to hospital.

The child with limited life experiences may well have preconceived ideas about hospital from friends, relatives, and the media. The aim of the admission process is not only to identify the alterations to the physical status of the child but, more importantly, to inform the child of all expected outcomes in order to allay fear and stress.

Children should only be admitted to children's wards, and the young person should be offered a choice of accommodation. The concept of family-centred care and partnership needs to be embraced as key principles when admitting a child to hospital. Parents know their child better that we ever can, so the need to involve the parents will serve to enhance their locus of control, thus having a more positive outcome for the child.

This may be achieved by:
- introductions to the ward team and fellow patients
- identifying what the child and family wish to know and allowing them time to question
- drawing on any previous experience of hospitalization
- orientation to the ward and hospital, outlining facilities available; this should be supported with written information
- consider the child's developmental stage at all stages of the hospitalization episode
- clarify the child's and family's understanding of the reason for hospitalization
- include other family members (if present)
- identify the impact of hospitalization on the child and family, and help them to comprehend their reaction. (e.g. reaction of siblings, behaviour of the sick child).
- identify normal routines and integrate into care plan; non-medical needs such as play and school work should not be overlooked
- negotiate care with parents and establish role of parents in care

Liz Gormley-Fleming, University of Hertfordshire

- establish preferred names
- identify who has parental responsibility
- recognize the terms the child and family may use for pain or their illness
- apply identification band and allergy band (if used) to child, having confirmed correct details with parent and child first
- including child and parent, perform nursing admission history and document
- record vital signs as a base line; this normally includes temperature, pulse rate, respiratory rate, blood pressure, weight, height, oxygen saturation level
- collect any specimens as required and manage as required
- support child and family during physical examination by medical colleagues, or other investigations such as venepuncture, ensuring adequate preparation prior to any procedure
- in the case of an emergency admission, care will be prioritized on physical need, with a nurse assigned to support the parents during this stage
- document admission process and findings before establishing nursing diagnosis and beginning to plan care with the child and parents
- ask the child and family to reiterate information to identify their understanding of it.

Parental participation in care

Parental participation in care is an essential aspect of partnership with parents and family-centred care. Care is planned and delivered in negotiation with parents, who enjoy an equal partnership with healthcare professionals in the care of the child.

Power in decision-making and care-giving is usually invested in the family, but in the hospital the nurse holds the balance of power. Parents may not see themselves as equal partners in care. The success of parental participation is dependent on a number of variables, but particularly on the willingness of nurses and parents to work together.

Although contemporary child care philosophy encourages parents to accompany their hospitalized children and to be actively involved in their care, this sometimes causes role stress for both parents and nurses:

- parents because of increased demands made upon them, or because they feel deskilled in their parental role
- nurses because of changes to their traditional caring roles, leaving them feeling threatened by parental participation in care.

Barriers to parental participation

- Role stress
- Nurses' attitudes, judgements, and beliefs
- Parental attitudes
- Poor communication skills
- Poor negotiation skills
- Poor documentation
- Poor information exchange
- Lack of commitment on either side
- Lack of clarity of the concept
- Lack of equal partnership
- Lack of parental control

Implications for practice

- Education to promote the concept
- Commitment to the concept
- Recognition of the barriers and strategies to overcome them
- Development of negotiation and communication skills
- Development of self-awareness
- Development of documentation to support practice
- Equal partnership
- Clear guidelines about expectations on both sides
- Respect, empowerment, and empathy

Evidence suggests that parents want to participate in their child's care. Nurses and healthcare organizations must adapt their practices to meet their needs.

Further reading

Coyne, I.T. (1995). Parental participation in care: a critical review of the literature. *Journal of Advanced Nursing*, **21**, 716–22.

Coyne, I.T. (1996). Parent participation: a concept analysis. *Journal of Advanced Nursing*, **23**, 733–40.

 http://pediatrics.families.com/family-centered-care-current-realities-in-parent-participation

Margaret Chambers, University of Plymouth

Preparing for discharge

A methodical approach to the discharge of a child and his/her family from hospital is necessary to ensure that a holistic family-centred approach is adopted.

- The child needs to undergo a physical examination by an appropriate professional to determine their suitability for discharge and to facilitate the identification and implementation of any interventions to ensure safe discharge and continuing care. The provision of any dressings, medication, or equipment deemed necessary to provide continuing care should be arranged prior to discharge.
- Any interventions planned should be negotiated with the child, family, and professionals to ensure they are realistic and practical and are fully understood. The discharge plan should be clearly documented in the child's hospital notes and a copy given to the family for reference. Written documentation regarding care following their surgery or treatment should be explained and clearly understood by the family. It may be necessary to demonstrate a procedure and assess the family's willingness and ability to undertake the intervention.
- Referral to colleagues in the community (e.g. health visitor, district nurse and CCN, dietician, social worker, etc.) may be necessary if continuing care is needed. A discharge summary from the hospital to the general practitioner (GP) and a referral letter to any relevant agency are necessary to ensure that any instructions are clear. A telephone call to relevant professionals may ensure that a seamless web of care is undertaken. Hospitals may have a Discharge Liaison Officer who is responsible for undertaking this task.
- Any follow-up appointments should be planned before discharge. Outstanding investigation results may be given to the family either via the GP or as an out-patient. Patients should be informed of any plan for follow-up.
- At discharge, families need to know how to get help if necessary after discharge. This may include the discharging ward name and telephone number, consultant secretary telephone number, or an out-of-hours contact number. Patients who do not require any follow-up or further treatment may be discharged back to their GP.

Further reading

📖 www.rcn.org.uk/publications/pdf/daysurgery_discharge.pdf
📖 www.dh.gov.uk/PublicationsAndStatistics/Publications/PublicationsPolicyAndGuidance/ PublicationsPolicyAndGuidanceArticle/fs/en?CONTENT_ID=4003252&chk=CKj7ss

Jan Walmsley, Royal Cornwall Hospital Trust

Care of the child/young person and family in the community

Effects of being a sick child or young person at home

As a result of the development of policy in the 1950s with regard to the care of sick children, professionals caring for children are generally of the mindset that acutely ill children are best cared for at home, and that any health problems a child encounters are likely to have an effect on the whole family system.

Parents have a sense of what is normal for their child, and use this knowledge as a reference point while monitoring the state of their child's health. When a child develops an acute illness, the carer is required to judge:
• if the child's illness is life threatening and therefore requiries hospital admission
• if they have enough information and confidence to cope with a child who may be fractious and frightened and refusing to cooperate
• if they have the patience and personal resources to care for a sick child.

The effects on parents of caring for a sick child at home include:
• overwhelming tiredness
• anxiety, especially if the child concerned is under 2 years old (this is appropriate as many physiological systems are not mature until the end of this period)
• fear they will not recognize or will misinterpret serious symptoms
• fear that they will be judged as inadequate or stupid
• lack of time to fulfil other roles and caring responsibilities
• time off work, which can result in financial hardship.

All these effects will be worsened; if there are other stressors, such as parental ill health, financial stress, other poorly siblings, a lack of emotional, social, and professional support, and unstable family functioning.

The role of the healthcare system is to ensure that the child is in a safe environment, where he/she will receive a reasonable standard of care. Parents will need to be reassured that any care or advice is approved, and health professionals need to be sure that the parents are able to respond to their child's symptoms, seek appropriate help, and work in partnership with staff to ensure the child does not suffer harm.

Further reading

Dimond, B. (2005). Legal aspects of the community care of the sick child. In *Textbook of children's community nursing*, 2nd edn, (ed. A. Sidey and D. Widdas). Elsevier, Edinburgh.

Neill, S. (2005). Caring for the acutely ill child at home. In *A textbook of children's and young people's nursing*, (ed. A. Glasper and J. Richardson). Churchill Livingstone, Edinburgh.

🖳 www.actionforsickchildren.org/

Sue Earney, University of Glamorgan

Managing long-term conditions in the community setting

Children with long-term health, educational, developmental, and social needs, may require additional support from services. The numerous agencies that could intervene are led by differing models of care, often funded from different government departments. These factors can result in territorial disputes, issues over 'ownership' of problems, and a lack of accountability for care. This can lead to a reactive service, which impacts on the quality of the child's life. Actively encouraging the child or young person to participate in decisions that affect his/her life, especially during transition, will deliver better outcomes.

Managing long-term conditions also requires caring for the family, who often perform many complex medical procedures, as well as facilitating the child's overall development and maintenance of family life.

The most responsive way forward is as follows:
- Build on the strengths of individuals and families to optimize health.
- Systematically assess the family's resilience, problem-solving skills, and adjustment and adaptation responses.
- Design, in collaboration, a health action plan to identify the level of support required.
- Establish a therapeutic relationships which recognizes boundaries, expectations, and the needs of the individual child within the context of family.
- Recognize that although caring can be a burden, this is often tempered by pride in caring and seeing improvements in the child. The family may not see the child's condition as a major source of stress, rather issues such as arrogant professional delivery.
- Identify the most appropriate key worker. Many 'expert' parents, if given the choice and authority, choose this role if they have control over care planning and services.
- Develop skills required for collaboration, negotiation, and partnership working—reciprocity, flexibility, and integrity—as children's needs and level of care varies over time, ranging from high-level management to supported self-care. One service may not meet all these needs.
- Get to know your 'patch' and where your organization 'sits' within the infrastructure of primary and community services.

These considerations, along with new pathways or models of care, will ensure that each child enjoys and achieves the most out of life, and that each family's success at parenting their child is optimized.

Further reading

Clarridge, A., Ryder, E. (2004). Working collaboratively. In *Nursing in the community: an essential guide to practice*, (ed. S. Chilton, K. Melling, D. Drew, and A. Claridge). Arnold, London.
Hudson, B. (2003). Working together in children's services: a time to be bold? *Journal of Integrated Care*, **11**(5), 3–12.
▣ www.kingsfund.org.uk/health_topics/managing.html

Sue Earney, University of Glamorgan

Communication with professionals

Good information sharing is the key to successful collaborative working and early intervention to help children and young people at risk of poor outcomes. The belief is that children, young people, and families who have multiple needs for which they require specialist help will achieve better outcomes, and have a better experience and engagement with services, through provision of integrated support.

Care agencies involved may include specialist consultants, paediatricians, social workers, occupational therapists, physiotherapists, and a primary care team, as well as others, and it is an excellent asset if a key worker can coordinate care.

While researching for the St Helen's Action Research Project in 2003, one parent documented the agencies involved in the care of his two children: nine health consultants; five therapists; a learning disability paediatric team; a school nurse; an orthotist; a wheelchair assessment team; a play, leisure respite support team; an education team. Over 7 years they had 774 contacts, spent 4942 hours on appointments and phone calls, and drove 11 004 miles to appointments.

He concluded that some stress could be removed if appointments were grouped, if a key worker system and coordination was the norm, and that a child should always be seen as an integral part of their family.

Key worker

It is good practice to have one of the multidisciplinary team to act as key worker and to be the lead professional, who will:

- act as a single point of contact, who children, young people, and families can trust, and who is able to support them in making choices and in navigating their way through the system
- ensure that children and families receive appropriate interventions when needed, which are well planned, regularly reviewed, and effectively delivered
- reduce overlap and inconsistency from other practitioners.

One poignant remark from a young adult who had undergone years of struggling in a family where her brother had cerebral palsy and she had juvenile arthritis, but was also one of his carers, was 'I felt let down by the system because I was never allowed to be a child. If we had had a key worker I would have had a brother not a responsibility.'

Further reading

 www.everychildmatters.gov.uk/deliveringservices/multiagencyworking/
Multi-agency working—a parent's view. www.cafamily.org.uk

Jackie Imrie, Central Manchester and Manchester Children's University Hospitals NHS Trust

Working with technology-dependent children at home

Advances in medical technologies have led to a number of children who require one or more medical devices to compensate for the partial failure or loss of a vital bodily function, in order to survive and/or to optimize health. The devices, which include ventilators, dialysis machines, and feeding pumps, enable the child to live in the community with the support of personnel who are technologically skilled. If the child is cared for at home, these personnel are primarily mothers, with a variable amount of family, professional, and voluntary support. Children living with life-threatening or life-limiting conditions may also have palliative needs requiring substantial and complex care for significant parts of the day and/or night.

An increasing weight of evidence is informing the commissioning, delivery, and funding of the management of their care. Studies describe parents wanting or experiencing the following.

- Professionals to acknowledge their expertise and to provide support to sustain their care-giving; to be easily accessible and approachable; acting as advocates; providing parents with relevant, timely, and robust information to enable them to feel in control.
- Respite services, both within the home and elsewhere for the child and/or family.
- A key worker whose skills involve diffusing emotional situations, identifying parents' strengths and weaknesses, and supporting appropriately and detailed knowledge of statutory and voluntary services.
- Negotiated rather than assumed responsibility; professionals generally supported parental care-giving rather than hands-on care; parents want choices regarding being the 'parent' or the 'nurse'.
- The emotional aspects of care—procedural pain, restraint, effects on parent–child relationship—to be acknowledged.
- Consideration of the effects of their home often resembling an intensive unit, complete with staff and alarmed machinery, resulting in a lack of privacy, sleep deprivation (equipment alarms and listening out for trouble), and extra household expense.

Parents suffer considerable strain in terms of resources, time, and emotional stress due to adapting to their child's circumstances and to the lack of suitably trained carers able to provide technical care. Better coordination of services and improvements in the design of devices would all help to reduce the stress. Paediatric nurses need to be fully informed regarding family resilience, adjustment, and adapting to living with a child who has a condition that results in him/her becoming dependent upon medical technology for survival .

Sue Earney, University of Glamorgan

Further reading

Kirk, S., Glendinning, C., Callery, P. (2005). Parent or nurse? The experience of being the parent of a technology-dependent child. *Journal of Advanced Nursing*, **51**(5), 456–64.

Margolan, H., Fraser, J., Lenton, S. (2004). Parental experiences of services when their child requires long term ventilation. Implications for commissioning and providing services. *Child: Care, Health and Development*, **30**(3), 257–64.

www.york.ac.uk/inst/spru/research/summs/techol_time.htm

Working with diverse communities

As the population of the UK is heterogeneous, practitioners working with diverse populations must surely investigate their own philosophical assumptions about diversity if they are to work within an ethos of justice, equality, and access. In the past, many nurses have worked with givens, often in an ethnocentric way, rather than theorizing about the factors that have influenced their approach with patients and clients somehow 'different' from themselves. This pragmatic non-reflective style may not be sensitive to the needs of those considered 'outsiders'.

British society has generally benefited from raised living standards, leisure, health, and education. However, there are many socially excluded groups who are prevented, either overtly or covertly, from all the benefits of British society that many enjoy and take for granted.

When we come into contact with a person perceived as different from ourselves, we socially construct this person as 'other'. This reconstruction occurs because, often hidden, stereotypes and prejudices come into play, and this can affect our behaviour, compassion, and commitment to relating to them, and them to us.

Requirements to promote inclusion, tolerance, and acceptance of 'difference' include the following.
• Open and critical debate about the concepts of belonging, 'active citizenship', diversity, community, and exclusion/inclusion.
• A philosophical debate regarding how practitioners perceive health work and how this influences the encounters they share with patients and carers, by exploring the ethics and the truth of what they believe are 'givens'.
• The ability, willingness, and skills to problem solve, challenge, engage with, and transform situations and services, recognizing power imbalances within society.
• Being aware of concept of 'rights', 'responsibilities', and how to hear 'hidden voices'.
• Advocating not only for individuals but working strategically and politically to oppose disadvantage.

Practitioners need to explore the dynamics of the exclusionary practices that affect many aspects of daily life and ultimately affect people's health and wellbeing. This is vital if we as a society wish to raise awareness and stimulate debate to overcome apathy and deep-seated suspicion of others, and to receive the support of the diverse communities that we serve.

Further reading

Davis, J., Hoult, H., Jones, M., Evans, M., Higgs, A. (2005). Working with socially excluded groups. In *Health visiting. Specialist community public health nursing*, 2nd edn, (ed. A. Robotham and M. Frost). Elsevier, Edinburgh.

Price, B. (2005). Practice, philosophy, culture and care. *Multicultural Nursing*, **1**(1), 21–6.

▣ www.rcn.org.uk/resources/transcultural/childhealth/index.php

Sue Earney, University of Glamorgan

NHS walk-in centres

Introduced in 2000, NHS walk-in centres have given nurses the opportunity to develop their skills as autonomous practitioners, providing nurse-led minor injury and illness treatment without appointment, 7 days a week. They formed a crucial part of the government's commitment to ensure everyone has access to a primary healthcare professional within 24 hours. More recently it has become commonplace for them to support local changes to out-of-hour's primary care provision, with the provision for 24-hour care no longer the responsibility of GPs but now with local primary care trusts.

National figures

Of the walk-in centre workload, 25–30% concerns children and young people. Supported by a small number of paediatric trained nurses, health visitors, and midwifes, the centres are prominently staffed by generic nurses from primary care or emergency department backgrounds.

Common presenting complaints

- Rashes
- Sore throat
- Earache
- Cough
- Fever
- Head injury
- Eye discharge
- Abdominal pain
- Headache
- Minor injuries.

Primary objectives of a paediatric consultation

- Identify those conditions that can easily be managed by the nurse
- Provide an accurate working diagnosis and management
- Avoid missed pathology
- Make appropriate and timely referrals as necessary

These consultations should always be carried out within the family context, while considering the child's developmental stage and needs.

History and examination

The systematic documentation within the majority of walk-in centres can be described as:
- presenting complaint
- history of presenting complaint
- past medical history
- social history
- examination
- impression
- plan.

Maureen Wiltshire and Penelope Aitken, Southampton University Hospitals NHS Trust

A thorough head-to-abdomen examination should be mandatory in all paediatric minor ailment examinations. Many walk-in centres have available to their staff 'computer-assisted software' similar to that used by NHS Direct, supporting the face-to-face consultation carried out by the nurse practitioner. This program can aid the practitioners' critical thinking and decision-making by offering a series of condition-based questions that will identify any important red flags, advising them on the most appropriate management.

Further reading

Department of Health (2004). *Spotting the sick child* (DVD) 💻 www.ocbmedia.com

Department of Health (2000) *The NHS plan*. HMSO, London.

Hsu, R., Lambert, P.C., Dixon-Woods, M., Kurinezuk, J.J. (2003). Effects of NHS walk-in centres on local primary healthcare services: before and after observation study. *British Medical Journal*, **326**, 530–7.

Assessing the sick child

Principles of physical assessment

The principles of paediatric physical assessment involve more than observation, palpation, percussion, and auscultation. It should be remembered that even though the examination of the child is relatively painless, interventions such as the introduction of an oroscope into the ear, the palpation of the abdomen, and a cold stethoscope on the chest might all be very stressful to the child. Consideration should always be given to the child's psychological needs.

General guidance for performing paediatric physical examination

• Perform the examination in an appropriate non-threatening area that provides privacy.
• Place all strange and potentially frightening equipment out of sight.
• Have some appropriate toys and games available to comfort or distract the child. Consider involving a play specialist if appropriate.
• Provide time for play and becoming acquainted.
• When appropriate, involve the child and parents in the examination process.
• Provide an explanation to the child and parent about the examination procedure.
• Use a quiet, calm, and confident voice.
• Begin the examination in a non-threatening manner.
• Examine the child in a secure and comfortable position.
• Proceed to examine the child in an organized sequence.
• Leave painful and unpleasant procedures until last.
• In emergencies examine Airway, Breathing, and Circulation (ABC) first.
• Reassure the child and family throughout the examination.
• Discuss the findings of the examination with the child and family at the end of the examination.
• Thank the child and family for their cooperation during the examination.

Examining the child

Usually the child is examined from head to toe by dividing the body into specific areas, so as to reduce the likelihood of omitting sections of the examination. When examining children, the order in which these sections are examined frequently changes to take into account the child's developmental needs.

When examining the child, remember the following four principles.
• *Rapport:* develop a rapport with the child in order to gain their confidence.
• *Observation:* gain information from informal observation while taking their history.

Stefan Cash, University of Central England Birmingham

- *Undress the child:* the child should be undressed down to his underwear to maximize the likelihood of finding physical signs; however, care should be taken to maintain the child's dignity.
- *Be systematic:* follow the order of
  - observation
  - palpation
  - percussion
  - auscultation.

Further reading

Rudford, M. (2004). *Clinical examination of the child*. University of Leeds.

Assessing a child's temperature

Indications

- To determine the child's temperature as a baseline for comparison with future measurements.
- To monitor fluctuations in temperature.

Methods of assessment

Rectal

A glass–mercury thermometer or electronic digital thermometer is inserted 2–4 cm into the rectum.

- *Advantages:* most accurate and reliable reflection of core temperature and the preferred means of assessing moderately or critically ill children and babies under 1 year.
- *Disadvantages:* invasive, potentially perceived as abusive. Risks include lower bowel perforation, breakage of glass thermometer, and exposure to toxic mercury, cross-infection, and reactionary diarrhoea (in babies).

Oral

An electronic digital thermometer or disposable chemical dot thermometer is placed in the sublingual pocket at the base of the tongue for 2 min.

- *Advantages:* provides the second most accurate and reliable readings; readings are commonly only 0.3–0.6°C lower than rectal measurements.
- *Disadvantages:* caution should be exercised with non-compliant children, those under 5 years, or those with a history of seizures, to avoid the hazards of biting the thermometer.

Axilla

An electronic digital thermometer or disposable chemical dot thermometer is placed in the clean dry armpit for 3 min.

- *Advantages:* safe and non-invasive and the preferred method for babies and small children (under 5 years) if the rectal method is not suitable.
- *Disadvantages:* relatively inaccurate and unreliable. Readings are up to 0.92°C lower than the rectal reading, commonly listed as the least accurate method. The time required to obtain an accurate reading can pose a problem with young active children.

Tympanic membrane

An electronic tympanic membrane thermometer is placed in the ear canal for 2–10 s.

- *Advantages:* very quick, safe, and non-invasive. This method is preferred by children.
- *Disadvantages:* some doubt exists as to reliability and accuracy. Least accurate for babies and young children and in detecting high fever. It cannot be used where the probe does not fit the ear canal, where ear problems exist, where accuracy is important, or within 20 min of a change in ambient temperature. High fevers need to be confirmed by another method.

Andrew J.S. Brown, Plymouth Hospitals NHS Trust

Normal core temperature by age	
Under 6 months	37.5°C
7 months–1 year	37.5–37.7°C
2–5 years	37.0–37.2°C
Over 6 years	36.6–36.8°C

Further reading

Huband, S., Trigg, E. (ed.) (2000). *Practices in children's nursing: guidelines for hospital and community*, pp. 45–54. Churchill Livingstone, London.

Rush, M., Wetherall, A. (2003). Temperature measurement: practice guidelines. *Paediatric Nursing*, **15**(9), 25–28.

Assessing a child's heart rate

Indications
- To determine the child's heart rate as a baseline for comparison with future measurements.
- To monitor fluctuations in the heart rate.

Methods of assessment
Infant
- Use a stethoscope to hear the sound of the heart beating—'apex beat'.
- Place the stethoscope head on the baby's chest, between the left nipple and the sternum, and establish the characteristic *'lub-dub'* sound of the heartbeat.
- The number of complexes heard over a full minute gives the heart rate.
- If the rate is very rapid (over 120 bpm), you may be able to count every other complex and double it to establish the actual rate.
- You may be able to palpate a pulse in an artery to verify the rate and observe the amplitude of the heartbeat.

Child
- Assess the heart rate by palpating the arterial pulse at any of a number of sites, including the radial, brachial, femoral, carotid, and temporal arteries.
- Consider the most appropriate site to be used with regard to privacy, dignity, and comfort.
- The radial artery pulse is the most common site and tends to cause the least discomfort; however, in shock it is likely to be one of the first pulses to become unpalpable.
- Place the pads of your first and second fingers over the pulse point and establish the pulse.
- Count the number of pulses over one full minute, giving the heart rate.
- Also note the characteristics of the pulse.

Pulse characteristics
When assessing the heart rate by either method, it is important to note the characteristics of the heartbeat.
- The amplitude of the beat gives a reflection of the pulse strength and elasticity of the artery wall and may be described as full or bounding, weak or feint.
- The rhythm may be noted as regular or irregular, and an irregular beat as 'regularly-irregular' or 'irregularly-irregular'. In these cases, an apex beat should also be observed for comparison.
- When recording the heart rate, it is also important to relate the observation to the activity level of the child and what rate might reasonably be expected.

Andrew J.S. Brown, Plymouth Hospitals NHS Trust

Normal heart rates		
	Awake (bpm)	**Asleep (bpm)**
Newborn	100–180	80–160
<3 months	100–220	80–180
3 months–2 years	80–150	70–120
3–10 years	70–110	60–100
10 years–adult	55–90	50–90

Further reading

Huband, S., Trigg, E. (2000). *Practices in children's nursing: guidelines for hospital and community*, pp. 45–54. Churchill Livingstone, London.

Mallett, J., Bailey, C. (ed.) (1996). Observations. In *The Royal Marsden NHS Trust manual of clinical nursing procedures*, 4th edn, pp. 395–9. Blackwell Science, Oxford.

Assessing a child's respiratory rate

Indications
- To determine the child's respiratory rate as a baseline for comparison with future measurements.
- To monitor fluctuations in the respiratory rate.
- To evaluate the child's response to respiratory medications or treatments.

Method of assessment
- Carry out this observation surreptitiously, to avoid the child being aware of the process and, either consciously or subconsciously, altering his/her breathing pattern.
- Count the number of complete inhale–exhale combinations over the course of a minute, observing the chest or abdominal movements and sounds as indicators.
- In babies and young children, it is important to count for a full minute as it is normal for the rate and pattern of breathing to change from one moment to the next, including pauses of up to 10 s.

Respiration characteristics
When assessing the child's respiratory rate, observe the following.
- The depth of respirations: gives an indication of the adequacy of the tidal volume.
- The quality of respiration: this can be indicated by use of muscles, breath sounds, and other body responses.

A baby normally uses its abdominal muscles, and a school-age child its costal muscles, to breathe.

Respiratory distress should be suspected in a baby who is breathing costally or a child breathing abdominally.

Normal respiration is quiet, but unusual sounds such as wheezing, crackling, grunting, crowing, or stridor may indicate respiratory distress.

If breathing is difficult, there may be evidence of accessory muscle use, including use of the intercostal muscles, shoulders rising on inspiration, or head-bobbing. Other signs such as tracheal tug, nasal flaring, restlessness, unusual posturing, intercostal, subcostal, or sternal recession, and peripheral or central cyanosis must all be taken as evidence of respiratory distress.

Normal respiratory rates	
Newborn	30–60
6 months	30–45
1–2 years	25–35
3–6 years	20–30
7–12 years	20–25
Adolescent	14–20

Andrew J.S. Brown, Plymouth Hospitals NHS Trust

Further reading

Huband, S., Trigg, E. (2000). *Practices in children's nursing: guidelines for hospital and community*, pp. 45–54. Churchill Livingstone, London.

Mallett, J., Bailey, C. (ed.) (1996). Observations. In *The Royal Marsden NHS Trust manual of clinical nursing procedures*, (4th edn), pp. 409–16. Blackwell Science, Oxford.

Assessing a child's blood pressure

Indications
- To determine the child's blood pressure as a baseline for comparison with future measurements.
- To monitor fluctuations in the blood pressure.

Methods of assessment
The blood pressure may be measured either directly or indirectly.
- *Direct* measurement is by far the more accurate method and involves placing a tiny pressure transducer into an artery, calibrating it, and reading the pressures on an electronic monitor.
- *Indirect* measurement can be carried out either by auscultation or oscillometry.

Auscultation
This method involves the use of an aneroid sphygmomanometer and stethoscope.
- Place the sphygmomanometer at the level of the child's heart and place the appropriately sized cuff snugly around the upper arm.
- Support the arm in a slightly flexed position and inflate the cuff rapidly while palpating the brachial pulse.
- When the pulse can no longer be detected, inflate the cuff by a further 20 mmHg and apply the stethoscope head gently over the brachial artery.
- Deflate the cuff at a rate of 5 mmHg/s while listening for Korotkoff's sounds.

Korotkoff's sounds				
Phase 1	**Phase 2**	**Phase 3**	**Phase 4**	**Phase 5**
Sharp thud	Blowing/swishing sound	Softer thud	Softer blowing/ swishing sound	Silence
Systolic			Diastolic	

- When the first 'sharp thud' is heard, this marks the systolic pressure.
- As the cuff is deflated further, the sound changes from a 'softer thud' to a 'softer blowing sound', which marks the diastolic pressure.
- Deflate the cuff rapidly and remove.

This method is very difficult to use reliably on infants and young children, especially if they are not cooperative.

Oscillometry
This involves the use of an electronic blood pressure machine to measure the pressures and can be advantageous for use on babies and young children.

The cuff can be applied to either the upper arm or the lower leg. However, there are limitations to its use; movement of the limb adversely affects accuracy and reliability, and the cuff inflation pressure may be excessive and painful.

Andrew J.S. Brown, Plymouth Hospitals NHS Trust

Factors to consider

- A child's blood pressure varies with age, is closely related to height and weight, and there is normal variability between children of the same age and build.
- Excitement, anxiety, discomfort, pain, and the process of measurement itself may all result in a rise in actual blood pressure.
- For these reasons, clinical decisions should never be based on a single blood pressure recording.
- Measurement should be carried out when the child is relaxed and has been sitting or lying quietly for at least 2 minutes.
- Korotkoff's sounds may not be reliably heard in children under 5 years of age.
- When measured in the legs, the blood pressure may be slightly higher than when measured in the arms.
- The widest possible cuff that can be applied to the limb should be used and the inflation bladder should be at least two-thirds of the circumference of the limb. An undersized cuff will result in a false high reading; an oversized cuff will give a false low reading. The cuff should be removed from the limb between use to prevent problems associated with ischaemia and neuropathy. Mercury sphygmomanometers are no longer considered acceptable for use because of the hazard that toxic mercury presents.

Normal blood pressure values		
	Systolic pressure (mmHg)	Diastolic pressure (mmHg)
Newborn	60–85	20–60
6 months	75–105	40–70
2 years	75–110	45–80
7 years	75–115	45–80
Adolescent	100–145	60–95

Further reading

Huband, S., Trigg, E. (2000). *Practices in children's nursing: guidelines for hospital and community*, pp. 45–54. Churchill Livingstone, London.

Mallett, J., Bailey, C. (ed.) (1996). Observations. In *The Royal Marsden NHS Trust manual of clinical nursing procedures*, 4th edn, pp. 402–409. Blackwell Science, Oxford.

Observation of the sick child

The European Resuscitation Council recommend using the ABC approach. This is a structured approach which is easy to remember, and the child should be constantly re-assessed using this system.

Airway and breathing

The rate and rhythm should be noted. Observe for:
• signs of recession
• inspiratory or expiratory noises
• grunting
• use of accessory muscles
• nasal flaring
• chest symmetry when auscultating the chest
• a silent chest is a worrying sign
• arterial oxygen saturation SaO_2 should be >98% in air; use of supplemental oxygen (O_2) will affect the reading
• child's ability to talk; severe breathlessness will affect this.

Respiratory rate by age at rest	
<1 year	30–40 rpm
1–2 years	25–35 rpm
2–5 years	25–30 rpm
5–12 years	20–25 rpm
>12 years	15–20 rpm

Circulation

• Note heart rate and pulse volume.
• Capillary refill should be <2 s and should be done on the sternum. A patient who is shocked or has hypothermia will give a false capillary refill time.
• If the capillary refill time is >2 s, give a fluid bolus of 20 ml/kg. Normal saline is the first bolus of choice. Repeat the fluid bolus until the capillary refill is <2 s.

Heart rate by age at rest	
<1 year	110–160 bpm
1–2 years	100–150 bpm
2–5 years	95–140 bpm
5–12 years	80–120 bpm
>12 years	60–100 bpm

Denise Toplis, Royal Devon and Exeter NHS Foundation Trust

Blood pressure

- Hypotension is a pre-terminal sign. Children maintain their blood pressure for a long period and respiratory arrest commonly follows a fall.
- The correct cuff size should be used for an accurate reading. The biggest size to fit the arm should be used—too small will result in a falsely raised reading. If the child is screaming, in pain, or fitting, this may also result in a falsely raised blood pressure.

Systolic blood pressure by age at rest	
<1 year	70–90 mmHg
1–2 years	80–95 mmHg
2–5 years	80–100 mmHg
5–12 years	90–100 mmHg
>12 years	100–120 mmHg

Disability

A rapid assessment can be made using:

A: Alert
V: Responsive to voice
P: Responsive to pain
U: Unresponsive

If a child has a score of P/U, consider intubation to maintain a secure airway.

After the initial assessment, use the Glasgow Coma Scale (GCS) with the appropriate age scale. There are two age scales: <4 years of age and >4 years of age.

All observations should be recorded in black ink and initialled by the professional recording them. It is important to look at the trend when recording observations and not isolated observations. The trend will show an improvement or decline in condition. Record observations as frequently as appropriate.

Recognition of the sick child

Recognition of the sick child can be difficult and clues can be missed, as infants/children are unable to describe their symptoms. The European Resuscitation Council recommends using the ABC approach.

Airway and breathing

- *Respiratory rate:* a raised rate may indicate lung or airway disease or metabolic acidosis
- *Recession:* may be intercostal, subcostal, or sternal
- *Inspiratory/expiratory noises:* stridor or wheeze
- *Grunting:* a sign of severe respiratory distress; it is an attempt to prevent airway collapse by generating a positive end expiratory pressure
- *Accessory muscle use:* in infants this may cause head-bobbing
- *Nasal flaring*

If a child is in respiratory distress for a long period, he/she will become exhausted and the signs of increased effort will decrease. Exhaustion is a pre-terminal sign and requires prompt attention.

Auscultation of the chest will indicate the amount of air being inspired and expired. Chest movement should be symmetrical and regular. A silent chest is extremely concerning.

Effects of respiratory distress on other organs

- Heart rate: initially produces tachycardia; prolonged hypoxia leads to bradycardia, a pre-terminal sign
- Skin colour: initially pale; cyanosis is a pre-terminal sign
- Mental status: hypoxia causes agitation and drowsiness

Circulation

- *Heart rate:* increases in shock
- *Pulse volume:* absent peripheral or weak central pulses are a sign of advanced shock
- *Capillary refill:* should be <2 s
- *Blood pressure:* children maintain their blood pressure for long periods; hypotension is a pre-terminal sign

When assessing a sick child, ABC takes priority and should be repeated until normal parameters are reached.

Disability

Conscious levels can be assessed rapidly using:

A   Alert
V   Responsive to voice only
P   Responsive to pain only
U   Unconscious

Level P/U equates to a GCS score of <8. If a child is at this level, intubation should be considered to protect the airway

Denise Toplis, Royal Devon and Exeter NHS Foundation Trust

Nursing care of the sick child

Management of procedural pain

Procedure-related pain is a major source of distress to the child and family. Poorly managed pain will result in the child continuing to display high levels of distress in future procedures. To a child there is no such thing as a minor procedure. Often the extent of tissue damage correlates poorly with the severity of pain that the child experiences.

Prevention and treatment of procedural pain should be multidimensional, involving both pharmacological and non-pharmacological interventions. The number of interventions required will depend on:
- invasiveness of the procedure
- level of child's anticipatory anxiety
- child's age and stage of cognitive development.

Pharmacological interventions

Use depends on the type of procedure:
- Emla®/Ametop®
- simple analgesics such as paracetamol and ibuprofen
- oral morphine or intranasal diamorphine have been used for more painful procedures
- non-nutritive sucking for infants
- Entonox©
- anxiolytics and sedatives

Non-pharmacological interventions
- Parental presence
- Hugging, holding
- Play, reading books, television
- Distraction, bubble blowing, singing, deep breathing
- Mind suggestion, e.g. 'putting on a magic glove'
- Guided imagery and relaxation

Management
- Plan ahead
- Justify the necessity of the procedure
- Provide step-by-step, honest, age-appropriate information to child and parent to increase their sense of control
- Use books or dolls to explain the procedure
- Maintain a calm environment
- Avoid delays and unnecessary distress by preparing all the equipment beforehand and keep covered
- Use a treatment room if possible and keep the child's room/bed-space as a 'safe area'
- Allow choices, e.g. which arm shall we use?
- Give the child a role, e.g. holding the tape
- Encourage use of distraction and play
- Ensure communication with the multidisciplinary team to reduce the number of procedures, e.g. taking all blood tests at once

Denise Jonas, University of Salford and Central Manchester and Manchester Children's University Hospitals NHS Trust

- For long procedures use time-out periods
- Use appropriate equipment, such as automatic lancets
- Limit the health professional to a number of attempts made for venepuncture
- Afterwards praise with an emphasis on the positive aspects of the experience, use reward stickers or certificates
- Always aim for a positive first experience

Further reading

Lossi, C. (2002). *Procedure related cancer pain in children.* Radcliffe Medical Press, Abingdon.
BOC Medical (2000). *Entonox. Controlled pain relief. Reference guide.* BOC Group PLC, Manchester.
www.us.elsevierhealth.com/WOW/
www.rcn.org.uk/members/downloads/restraining-holding-still-cyp.pdf

Pain assessment tools

Pain is difficult to measure precisely and accurately in children. Many pain measurement tools and scores have been developed for use with children. Their use depends upon the child's verbal and cognitive ability. Additionally, consider the severity of the child's illness, the surgical or medical procedure, and the medical environment. It is also vital that you are completely familiar with the use of the selected pain assessment scale.

Whichever scoring system is used, repeat pain assessment regularly, prescribe appropriate intervention, and record their effectiveness.

Selecting a pain assessment tool: points to consider

- Condition of child: a very sick child may be too ill to comprehend instructions regarding the use of a pain scale.
- Age of child: behavioural measure or self-report measure.
- Time available to teach child to use selected tool.
- Interventions that may be necessary: pain assessment must be linked to interventions, with the aim of ensuring that the child experiences no pain or only mild pain.
- Culture can influence an individual's perception and response to pain.
- History taking: vital on admission to record child's usual reaction and normal responses to pain at home, e.g. behaviour, words used to describe pain. Include this information in the nursing care plan.
- Special needs: parents can be a valuable resource with children with complex needs.
- Parent involvement: parents can be involved in identifying a pain assessment scale appropriate for their child.
- Type of pain: acute, chronic, or recurrent.

Pain scales

Usually incorporate one or more of the following:
- self-reported assessment
- physiological assessment
- behavioural assessment.

Self-reported assessment

- Examples of self-report assessment scales include visual analogue scales, verbal rating scales, and facial expression scales.
- As pain is a subjective experience, self-reporting techniques are acknowledged as the most accurate indicators of pain.
- Self-report is usually possible by 4 years of age, but will depend on the cognitive and emotional maturity of the child.
- At 4–5 years of age children can differentiate 'more', 'less', or 'the same'.
- Indicating severity using a faces pain scale can work well. Some children are unable to relate the faces to their own pain experiences, while others tend to choose those at the extremes of the scale.

Catherine Trower, Royal Hospital for Sick Children, Glasgow

- Between 7 years and 10 years of age children develop skills with measurement, classification, and putting things in order. Hence, visual analogue scales can be used to describe pain intensity, location, and quality.

Physiological assessment

- Physiological changes associated with pain include increased heart rate, respiratory rate, blood pressure, intracranial pressure, cerebral blood flow, and palmar sweating; decreases in SaO_2.
- Care must be taken because not all of the variability they show may be specifically related to pain. One measure may not be an accurate indicator of pain; therefore, a good approach to pain measurement may be multidimensional.

Behavioural assessment

- Examples of behavioural assessment scales include FLACC, PIPP, and PPP.
- For children younger than 3 years, a tool that includes observation of behaviour can be effective in scoring pain accurately.
- Observations of behaviour include facial expression, body position, mobility, crying, sleep pattern, skin colour, and vital sign measurement.
- Caution should be taken when relying solely on behavioural responses with neonates, because they may be physically incapable of crying or body movement, and their stillness may not indicate that they are pain free.

Further reading

Howard, R.F. (2003). Current status of pain management in children. *Journal of the American Medical Association*, **290**(18), 2464–9.

Morton, N.S. (2001). Assessment of pain in children. *Anaesthesia and Intensive Care Medicine*, **1**(4), 138–40.

Pre-operative care

Pre-operative preparation is important for both the child and the family. Effective and appropriate physical and psychological preparation of the child and the psychological preparation of the family are necessary to ensure both the safety of the child and reduce the anxiety of the family experience.

Psychological preparation and support

- Must be age appropriate.
- If surgery is electively planned, then ideally preparation should start prior to admission via a pre-admission programme visit, where staff can explain and discuss what will happen with both the child and his/her parents.
- Parents can begin to explain about hospitals and operations prior to admission using age-appropriate books and audiovisual aids, available from local libraries.
- Parents should receive both verbal and written information.

Physical preparation

- Explain the procedure to child and parents.
- Ensure that the doctor has explained the procedure to parents and child and that the consent form has been completed correctly and signed.
- Record baseline observations: temperature, pulse, respiration, and blood pressure.
- Obtain and record current weight and height.
- Ensure that the identity wrist band with name, age, date of birth, ward, and weight is in place and legible.
- Ensure allergies are recorded clearly in notes and apply a second armband identifying the allergies.
- Identify and clearly record any loose teeth.
- Ensure specific pre-operative investigations have been obtained and results recorded in notes, e.g. chest X-ray, urinalysis, blood samples.
- Ensure child has had a bath and is wearing appropriate clothing.
- Remove any nail varnish.
- Remove all jewellery; give to parents for safe keeping.
- Tie long hair back with a non-metallic bauble.
- Ensure child has been fasted for the specified time identified in the trust policy.
- Ensure child has emptied his/her bladder, or infant has had a dry nappy put on, before giving premedication.
- Administer premedication as prescribed.
- Ensure medical staff have clearly marked operation site if necessary, e.g. leg or arm.
- Ensure notes, nursing documentation, and X-rays are ready and available.
- Complete theatre checklist according to trust policy.

Pauline Carson, University of Wolverhampton

- Accompany child and parents to theatre with porter when advised by theatre.
- Check child into theatre with theatre staff and advise regarding specific issues such as allergies or loose teeth.

Further reading

Huband, S., Trigg, E. (2000). *Practices in children's nursing guidelines for hospital and community.* Churchill Livingstone, London.

Royal College of Nursing (2005). *Peri-operative fasting in adults and children.* A national guideline developed by the Royal College of Nursing. Royal College of Nursing, London.

Fundamental skills

Handwashing

Handwashing is a process that removes potentially pathogenic organisms from hands, prevents cross-infection, protects the patient and nurse, and can reduce high rates of hospital-acquired infection. The principle of handwashing is to remove dirt and reduce the levels of transient and resident organisms on the hands.

Wash your hands:
- on entering and before leaving the work area
- before and after
  - patient contact
  - contact with body fluids, your own or patients'
  - wearing gloves
  - isolation nursing
  - food handling
  - invasive procedures
  - contact with contamination sources
  - caring for susceptible/high-risk patients.

Types of handwash
- Social handwash: 10–15 s
- Hygienic/antiseptic hand disinfection: 15–30 s
- Surgical scrub: 2–5 min

Equipment requirements
- Easy access to handwashing instructions
- Easy access to sink
- Hot and cold running water
- Liquid soap
- Antiseptic handwash if required
- Paper towels
- Bin with foot pedal

Points to consider
- Wetting of hands before applying soap
- Working up a soapy lather before commencing procedure
- Complete coverage of all areas of both hands
- Removal of debris from under the finger nails (do not use nail brush)
- Short finger nails
- Removal of rings and wrist items

Leyonie Higgins, Central Manchester and Manchester Children's University Hospitals NHS Trust

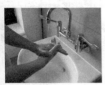

1. Palm to palm

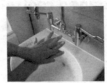

2. Right palm over left dorsum and left palm over right dorsum

3. Palm to palm fingers interlaced

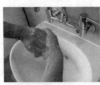

4. Backs of fingers to opposing palms with fingers interlocked

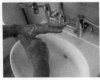

5. Rotational rubbing of right thumb clasped in left palm and vice versa

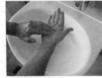

6. Rotational rubbing, backwards and forwards with clasped fingers of right hand in left palm and vice versa

Keeping hands up, rinse hands under running water and dry thoroughly with a *minimum* of two paper towels.

Effective handwashing

Further reading

Department of Health (2003). *Winning ways: working together to reduce healthcare associated infection in England.* DOH, location.

Storr, J., Clayton-Kent, S., (2004). Hand hygiene. *Nursing Standard*, **18**, 40, 45–51.

🖳 www.cdc.gov/handhygiene

Prevention and control of infection

Many healthcare-associated infections (HAIs) are potentially life threatening.

Little work has been carried out on paediatric patients and much of the evidence on HAI and how to reduce the risk to patients is extrapolated from adult or mixed adult–paediatric studies.

Approximately 10% of patients will acquire an infection as a direct result of receiving healthcare. Nurses must have a basic understanding of:
- the epidemiology of diseases causing infections
- the factors that put patients at increased risk of acquiring these infections
- the best evidence-based guidance for practice.

Micro-organisms

Potential pathogens are micro-organisms that can bypass the body's natural defence mechanisms and cause infection. They include bacteria, viruses, fungi, and protozoa.

Resident/endogenous micro-organisms

The human body already has its own population of microbes that are not easily removed. If they do not enter sterile body sites, they cause no harm.

Area of body	Micro-organisms commonly resident
Skin	Staphylococci, diptheroids, *Candida*
Respiratory tract	Staphylococci, streptococci, *Haemophilus*
Gastrointestinal tract	*Enterococcus, Enterobacter, Lactobacillus, Escherichia coli, Klebseilla, Serratia*

Transient/exogenous micro-organisms

Transient micro-organisms are those that are acquired by the body from an external source, i.e. other people or the environment.

Route of transmission

Route of transmission	Micro-organisms
Direct/indirect contact	Staphylococci
	Most pathogens can be spread by contamination of hands or the environment
Aerosol droplets	Respiratory syncytial virus
Airborne	Chickenpox, measles
Faecal–oral	Rotavirus
Blood-borne	Hepatitis C and B, human immunodeficiency virus (HIV)

Pamela Joannidis, Hospital for Sick Children Glasgow

Risk of infection

The risk of acquiring an infection will increase with:
- prematurity of age
- impaired immunity
  - chronic disease
  - treatment, e.g. cytotoxic therapy or steroids
- break in the skin, i.e. trauma, surgical wound, or invasive device.

Standard infection control precautions

Standard infection control precautions (SICP) are a series of actions designed to reduce the transmission of micro-organisms. They include:
- hand hygiene
- personal protective equipment
- decontamination of medical equipment
- environmental cleanliness
- safe use and disposal of waste
- patient placement
- safe handling of laundry.

Further reading

Jarvis, W.R. (2004). The state of the science of health care epidemiology, infection control, and patient safety, 2004. *American Journal of Infection Control*, **32**(8), 496–503.

Wilson, J. (2002). *Infection control in clinical practice*, 2nd edn. Ballière Tindall, London.

Pittet, D. (2004). The Lowbury lecture: behaviour in infection control. *Journal of Hospital Infection*, **58**(1), 1–13.

Pratt, R.J., Pellowe, C., Loveday, H.P., *et al.* (2001). The EPIC Project: developing national evidence-based guidelines for preventing healthcare associated infections. Phase 1: guidelines for preventing hospital-acquired infections. *Journal of Hospital Infection*, **47**(suppl. A).

Personal protective equipment

Employes have a duty to provide healthcare staff with PPE that is intended to protect them from exposure to microbial agents, where there is a risk to health and safety.

Risk assessment

All procedures to be carried out by healthcare staff must be risk assessed for potential exposure to patient blood, body fluids, and potentially pathogenic micro-organisms.

Procedure to be
carried out

↙ ↓ ↘

No contact with
body fluids

Contact with body fluids (low
risk of splashing)

Contact with body fluids
(high risk of splashing)

↓ ↓ ↓

No protective
clothing required

Gloves and aprons

Gloves apron, mask, and
eye protection

Healthcare managers have a duty of care to provide staff with the appropriate equipment and nurses should understand when they should be worn.

Examples of PPE

Procedure	Potential exposure	PPE required
Changing a nappy, stoma bag	Exposure to urine and faeces	Vinyl gloves, plastic apron
Venepuncture	Exposure to patient's blood on hands	Nitrile gloves
Care of patient with infectious agent, e.g. rotavirus	Exposure to virus on the patient and in the patient's immediate environment	Aprons and gloves
Theatre procedures where there is a risk of blood splash	Exposure to patient's blood on face, hands, and clothing	Theatre gown, nitrile or latex gloves, full visor

Further reading

UK Health Department (1998). *Guidance for clinical health care workers: protection against blood-borne viruses.* Department of Health, London.
Wilson, J. (2002). *Infection control in clinical practice*, 2nd edn. Ballière Tindall, London.
www.dh.gov.uk/assetRoot/04/01/474.pdf

Pamela Joannidis, Hospital for Sick Children Glasgow

Patient equipment

Patient equipment must be decontaminated appropriately. The level of decontamination will depend on:
- the level of contamination
- manufacturer's instructions for re-use ('single-use' must not be re-used; 'single-patient use' can be re-used on the same patient only).

Risk categories for medical devices and method of decontamination

Risk category	Level of contamination	Equipment	Recommendation
High risk	Penetrate skin or mucous membranes; enter sterile body area	Surgical instrument	Sterilization by autoclave; single use
Medium risk	Contact with mucous membranes	Laryngoscope blades	Sterilization or disinfection
Low risk	Contact with intact skin	Stethoscope; mattress	Cleaning

There are three levels of decontamination for medical equipment.
- Cleaning: the physical removal of dirt, soil, grease, body fluid, and many micro-organisms.
- Disinfection: kills a large number of micro-organisms but not spores.
- Sterilization: kills all micro-organisms, including spores.

Cleaning

Cleaning with neutral detergent and water is an effective way to decontaminate low-risk items. It is important to dry items thoroughly prior to storage. Fresh warm water should be used with a neutral detergent and disposable cloth (or detergent wipes).

Fit for purpose

All medical equipment being cleaned must be inspected to ensure it is fit to be re-used. Equipment that cannot be adequately decontaminated should be replaced.

Disinfection and sterilization

These procedures are carried out in approved facilities specializing in the decontamination of medium- to high-risk equipment. Please refer to local policies for further information.

Purchase or loan

Medical equipment purchased or on loan must only be used after consideration of the following.
- Is it re-usable?
- Manufacturer's instructions for cleaning.

Seek the advice of the local infection control team if unclear about decontamination of re-usable items.

Pamela Joannidis, Hospital for Sick Children Glasgow

Toys

Studies have linked toys to outbreaks of rotavirus and *Pseudomonas*, while *Aspergillus* and other fungal spores have been isolated from teddy bears and soft toys.

Choose toys that can be cleaned (hard surface, e.g. vinyl, metal, or plastic) or laundered between patients. Try to avoid soft toys for decoration.

Children may be allowed to bring their own toys into hospital but must not share them with other children.

Further reading

Ayliffe, G.A.J., Lowbury, E.J.L., Gedde, A.M., Williams, J.D. (2000). *Control of hospital infection: a practical handbook.* Chapman & Hall, London.
Wilson, J. (1995). *Infection control in practice.* Ballière Tindall, London.

Patient placement

When patients present with signs and symptoms suggestive of an infectious aetiology, consideration must be given to the most appropriate accommodation to optimize care while reducing the risk of transmission of that agent. (Please refer to the appropriate sections of the handbook for presenting symptoms for infectious agents, e.g. respiratory syncytial virus (RSV).

Single room accommodation should be considered for children presenting with the following:
• fever, cough, wheeze, and increased mucus production
• undiagnosed rash
• diarrhoea and vomiting
• bacterial meningitis (first 24 hours of antibiotic therapy)
• previous/current MRSA.

Patents admitted to high-risk areas such as paediatric intensive care, high dependency, neonatal unit, or burns unit should be screened for resistant mico-organisms such as MRSA.

Standard infection control precautions are sufficient to reduce the risk of transmission of the majority of micro-organisms. However, there are a number of recognized infectious agents for which additional precautions are recommended to further reduce the risk to patients, staff, and visitors.

Transmission-based precautions are linked to what is understood about the route of transmission of the micro-organism. The recognized transmission routes for common infectious agents and the recommended precautions to take are given in the table opposite.

Resident parents

Parents must be allowed to stay with their sick child. Nursing staff must take the opportunity to explain to parents the importance of:
• hand hygiene
• other standard infection control precautions as appropriate
• adherence to isolation procedures
• not touching other patients
• not sharing toys between patients
• not visiting if they have an infection (check with local infection control team).

Further reading

Haley, R.W., Culver, D.H., White, J.W. *et al.* (1985). The efficacy of infection surveillance and control programs in preventing nosocomial infections in US hospitals. *American Journal of Epidemiology,* **121**(2), 182–205.

Pratt, R.J., Pellowe, C., Loveday, H.P. *et al.* (2001). The epic project: developing national evidence-based guidelines for preventing healthcare associated infections. Phase 1: Guidelines for preventing hospital-acquired infections. *Journal of Hospital Infection,* **47** (suppl. A).

Pamela Joannidis, Hospital for Sick Children Glasgow

Route of transmission of common pathogens.

Micro-organism	Route of transmission	Recommended precautions
RSV	Aerosol droplet	Isolation in single room or cohort a group of patients with RSV
	Contact with items contaminated by droplets	Apron and gloves for direct contact with patient
Rotavirus	Ingestion of contaminated food	Isolation in a single room
	On hands via contaminated items	Apron and gloves for direct contact with patient
MRSA	Direct contact with patient	Isolation in a single room
	Indirect contact via contaminated equipment and environment	Aprons and gloves for direct contact with patient
Chickenpox	Airborne spread of fine respiratory secretions	Isolation in a single room
	Direct contact with vesicular fluid	Apron and gloves for direct contact with patient
		Only staff that have immunity to chickenpox should care for the patient

Safe handling and disposal of clinical waste

Clinical waste is divided in to five main categories.
- Group A: Human or animal tissue, soiled surgical dressings, and swabs
- Group B: Sharps: discarded syringes, needles, broken glass, and other sharp surgical instruments
- Group C: Laboratory or postmortem waste
- Group D: Drugs and chemical waste
- Group E: Other wastes arising from healthcare, e.g. bed pans, and stoma bags

The responsibility and duty of care of those who produce clinical waste and those who are responsible for the transfer of the waste from the healthcare premises is described in the Environmental Act 1999 and the Environmental Protection (Duty of Care) Regulations 1991. Previously, clinical waste was incinerated, but new methods being considered include microwave and autoclave technologies.

Always decontaminate hands after handling clinical waste.

Safe use and disposal of sharps

Healthcare staff are encouraged to segregate clinical waste from domestic waste to ensure appropriate treatment prior to disposal and to reduce the cost of treating non-hazardous waste. Colour-coded systems are in place in all healthcare facilities and nursing staff must be aware of local protocols for the safe disposal of waste in their facility.

Routine safe practice with sharps should be observed with all patients:
- Place all disposable sharps into an approved sharps bin immediately after use. Do not delegate this task to someone else, but dispose of sharps you have used yourself.
- Take sharps containers to the point of use.
- Ensure all sharps bins are out of reach of children.
- Never overfill a sharps container. When three-quarters full or less, close securely and tag with a yellow clinical waste tag. It is not necessary to label the bin with 'Danger of Infection' or 'Biohazard' labels.
- Avoid manual resheathing of used needles.
- Dispose of a used needle and syringe as a single unit into the sharps bin where possible.

Further reading

Department of the Environment (1991). Environmental Protection Act 1990. *Waste management: the duty of care*. A code of practice. HMSO, London.

Pamela Joannidis, Hospital for Sick Children Glasgow

Laundry

Laundry used in healthcare can become a potential source of micro-organisms from the patient. The route of transmission of these can be by direct contact with contaminated items or dispersal into the environment during handling.

Handling used linen
- A plastic apron should be worn
- Have a laundry bag available at the bedside
- Remove apron and decontaminate hands after contact with used items
- Secure laundry bags in preparation for transport.

Laundering process
- Laundering should be carried out in an approved healthcare facility.
- Used laundry will undergo a process of disinfection by heat. Within the wash cycle, laundry is held at a temperature of either 65°C for 10 min or 71°C for 3 min to achieve an acceptable level of decontamination.
- Tumble drying and ironing will also help to kill any residual micro-organisms.

Duvets are being used increasingly in healthcare premises. PVC-coated duvets, which can be cleaned with detergent and water between patients, are preferred.

Pillows should have a PVC cover which can be wiped with detergent and water once pillow cases have been removed.

Infected (contaminated) laundry
Laundry that has been contaminated with blood or body fluid, or which has been used by a patient with a particular infectious agent, is bagged into a water-soluble bag (usually red). This bag will be placed unopened into the washing machine, to reduce the risk of exposure to laundry staff.

Laundry that may remain hazardous after normal processing
In many health boards, staff are recommended to incinerate laundry contaminated with any of the following pathogens:
- *Bacillus anthracis*
- viral haemorrhagic fevers
- rabies
- tropical pyrexia of unknown origin
- lepromatous leprosy
- CJD where CSF fluid has leaked on to linen.

Further reading
NHS Executive (1995). *Hospital laundry arrangements for used and infected linen.* HSE(95)**18**. HMSO, London.

Pamela Joannidis, Hospital for Sick Children Glasgow

Meeting children's hygiene needs

Hygiene is one of the fundamental requirements of any child in any educational establishment, at home, or in hospital.

The skin has many different functions and therefore it is imperative that it is cared for and kept clean:
- protects deeper and more delicate organs
- acts as barrier against invasion of micro-organisms
- forms vitamin D from the sun
- regulates temperature
- produces sweat when body temperature rises

Benefits of good hygiene
- Makes the child feel good, giving a positive self-image.
- Washing is a tonic, making the child feel healthy.
- Prevents infection and infestation by parasites.
- Promotes independence, forming good habits later on in life.
- Stimulates the physical, emotional, and cognitive areas of development by involving pouring games.
- Treats skin problems such as eczema, sweat rash, and sore skin, which can make the child irritable.

Main areas for consideration
When meeting hygiene needs, the main areas for consideration are:
- skin: some cultures use certain moisturizer creams to soften the skin
- nails: keep short and cut horizontal, not digging into the corners
- genitalia: do not push back the foreskin, simply wash the glans
- hair: brushed with a soft brush
- mouth: brush teeth as soon as teeth are apparent and avoid sugary drinks to prevent tooth decay
- eyes: use clean cotton wool balls and clean water; clean eyes from edge of nose outwards, using two clean pieces for each eye and clean, dry pieces for drying
- ears: to prevent perforation of eardrums and pushing wax further down the ear, do not use cotton buds to clean ears
- umbilicus: use clean water or prescribed cream to clean

Factors influencing children's hygiene requirements
- Age
- Culture
- Ethnicity
- Child and parental preference
- Economics
- Media
- Social influence
- Education

Martin Firth, University of Nottingham

Oral hygiene

General principles

- Inspect the mouth at least daily, noting the presence of *Candida*, ulcers, breaks in oral mucosa, saliva consistency, condition of teeth, tongue, gingival, and lips.
- Note pain or difficulty in using voice or swallowing.
- Consider using an assessment tool.
- Commence brushing routine with eruption of first tooth.
- Brush child's teeth at least twice a day.
- Help and supervision will be required until around the age of 7 years.
- Antibacterial mouthwashes and antifungal preparations may be necessary for some children.

Further reading

Hanson, C., (2004). Mouth care: how important is it? *Journal of Community Nursing*, **18**(8), 4–8.

Sgan-Cohen, H.D. (2005). Oral hygiene: past history and future recommendations. *International Journal of Dental Hygiene*, **3**(2), 54–8.

Paula Dawson, Nottingham University Hospitals NHS Trust

Action	Rationale
1. Assess need Age and development NBM Child receiving chemotherapy, corticosteroids, antibiotics, or O_2 Child requiring oral suction Intubated child Fluid-restricted and dehydrated child	To prevent infections, dental and systemic diseases, distress, and discomfort
2. Explain procedure Encourage involvement and/or self-care where appropriate	To gain cooperation and minimize distress and anxiety; to promote partnership in care
3. Gather supplies and wash hands Soft paediatric toothbrush Fluoride toothpaste Tap water Sterile water (babies <1 year) Mouthcare pack from sterile supply service Foam sponges Yellow soft paraffin	To prevent cross-infection; to avoid unnecessary interruption in procedure
4. Assess current mouth condition	To determine required intervention
5. Gently brush teeth and gums with paediatric head toothbrush and fluoride toothpaste for at least 2 min; use tiny smear of toothpaste for babies and pea-sized amount for children	Only toothbrush is effective in removing plaque formation
6. Encourage the child to spit after brushing; If they are able to, do not rinse	Rinsing reduces the benefit of fluoride toothpaste
7. Rinse mouth with water (use sterile water for babies <1 year) if child is unable to spit Foam swabs may be used for this purpose, or for moisturising the mouth	 Foam swabs are not effective for mouth cleaning
8. Orally intubated children should, where possible, have ET tube moved to alternate sides of the mouth daily	To prevent ulceration at pressure points
9. Apply yellow soft paraffin to lips	To prevent lip dryness and cracking

Assessment of a child with a wound

- Healing process: complex and affected by general and local factors.
- Essential to treat the whole child and not just the wound.

Factors to be considered

- Skin appearance
- Mobility
- Continence
- Nutritional status
- Sensory function
- Cardiovascular status
- Conscious state and level of comprehension according to age
- Physical and social environment
- Fear, causing stress

Assessment of the wound

- Systematic assessment of a wound is essential
  - provides data to evaluate healing rates and efficacy of the treatment regimen
  - carried out at regular intervals
- Process should be clearly documented.

The following should be included:
- type of wound: surgical, traumatic, pressure ulcer, etc
- site of wound: area of body
- wound measurement: width, depth, and length
- wound bed: amount of granulation, slough, and necrotic tissue
- condition of peri-wound: signs of infection
- exudate: amount and colour
- odour: is it offensive?
- pain: site, scale, and exacerbating factors
- infection: if suspected, send swab.

Planning and implementing care for a child with a wound

- Identify actual and potential problems.
- Factual statements, including accurate measurements and descriptions, are essential to ensure that an objective assessment is obtained which can be evaluated.
- Provide a good wound-healing environment with the use of evidence-based practice and clinical judgement.
- Adhere to local policies.
- You are accountable for any plan of care.

Linda Gibson, Royal Devon and Exeter NHS Foundation Trust

Selecting a wound dressing for a child

Criteria
- Remove excess exudates and toxic components
- Be impermeable to micro-organisms
- Be suitable for age of child, i.e. able to be appropriately secured
- Be atraumatic at dressing change, i.e. easily removable
- Maintain a high humidity at the wound dressing interface

Aims
- *Necrotic and sloughy wounds:* to remove devitalized or contaminated tissue from a wound until healthy tissue is exposed.
- *Infected wounds:* to rid the wound of infection and to prevent tissue damage and delayed healing.
- *Cavity wounds:* to provide a moist wound-healing environment to aid the wound-healing process.
- *Granulating wounds:* the management of a clean granulating wound depends on the amount of exudate. The aim is to select a dressing which can be left *in situ* as long as possible so as not to disturb the delicate healing process at frequent dressing changes.
- *Epithelializing wounds:* to protect and encourage a moist environment for optimal healing.

Further reading
Pudner, R. (1997). Assessing a patient with a wound. *Journal of Community Nursing.*, **11**(5), 28–30.
⌕ www.nurse-prescriber.co.uk/journals
⌕ www.shrinershq.org

Linda Gibson, Royal Devon and Exeter NHS Foundation Trust

Eye care

Eye care is necessary to help maintain hygiene, prevent drying of the cornea, treat infection, and administer required medication. How often eye care should be performed is variable and depends upon an individual's needs/circumstances.

The production of tears and blinking help wash away irritants and keep the eyes healthy. However, children may require eye care for various reasons, including:
• infection
• immunosuppression
• congenital abnormality
• post-operative surgical requirement
• poor blinking reflexes
• inability to close the eyes completely.

Newborn babies and infants are prone to getting sticky eyes because they have underdeveloped lacrimal drainage systems and therefore they may also require eye care.

Equipment required
• Prescribed medication
• Sterile dental rolls or gauze
• Sterile water
• Basic dressing pack
• Alcohol hand rub
• Gloves (if indicated)

Jacqueline Ulyatt, Nottingham University Hospitals NHS Trust

Eye care

Action	Rationale
Explain procedure to patient and carer	Alleviates anxiety, promotes cooperation
Swaddle babies and toddlers in a blanket; position with head/back supported, either lying or sitting	Restricts movement; promotes feeling of comfort and security; expedites procedure
Wash hands	Minimizes risk of cross-infection
Prepare surface	
Open basic dressing pack	
Apply alcohol hand rub and non-sterile gloves if indicated	
Dip dental roll into sterile water and gently wipe along closed eyelid from inner to outer canthus	Avoids corneal trauma during cleaning; reduces risk of infection
Discard dental roll and repeat as necessary, using a new dental roll each time	Reduces risk of cross-infection
Wash hands, re-apply hand gel, and repeat procedure on other eye	Reduces risk of cross-infection
If eye drops required, wash hands, gently retract lower eyelid and insert one eye drop	Exposes lower fornix; ensures correct delivery of medication
Avoid contact between dropper and eye	Reduces risk of accidental trauma
If ointment prescribed, wash hands, gently retract lower eyelid, apply small line of ointment into lower fornix	Exposes lower fornix; ensures correct delivery of medication
Avoid contact between tube with eye	Reduces risk of accidental trauma
Dab away any excess medication from skin	Prevents skin irritation
Social hand wash	Minimizes risk of cross-infection

Further reading

Kay, J. (2000). Eye care. In *Practices in children's nursing: guidelines for hospital and community*, (ed. S. Huband and E. Trigg), p.103. Churchill Livingstone, London.

Rowley, S. (2001). Aseptic non-touch technique. *Nursing Times*, **97**, VI–VIII.

Ear care

- It is advisable to keep children's ears dry when washing their hair, showering, or swimming, especially if they are known to have ear problems. The use of swimming plugs, which can be purchased in a chemist, or a plug of cotton wool smothered in vaseline will keep the ear canals dry.
- Some wax in the ears is normal. Glands in the inner one-third of the ear canal produce wax. As the squamous cells in the ear canal migrate outwards from the eardrum, wax is normally shed with these cells. It is not advisable to use cotton buds, matches, or hairgrips to clean or to dry the child's ears. These items can damage the lining of ear canal and, if pushed in far enough, can damage the child's eardrum. Rule number one is never put anything smaller than your elbow in your ear!
- Some children do have a build up of wax, for example those wearing hearing aids. Olive oil drops can be used to keep the wax soft, in the hope that it will be expelled naturally. If the child needs to have the wax removed, it is advisable to see an experienced practitioner.
- Refer to a doctor if a discharge or bleeding is seen coming from the child's ear.
- Please remember to apply sunscreen to the ears when the child is exposed to sunlight. Exposure to excessive sunlight can lead to basal cell carcinoma. It is also advisable for the child to wear a hat when in the sun.
- Avoid spraying anything into the ears, e.g. hair spray or any other cosmetic preparations.
- Always protect against, and preferably avoid, exposure to loud noise.

Further reading

Kaufman, G. (1998). Ear problems: care and prevention. *Practice Nurse*, **15**, 338–42.
Rodgers, R. (2000). Understand the legalities of ear syringing. *Practice Nurse*, **19**(4).
🖥 www.entnursing.com

Pressure ulcers

Pressure ulcers, formerly known as decubitus ulcers or pressure sores, are areas of tissue death, often, but not always, over a bony prominence which correlates with the positioning of the infant or child and/or their equipment. Areas at risk include occiput, nose, ears, sternum spinal processes, scapula, sacrum, buttocks, ischial tuberosities, iliac crest, knees, heels, and any area of pressure through equipment, e.g. endotracheal tubes, splints.

Pressure ulcers do occur in children and young people and may result in medical or body image consequences.

Prevention is better than cure

Principles of care	Rationale
Risk assessment within 6 hours of admission and if condition alters	Identify risk: **intrinsic risk factors**, e.g. age, skin integrity, underlying medical condition, medication, nutritional status, reduced mobility, and pain; **extrinsic risk factors**, e.g. pressure, anaesthesia, length of stay, severity of illness, and equipment *in situ*
Clinical judgement important; risk assessment tools aides-memoires	Tools: modified adult or PICU
Suitable positioning; correct use of manual handling devices as per local guidelines	Eliminate pressure/friction/shearing force
Maintain normal skin integrity, personal hygiene; clean immediately when soiled using mild non-alkaline cleansing agents	Minimize moisture as risk factor; maintain normal skin pH
Soft smooth bed linen	Avoid unwarranted pressure
Ongoing assessment and documentation of skin integrity as condition warrants	Non-blanching hyperaemia (discoloration in dark skin) blisters, warmth, oedema, and indurations are indicators of skin damage
Repositioning schedule dictated by risk assessment	Based on skin inspection and individual needs, not a ritual turning schedule
Observation of site of any equipment and reposition regularly wherever possible	Plaster casts, splints, saturation probes, nasogastric NG and ET tubes can cause pressure ulcers
Ensure free of pain	Increase mobilization in bed/chair
Educate children and young people and family	Encourages understanding and participation in care
Appropriate use of adjuncts for at-risk patients	Special beds, bed aids, chair aids, and local aids. Note: sheepskins, water-filled gloves, and doughnuts are not advised

Above all eliminate/diminish pressure, friction, and shearing. In the event of any loss of skin integrity, follow local wound care guidelines.

Rosemary Smith, Robert Gordon University, Aberdeen
Donald Todd, Royal Aberdeen Children's Hospital, Aberdeen

Further reading

National Institute for Clinical Excellence (2003). *Pressure ulcer prevention. Clinical guideline 7*. NICE, London. ▣ www.nice.org.uk/pdf/CG7_PRD_NICEguideline.pdf (accessed 7 July 2005).

Nursing and Midwifery Practice Development Unit (2002). *Pressure ulcer prevention: best practice statement*. NMPDU, Edinburgh. ▣ www.nhshealthquality.org/nhsqis/files/BPSPressureUlcer Prevention.pdf

Willock, J. (2004). Pressure ulcers in infants and children. *Nursing Standard*, **18**(24), 56–8, 60, 62.

Fluid requirements in children

Young children and infants have a greater fluid intake and output than adults and older children. This fluid requirement is relative to their size and several physiological characteristics; blood volume is greater in the neonate and decreases with age, as does the infant's extracellular fluid.

They have a greater need for water and can be susceptible to alterations in fluid balance. Water and electrolyte disturbances can occur often and progress rapidly. When there is a disturbance in fluid balance, infants and young children slowly re-adjust to these alterations.

The table below shows a simple formula for calculating normal fluid requirements in kilograms. This is useful when assessing the total daily fluid requirement for different age ranges:

Body weight	Fluid requirement/day	Fluid requirement/hour
First 10 kg	100 ml/kg body weight	4 ml/kg body weight
Second 10 kg	50 ml/kg body weight	2 ml/kg body weight
Subsequent kg	20 ml/kg body weight	1 ml/kg body weight

For example:
5 kg infant would require 500ml/day
15 kg child would require 1000 + 250 = 1250 ml/day
25 kg child would require 1000 + 500 + 100 = 1600 ml/day

Neonate fluid requirement

Fluids are prescribed as 150 ml/kg body weight/day. This fluid requirement is calculated on the volume of standard formula milk required, this is in relation to the protein and calorie intake required.

Further reading

Advanced Life Support Group (2001). *Advanced paediatric life support; The practical approach,* 3rd edn. BMJ Books, London.

Fluid balance monitoring

This is an essential part of caring for a sick child, but can be hard to understand.

Infants have a higher risk of fluid loss, because of a higher metabolic rate, larger surface area, a greater percentage of total body water, and an inability to concentrate urine. This makes infants more susceptible to developing a fluid imbalance as a result of:
• respiratory infection
• diarrhoea and vomiting
• sepsis
• burns.

A simple formula for working out fluid requirements	
Newborn infants	60 ml/kg body weight/24 hours Increase by 10 ml/kg body weight/24 hours for 4 days
<10 kg	100 ml/kg body weight/24 hours
11–20 kg	1000 ml plus 50 ml for each kg body weight over 10 kg
21–30 kg	1500 ml plus 25 ml for each kg body weight over 20 kg

• Insensible losses can be calculated by: 300 ml/m^2 BSA/24 hours.
• It is therefore important to monitor all input and output. Nappies can be weighed to assess losses due to urine output and diarrhoea (1 oz = 30 ml) to enable an accurate total in children unable to use the toilet/potty.
• A minimum output of 2 ml/kg body weight/hour in infants and 1 ml/kg body weight/hour in children indicates adequate renal perfusion.
• When assessing fluid status, also assess the following:
  • abnormal blood losses
  • heart rate
  • core–toe gap and capillary refill time
  • blood pressure (remember—a falling blood pressure is a pre-terminal sign)
  • conscious level by assessing AVPU
  • U&Es.

Signs of dehydration	
<5% dehydration	Thirst, decreased urine output, and dry mouth
5–10% dehydration	Dry soft anterior fontanelle and mucosa, dry skin with tenting, dark rings around the eyes, loss of body weight, tachycardia, oliguria <1 ml/kg body weight/hour
10–15% dehydration	Dry mucosa, poor skin turgor with clamminess, sunken anterior fontanelle and eyes, anuria, reduced blood pressure, and reduced conscious level

Further reading

William, C., Asquith, J. (2000). *Paediatric intensive care nursing*, pp.14–15. Churchill Livingstone, London.

Denise Toplis, Royal Devon and Exeter NHS Foundation Trust

Assessing dehydration

The initial assessment of the child focuses upon determining the extent of dehydration and electrolyte imbalance, in addition to monitoring the effect of interventions. By taking an accurate history from the child and parents, you can gauge the success of previous interventions, in particular the nature and amount of recent drinking. The older child who continues to have diarrhoea and vomiting, but has been able to drink fluid over the previous 24 hours, is less cause for concern than the younger child who has refused drinks or who is unable to tolerate fluids.

The assessment of the extent of dehydration in a child includes measurements of serum electrolyte levels in the blood along with an accurate nursing assessment, which will include:

- the child's behaviour
- skin: colour and condition
- capillary refill time (CRT)
- temperature, pulse, and respiration
- blood pressure

The key electrolytes involved are sodium, which is present in gastric secretions and lost through vomiting, and potassium, which is lost through diarrhoea. The loss of these electrolytes creates a major shift of fluid from the intracellular to extracellular fluid compartments, and also alters the acid–base balance.

The dehydrated infant often appears:
- pale
- lethargic and listless: probably because of the effects of electrolyte imbalance and ensuing acidosis
- sunken eyes due to loss of intra-occular fluid
- sunken fontanelle due to a reduction in cerebral spinal fluid volume
- the skin will lack elasticity due to loss of intracellular fluid into the extracellular fluid compartment to maintain blood volume
- cold extremities due to peripheral vasoconstriction
- reduced urinary output, as antidiuretic hormone is produced as a response to changes in plasma osmolarity, and urine output will be reduced in an attempt to conserve fluid.

An older child may present as irritable, restless, or weak, pale with sunken eyes, and with reduced skin elasticity.

All of the above are adaptive mechanisms that will come into play in an attempt to compensate for the effects of fluid loss. Eventually, if there is delayed or inadequate intervention, the pulse rate will rise and the blood pressure fall as a result of hypovolaemic shock.

Elaine Mahoney, University of Glamorgan

Further reading

Lockyer-Stevens, V., Francis, A. (2003). *Insights into meeting hydration needs*. In *Foundation studies for nursing; using enquiry-based learning*, (ed. S. Grandis, G. Long, A. Glasper, and P. Jackson). Palgrave Macmillan, Basingstoke.
Neill, S., Knowles, H. (2004). *The biology of child health*. Palgrave Macmillan, Basingstoke.
☐ www.rehydrate.org.dehydration

Assisting with taking a blood sample

Preparation

- Successful venepuncture ideally requires advanced notice.
- The use of anaesthetic gels and creams is vital to minimize pain and distress during the procedure, and these must be applied in advance.
- If the procedure is urgent, then ethyl chloride spray is very useful. Follow the manufacturer's instructions.
- If you are not used to choosing venepuncture sites, then ask advice from the person who is going to perform the procedure.
- Depending on age and understanding, as much as possible should be explained to the child and parents. Parents should be offered the choice of whether to be involved in the procedure and reassured either way.

Positioning

- If the child is of an age and understanding where he can give consent and be cooperative, then let him choose sitting or lying down.
- However, the younger child may not have so much of a choice because of the need for supportive holding and restraint.
- With clever positioning, anxiety can be minimized and, in combination with other techniques, such as distraction, children may even be unaware that the procedure has taken place.
- For babies up to 9–12 months: swaddle them to include the three limbs not being used. This can help them feel more secure.
- For children who can sit on a parent's or a nurse's lap, cuddle them by putting the arm that you are using under the 'cuddler's' arm. The child cannot see what is happening, and he/she can be reading a book while it is happening.

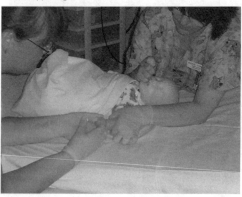

oyal Devon and Exeter NHS Foundation Trust

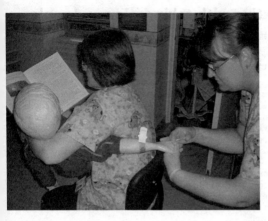

Procedure

- It is common practice with younger children needing support for venepuncture for an assistant to provide circumferential pressure instead of using a tourniquet. Pressure is applied more gently and can be released immediately, and it also helps to hold the limb still. If you are inexperienced, then ask the person doing the procedure to be explicit in their instructions to you. They can tell you if you are holding too tightly or not tightly enough.
- It is vital that calming and reassuring words are used throughout the procedure and lots of praise used once procedure is finished.

Role of the nurse as advocate; restraint/supportive holding. Read these before attempting to assist with venepuncture.

Further reading

Courtenay, M. (2000). *Advanced nursing skills: principles and practice.* Greenwich Medical Media, London.

📖 www.clinicalevidence.com/ceweb/conditions/chd/0313/0313.jsp

Assisting with cannulation and cannula care

Please read **Assisting with taking a blood sample**, as the information is exactly the same for assisting with cannulation, with the following added points.

Before assisting with cannulation:
- Ensure your colleague performing the procedure has everything he/she needs, as trying to find things halfway through is distressing for the patient and potentially unsafe.
- You should be familiar with the dressings designed for securing cannulae. There are various types available:
  - non-occlusive, allowing the insertion site to be viewed at all times.
  - semi-permeable, to prevent moisture build-up underneath and to reduce infection rates.
- Ensure you can apply them, as this may be required during the procedure if your colleague is unable to let go the limb because the child is distressed.
- Avoid the use of non-sterile tape directly over the site.
- Good cannula care relies on a clear view of the insertion site to check for redness.

Ensuring the cannula is secure

In children, the hands and feet are often the chosen sites for cannulation. There is then the problem of protecting the cannula and surrounding tissues from trauma, so splinting is used.
- Always use a specially designed splint, not a 'home-made' one as these can cause more damage.
- If possible, only use a bandage to attach splint to limb.
- If tape must be used, then ensure it does not irritate skin (touch cotton wool to the sticky surface of tape that will be next to skin), and make sure it does not form a circumferential band around the limb, acting as a tourniquet.
- Bandaging is to be used to protect the cannula between usages, but must be removed to enable a clear view of the entry site and surrounding tissues at each usage—at least every 8 hours.
- Ensure fingers and toes are visible to keep a check on circulation.

Courtenay, M. (2000). *Advanced nursing skills: principles and practice*. Greenwich Medical Media, London.
 www.clinicalevidence.com/ceweb/conditions/chd/0313/0313.jsp

Elizabeth Lane, Royal Devon and Exeter NHS Foundation Trust

Site management of a peripheral cannula

Close observation and a high standard of nursing care is essential to prevent and detect complications caused by a peripheral venous catheter.

Insertion of cannula

- Local anaesthetic cream should be offered.
- Diversional therapy should be employed where appropriate.
- Preferable sites of insertion: dorsal veins in hands or feet, basilic and cephalic veins in forearm and antecubital fossa, saphenous vein. Scalp veins can be considered, difficult to secure.
- Non-dominant arm/hand where possible.
- Avoid points of flexion.
- Smallest gauge cannula to facilitate flow rate and viscosity of fluid.
- Protect skin underneath hub of cannula.
- Non-winged cannula to protect skin integrity.
- Electronic volumetric pumps/syringe drivers. Set pressure alarm to 30 mmHg above pressure reading at initiation of infusion.

Complications

The bandage and splint should be removed every hour to observe the cannula site and whole limb for complications.

Phlebitis

Venous inflammation. Three types: mechanical (irritation from the cannula), chemical (irritation from medications), and bacterial (localized infection of the vein).

Signs and symptoms:

- swelling
- redness/erythema at intravenous IV site/along path of cannula
- pain at IV site/along path of cannula
- induration
- palpable venous cord
- increase in volumetric pump pressures
- pyrexia

Infiltration/extravasation

- Infiltration is the leakage of the infusion fluid into surrounding tissues
- Extravasation is the inadvertent administration of vesicant medication or solution into the surrounding tissue. If extravasation has occurred, the patient may complain of severe pain/burning at the site, erythema.

Signs and symptoms of infiltration:

- increasing pressure recordings, may drop suddenly
- leakage at the site
- cool to touch
- tenderness
- swelling/oedema (may be pitting)
- taut/hard skin
- blanching
- pain/numbness

Occlusion

A blocked catheter can be caused by incorrect flushing of the device or precipitate formation.

Jo Rothwell and Alison Hegarty, Central Manchester and Manchester Children's University Hospitals NHS Trust

Prevention of complications
- Restrict movement of cannula:
  - fix cannula firmly
  - attach short extension set and secure with a safety loop
  - consider the use of a splint.
- Reduce irritation/blockage from particles/medications/blood:
  - small cannula, large vein
  - administer drugs slowly, dilute where possible
  - inspect equipment for particulates
  - filter needles for glass ampoules
  - flush cannula with 0.9% saline before, in-between, and following drug administration with a stop–start motion and clamp under positive pressure
  - flush cannula every 12 hours if not in use.
- Prevent transmission of organisms:
  - handwashing and aseptic non-touch technique at insertion and at every manipulation of the line/equipment
  - cleanse skin with 70% alcohol prior to insertion (use with care on premature babies)
  - maintain a closed system
  - sterile semi-permeable dressing
  - clean access ports with 70% alcohol, allow to air dry
  - change IV lines every 72 hours (24 hourly if used for continuous administration of medications), change immediately following blood and blood-component administration
  - discard IV lines if disconnected or contaminated
  - change injectable bungs/needleless systems as per manufacturer's guidelines.

Documentation
Record the following:
- date and time of cannula insertion, device, site, and immobilization of the cannula/protection of the site
- serial number of infusion pump, hourly pressure readings
- hourly observation of the cannula site, including phlebitis score
- record of flushes administered
- date and time lines/bungs changed.

Further reading
Dougherty L., Lamb J. (ed.) (1999). *Intravenous therapy in nursing practice*. Churchill Livingstone, Edinburgh.
📖 www.omni.ac.uk/browse/mesh/D007262.html

Tunnelled central intravenous line care

Central venous access devices (CVADs) are totally implanted venous devices/catheters that can have either single or multiple lumens. They should only be accessed when the appropriate training and assessment has been undertaken. Users should refer to the manufacturer's instructions. A CVAD is inserted into a large vessel, e.g. the internal/external jugular vein or the subclavian vein. In long-term use, where growth may result in frequent line changes, the tip may be placed in the right atrium (this is not recommended in neonates). When access to the superior vena cava is not possible, the femoral vein may be used.

Indications for use

- Difficult or impossible peripheral access requiring prolonged drug treatment, e.g. chemotherapy.
- Regular transfusion requirements, e.g. blood or blood products, parenteral nutrition (PN), IV fluids.
- Repeated intermittent drug therapy requiring easily accessible, reliable access, e.g. IV antibiotics, factor VIII, and haemodialysis.
- Drugs that would have adverse effects to the patient if given peripherally, e.g. cytotoxic drugs.
- Repeated blood sampling, except cyclosporin drug levels and coagulation testing.

Specific pre-operative care

- Educate child and carers so they are aware of what a CVAD looks like, where it will go, and what to expect post-operatively, e.g. incision sites and pain.
- Obtain informed consent, ensure that the child and carers are aware of how long the line is to stay in, possible short- and long-term post-operative complications, and any aftercare the CVAD will require.
- Ultrasound of neck veins might be necessary.

Specific post-operative care

- Analgesia as prescribed.
- Dissolvable sutures should be used at both incision sites.
- Remove any dressings over neck incision site 5 days after operation, no further dressing is required.
- Remove exit site dressing 14 days after operation; leave uncovered, or cover with a film dressing that has moisture vapour transmission.
- Observe both incision sites for swelling, temperature, bruising, or haemorrhage.
- Before the CVAD is accessed, an X-ray should have been performed to ensure correct positioning of the catheter tip and to exclude pneumothorax. This should be documented in the patient's medical records by the surgeon.

Immediate post-operative complications

- Pneumothorax
- Haemothorax
- Air embolism

Leyonie Higgins, Central Manchester and Manchester Children's University Hospitals NHS Trust

- Cardiac tamponade
- Cardiac arrhythmias
- Haemorrhage
- Haematoma

Nursing management

- Observe the exit site for signs of infection; neutropenic patients do not produce any pus. Remove debris from site before taking a swab.
- If infection is suspected, obtain blood cultures; commence antibiotics via the CVAD if possible.
- Observe the patient for signs of venous thrombosis.
- Observe for signs of CVAD dislodgement.
- Report any pyrexia or rigors following use of CVAD.
- Encourage daily showers to clean exit site.
- Ensure a safety loop is *in situ* at all times.

Maintaining patency

- Use injectable bung unless the CVAD is being used for blood sampling or is not required for intermittent use.
- Flush weekly with 5 ml of heparinized 0.9% sodium chloride 10 U/ml.
- A CVAD smaller than 6FG, one used for PN, or a multiple lumen device may require more frequent flushing.
- A 5 ml 0.9% sodium chloride flush should be administered between medications.
- Always clamp the line as the last 0.5 ml of solution is instilled.
- Always flush the line using a push–pause technique.
- Press the end of the plunger on the syringe using your thumb as the needle is withdrawn from the bung.
- Respond promptly to pump alarms, increase in pump pressure, or sudden drop in pump pressure.
- Set a minimum infusion rate of 10 ml/h.
- Flush any blood seen in the lumen of the catheter immediately.

Occlusion

- *Types:* persistent withdrawal or total occlusion
- *Causes:*
  - fibrin sheath
  - lipid deposits
  - drug precipitation
  - malposition of catheter tip
  - pinch syndrome.

Futher reading

Department of Health (2001). Guidelines for preventing infection associated with the insertion and maintenance of central venous catheters. *Journal of Hospital Infection*, **47** (suppl.), 47–67.

Dougherty, L. (2000). Central venous access devices. *Nursing Standard*, **14** (43), 45–50.

Drewett, S.R. (2000). Complications of central venous catheters: nursing care. *British Journal of Nursing*, **9**, 8.

Safe administration of blood products and blood transfusion

Action	Rationale
1. Inform child/carer about intended therapy, risks/benefits	
Provide written information	Child/carer are fully informed
2. Pre-administration checks	
Prescription correct and documented in child's medical notes	Promotes patient safety
Any special requirements, e.g. irradiated blood or diuretic	To reduce clinical risk and error rates
ABO and RhD group, donation number, and child's identity details all identical on:	Severe or fatal reactions can occur if incorrect blood is transfused
blood pack	If discrepancies found, unit must not be transfused; contact blood bank for advice
compatibility label	Pack in date?
blood bank form	Any sign of leakage?
Check the name band and ask the child/carer to state child's full name and date of birth	Unusual colour?
	Signs of haemolysis?
	Signs of possible contamination, pack should be returned to blood bank
3. Technical aspects	
Wash hands and wear gloves	Prevent cross-infection
Set blood up within 30 min of being removed from refrigerator	Risk of bacterial proliferation once out of refrigerator
Blood components must be transfused through a sterile blood administration set with an integral mesh filter. If given by syringe to an infant, a screen filter must be used	Filters any unwanted cells and prevents bacterial contamination
Ensure correct flow rate is set	Fluid overload or transfusion reaction can occur if transfusion is too rapid
Sign and record blood transfusion administration	Permanent record required of all blood products transfused

Celia Charlton, Royal Devon and Exeter NHS Foundation Trust

Contd.

4. Patient monitoring	
Record temperature, pulse, and blood pressure pre-transfusion, 15 min after start, and at end of transfusion	Severe reactions are most likely to occur in the first 15 min
Additional observations as indicated by patient's condition	
Advise child/carer to report immediately if they feel unwell or are aware of any adverse reaction	To detect any adverse events or reactions
Record volume of blood transfused on fluid balance chart	Monitor fluid balance and record kept of amount of blood transfused
If transfusion reaction is suspected:	
stop transfusion and inform doctor immediately	
if life-threatening reaction, call paediatric resuscitation team	Emergency support will be necessary
5. Document start and finish time of each unit	Each unit should be transfused within 4 hours of spiking the pack

Further reading

Royal College of Nursing (2004). *Right blood, right patient*, right time. RCN, London.

Caring for an indwelling urethral catheter

Action	Rationale
1. Assess need: inability to void/urine retention strict fluid balance	To avoid unnecessary catheterization: catheterization increases risk of infection; can cause urethral trauma and increase psychological distress
2. Explain the need for a catheter in age-appropriate language to meet child's understanding	To promote effective communication; to build a trusting relationship; to work in partnership with child and family
3. Once *in situ*, the catheter should be connected to a sterile drainage bag	To ensure a sterile closed system, to reduce the introduction of bacteria and infection
4. To empty urine bag: wash and dry hands use disposable gloves wear a disposable apron clean tap with 70% isopropyl alcohol before and after emptying	To reduce risk of introducing infection and maintain the sterility of the closed system
5. Maintain good levels of personal hygiene by daily washing/bathing where possible	To prevent infection and maintain good skin integrity
6. The drainage bag should be changed every 5–7 days, according to the manufacturer's guidelines	To reduce susceptibility to colonization of bacteria
7. Utilize appropriate tape/strapping to secure catheter, ensuring safe pressure area monitoring	To reduce the risk of trauma and accidental removal
8. Aim to increase fluid intake	To aid in keeping the indwelling catheter patent
9. The catheter bag should be positioned 5–30 cm below the bladder for optimal drainage	If the bag is placed too low, negative pressure can create a vacuum which pulls the bladder mucosa into the drainage holes at the end of the catheter, blocking it off If the bag is placed too high, drainage will not occur Poor positioning can increase the risk of infection

Sarah Doyle, Royal Liverpool Children's Hospital NHS Trust

Contd.

10. Ensure continuous drainage and observe for kinks or twisting in tubing	To monitor for any blockage and to promote continuous flow
11. Assess for normal bowel motion and avoid constipation	Constipation can cause internal blockage of the catheter, poor drainage, and increases the risk of infection
12. If blockage occurs: using a sterile procedure, flush the catheter with saline if undue force is required or if the blockage does not clear, contact medical staff	To maintain patency of catheter; undue force could potentially cause damage to the urethral tissues and bladder mucosa
13. Observe for bladder spasms caused by irritation to the trigone area of the bladder	Bladder spasms are particularly painful; incidence can be reduced by anticholinergics
14. Document the rationale for catheterization, daily activity, and any difficulties	To maximize safe practice, minimize risk, and maintain NMC standards for documenting practice

Further reading

Pomfret, I. (2000). Catheter care in the community. *Nursing Standard*, **14**(27), 46–51.
Simpson, L. (2001). Indwelling urethral catheters. *Nursing Standard*, **15**(46), 47–53.
www.nice.org.uk

Care of a child with raised body temperature

In children a common cause of a raised body temperature is fever. Most clinicians define fever as an oral temperature above 38°C.

Increase of the body temperature to a higher level during fever is a normal process. Fever is not harmful and has many immunological benefits. It is only when the body temperature exceeds 42°C that tissue damage is likely to occur. In such cases the condition is referred to as hyperthermia, a serious condition not regulated by the hypothalamus and thus requiring quite different management.

Fever often has distinct stages, and the child fluctuates between the first two stages; hence the peaks seen on a temperature chart, before reaching the final defervescence stage.

First stage

Physiological rationale
- The thermoregulatory centre in the hypothalamus changes its set point so the body temperature will rise.
- The sympathetic nervous system is activated to increase body heat. This includes peripheral vasoconstriction, a means to conserve and retain heat.
- To allow body temperature to rise, more energy is required, involving activation of endocrine system. There is a 10–12% increase in energy demand with every 1°C rise in temperature. More O_2 and glucose will be required, the first through increased respirations, and the second by the liver mobilizing energy stores.
- The liver also releases substances such as C-reactive protein (CRP), an important molecule in immune defence.
- Shivering (muscle activity) occurs to create heat.
- The hypothalamus initiates change in its set point in response to cytokines and polypeptides released from immune cells.

Signs and symptoms
- Discomfort and general misery.
- Pallor owing to peripheral vasoconstriction. The child will feel cold and shiver and adopt the fetal position.

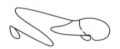

Maureen Harrison, University of Southampton

- Temperature receptors in the skin inform the hypothalamus whether the set temperature has been reached. As the temperature rises haemoglobin loses its affinity for O_2, hence the mottled, slightly cyanosed look that some children have. For every 1°C rise in temperature, the pulse rate increases by approximately 10 bpm, and respiratory rate increases by 2.5 breaths. The child may have a slight cyanotic discoloration around his/her lips.
- Sympathetic nervous system activation—reduced circulation to peripheral organs such as the gut. The appetite is also suppressed.
- Sleep is induced, a symptom seen in particular in younger children.
- There is often mild muscular pain.
- Most children have behavioural changes with reduced coping.

Actions
- Parents are always the first to detect that their child is unwell and this may cause anxiety.
- Keep the child covered with loose clothes or light covers. Removing clothes will make the child shiver more, and will make him/her feel more uncomfortable. Never use a fan to cool the child down during this stage, even if the temperature is already raised.
- Monitor all vital signs and body temperature. Monitor the child's SaO_2 if any suspicion of compromised respiratory status.
- When the child's appetite is suppressed, limit fluids or food because digestion and absorption is reduced.
- Minimizing activity is beneficial so that energy can be channelled into immunological actions.
- If the child is very uncomfortable, mild analgesics (such as paracetamol) can be offered, but evidence suggests that that their benefits are exaggerated.
- In such situations, promoting sleep is a useful strategy.

Second phase
Physiological rationale
- This stage is controlled predominantly by the parasympathetic nervous system. The body temperature has reached, and often rises above, the new set point. The hypothalamus will now initiate heat-loss mechanisms until the temperature has dropped back the adjusted set point.
- Heat is lost from the body through radiation (60%), convection, conduction, and evaporation (20–25%). This is aided through vasodilatation of the arterioles in the skin and through sweating.
- The regulation of heat loss is reliant on fluid and electrolytes.
- Digestion and absorption from the gut improve during this phase.
- If the fever has been caused by sepsis or other serious infections, sympathetic activation is maintained owing to shock factors. In these circumstances it is difficult to differentiate between the phases of fever.

Signs and symptoms
- Whereas the first stage was characterized by misery, in this stage many children feel a bit better.
- Face red and flushed. Skin, in particular on the face and top of shoulders, will feel hot. The child will often adopt a splayed out position.

- Heat loss through evaporation is from the skin and lungs. The child may start to appear dehydrated; dry lips and mucous membranes.

Action
- Child is more alert and playful, although some children will still feel unwell.
- If the child has not already kicked off his/her covers, remove them. The child may welcome sponging of the face and under arms with tepid–warm water. If the child wishes, use fan to help them cool down. This is the only time when physiologically it is appropriate to use fan therapy.
- Maintain hydration and replace fluid loss through oral fluids.

Defervescence
- The raised set point returns to normal (36.5–37.3°C). Children are often feeling much better by this stage, and behaviour returns to normal patterns. Heat-loss mechanisms continue until temperature is normal.
- Return to the child's normal daily routine.

Further reading
- www.nice.org.uk/page.aspx?o=guidelines.inprogress.feverishchildren
- www.mrw.interscience.wiley.com/cochrane/clsysrev/articles/CD003676/frame.html
- www.mrw.interscience.wiley.com/cochrane/clsysrev/articles/CD004264/frame.html

Manual handling and children

The Manual Handling Operations Regulations 1992 (amended in 2002) define manual handling as 'any transporting or supporting of a load (including the lifting, putting down, pushing, pulling, carrying or moving thereof) by hand or bodily force'.

The Health and Safety Executive (HES 2005) have identified that manual handling is a major cause of back injury. Owing to the high incidence of back injuries in the health services, many Trusts have a 'no-lifting policy', but what about the nurse needing to lift distressed babies and toddlers? If you undertake this task, you must comply with good handling techniques and avoid all high-risk activities.

Techniques in lifting children

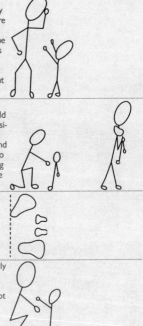

1. Think before you lift. Does the child really need lifting? Can the child help by standing, to raise his position, so you are not lifting from the floor? Where does the child need to be moved to? If he/she is picked up, are there any obstructions on the floor that may trip you? When picking up the child will his/her movements be unpredictable? If so, this might be unsafe for you.

2. Hug the load—the child—close to your waist. Does this mean you would be better off in a partial squatting position before you lift? It is always safer carrying 'loads' close to your waist and trunk. Are your legs strong enough to allow you to move from the squatting to standing position while holding the child?

3. Adopt a stable position: the feet should be a shoulders-width apart, with one foot in front of the other. Is your footwear suitable? Are your clothes suitable for a full range of movement?

4. Start the lift in a good position. Slightly bending the back, hips, and knees is better than bending the back fully, a stooping position. While lifting, do not bend the back further.

Maureen Harrison, University of Southampton

5. Avoid twisting the back. Children can be unpredictable with their movements while they are being held. The child may lean to the side or forward, which might mean the person holding the child will twist their back. This is a hazardous move.

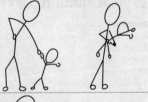

6. Do not handle more than can be easily managed, so do not be tempted to hold the child and another heavy object at the same time. If a child is holding something, like a teddy, this will make the 'load' safer rather than more risky because the child is less likely to move about in your arms.

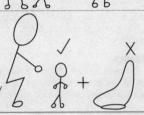

Lifting children will never be completely safe, but working with the following weight guidelines will cut the risk and reduce the need for a more detailed assessment. Thus these guidelines are for infrequent operations, <30 lifts an hour, and thus compatible with your day-to-day work. The two positions are close to or away from the body.

WOMEN							MEN
	3kg	7kg		10kg	5kg		
Shoulder height	7kg	13kg		20kg	10kg		Shoulder height
Elbow height	10kg	16kg		25kg	15kg		Elbow height
Knuckle height	7kg	13kg		20kg	10kg		Knuckle height
Mid lower leg height	3kg	7kg		10kg	5kg		Mid lower leg height

Interpreting 'safe' weights into age groups of children

Average age of child	Weight	Comments
Birth–1 month	3 kg	Before lifting a child make a quick assessment. If a child is lifted between zones, e.g. from floor to waist, the smallest weight should be the guide weight. If the weight involves any twisting, such as getting a child out of a car, the weight needs reducing further.
4–6 months	7 kg	
11–13 months	10 kg	
22–25 months	13 kg	
3 years	15–16 kg	
5.5–6 years	20 kg	
8 years	25 kg	

Cervical spine injury

Causes
- Road traffic accidents (most common)
- Falls
- Diving and sporting injuries
- Non-accidental injuries
- Self-harm (hanging)

Excessive force may result in subluxation, contusion, laceration, transection, haemorrhage, oedema, damage to blood vessels supplying the cord, and spinal shock.

Incidence
Cervical spine injury in children is relatively rare. Less than 10% of all UK spinal injuries occur in children <14 years of age. Of these, at least 40% are associated with severe head injury.

Clinical signs and symptoms
- Injury above C3 usually results in respiratory arrest at the scene
- Paradoxical breathing and respiratory muscle fatigue (C3–C5 injury)
- Total/partial loss of voluntary movement and sensation
- Neck pain/stiffness
- Absent reflexes to stimuli
- Flaccid rectal muscles, retention of urine, priapism
- Signs of spinal shock

Andrea Macarthur, Central Manchester and Manchester Children's University Hospitals NHS Trust

Care of the child with potential cervical spine injury: moving and handling

Immobilization

Effective immobilization of the cervical spine is essential in order to prevent further neurological damage. Head and neck should be immobilized in a neutral position with a hard cervical collar, sandbags, and tapes if indicated.

Collars

Correctly fitted and sized collars restrict only 80% of movement at best. The cervical spine must be manually immobilized during all turns/transfers/removal and reapplication of collars. The collar may be removed if the child is receiving muscle relaxants, but must be re-applied if the child is capable of spontaneous movement. Sandbags and tapes should remain in place.

Sandbags

Sandbags should be used to minimize the risk of movement of the head and neck. Avoid other devices such as bags of fluid, towels, etc.

Tapes

For a child receiving muscle relaxants and incapable of spontaneous movement, non-elastic tape should be applied from the rigid bed frame, across the child's forehead, to the opposite rigid frame of the bed.

Tapes are contraindicated in children who are able to move spontaneously.

Log rolling

Log rolling must be performed for all manoeuvres. The basic requirements are an adequate number of carers and good control in order to immobilize the spine.

Method

- Prepare the child and family: explain the procedure.
- Gather staff: four people (three for a small child/infant).
- Position staff as shown in the first table.
- Ensure that staff are clear about what to do (second table).
- Assess child's neurological function before and after the procedure.

Positioning of staff for log rolling		
Staff member	Position of staff for smaller child and infant	Position of staff for larger child
1	Head	Head
2	Chest	Chest
3	Legs and pelvis	Pelvis
4	—	Legs

Andrea Macarthur, Central Manchester and Manchester Children's University Hospitals NHS Trust

Tasks of individual members of staff

Staff member	Position	Task
1	Head	Lead the log roll. Tell other staff when to roll. Clear instructions, e.g. 'Roll on the count of 3'. Maintain head and neck immobilization at all times
2	Chest	Roll the chest at the same rate as the head. Sternum must be aligned with nose
3	Pelvis and top leg (small child/ infant)	Roll pelvis and legs together, at the same rate as chest and head. Symphysis pubis must be aligned with sternum and nose
	Pelvis large child	Roll pelvis at the same rate as chest and head. Symphysis pubis must be aligned with sternum and nose
4	Legs	Roll far leg at same rate as pelvis, chest, and head

Surface-to-surface transfers
Log roll the child onto pat slide/spinal board. The lead person should continue to immobilize the cervical spine throughout the procedure.

Pressure area care
Log roll child at all times, maintaining mid-line alignment. When nursed on side, place padding under head to maintain neutral alignment of the cervical spine. A firm mattress minimizes risk of flexion of the cervical spine. Avoid low-air-loss/Spenco mattresses. The child's position should be changed regularly and pressure areas inspected, particularly the occipital area and skin in contact with the collar.

Radiological and clinical clearance of potential cervical spine injury

Radiological screening

NICE guidelines: the cervical spine/whole spine should be radiologically cleared at the same time as any other injury, wherever possible.

Children over 10 years

- Anterior/posterior and lateral views of the whole cervical spine and multiplanar CT imaging of the cervical spine from C1 to the base of C2.
- CT of the whole cervical spine if a plain film series is technically inadequate, suspicious, abnormal, or if there is suspicion of injury despite normal study.
- Consider CT imaging of the cervical spine if other body areas are being scanned.
- MRI scan if neurological signs of cervical spine injury and suspicion of vascular injury.

Children under 10 years

- Anterior-posterior and lateral views should be performed.
- Abnormalities or uncertainties should be clarified by CT imaging.

General information

- Consider CT of C7 to T1 at the same time as head, if not clearly seen on plain film.
- A multiplanar view should be requested.
- CT of C1 and C2, and any other appropriate views should be done at the same time as CT of the head.

Avoid CT imaging of cervical spine alone. If it is not done with the initial CT of the head, it should be performed with repeat head CT scans.

The child should be referred (consultant to consultant) to a spinal injuries centre within 24 hours of diagnosis of cervical spine injury.

Interpreting radiology

Radiology should be cleared by someone qualified to do so, ideally a consultant radiologist.

Clinical clearance

The cervical spine must be cleared radiologically and clinically, because of the potential for spinal cord injury without radiological abnormality (SCIWORA). Normal radiology found in up to 75% of children with spinal cord injury. The cervical spine should be cleared clinically by a consultant or designated registrar (usually neurosurgery). Clearance may have to be based on the best clinical information available, as development and cooperation allow.

Andrea Macarthur, Central Manchester and Manchester Children's Hospitals NHS Trust

Criteria for clinical clearance

Central nervous system: tone, power, reflexes, plantars, and sensation.

- If the above are normal, and radiology has been cleared, the collar can be removed.
- Inspect the neck for bruising, swelling, tenderness, and deformity.
- Make sure there is no pain or paraesthesia with movement of the neck.
- Gradually raise child to a sitting position. If still symptom free, the child can then be mobilized.
- If at any time there is altered neurology, replace the collar, lay the child flat, and immobilize the cervical spine. Seek advice from the surgical speciality involved.

The child should be referred to a spinal injuries centre within 24 hours of diagnosis of cervical spine injury.

Further reading

National Institute for Clinical Excellence (2003). *Head injury: Triage, assessment, investigation and early management of head injury in infants, children ands adults.* Clinical Guideline 4. Developed by the National Collaborating Centre for Acute Care.

Supportive holding and restraint

Definitions

Restraint is defined as the positive application of force with the intention of overpowering the child.

Supportive holding, or holding, still means immobilization by using limited force or by splinting to manage a painful procedure quickly and effectively.

Hazard

With regard to the registered nurse's accountability to promote and protect the rights and best interest of their patient, consideration must be given to the rights of the child and legal frameworks surrounding this before using restraint or supportive holding.

Restraint of a child/young person may be required to prevent significant harm to themselves, healthcare workers, or others, e.g. in situations where the child is under the influence of alcohol or drugs and is violent or aggressive as a result. If restraint is required, the degree of force must only be that necessary to hold the child/young person while minimizing injury to all involved.

Nursing management

Local policy

Each healthcare provider should have a local policy. The policy should include children's rights, privacy, dignity, risk assessment, family-centred care, and staff education and support.

When to intervene

- Consider whether the procedure is really necessary and if there is an alternative way.
- Give the child information, encouragement, and distraction. This could prevent the need for holding.
- Obtain consent in all children old enough and able to understand. Consent must also be obtained from their parent/guardian or an independent advocate.
- Plan and agree an action plan with the child and their parent/guardian. Include other healthcare professionals, such as play specialists. Document the process.
- Involve the parent/guardian if they wish, but do not make them feel guilty if they do not want to be present.
- Comfort the child/young person when it has not been possible to obtain consent and explain clearly why it was needed.
- Ensure that all healthcare workers have access to support networks to reflect on the situation afterwards, as it can be upsetting.

Further reading

Royal College of Nursing (2003). *Restraining, holding still and containing children and young people. Guidance for nursing staff.* RCN, London.

Lambrenos, K. McArthur, E. (2003). Introducing a clinical holding policy. *Paediatric Nursing,* **15**(4), 30–3

Jan Orr, Royal Cornwall Hospital Trust

Skin problems and communicable diseases

Anatomy and physiology of the skin

The skin is the largest organ of the body, by area and weight; it covers the outside of the body.

It measures between 0.5 mm and 4.0 mm at different parts of the body.

The structure of the skin

The skin is composed of two layers of tissue: the epidermis and the dermis.

The epidermis

This tissue:
- is the outer and thinner section of the skin and is compiled of stratified squamous epithelial tissue
- provides protection and prevents micro-organisms and other contaminants from entering or damaging the body
- measures between 0.5 mm and 1.5 mm
- is divided into four to five further layers:
  - stratum corneum (outermost): contains dead keratin, a waterproofing protein, which is continually shed and is replaced from the layers below
  - stratum lucidum: contains keratin and is only found in areas of the body that have thicker skins, e.g. hands or soles of feet
  - stratum granulosum: contains keratohyalin, which is involved with the first stage of keratin development
  - stratum spinosum: rows of closely fitting keratinocytes
  - stratum basale (innermost): cell division to produce keratinocytes.

The dermis

This is the inner and thicker section of the skin, compiled of connective tissue, and lies under the epidermis. It:
- measures between 1.5 mm and 4 mm
- contains blood vessels and accessory structures such as:
  - hair, nails, sweat, and sebaceous glands, nerve endings, collagen fibres, and elastin.

The hypodermis (subcutaneous layer)

Although not technically part of the structure of the skin, it links the skin to its underlying structures. The hypodermis acts as a fat storage unit and carries blood vessels that supply the skin.

The functions of the skin

- Temperature regulation
- Protection of underlying structures from mechanical damage
- Excretion of salts, water, and urea during sweating
- Maintains body shape
- Protection against excessive loss of water
- Protection against micro-organisms
- Detection of stimuli
- Vitamin D synthesis
- Protection from radiation

Angela Waddell, Royal Hospital For Sick Children, Edinburgh

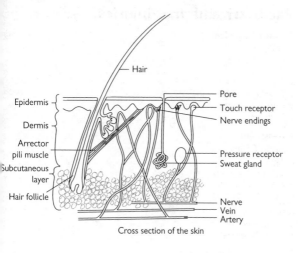

Cross section of the skin

Further reading

Tortora, G.J., Grabowski, S.R. (2003). The integumentary system. In *Principles of anatomy and physiology* (ed. B. Roesch *et al.*), pp. 140–3. John Wiley, New York.

Johnstone, C.C. *et al.* (2005). The physiological basics of wound healing. *Nursing Standard*, **19**, 59–65.

http://training.seer.cancer.gov/ss_module14_melanoma/unit02_sec01_anatomy.html

Paediatric thermal injuries

Types of injuries
- Scalds
- Contact burns
- Flame burns
- Sunburn
- Chemical burns
- Electrical burns
- Flash burns.

Assessment
History of injury
- Type
- What first aid was given
- Associated trauma
- Consider non-accidental injury.

Risk factors
- Current health
- Other health-related problems.

Severity of injury (depth)
Superficial injury
- Epidermis only involved
- May result in serous fluid-filled blisters
- Appears red in colour
- Skin blanches on pressure
- Painful
- Heals within 7 days, no scarring.

Partial thickness
- Epidermis and part of dermis lost
- May result in serous fluid-filled blisters
- Usually pink with paler areas
- May blanch on pressure
- Potentially reduced sensation
- Heals within 2–3 weeks
- Scarring may occur
- May require skin grafting.

Full thickness
- Epidermis and dermis are destroyed
- Blisters absent
- May appear white in colour
- Does not blanch on pressure
- Sensation is absent
- Without grafting healing will occur but will take longer than 3 weeks.

Angela Waddell, Royal Hospital For Sick Children, Edinburgh

Extent of burn

The total body surface area (TBSA) affected can be estimated using a chart developed by Lund and Browder.

Age (years)	0–1	1–4	5–9	10–14	15
A—half head	9 ½ %	8 ½ %	6 ½ %	5½ %	4½ %
B—half one thigh	2¾ %	3¼ %	4%	4½ %	4½ %
C—half one leg	2 ½ %	2½ %	2¾ %	3%	3 ¼ %

- An injury <10% of the TBSA is classed as a minor thermal injury unless smoke inhalation is present. If a thermal injury is >5%, the child must be assessed, preferably at a specialized paediatric burn care hospital, and admission may be considered.
- An injury >10% of the TBSA is classed as a major thermal injury and will require fluid resuscitation within a specialized paediatric burn care hospital.

Management

- Administer adequate analgesia
- Blister debridement
- Take wound swab, if indicated
- Take photograph for medical notes, ensuring consent obtained
- Complete wound chart
- Cleanse wound with warm water and mild soap
- Dress appropriately as per hospital wound management guidelines
- Ongoing assessment depends on healing and amount of exudates
- Ensure parents/guardians have been given information on discharge:
  - dressing care advice leaflet
  - hospital contact details
  - follow-up appointment

Further reading

Herndon, D.N. (2002). *Total burn care.* Harcourt, London.

Fluid resuscitation in paediatric thermal injury

Indication
An injury >10% of the TBSA.

Burn shock
Burn shock is both hypovolaemic and cellular. In response to the thermal injury, inflammatory mediators, which are essential for wound healing, are released at the injury site. In a major burn the systemic inflammatory response may be triggered by the amount of these mediators entering the circulation. This increases the whole body permeability, thus resulting in large fluid shifts between the interstitial space. In addition to oedema formation, fluid exuding from the wound also contributes to burn shock.

Fluid resuscitation
- Intention: to prevent burn shock.
- The resuscitation fluid must be commenced immediately.
- It is essential that the fluid resuscitation be calculated from time of injury, rather than presentation at accident and emergency.
- Two large-bore cannulae must be inserted as soon as possible to administer fluid.
- In children, IV maintenance is also administered over and above the resuscitation fluid, because of a child's higher surface area to body mass ratio.
- There are many formulae used to calculate amount of fluid to be administered. The two most used are Muir and Barclay Formula and the Parkland Formula.
- The formulae take into account the child's weight and the TBSA affected.

Monitoring
- Observe closely in a warmed cubicle (>29°C).
- Saturation monitor, skin temperature probe, and cardiac monitor (if electrical burn) *in situ*.
- Record fluid input and output accurately.

Vital signs
Record 1–2 hourly, to detect signs of burn shock.

Urinary output
- Insert urinary catheter—record volumes hourly.
- Ensure output is 0.5–2.0 ml/kg body weight/hour.
- 4-hourly urinalysis and observe for haemoglobinuria (dark red pigment).

Nutritional support
- Oral/NG feeding should be commenced as soon as possible.
- The benefits include:
  - increases both immune deficiency and mortality
  - accelerated healing
  - prevention of Curling's (peptic) ulcer.
- Reduce IV maintenance as oral/NG intake increases.

Angela Waddell, Royal Hospital For Sick Children, Edinburgh

Blood tests

- Baseline bloods must be obtained: full blood count, urea and electrolytes, blood glucose, and a group and save.
- Subsequent bloods to be obtained as clinically indicated.

Medications

- Regular analgesia.
- Sytron and zinc.

The formulae

Muir and Barclay (using a colloid)

The formula is

$$0.5 \text{ ml} \times \text{weight in kg} \times \%\text{TBSA.}$$

The resuscitation period is 36 hours divided into six blocks. Three blocks of 4 hours, two blocks of 6 hours, and one block of 12 hours. The result from the formula is given during each of the blocks.

Parkland (using a crystalloid)

The formula is

$$4 \text{ ml} \times \text{weight in kg} \times \%\text{TBSA.}$$

The resuscitation period is 24 hours divided into two blocks. Half the fluid is given over the first 8 hours and the rest given over the remaining 16 hours.

Further reading

Herndon, D.N. (2002). *Total burn care*, pp. 4, 6, 93–5, 271, 279, 423, 428–9, 436,445. Harcourt, London.

Hemington-Gorse, S. J. (2005). Colloid or crystalloid for resuscitation of major burns. *Wound Care*, **14**(6), 256–8.

www.burnsurgery.org

Burns: reconstructive surgery

Reconstructive surgery following a burn injury is orientated towards restoring form and function to the affected part. In most cases the person's expectations of the results of reconstructive surgery will far exceed what is possible.[1]

Timing

The timing of the initial surgery for burns reconstruction will be determined by the depth of the wound and/or its location. Generally, early intervention is indicated when the wound is clearly full thickness. Injuries of mixed or indeterminate depth may be left to see if partial thickness areas will heal spontaneously.

Method

Split-skin grafting is the method of choice, as opposed to full thickness graft, given the ability for meshing and expansion to cover relatively large areas. The area to be grafted is judged by its clinical appearance and, apart from the presence of *Streptococcus pyogenes,* other bacteria may be regarded as flora.

The child and family should be prepared for surgery in the accepted way.

Dressings

Dressings are applied to ensure that the newly applied graft does not move around, as shearing pressures will disrupt the process of 'take'. This is especially important with children, who may find it difficult to understand the necessity of minimizing mobilization.

First dressing change is usually performed on day 5 post-operatively and the graft is inspected to ascertain the extent of the take. The appearance of the graft is noted and recorded, with particular attention paid to areas that have either necrosed or demonstrate the presence of haematoma. Necrosed areas may be removed carefully. Discussion with the medical team will indicate the best way to manage the haematoma if present. The graft may be re-dressed (☐ *Burns dressings*).

Donor sites

Donor sites are usually left for the dressing to separate spontaneously, but this can be difficult if the site gets wet. Donor sites may, on occasion, be more painful than the graft and as healing progresses itching and subsequent scratching may cause significant problems to be overcome.

Long-term care

As the grafts heal they contract and can cause significant contractures. Early intervention by the multidisciplinary team with particular reference to physiotherapy and occupational therapy may minimize the effects of these.

Brian McGowan, University of Ulster

Once the wound-healing process has resolved, further surgery may be indicated to release contractures or to achieve a more satisfactory cosmetic result.

1 Barret, J.P. (2004). ABC of burns: Burns reconstruction. *British Medical Journal* **329**, 274–6.
2 McGregor, A.D., McGregor, I.A. (2000). Fundamental techniques of plastic surgery, 10th edn. Churchill Livingstone, Edinburgh.

Scabies

Scabies is an allergic response to the *Sarcoptes scabiei* mite. The mite tunnels into the epidermis and deposits eggs along the burrow.

Symptoms

- Itching: particularly at night.
- Symmetrical rash: small, red papules or vesicles.
- Burrows: found on finger webs, wrists, and elbows; appear as fine wavy greyish dark or silvery lines 2–15 mm long; may be difficult to identify, as they are easily distorted or destroyed by scratching.
- In infants, young children, the elderly, and the immunocompromised: mites may infect face, neck, scalp, and ears.
- Scabies persists indefinitely unless treated; itching persists for up to 3 weeks after successful treatment.

Transmission

- Transferred by direct skin contact.
- Incubation period is up to 6 weeks before onset of itching. If a person is re-exposed, incubation period is ~1–4 days.

Diagnostic tests

Diagnosis can be confirmed by microscopic examination of skin scrapings.

Treatment

- Do not delay treatment. *All* close contacts should be treated with an acaricide simultaneously to minimize re-infestation.
- Apply treatment to whole body, including scalp, neck, face, and ears, especially between fingers and toes and under nails.
- Do not apply treatment after a hot bath, because this increases systemic absorption and removes drug from its treatment site.
- Two applications of treatment are used, 7 days apart:
  - first-line treatment—permethrin 5% dermal cream
  - second-line treatment—malathion 0.5% aqueous liquid.
- Children under 2 years of age should be treated only under medical supervision. A single application is usually effective.

Treatment of itch

- A sedative oral antihistamine at night may help with sleeping and to break the itch–scratch cycle.
- If creams for itching need to be applied during the application time of acaricide, allow acaricide to disappear into skin before antihistamine cream is applied.

Gilli Lewis, Queen's University Belfast

Nursing management

- Reassure family to relieve anxiety regarding diagnosis.
- Children infected with scabies do not normally require isolation.
- Educate family (and provide written advice) regarding correct application of acaricide and prevention of transmission.
- Prevention: clothes, towels, and bed linen should be machine-washed (≥50°C) after first application of treatment to prevent re-infestation and transmission to others.
- Children can return to school after the first application of treatment.

Further reading

Chouela, E., Abeldano A., Pellerano, G., Hernandez, M.I. (2002). Diagnosis and treatment of scabies: a practical guide. *American Journal of Clinical Dermatology*, **3**(1), 9–18.

www.prodigy.nhs.uk/guidance.asp?gt=Scabies (accessed 30 June 2005).

www.dermis.net/index_e.htm (accessed 30 June 2005).

1 Walker, G.J.A., Johnstone, P.W. (2000). Interventions for treating scabies. *Cochrane Database of Systematic Reviews*, Issue 3, Art. No. CD000320.

Impetigo

Common skin infection in young children (because of immature immune systems and grouping in nursery or school). Caused by streptococcal or staphylococcal bacteria.

Symptoms
- Skin lesions appear 4–10 days after exposure, often 2–3 days after an upper respiratory tract infection.
- Commonly seen on the face and perineal area, but can occur anywhere on the skin.
- Lesions are erythematous, inflammatory, and infectious.
- Lesions develop into small vesicles or pustules (*Impetigo contagiosum*) that expand into thin-walled blisters.
- Larger thicker blisters may develop (*Bullous impetigo*).
- Blisters erupt leaving characteristic honey- or brown-coloured crusts, which are friable but adherent.
- Crusts eventually exfoliate, leaving behind an erythematous lesion, which generally does not result in scarring.
- Although rarely painful, the affected area may be itchy and sore.

Transmission
- Physical contact; person to person.
- Broken skin usually required for development of streptococcal impetigo.
- Possibly through contaminated articles (e.g. bedding, towels, etc.).

Staphylococcal impetigo
- *Staphylococcus. aureus* is the predominant cause of impetigo in the UK.
- Risk of transmission: low.

Streptococcal impetigo
- 10% of impetigo cases in UK result from group A haemolytic streptococcus infection.
- Risk of transmission: high (up to 100%) among household childhood contacts during epidemics.

Treatment
- Maintain a high standard of hygiene.
- Topical and/or systemic antibacterials.
- Exclusion period: until lesions healed/crusted.

Nursing management
- Early active (antibacterial) treatment:
  - may reduce absenteeism from school/nursery and prevent outbreaks
  - may reduce risk of glomerulo-nephritis in streptococcal-mediated impetigo.
- Reduce anxiety:
  - treatments reduce anxiety of visibly unpleasant lesions

Gilli Lewis, Queen's University, Belfast

- educate regarding diagnosis; dispel myths surrounding infectious skin disorders
- provide active listening to anxious frustrated children and guardians.
- Education:
  - educate child and family regarding care and treatment
  - educate child and family regarding prevention of transmission.
- Prevention:
  - wash infected area with soap and water
  - cover lesions loosely with gauze, bandages, or clothing
  - wash hands thoroughly, especially after touching an infected area
  - use separate towels and washcloths
  - avoid contact with newborn babies
  - exclude from school or child care, or food handling, until 24 hours after start of treatment.
  - apply emollient moisturizers to dry skin frequently.

Further reading

Malcolm, B. (2001). *Core tutorials in dermatology for primary care series*. Dermal Laboratories, Hitchin.

Watkins, P. (2005). Impetigo: aetiology, complications and treatment options. *Nursing Standard*, **19**, **36**, 51–4.

Eczema (atopic dermatitis)

Inflammatory skin disease → itchy, erythematous eruptions.

Incidence
- 15–20%, 1 : 7 children under the age of 7 years in UK.
- All ages, predominantly infants. Affects all races and both sexes.

Prognosis
No cure. Control symptoms. 60–70% outgrown by mid-teens.

Aetiology
- Multifactoral: immunological, environmental, genetic (two-thirds associated with family history of atopy).
- Aggravating triggers: animal dander, pollens, soaps, detergents, house dust mite, stress, infection, heat, and dairy products.

Diagnostic criteria
Intensely itchy dry inflamed skin plus three of the following:
- onset in first 2 years of life
- history of itchiness in skin creases
- personal or immediate family history of atopy
- tendency towards dry skin
- flexural eczema.

Child and parental distress due to persistent scratching, resulting in raw bleeding skin. Sleep disturbance affects the quality of life for the whole family. Persistent long-term scratching results in lichenification (thickening), usually in the flexures.

The natural protection of the skin against the environment is compromised by a reduction of natural moisturizers → dryness = itch = scratch = skin damage and fluid loss = dryness →

Mainstay of controlling eczema is to break the itch–scratch cycle by education about keeping skin clean and hydrated with total emollient therapy.

Total emollient therapy
- A warm daily bath/shower with bath oil and soap substitute to reduce risks of secondary infections, help hydrate the skin, and enhance penetration of topical agents applied immediately afterwards. Some oils and soap substitutes such as Emulsiderm and Dermol 500 contain antimicrobial agents.
- Emollients soothe and soften the skin, reduce irritation, inflammation, and itch by restoring the skin's natural barrier function against allergens and irritants, and provide an oily surface film that slows water loss. Effects are short lived so apply liberally and at least 3–4 times a day, smoothed on in the direction of hair growth to reduce risk of folliculitis; 'rubbing in' causes heat and irritation.
- Tubifast garments/wraps (wet or dry) will intensify emollient therapy and protect the skin from scratching (📖 Wet wrapping).
- Coal tar impregnated bandages such as Icthopaste, left in place for 3 days at a time, along with emollient and steroid therapy, can be very helpful for treating severe excoriations and lichenification.

Di Keeton, Southampton University Hospitals NHS Trust

SOUTHAMPTON PAEDIATRIC ATOPIC ECZEMA TREATMENT GUIDELINES

FIRST LINE TREATMENTS

EMOLLIENTS

- Prescribe 'Total Emollient Therapy' always = bath oil + soap substitute + emollient
- Recommend daily bath (up to 20 minutes) with warm water using bath oil and soap substitute pat skin dry and apply bath an emollient
- Apply emollients liberally and frequently in the direction of hair growth at least 3–4 times a day (250g/week of emollients are needed for generalized eczema in a child)

BATH OILS	SOAP SUBSTITUTES	EMOLLIENTS
Dermalo bath emollient (fragrance free) *Contains lanolin *Emulsiderm liquid emulsion (antimicrobial) If repeated skin infections* *Oilatum fragrance free bath additive* *Contains lanolin	*Epaderm ointment Dermol 500 lotion (antimicrobial) If repeated skin infections Aqueous cream Emulsifying ointment Diprobase cream*	Will depend on personal preference and skin dryness *Epaderm ointment Diprobase cream Doublebase Unguentum M (There is evidence that Aqueous cream causes problems if used as an emollient)*

Epaderm ointment and Diprobase cream can be used as both a soap substitute and an emollient

TOPICAL CORTICOSTEROIDS

- Intermittent use as required. Use ointments unless 'wet' eczema
- There is evidence to show that short bursts of a potent topical corticosteriod are as safe and effective as long-term use of hydrocortisone
- Studies have found little difference between once and twice daily application of potent topical corticosteroids
- 1% Hydrocortisone can be used at night intermittently for as long as neccessary (Suggest 10–14 days continuous use then 1–2 days off)

FACE	BODY INFANT	BODY > 1 YEAR OLD
1% Hydrocortisone ointment Apply at night	0.5 % 1% Hydrocortisone Ointment Apply at night	1% 2.4% Hydrocortisone ointment Apply at night
	MILD FLARE	**MILD FLARE**
	Clobetasone butyrate 0.05% (Eumovate ointment) Apply at night for up to 7 days	*Clobetasone butyrate 0.05% (Eumovate ointment)* Apply at night for up to 7 days
	SEVERE FLARE	**SEVERE FLARE**
	Fluticasone propionate 0.005% (Cutivate ointment) Apply at night for 3 days up to 3 times a month	*Mometasone furoate 0.1% (Elocon ointment)* Apply at night for 3 days up to 3 times a month

Written by Dr Keefe, Consultant Dermatologist, and Helen West, Dermatology Liaison Nurse Specialist. Approved by Winchester and Southampton District Prescribing Committee September 2004. Reproduced by kind permission of Dr Keefe.

Topical steroids

- An important anti-inflammatory element of treatment. An ointment base provides better penetration than a cream and has lower risk of irritation. Used intermittently in combination with emollient therapy. Skin thinning can occur with long-term use of potent topical steroids.
- Applied in adult finger tip units.
- Finger-tip units (FTU): recommended prescribing quantities for applying topical steroids—2 adult FTU = 1 g
- 1% Hydrocortisone ointment is mild and safe to use on face and body for as long as necessary. Most effective with a 2-day break every 10–14 days.
- Eumovate ointment, twice daily 7–10 days, is moderately potent for use on body only.
- Elocon ointment, potent treatment for severe flares on the body, used at night only, 3–5 days up to 3 times a month maximum.

▶Not routinely recommended under occlusive bandages as potency enhanced up to 10-fold.

Antihistamines

Sedative syrups at night may help with sleep pattern.

Topical immunosuppressants

Tacrolimus (Protopic®) and pimecrolimus (Elidel®) reduce inflammation without skin thinning, but may increase risk of infection.

Criteria for use

Eczema requiring frequent and long-term use of potent topical steroids.

Secondary infection is a common cause of flare

- Bacterial: crusty/weepy areas are best treated with oral/IV antibiotics + above treatment. Topical antibiotics can cause sensitivity and resistance.
- Viral: mulloscum contagiosum (MCV): groups of small, skin-coloured, raised lesions, not itchy. Usually self-limiting; no active treatment required.
- Eczema herpeticum (cold sore virus): rapid onset, crusty vesicles, systemically unwell, treat with oral/IV aciclovir.

Further reading

▣ www.eczema.org.

Long, C.C., Mills, C.M., Finlay, A.Y. (1998). A practical guide to topical therapy in children. *British Journal of Dermatology*, **138**, 293–6.

Williams, H.C., Robertson, C., Stewart, A. *et al.* (1999). Worldwide variations in the prevalence of symptoms of atopic eczema in the international study of asthma and allergies in childhood. *Journal of Allergy and Clinical Immunology*, **103**,125–38.

Shingles

Causes
- Shingles, like chickenpox, is caused by the herpes zoster virus.
- It is rare in children.
- After infection with the virus and the development of chickenpox, the virus remains in the nervous system, inactivated by the immune system.
- However, in late childhood and adulthood, particularly late adulthood, when the effectiveness of the immune system is reduced, the virus reactivates, causing a rash that often rings around one side of the body (looking like a girdle), closely following a nerve tract.

Characteristics of shingles
- Tingling sensation in the affected area
- Pain in the area
- Fever
- Feeling of being unwell
- Rash after 5 days, consisting of blisters containing the virus, usually on the part of the body covering the nerve supply to that area of skin
- The rash turns yellow, flattens, dries out, and crusts over 3 days later
- Lasts for 2–4 weeks
- Episodic pain may be experienced for years because of nerve damage
- The person is contagious until the last blister scabs over
- A person cannot give another person shingles, but can give someone else chickenpox

Treatment
- Give antiviral drugs to reduce the severity and length of symptoms and to reduce nerve damage.
- Give paracetamol or ibubrofen for pain relief and fever control.
- Give plenty of fluids to control fever and distract from the pain.

Complications
- Persistent pain in the area of the rash, because of nerve damage
- Bacterial infection of the rash
- Involvement of the middle and inner ear if the facial nerve is affected, causing deafness and vertigo
- Ulceration or inflammation of the cornea, iris, or ciliary body [1]

Further reading
- www.prodigy.nhs.uk/guidance.asp?qt=chickenpox
- www.nhsdirectonline.nhs.uk

Martin Firth, University of Nottingham

Acne

Acne: disease related to sebaceous glands and ducts, which occurs mainly on the face, back, and chest.

Incidence
- Usually begins in early teenage years
- Peaks between 17 years and 21 years
- Declines after 25 years
- Can persist to 40+ years

Causes
- Sebaceous glands controlled by sex hormones.
- Acne is not due to excess of hormones but to an over-reaction to the hormones.
- Normal skin bacteria includes *Propionibacterium acnes* → thrive on excess sebum → chemical breakdown → free fatty acids → redness and inflammation of deep layers of the skin.
- Therefore not related to poor hygiene.
- Females:
  - acne is more active before menstrual periods.
  - is not influenced by pregnancy.
- Not affected by diet.

Signs and symptoms
- Blackheads: thickening of the surface of the skin (horny layer) that builds up around pores.
- Whiteheads: blockage of sweat glands due to build up of horny layer.
- Yellow heads: blocked sebaceous glands, leakage of the sebum into deeper tissues causes redness and inflammation, can take months to resolve, leaving purple marks.
- Severe acne: cysts → physically unwell + scarring.

Complications
Psychological: depression and suicide.

Treatment
Topical
- Apply to affected areas—20% reduction of spots in 8 weeks.
- Mild acne: benzoyl peroxide, buy from chemist.
- GP-prescribed retinoic acid, topical antibiotics, and azelaic acid.
- Side effects: mild irritation and scaling redness. Moisturizers can reduce dryness.

Oral
- GP-prescribed antibiotics—20% reduction in 8 weeks:
  - oxytetracycline, erythromycin, doxycycline, trimethoprim, and minocycline.
  - side effects: thrush, nausea, colic, slight increase in contraceptive pill failure.
- Hormonal treatment: Dianette, not appropriate for all patients.

Gill McEwing, University of Plymouth

• Severe acne: consultant dermatologist may give isotretinoin, but only for patients who have not responded to several different high-dose antibiotics, or acne persisting beyond 25 years
  • 4 month course
  • side effects: dry lips and skin, joint/muscle pain, headaches, liver damage, depression, and suicide. Severe teratogenic effects.

Surgical
Treatment for scarring: YAG laser.

In most cases a combination of topical and oral treatments is successful but slow to respond and long term.

Further reading
MacKie, R. (2003). *Clinical dermatology*, 5th edn. Oxford Medical Publications, Oxford.
www.medicdirect.co.uk/diseases/
www.acne.org/

Mumps

Mumps is a generalized infection caused by the para-influenza virus of the paramyxus group. It may cause inflammation of the salivary glands, testes, pancreas, or central nervous system.

Characteristics

- Mainly a disease of children and young adults, mumps is acquired by droplets, saliva, and possibly urine.
- Highest incidence occurs between the ages of 5 years and 10 years.
- Incubation period is 15–25 days.

Clinical features

- Prodromal symptoms are non-specific, but include myalgia, anorexia, malaise, headache, and a low-grade temperature.
- Bilateral or unilateral parotitis is the most common manifestation (occurring in 30–40% of infected children).
- Swelling within 2 days and usually lasts about 7–10 days.
- Parotitis may first be noticed as earache and tenderness at the angle of the jaw.

Management

- The management of parotitis and meningitis is symptomatic.
- Orchitis, if it appears, may be very painful and require analgesics, with support of the scrotum.

Prevention

Vaccination.

Complications

- Involvement of the central nervous system is common.
- Headache and meningism may occur 1 week before the involvement of the parotid glands until 1 week after.
- Meningoencephalitis is also a possible complication, and, rarely, facial paralysis, deafness, cerebellar ataxia, and polyneuritis.
- Orchitis: about 20% of post-pubertal males, but very few children, may develop orchitis. Even if bilateral, cases of sterility are rare.
- Pancreatitis, if it occurs, is mild.
- Other inflammatory complications include oophoritis, mastitis, thyroiditis, nephritis, myocarditis, and thrombocytopenic purpura. All these are self-limiting.
- During pregnancy, possible increased chance of abortion.
- Neonatal mumps possible if mother infected around the time of delivery. [1]

Further reading

Emond, T.D., Welsby, P.D., Rowland, H.A.K. (2003). *Colour atlas of infectious diseases*, 4th edn. Mosby, Edinburgh.

⌕ www.nlm.nih.gov/medlineplus/mumps.html
⌕ www.emedicine.com/med/INFECTIOUS_DISEASES.htm

Peter Vickers, University of Hertfordshire

Measles

Measles is a highly infectious disease and is caused by a paramyxovirus of the genus *Morbillivirus*. It is a notifiable disease in the UK. Before a vaccine was available, measles infection was almost universal during childhood. Measles is a common and often fatal disease in developing countries, with an estimate from the World Health Organization (WHO) of 30–40 million cases of measles in 2001, with 745 000 deaths. However, another estimate puts the number of deaths from measles annually as 1–2 million.

Characteristics
- Humans are the only host of the measles virus.
- The virus is spread primarily from person to person by droplets.
- It is a systemic infection, with the primary site of infection being the nasopharynx.
- From exposure to the virus until the prodromal stage, the incubation period of measles averages 10–12 days.
- The child is infectious from the start of the prodromal stage until 3–4 days after the rash has commenced.

Clinical features
- The prodromal stage lasts for 2–4 days, and is characterized by a high temperature.
- The fever is followed by the onset of a cough, coryza, and/or conjunctivitis, with a mild generalized lymphadenopathy.
- Child is usually miserable and anorexic.
- Koplik's spots (white spots) appear in the mouth 1–2 days after the fever appears, followed within 2 days by a maculopapular rash that appears initially at the hairline, often behind the ears, and then spreads over the face and body.
- After 3–4 days, the rash may become brownish before beginning to fade in the same order that it appeared.
- Usually the temperature begins to settle down before the rash fades.

Management and treatment
- No need to isolate.
- Symptomatic treatment is all that is necessary for uncomplicated measles.
- Any complications are managed as necessary.
- If secondary bacterial infection, give antibiotics.

Prevention
Vaccination.

Complications
- Otitis media
- Pneumonia
- Croup
- Convulsions and encephalitis
- Subacute sclerosing encephalitis
- Death

Peter Vickers, University of Hertfordshire

Further reading

Davies, E.G., Elliman, D.A.C., Hart, C.A., Nicoll, A., Rudd, P.T. (2001) *Manual of childhood infections*, 2nd edn. Saunders, Edinburgh.

www.nlm.nih.gov/medlineplus/measles.html
www.emedicine.com/med/INFECTIOUS_DISEASES.htm

Rubella

Rubella is a viral disease (togavirus) with a worldwide distribution. Also known as 'German measles' because it was first described as a separate disease in Germany. In the UK it is a notifiable disease.

Epidemiology
- Humans are the only host.
- In countries without vaccination, it occurs in epidemics every 6–9 years.
- In temperate climates, the peak times for infection are late winter and early spring.
- Transmission is by direct contact or by droplets.
- The incubation period is 15–20 days.

Clinical features
- 25–50% of cases are asymptomatic, and any symptoms that do occur are rarely serious in children.
- There is rarely a prodromal stage in children, but adolescents may have a low-grade temperature, malaise, headache, conjunctivitis, coryza, sore throat, and cough preceding the rash by 1–5 days.
- In children a rash is usually the first symptom.
- Children and adolescents will have a generalized lymphadenopathy that may precede the skin rash; there may also be small red spots in the mouth just before the skin rash.
- A faint rash, which may cause itching, occurs on the face and then spreads from head to toes, lasting about 3 days.

Management
Symptomatic.

Prevention
Vaccination.

Complications
- Rare in children, although adolescents may develop an arthralgia or arthritis.
- This arthritis usually affects the small joints of the hands, but rarely any long-term problems.
- Idiopathic thrombocytopenic purpura may occasionally follow.
- Very rarely (1 in 6000 cases), an encephalitis may occur.
- Other complications may include orchitis and neuritis.
- A major complication is congenital rubella syndrome in neonates as a result of the mother becoming infected with rubella during pregnancy, particularly in the first 6–8 weeks, although rubella up to the 16th week may cause deafness.

Further reading
Davies, E.G., Elliman, D.A.C., Hart, C.A., Nicoll, A., Rudd, P.T. (2001). *Manual of childhood infections*, 2nd edn. Saunders, Edinburgh.

Peter Vickers, University of Hertfordshire

Emond, T.D., Welsby, P.D., Rowland, H.A.K. (2003). *Colour atlas of infectious diseases*, 4th edn. Mosby, Edinburgh.
- www.cdc.gov/nip/publications/pink/meas.pdf
- www.nlm.nih.gov/medlineplus/rubella.html
- www.emedicine.com/med/INFECTIOUS_DISEASES.htm

Chickenpox

- Varicella-zoster virus (VZV): highly contagious in childhood.
- Viral infection:
  - transferred by direct contact with the broken chickenpox blisters and through airborne droplets
  - infectious period lasts from about 3 days before the rash appears until all the blisters have formed scabs.
- Incubation period: 10–20 days.

Characteristics of chickenpox

- The rash generally begins on the scalp, face, and back. Rarely seen on the palms of the hands or soles of the feet, it can spread to the mucous membranes, especially in the mouth and on the genitals.
- The rash is often itchy and begins as small red spots, which develop into blisters in a couple of hours, after 11 or 12 days they turn into scabs.
- New blisters may appear after 3–6 days; the number of blisters differs greatly from one person to another.
- The infected person may spike a temperature.
- These symptoms are mild in young children.
- Chickenpox lasts 7–10 days in children and longer in adults.
- Adults can feel very ill and take longer to recover. They are also more likely than children to suffer complications.

Treatment, advice, and nursing care

- The infected child will be contagious until new blisters have stopped appearing and until all the blisters have scabs. They should stay at home while they are infectious to reduce the infection spreading.
- In hospital barrier nursing is essential; wear gloves and apron, wash hands thoroughly, and remove apron before leaving the cubicle.
- To reduce risk of infection, prevent child from scratching blisters by cutting nails short or giving them mittens to wear.
- Pay attention to child's personal hygiene.
- Calamine lotion has a cooling effect to help relieve itching.
- Keep the child cool; heat and sweat make the itching worse.
- If itching is so serious that the child's sleep is totally disturbed, anti histamine medicines with a heavily sedative effect can be used.
- Give paracetamol to reduce the fever symptoms.
- Cool baths help reduce temperature and irritation of blisters.
- Aciclovir can be administered in serious cases of chickenpox in children with a weak immune system.

Possible complications

- Bacterial infection of blisters
- Scars at site of blisters
- Conjunctivitis
- Pneumonia
- In very rare cases, chickenpox can result in complications such as meningitis, encephalitis, inflammation of the heart (myocarditis), or Reye's syndrome

Kathryn Summers and Rebecca Batrell, Canterbury Christ Church University

Future prospects

Infection → lifelong immunity exists. However, the virus may return later in life as shingles. Active shingles can infect others with chickenpox, but not with shingles.

Further reading

Issauer, T., Clayden, G. (1997). *Paediatrics*. Mosby, London.
www.netdoctor.co.uk/diseases/facts/chickenpox.htm

Herpes simplex

Herpes simplex is a viral infection arising from a double-stranded DNA virus, which causes two different viruses: type 1 herpes simplex virus (HSV-1) and type 2 herpes simplex virus (HSV-2). These viruses cause the formation of blisters on the lips, mouth, face, and eyes (also known as cold sores) or in the genital areas (known as genital herpes).

- Both viruses are highly contagious and herpes simplex can be a sexually transmitted disease, which causes genital herpes to develop.
- In rare cases, the virus can also infect the brain, causing herpes simplex encephalitis to occur.
- HSV-1 infection causes oral lesions in approximately 80% of patients and genital lesions in 20% of patients. It is contracted by direct contact with infective saliva, e.g. from kissing or by droplet infection.
- HSV-2 infection causes genital lesions in 80% of patients and oral lesions in 20% of patients. The usual route of infection is via genital contact.
- Newborn infants can become infected if the mother has active genital herpes at the time of vaginal delivery.

Signs and symptoms

- Itching, tingling, or burning sensation prior to the eruption of the blisters.
- Often very uncomfortable and painful.
- Oral intake of diet and fluids may be impaired if blisters are present around the mouth.
- Passing urine may be difficult with genital blisters.
- Pyrexia, headache, and confusion with herpes simplex encephalitis.
- General feeling of being unwell with reduced appetite and lethargy.
- Incubation period: 2 days to 2 weeks.
- Fresh outbreak may be triggered by sunlight, stress, or illness.
- Patients with compromised immune systems, e.g. HIV, AIDS, or those receiving chemotherapy, are particularly at significant risk, and require prompt assessment and treatment to prevent overwhelming infection from developing, with associated potential morbidity.

Treatment

- IV, oral, or topical treatment with antiviral drugs, e.g. aciclovir.
- Regular analgesia to control pain and discomfort.
- Careful attention to handwashing and hygiene techniques to minimize the spread of infection.
- Informing patients of the route of transmission, e.g. kissing when active blisters are present, to reduce the spread of infection to others.
- Consider mode of delivery for unborn infant if the mother has active genital herpes.
- Appropriate use of condoms and protection to prevent spread of genital herpes during sexual intimacy.
- Consider sexual abstinence if active genital lesions are present.

Laura Gilbert, Canterbury Christ Church University

Further reading

ames, K. (2003). *Paediatrics. A clinical guide for nurse practitioners.* Butterworth Heinemann, Edinburgh.

Wong, D. (2003). *Nursing care of infants and children,* 7th edn. Mosby, St. Louis.

www.herpes.org.uk

www.emedicine.com/EMERG/topic246.htm

Fifth disease

- Refers to the fifth of six classic exanthems (rash-associated diseases) of childhood.
- Also called erythema infectiosum or slapped cheek.
- Viral illness caused by parvovirus B19.
- Common in children <10 years old.
- Short-lived (rash may take 1–3 weeks to clear) with no complications.
- Outbreaks tend to occur in late winter/early spring.

Symptoms

- Begins with low-grade fever, headache, and coryzal symptoms.
- Rash appears after initial symptoms are over, a few days later.
- Bright red rash appears on face—child appears to have a 'slapped cheek'.[1]
- A more mottled rash then spreads to trunk, arms, and legs, usually sparing palms of hands and soles of feet.
- Older children and adults complain rash is itchy.
- Certain stimuli (e.g. sunlight, heat, exercise, and stress) may reactivate rash.
- Swollen glands, red eyes, sore throat, diarrhoea, unusual rashes, blisters, or bruises may also occur.

Transmission

- Physical contact: person to person.
- Droplet: spreads easily in nasopharyngeal fluids.
- Incubation period (4–28 days) between infection and the onset of symptoms. Child is not usually contagious once the rash appears.
- *Not* the parvovirus affecting animals; cannot be transmitted from animals to humans or vice versa.

Treatment

No treatment available or required.

Nursing management

- Reduce anxiety: educate and reassure regarding diagnosis.
- Educate child and family regarding good hygiene.
- Care of vulnerable children: children with weakened immune systems (e.g. with AIDS or leukaemia) may become significantly ill if infected. Parvovirus B19 can temporarily slow down or stop the body's production of red blood cells, causing anaemia. These children may be pale, lethargic, have a fever, rapid pulse, and abnormally fast breathing. May require blood transfusions and O_2.
- Care of pregnant women: infection during pregnancy may affect the fetus. Some fetuses may develop severe anaemia, especially if infection occurs during first half of pregnancy. If anaemia is severe, the fetus may not survive. Fortunately, half of all pregnant women are immune from previous parvovirus infection. Serious problems occur in <5% of infected pregnant women.

Gilli Lewis, Queen's University Belfast

Prevention
* No vaccine.
* Difficult to isolate, because once diagnosed it is no longer infectious.
* Good hygiene practices help prevent spread of infection.

Further reading
Cohen, B. (1995). Parvovirus B19: an expanding spectrum of disease. *BMJ* **311**(7019), 1549–52.
🖳 www.hpa.org.uk/infections/topics_az/parvovirus/gen_info.htm (accessed 1 August 2005).
Crowcroft, N.S., Roth, C.E., Cohen, B.J., Miller, E. (1999). Guidance for control of parvovirus B19 infection in healthcare settings and the community. *Journal of Public Health Medicine*, **21**(4), 439–46.

1 🖳 http://dermnetnz.org/viral/fifth.html (accessed 1 August 2005).

Glandular fever (infective mononucleosis)

Glandular fever is usually caused by the Epstein–Barr virus, but may be caused by cytomegalovirus (CMV), adenovirus, or human herpes 6 virus (HHV-6). Viral illness associated with a high temperature. Commonly seen in adolescents and young adults, although it can occur in younger children.

It is also known as 'infective mononucleosis', as it is passed on by contact from infected saliva, e.g. from kissing.

Signs and symptoms
- Sore throat
- May develop tonsillitis
- Enlargement of the lymph glands in the neck, armpits, and groin
- Occasionally a faint red rash
- Lack of energy and tiredness are common
- High fever
- Headache
- Muscle pains
- Hepatitis may result from inflammation of the liver
- Loss of appetite
- Spleen may become enlarged
- Sore or swollen eyes

Diagnosis
- Heterophil antibody test (Mono spot or Paul–Bunell) will identify 90% of cases in those aged over 4 years.
- Can have false-negative result; if repeated after a few days may yield a positive result.

Treatment
- For the majority of patients, symptomatic relief of pyrexia, sore throat, and any other symptoms is all that is required.
- Adequate food and fluid intake should be maintained and prevent dehydration. If severe tonsillitis is present, IV fluids may be required to maintain hydration.
- Throat swabs → to exclude group A β-haemolytic streptococci (GABHS) infection, which, if present → antibiotic therapy—erythromycin or phenoxymethylpenicillin (penicillin V).
- If severe abdominal pain is reported, rupture of the spleen should be considered; this occurs in approximately 1 in 1000 cases.
- Many patients recover within 4–6 weeks; however, lack of energy and depression are common residual symptoms for some weeks after the acute episode has passed.
- Patients and their families should be informed that recovery may be biphasic, where symptoms may briefly become worse after a period of improvement, but the self-limiting nature of the condition should be emphasised.

Laura Gilbert, Canterbury Christ Church University

Further reading

Maill, L., Rudolf, M., Levene, M. (2003). *Paediatrics at a glance*. Blackwell Science, Oxford.

Barnes, K. (2003). *Paediatrics. A clinical guide for nurse practitioners*. Butterworth Heinemann, Edinburgh.

Scarlet fever

- Scarlet fever is an infectious disease caused by GABHS bacteria (which are normal flora of the nasopharynx).
- Usually associated with pharyngitis.

Characteristics

Initial symptoms include:

- fever/chills
- sore throat
- headache
- vomiting
- abdominal pain
- coated white tongue ('white strawberry tongue')
- followed by a red fine sandpaper rash (erythematic, blanches with pressure).

Physical findings

- Flushed cheeks with circumoral pallor.
- Tachycardia.
- Tonsils oedematous, erythematous, and covered with a yellow, grey, or white exudate.
- After 2 days, the tongue desquamates, resulting in a red tongue with prominent papillae, called 'red strawberry tongue'.
- Skin may be pruritic but is not usually painful.
- After a few days, rash becomes more intense along the skin folds and produces lines of confluent petechiae, known as 'Pastia's lines'.
- After 3–4 days, desquamation begins and lasts for about 1 month.

Transmission

- Person-to-person spread by respiratory droplets.
- Incubation: 12 hours to 7 days.
- Contagion: contagious during both acute illness and subclinical phase.

Diagnostic tests

Throat swab for culture and sensitivity.

Treatment

Pharmacological intervention:

- antipyretic for fever
- antibiotic (penicillin V) therapy for 10 days.

Nursing management[1]

- Reduce anxiety: provide child and family with clear information about progress of infection.
- Encourage rest with play for distraction.
- Ensure fluid intake in adequate amounts to maintain hydration.
- Monitor for signs of complications:
  - otitis media
  - sinusitis
  - peritonsillar abscess

Gilli Lewis, Queen's University Belfast

- pneumonia
- septicaemia
- meningitis
- osteomyelitis/septic arthritis
- rheumatic fever
- acute renal failure from post-streptococcal glomerulonephritis.

Instruct guardians that child must complete the entire course of antibiotics, even if symptoms resolve.

Warn guardians of generalized exfoliation over the next 2 weeks.

Emphasize the warning signs of complications of the streptococcal infection, such as persistent fever, increased throat or sinus pain, and generalized swelling.

- Children should not return to school or day care until the first 24 hours of antibiotic therapy is complete.

Further reading

Hockenberry, M. (2004). Wong's *Essentials of pediatric nursing*, 7th edn. Mosby, St Louis.

Watkins, J. (2004). Dermatology differential diagnosis. Scarlet fever and fifth disease. *Practice Nursing*, **15**(5), 237–8, 240.

www.dermis.net/index_e.htm (accessed 1 August 2005).

Hand, foot, and mouth disease

Definition

Hand, foot, and mouth disease is a common viral childhood disorder causing sores to the mouth, with oval vesicles appearing on the hands and feet.

Epidemiology

Most common in children under 5 years, and can occur in epidemics therefore outbreaks in nurseries and play schools are common. Commonly caused by Coxsackie A16 virus, which is an enterovirus.

History and examination

Incubation period 3–6 days. Can be contracted by young children without any obvious presenting signs and symptoms. Examination includes monitoring the child's temperature, inspection of the throat and mouth for small blisters, and observation for outbreaks of vesicles on the hands and feet. Any recent contact with children with infections, or any known outbreaks of hand, foot, and mouth disease, would be significant.

Symptoms and signs

Early symptoms and signs would include pyrexia, loss of appetite, sore throat, and general malaise. Initially yellowy-red lesions will appear in the mouth; loss of appetite is due to these lesions causing discomfort. Within 24 hours 3–8 mm vesicles appear on the hands and feet. The outbreak of vesicles lasts between 3 and 5 days and may cause itching.

Treatment

Largely symptomatic; will include the use of antipyretics such as paracetamol. Analgesia in the form of paediatric paracetamol preparations can be administered to control painful lesions. Encourage fluids and observe for signs of dehydration, particularly when caring for the infant; consult with a doctor if dehydration is a concern. Do not offer juice, as its acidity can cause further oral discomfort; water or milk is preferable.

Prevention

The virus is contagious and can be spread in the faeces; therefore careful disposure of soiled nappies and handwashing by the child after using the toilet are essential.

Further reading

Ashton, R., Leppard, B. (2005). *Mouth, tongue lips and ears. Differential diagnosis in dermatology,* 3rd edn. Radcliffe, Medical Press, Abingdon.
White, G. (2004). *Childhood rashes. Colour atlas of dermatology,* 3rd edn. Mosby, London.

Mary Donnelly, University of Hertfordshire

Molluscum Contagiosum Virus (MCV)

Definition
MCV is a member of the poxvirus family. It is a harmless viral skin infection which usually resolves over a period of approximately 18 months.

Epidemiology
The virus occurs in children and young people, being transmitted by close direct contact. The virus can appear in well children, but can also be associated with immunocompromised individuals, such as those being treated for HIV.

History and examination
- Children present with white or pink umbilicated papules (dome-shaped with a dimpled centre) approximately 1–5 mm in diameter.
- The first papules appear within 2–3 weeks of infection; the child may complain of an itchy spot.
- Outbreaks of these lesions occur in a scattered manner over the body; the number of lesions varies between two and 50.
- There may be a history of these children spending considerable time in swimming pools.
- The papules may become inflamed and red in colour, but they will disappear over a period of several months.

Risk factors
The virus is highly contagious through direct contact.

Symptoms
Asymptomatic; the diagnosis is made on the presenting lesions.

Management
Cases in otherwise well children resolve over a period of 12–18 months.

Treatment
More troublesome lesions can be treated with curettage or cryotherapy under topical local anaesthetic such as EMLA.

Prevention
- Careful handwashing and washing of towels and clothing at high temperatures.
- Each child should have his/her own towels and flannels.

Further reading
Ashton, R., Leppard, B. (2005). *Mouth, tongue and ears. Differential diagnosis in dermatology*, 3rd edn. Radcliffe Medical Press, Abingdon.

Hughes, E., Van Onselen, J. (2001). *Infections and infestations. Dermatology nursing*. Churchill Livingstone, London.

White, G. (2004). *Childhood rashes. Colour atlas of dermatology*, 3rd edn. Mosby, London.

Mary Donnelly, University of Hertfordshire

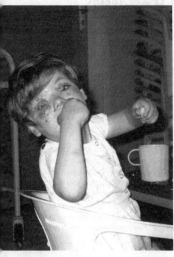

MCV before treatment

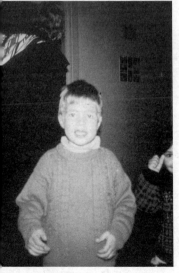

MCV after treatment.

Whooping cough (pertussis)

Whooping cough (pertussis) is an acute respiratory infection caused by *Bordetella pertussis*, a bacterium that is transmitted by direct contact or by droplets spread from an infected person. These become airborne when the person sneezes, coughs, or laughs.

Whooping cough occurs chiefly in small children, younger than 4 years of age, who have not been immunized. The incidence is higher in winter, occurring in cycles with average intervals of 4 years.

The disease is characterized by severe coughing spells that end in a whooping sound when the child breathes in.

Characteristics

- The first symptoms of whooping cough are similar to those of a common cold: runny nose, sneezing, mild cough, and a low-grade fever (at this stage, culture of a pernasal swab may detect pertussis bacteria).
- After 1–2 weeks, the dry irritating cough evolves into coughing spells. During a coughing spell, which can last for more than 1 min, the child may turn red or purple. At the end of a spell the child may make a characteristic whooping sound when breathing in or vomit.
- High fever, rapid pulse and respirations, systematically unwell—pale and lethargic.
- Extreme anxiety and agitation.

Hazards

- It is important to realize that not all children who are infected with whooping cough bacteria will develop the characteristic cough, with the accompanying whoop.
- The child may look as if he/she is gasping for air, turning red in the face, and may actually stop breathing for a few seconds during a particularly bad spell. Therefore it is important to nurse these children near O_2 and suction.

Complications

- Pneumonia
- Bronchiolitis
- Convulsions
- Atelectasia
- Otitis media
- Weight loss and dehydration
- Hernia
- Prolapsed rectum

Treatment

- If whooping cough is suspected, take a pernasal swab to detect pertussis bacteria.
- Isolate the child as soon as possible.
- Children who are dehydrated or who are suffering any complications may need to be admitted to hospital.
- Antimicrobial therapy may be required, e.g. erythromycin.

Kathryn Summers and **Hannah Selway**, Canterbury Christ Church University

Some children may require increased O_2 and humidity.
In the most severe cases, intubation may be necessary.

Nursing management

Reduce anxiety

Whooping cough can be extremely frightening for the child,
as well as his/her parents. Act quickly and calmly to provide
support and guidance.
- Provide a suitable environment to allow the child to rest.
- Give clear explanations to the child and parents before any
procedure is carried out.

Maintain airway

Increased O_2 and suction may be required.
Pain management.
Keep emergency equipment available.

Maintain and monitor respiratory function

- Allow the child to adopt a position in which he/she feels comfortable.
- Continue monitoring of respiratory status.
- Pulse oximetry to monitor O_2 status.
- Use an appropriate O_2 delivery system if required.

Nutrition

- Encourage fluids; offer small amounts of fluid regularly.
- Re-feed the child after vomiting.

Prevent spread of infection

- Use standard precautions, for example handwashing, gloves, and
aprons.

Prevention

Routine pertussis vaccine at 2, 3, and 4 months of age, and later at
3 years and 4 months to 5 years old.

Further reading

Campbell, S. and Glasper, E. (2001). *Whaley and Wong's Children's nursing*. Mosby, London.
Huband, S., Trigg, E. (2000). *Practices in children's nursing Guidelines for hospital and community*.
   Churchill Livingstone, Edinburgh.
⌐ www.immunisation.org.uk

Ringworm

Causes

Ringworm or tinea is not actually a worm but a fungus of the skin caused by dermatophyte fungi. These fungi live in soil, on animals such as puppies and kittens, and on humans, and invade the skin, hair, and nails. Ringworm is mostly seen in schoolchildren.

Different dermatophytes affect different areas of the body and cause different types of ringworm:
• the scalp: tinea capitis
• the body: tinea corporis
• the feet: tinea pedis (athlete's foot)

Signs and symptoms

• Round ring-shaped patch
• Maybe silvery and scaly
• Edge is raised and red
• Ring spreads outwards and may blister and ooze
• Scalp infections may cause some bald patches and swollen lymph nodes at the back of the neck

Treatment

• Topical selenium sulphide or povidone iodine shampoos twice weekly.
• Topical treatments are not effective alone.
• An antifungal, griseofulvin, available as an oral mixture or tablets, arrests fungal cell division and is also anti-inflammatory.
• A larger selection of treatments can be prescribed by a GP than a pharmacist.
• If the patch of ringworm is severe, inflamed, or infected, the GP may prescribe a corticosteroid cream, such as hydrocortisone.
• Treatment for inflamed or infected ringworm may have to be continued for 4 weeks.
• Keep infected skin clean and dry, taking care following washing and drying.
• Wash bedding and towels daily if possible.
• Change underwear and socks daily.

Prevention

• Take pets that are scratching themselves, or with skin lesions, to the vet.
• Check all other members of the family.
• Do not share towels, combs, and brushes; avoid contact with the affected area.
• Wash hands frequently.
• Once treatment has begun, do not exclude children from school.

Further reading

📖 www.nhsdirectonline.nhs.uk
📖 www.kidshealth.com

Martin Firth, University of Nottingham

Threadworm

Description

- Threadworms are small intestinal worm parasites and are the most common parasite of children in northern Europe.
- They can be as small as 2 mm as long as 13 mm, and look like thin white cotton threads with a blunt head.
- Adult worms can live up to 6 weeks in the intestine.

Symptoms

- Intense itching around the anus (or the vagina and urethra in girls), especially at night when the worms are actively laying eggs.
- Lack of sleep and irritability.
- May cause loss of appetite, weight loss, or insomnia.

Treatment

- The treatment of choice is mebendazole, but it is not licensed for children under 2 years of age.
- Treat all people in the household, as some people can be asymptomatic.
- Strict hygiene measures, including:
  - daily vacuuming of carpets and damp-dusting all flat surfaces
  - disinfect bathroom surfaces daily
  - wear fitted underwear at night, not boxer shorts or nightgowns
  - change all nightwear and bed linen daily if possible
  - wash the anal area every morning
  - discourage sucking of thumbs or fingers
  - wash hands and scrub nails frequently
  - rinse toothbrushes daily
  - each family member should have their own facecloth and towel
  - discourage eating in the bedroom, as eggs can be shaken off bedclothes and survive in dust.

Further reading

National Prescribing Centre (1999). *National Prescribing Centre Bulletin* **1**(3).
Tassoni, P., Beith, K. (2002). *Diploma in childcare and education*. Heinemann, Oxford.
🖳 www.nhsdirectonline.nhs.uk

Martin Firth, University of Nottingham

Head lice

Head lice are the most common form of louse infestation to affec
children. They are an almost microscopic blood-sucking insect, presen
on body hair.

Characteristics

Usually recognized by the presence of lice eggs, commonly
known as nits, which are laid within 24–48 hours of infestation
and hatch within 7–10 days.

Spread

- Personal contact
- By infested combs or brushes

Management and treatment

- Encourage parents to check for nits or lice every time their child's
  hair is washed and conditioned, using a special comb to collect the nits
  or lice.
- All members of the family must be checked in this way to reduce
  spread among family members.
- It is not necessary to exclude children from school.
- All contacts and their families should be requested tactfully to check
  their child's hair, and to treat it if nits or lice are identified.
- Most health authorities have a rolling programme for head lice
  treatment to prevent the development of resistance to treatment
  of the strain of head lice.
- Treatments may include malathion and carbaryl lotions.
- Usually treatments have to be repeated 7 days after the initial
  treatment to kill all the nits, as some may be strong enough to
  resist one treatment.
- Above all, stringent checking, conditioning, and combing of hair will be
  sufficient to stop the spread of the nits and thus infestation by lice.

Further reading

 www.surgerydoor.co.uk

Martin Firth, University of Nottingham

Ammoniacal nappy rash

- A nappy rash appears as a red rash on the area covered by a terry towelling or disposable nappy.
- It can be caused by irritation of the skin by urine or infection.
- This is a very uncomfortable experience for the baby and can cause immense pain when washing the skin and changing the nappy.

Characteristics

- The skin appears chapped and sometimes spotty.
- If the area is infected, it is likely to be blistered and may produce clear or yellow-coloured fluid.

Treatment

- It is vital to change the baby's nappy frequently to minimize further irritation by urine and/or faeces.
- Use cotton wool with warm water, rather than baby wipes, to clean the skin to reduce further irritation.
- Pat the skin dry, rather than rubbing, prior to applying a further nappy.
- Apply barrier creams, such as zinc and castor oil or Vaseline, to the dry skin to discourage passage of urine on to the sore skin.
- Exposing the skin to the environment frequently can be as beneficial as any barrier cream, as long as the skin is dried when the baby urinates or defecates.

Prevention

- Change nappies regularly and wash the nappy area when changing.
- Change to a different soap powder if the skin is sensitive to biological washing powders.
- Give the child plenty to drink to reduce the acidity of the urine.
- Avoid talcum powder, as this can clog and cause further irritation.

Note

Some nappy rashes may be caused by fungal infections, which may need GP-prescribed treatment if other measures are not effective.

Further reading

Tassoni, P., Beith, K. (2002). *Diploma in child care and education.* Heinemann, Oxford.
🖳 www.nhsdirectonline.nhs.gov.uk

Martin Firth, University of Nottingham

Candida of the mouth and nappy area

Candida (thrush) is a fungal infection. Found in any age group, it is common in the newborn, immunocompromised children, and those on long-term antibiotic therapy.

Characteristics of oral *Candida*

- Can be asymptomatic
- White adherent patches on tongue, inside of cheeks, and palate, which are difficult to remove
- Difficult to distinguish from milk
- Infant refusing to feed
- If breastfeeding, the mother may have sore, red nipples
- Complaints of a sore mouth in older children

Characteristics of nappy *Candida*

- Red erythema
- Pustules
- Soreness
- Not healing

Hazards

- Dehydration due to refusal to feed or drink
- Spread of infection
- Neonatal sepsis
- Endocarditis

Treatment

- Give oral antifungal.
- Apply topical antifungal to nappy area, and mother's nipples if breastfeeding. Nystatin® or Daktarin® are commonly used.
- Give prophylactic antifungal agents to children at risk.
- Maintain normal gut flora:
  - *Lactobacillus acidophilus* capsules
  - brewer's yeast
  - live natural yoghurt.
- IV aciclovir in systemic infections.

Nursing management

Recognition

- Assessment of the child's mouth.
- Inspection of the nappy area.
- A crying fretful baby having difficulty feeding.
- A breastfeeding mother complaining of sore nipples.

Support and education

- Educate the mother about the treatment of *Candida*.
- Provide support for the mother and encourage her to continue breastfeeding.
- If necessary, involve the midwife, health visitor, or breastfeeding counsellor.

Sue Mason, Royal Devon and Exeter NHS Foundation Trust

• Educate the parents and those at risk about good oral hygiene and preventive treatment of *Candida*.

Nutrition

• Give analgesia if required to help prevent discomfort when feeding/eating.
• Provide breastfeeding advice to ensure that the baby is latched on correctly, to prevent discomfort to the mother.
• Ensure adequate fluid intake.

Promote healing of nappy rash

• Change nappies regularly.
• Keep the area clean and dry.
• Apply prescribed antifungal treatment.
• Use barrier creams between treatments if necessary.

Prevent the spread of infection

• Wear gloves when performing oral hygiene.
• Use standard precautions when changing nappies.
• Educate parents about infection control precautions.
• Ensure bottles, teats, and breast shields are being sterilized correctly.
• To help prevent re-infection, do not use expressed breast milk during an episode of thrush.
• Each family member should use their own towels.

Prevention

• Oral assessment and inspection of nappy area.
• Recognition of *Candida* in, and treatment of, breastfeeding mother.
• Preventive treatment of those at risk.

Further reading

Husband, S., Trigg, E. (2000). *Practices in children's nursing. Guidelines for hospital and community.* Churchill Livingstone, London.

Wong, D. (1999). *Whaley and Wong's Nursing care of infants and children,* 6th edn. Mosby, St. Louis.

⊞ www.lalecheleague.org

Seborrhoeic dermatitis

'Dermatitis' is inflammation of the skin and 'seborrhoeic' means that that the inflammation commonly occurs in areas rich in sebaceous glands which are normally the scalp, face, trunk, and flexures.

Cause

Not fully understood—many factors, including hormonal influences, have been suggested. Because seborrhoeic dermatitis is common in babies usually disappearing by 6–12 months, this could suggest a response to maternal hormone stimulation. It is also common after puberty.

Seborrhoeic dermatitis responds better to treatments that attack the yeasts that live on the surface of everyone's skin; this suggests that these skin yeasts are involved.

Characteristics

• Red rash covered with greasy-looking white or yellowish scales
• Can be itchy or sore
• Seborrhoeic dermatitis of the scalp can produce embarrassing dandruff
• Can cause stress and anxiety

It occurs most often:
• On the scalp, which ranges from mild dandruff to a very red, scaly rash, which can sometimes ooze; babies have cradle cap.
• On the face, common areas are eyebrows; creases beside the nose and eyelids can be red and irritated.
• Around and inside the ears, the skin can ooze and crust in this area, this in turn can cause swelling and inflammation of the ear canal.
• On the trunk, it appears as red scaly patches.
• In the flexural areas that are prone to sweating and that retain moisture; in babies this could be the nappy area.

Treatments

The treatment involves control rather than cure. Treatments are applied in the long term to keep the condition under control.

For the scalp

A medicated shampoo containing agents such as ketoconazole, selenium sulphide, and zinc pyrithione. The shampoo should be left on for 5–10 min, massaged gently into the scalp, and then rinsed off. A scalp application that contains a steroid can help with inflammation and itching. Salicylic-acid-based ointment can also used to reduce scales; this is applied at night and then rinsed off in the morning.

For face, trunk, and flexural areas

A mild steroid cream that has either antibacterial or antifungal properties is the most effective.

Management issues

Seborrhoeic dermatitis is a visible condition and this can cause stress and anxiety for sufferers and their families. Treatments can be time consuming and long term.

Lizanne McInnes and Anne Speirs, Royal Hospital For Sick Children Glasgow

Management
- Provide education and information on the topical treatments available.
- Reassure and support the patient and their families, and offer any support groups available to them.
- Work in partnership with the patient and family to develop a treatment plan appropriate to their needs.

Further reading
- www.dermnet.org.nz

Psoriasis

- Inherited chronic inflammatory non-infectious scaling skin condition that recurs throughout life.
- Specific immune response in individuals who are genetically predisposed, which is triggered by a number of factors: streptococcal infection (usually of the throat), trauma, drugs, and stress.

Characteristics

- Red/pink raised plaques with a well-defined edge that are covered in a white/silvery scale.
- The plaques are typically disc shaped, although the shape can vary and when plaques are joined together they form more irregular shapes.
- The plaques thicken and are often uncomfortable, itchy, and painful.
- Plaques can appear anywhere on the skin, including the scalp.

Pathology

- Keratin cells reproduce rapidly and move up to the surface of the skin at around seven times the normal rate, resulting in the loose silvery scale.
- Rapid cell reproduction causes the epidermis to thicken and, as keratin cells have an immunological function, the skin becomes inflamed, resulting in increased blood flow to the skin at these sites.

Types

Plaque

- Most common type, affecting the knees, elbows, trunk, and scalp.
- Well-defined disc-shaped plaques with sharp borders.
- Often has a symmetrical distribution.

Guttate

- An acute form of psoriasis that occurs following a streptococcal throat infection.
- Round 'drop-like' lesions between 2 mm and 1 cm in diameter.
- Scattered, usually symmetrically, over the trunk, face, and scalp.
- Present for 3–4 months but can persist for more than 1 year.
- Can precipitate chronic plaque psoriasis.

Flexural

- Most frequently affected sites in children are the axillae and napkin area.
- Plaques are well defined and shiny, with little or no scaling as friction removes the scale.

Rare presentations in childhood

- *Generalized pustular psoriasis:* small sterile pustules develop on an erythematous background; spread rapidly.
- *Erythrodermic psoriasis:* erythema may spread rapidly to trunk and limbs.

Lizanne McInnes and Anne Speirs, Royal Hospital For Sick Children Glasgow

These are dermatological emergencies and require hospital admission as they can be life threatening.

Treatment

There is no cure for psoriasis; the treatments available only suppress the disease.

Topical treatment

- Emollients: bath oils and moisturizers are simple yet effective treatments:
  - soften skin
  - minimize scaling and flaking
  - prevent the plaques cracking
  - help alleviate the itch.
- Coal tar: can be used on the face and body.
- Vitamin D analogues: can only be used on the body.
- Dithranol: can only be used on the body.
- Topical steroids: mild/moderate steroids mainly used for the treatment of psoriasis on the face, flexures, and genitalia. Care must be taken if used elsewhere as psoriasis can become unstable when steroids are withdrawn.
- Keratolytics: help remove excess scaling.

Systemic treatment

- Oral therapy: methotrexate, retinoids, cyclosporin.
- Phototherapy: UVB light treatment.

Not routinely used in children.

Management issues

Psoriasis has both a physical and emotional impact, as well as practical issues.

- Physical discomforts include pain, itching, stinging, cracking, and bleeding of the skin.
- Emotional impact includes embarrassment, fear of the disease flaring, low self-esteem, and depression.
- Practical issues are that the treatments are often messy, strong smelling, and time consuming to apply.

Holistic management

- Provide education and information on the use of the topical treatments.
- Reassure and support the patient/parents and provide information about the disease and any support groups available.
- Work in partnership with the patient/parents to develop a plan of treatment, which is acceptable and effective.

Further reading

Harper, J., Oranje, A., Prose, N. (2000). *Textbook of paediatric dermatology*, vol. 1. Blackwell Science, Oxford.
Gawkrodger, D.J. (2001). *Dermatology: an illustrated colour text*, 2nd edn. Churchill Livingstone, Edinburgh.
▣ www.dermatology.co.uk

Urticaria (nettle rash or hives)

- Erythema: weals or raised red itchy bumps in the skin, a few millimetres or several centimetres diameter, coloured white or red, often surrounded by a red flare.
- May appear rapidly, can be round, form rings, map like, can change shape.
- Swelling of eyelids and lips.
- Transient: few minutes to several hours.
- Recurrent.
- Due to fluid transfer from blood capillaries in the dermis.
- Swelling around the mouth should be considered a dermatological emergency (danger of respiratory obstruction).

Causes

- Immune reaction to medicines such as antibiotics, or food, including even tiny amounts of fish, eggs, nuts, or chocolate.
- Histamine-liberating drugs: salicylates, aspirin, codeine, morphine, indomethacin.
- Food additives: tartrazine (yellow/orange dye) and benzoates (preservative).
- Contact urticaria: lesions develop at site of contact, e.g. dog hair or on lips after ingestion of protein foods.
- Physical urticaria: due to pressure, heat, cold, or sunlight.
- Hereditary angio-oedema: autosomal dominant, basic biochemical defect, can present with gross swellings and internal swelling of the intestine → intestinal obstruction.
- Related to other medical problems such as parasite infection, chronic bacterial infection, thyrotoxicosis, and lupus erythematosus.

Usually a mild reaction affecting only the skin; rarely, very allergic individuals develop anaphylaxis. The cause is usually obvious—an antibiotic injection, a bee sting, ingestion of peanuts—a few minutes earlier. The urticarial rash is accompanied by a tight chest, wheezing, faintness, and collapse. Medical attention must be sought urgently. An epinephrine injection may be required.

- Acute urticaria: usually resolves in a few hours or days.
- Chronic urticaria: persists for several months or years and may be due to an autoimmune disease.

Diagnosis

- Self-evident, only investigate if recurrent attacks over 9 months.
- Careful history may reveal cause.

Treatment

- Usually resolves spontaneously
- Non-sedating antihistamines
- Acute cases subcutaneous epinephrine
- Elimination diets if persistent

Gill McEwing, University of Plymouth

Further reading

MacKie, R. (2003). *Clinical dermatology*, 5th edn. Oxford Medical Publications, Oxford.

www.allergyhospital.co.uk/anaphylaxis.htm

http://urticaria.co.uk/index.html

Burns dressings

Action	Rationale
1. Preparation. You will need: Dressing trolley Dressing pack + sterile gloves Sufficient area of wound contact layer as prescribed, e.g. paraffin gauze Topical antimicrobial (if prescribed) Sterile gauze Wool bandage Crêpe bandage Tape (may be waterproof, depending on site) Wound swabs McIndoe forceps Scissors (bandage and sterile)	The key to a smooth and measured procedure is to be adequately prepared beforehand, ensuring that the supplies you need are to hand. This will also reduce the time required to carry out the dressing, thus reducing the time the patient is exposed
2. Ensure that the procedure has been adequately explained to the child and family	Involving the child and family in the procedure through adequate explanation will increase their willingness to take part. This will potentially reduce the length of the procedure, with the knock-on effect of potentially reducing the pain and anxiety associated with the dressing
3. Involve the parents Involve the play specialist	Allow time for the pain relief to take effect, thus reducing trauma. Involving play specialists[1] and parents helps to normalize the environment and thus reduce anxiety
4. Wash hands, remove the old dressings and dispose of appropriately	Infection control is paramount
Do not force dressings off	Forcing off old dressings can remove granulation tissues, cause bleeding, and increase the pain and anxiety being experienced by the child
The child may be bathed to assist in the removal of dressings	
5. Clean the wounds using tap water or saline, according to local policy guidelines	Literature to date has been inconclusive, either in support of or in opposition to the use of tap water in wound cleansing[2]

Brian McGowan, University of Ulster

Contd.

6. Assess the wounds for signs of:	
Healing/graft take	Assessing the wound will give an indication of how effective the burn care is
Deepening	Over time burns of an indeterminate depth on admission will 'declare' so that a definitive decision can be made about their management
Infection	Infection of the wound can be detected through direct observation and smell
7. Provide feedback to the child and his/her parents about how the wound is progressing and possible course of action to take from this point	Constant information flow will keep the child and family engaged in the process and help to make them feel like contributing members of team as opposed to observers
8. Apply topical antimicrobial if prescribed	Topical applications may mask the extent of the burn and therefore should only be used after a definitive decision about wound management has been made
9. Apply wound contact layer as discussed and prescribed	Wound contact layers should be non-adherent and promote an environment that is conducive to wound healing
10. Apply layers of gauze	
11. Apply layers of wool or gamgee	Gauze, wool, and gamgee absorb exudate and provide support for the affected area
12. Apply layers of crêpe and secure with tape, ensuring that it does not constrict and impair circulation	Crêpe provides support and can expand if there is any swelling present
13. Provide positive feedback and reassurance to the child and family. Check that dressings are secure and that pain levels are within an acceptable level	Reassurance will ensure that anxiety levels are kept manageable, bearing in mind that this procedure will be repeated many times
14. Dispose of soiled dressings appropriately and safely, and clean up the area in preparation for the next procedure	The procedure is not complete until the area is cleaned and prepared for the next procedure/patient. Minimizing the risk of cross-infection is paramount
15. Document the appearance of the wound, its size, and any change since it was last dressed	Clear documentation can help to establish a pattern of healing for the wound, thus identifying the child's overall response to treatment and care

1 Webster, A. (2000). The facilitating role of the play specialist. *Paediatric Nursing*, **12**(7), 24–7.
2 Patel, S., Beldon, P. (2003). Examining the literature on using tap water in wound cleansing. *Nursing Times*, **99**(43), 22–4.

Gluing wounds

Wound glue has been used to close superficial wounds on faces and scalps for over 15 years and is an established method for closing appropriately sized wounds.

Application

- Clean wound thoroughly; if the wound is in the scalp, ensure that the patient's hair is not in the wound before closure.
- Achieve haemostasis.
- Hold the wound edges together, ensuring good opposition.
- Place the glue along the wound edges, either by using the spot welding method or by one continuous thin line.
- Hold the wound edges together for approximately 30–60 s.
- Ensure that good closure has been achieved.

Advice on discharge

- Keep wound clean and dry for 5 days.
- Avoid picking or touching wound.
- The glue will form a scab and will flake off after 5–10 days.
- If bleeding recurs, seek medical advice.

Tips for gluing wounds

- Do not apply glue directly into the wound.
- Avoid use excessive amount of glue, thin layers are most effective.
- Avoid gluing yourself to the patient.

Further reading

Elmasahne, F.N., Matbouli, S.A., Zuberi, M.S. (1995). Use of tissue adhesive in the closure of small incisions and lacerations. *Journal of Pediatric Surgery*, **30**, 837–8.

Quinn, J.V., Drzewiecki, A., Li, M.M., *et al.* (1993). A randomized controlled trial comparing a tissue adhesive with suturing in the repair of pediatric facial lacerations. *Annals of Emergency Medicine*, **22**, 1130–5.

Wang, M.Y., Levy, M.L., Mittler, M.A., Liu, C.Y., Johnston, S., McComb, J.G. (1999). A prospective analysis of the use of octylcyanoacrylate tissue adhesive for wound closure in pediatric neurosurgery. *Pediatric Neurosurgery*, **30**, 186–8.

Alan Charters, Portsmouth Hospitals Trust

Suturing wounds

When suturing children's wounds, careful consideration must be made as to whether the wound really requires suturing. Modern more appropriate wound closure measures have been developed in order to reduce scarring, pain, and anxiety, both for the child and his/her parents. However, one must not avoid suturing an appropriative wound simply because other methods are easier. The object of suturing a wound is to oppose the skin, aiming for slight eversion of the wound edges. Before suturing a child, he/she needs to be prepared both physically and mentally for the procedure (play and analgesia). This should involve an explanation of the procedure and the risks associated with it.

Procedure

- Prepare a clean field by opening a suturing pack over a clean dressing/suturing trolley.
- Infiltrate around the wound with local/topical anaesthetic: 1% lidocuine or lidocaine–epinephrine–tetracaineqel.
- ▶ Do not use epinephrine on wounds involving digits, genitalia, or mucous membranes.
- Decide on the appropriate suture material.

Wound site	Which material and size	When to remove
Face	5/0 or 6/0 non-absorbable	3–5 days
Scalp	3/0 non-absorbable	7 days
Hand	5/0 or 4/0 non absorbable	7–10 days
Small wounds	4/0 non absorbable	7 days
Large wounds	4/0	10–12 days
Over joints	4/0	10–12 days

- The wound must be thoroughly cleaned with normal saline and all debris irrigated out of the wound. This is best achieved using a 10 ml syringe.
- The wound must be closed using the appropriate sutures according to the technique.

Key points for suturing

- Do not be afraid to remove sutures, especially the first one applied.
- Do not close dirty wounds.
- Fully explore wounds. If not confident or competent to know what you are examining, seek more senior help.
- Do not close wounds under too much tension.
- Do not over tighten suture knots.
- Always ask for help when unsure.

Alan Charters, Portsmouth Hospitals Trust

Further reading

ano, K., Yoshizu, T., Maki, Y., Tsubokawa, N. (2005). Easy-removal 'ribbon-knot suturing' for pediatric wound care. *Plastic and Reconstructive Surgery*, **116**(2), 694–5.

onadio, W.A., Carney, M., Gustafson, D. (1994). Efficacy of nurses suturing pediatric dermal lacerations in an emergency department. *Annals of Emergency Medine*, **24**(6), 1144–6.

Wet wrapping with Tubifast

Warm wet occlusive dressings for treatment of poorly controlled eczema that is dry, red, and itchy. Available in age-specific garments for home use and tubular bandages for hospital use. Usually used at night after bathing with regular emollients, but initially may also be needed during daytime. Suitable for all ages. Most children find them very soothing. Thick greasy emollients such as Epaderm are most effective under wraps.

They should not be used while the skin is infected, open, and weeping, because they may stick.

How do they work?
- Aid rehydration: large quantity of emollients, moisturize deeply rather than superficially, absorbed slowly over a long period.
- Steroid absorption is enhanced, allowing weaker strengths for shorter periods and faster control of eczema.
- Cooling effect on skin, reducing the itch and increasing comfort and improved sleep patterns.
- Skin healing is promoted because bandages protect skin from scratching.

For wet wrapping, you need two layers for each part of the body.

Measuring Tubifast
- Legs: top of thigh to tip of toes + 8 cm × four lengths
- Arms: top of shoulders to tip of fingers + 8 cm × four lengths
- Body: top of neck to base of bottom × two lengths
- Ties: eight 2–3 cm strips from left over bandages

Tubifast garments are age specific: two vests + two leggings or two tights + socks

Application
- After bathing, place one complete body suit in very warm water.
- If whole body is being wrapped, it is best to do one area at a time. Apply a small amount of topical steroid to affected areas if needed.
- Emollients should be applied copiously.
- Squeeze out wet Tubifast layer, apply, and cover immediately with dry layer.
- Repeat for all areas.
- Bandages are kept in place by making small holes and tying together at shoulders and top of thighs.
- Once skin is settled, wraps may be used ad hoc, with emollients only once or twice weekly to keep skin well hydrated. Wraps may also be used as single dry layer to protect skin from scratching, improve treatment absorption, and protect clothes, especially during day.

Further reading
National Eczema Society. ⬚ www.eczema.org
SSL International plc. ⬚ med-marketing@ssl-international.com

Di Keeton, Southampton University Hospitals NHS Trust

Neurological problems

The role and function of the nervous system

The primary role of the nervous system, in conjunction with the endocrine system, is to maintain homeostasis. In contrast with other body systems that grow following birth, the nervous system grows more rapidly before birth, with two distinct growth spurts: between 15 weeks and 20 weeks gestation, and between 30 weeks' gestation and 1 year.

The neuron is the structural unit of the nervous system; it conducts impulses from one part of the body to another. This is a two-way process, with impulses moving from the periphery to the brain via the spinal cord, and impulses originating in the higher centres of the brain transmitted via the spinal cord to the muscles to enact a response.

Functions of the nervous system

- Sensory function: internal management and analysis of body functions to maintain homeostasis. An external function conveys environmental information through sensory neurons to the central nervous system CNS.
- Integrative function: processes assimilated information for immediate use or storage for the future through a series of interneurons that connect and communicate with many areas within the brain. This promotes a conscious awareness of the sensory information (perception).
- Motor function: once analysed, an action is needed; this could involve glandular secretion or the use of efferent (motor) neuron activity, resulting in muscular contraction.

Organization of the peripheral nervous system

The peripheral nervous system has afferent pathways (ascending) transmitting sensory information to the CNS, and efferent pathways (descending) conveying commands from the CNS to the efferent organs, e.g. cardiac, skeletal, and smooth muscle. The peripheral nervous system can be further subdivided into:

- Somatic nervous system: provides voluntary control of skeletal muscle through the combined effect of the afferent and efferent pathways.
- Autonomic nervous system: the combined effects of the afferent and efferent pathways control involuntary internal body functions.
  This system can be further divided:
  - sympathetic nervous system: in general terms, processes and prepares the body for exercise or emergency action.
  - parasympathetic nervous system: prepares for rest and digestion.
- Enteric nervous system: monitors the control and management of the gastrointestinal tract, communicating with the CNS through the autonomic nervous system.

Mark Broom, University of Glamorgan

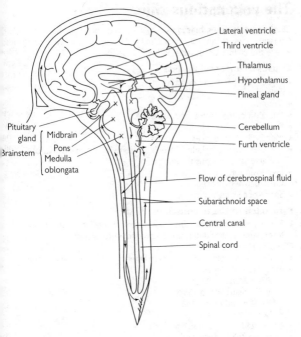

The brain and spinal cord

Further reading

Martini F.H. (ed.) (2005). *Fundamentals of anatomy and physiology*, 7th edn. Benjamin Cummings, San Francisco.

Montague, S.E., Watson, R., Herbert, R.A. (ed.) (2005). *Physiology for nursing practice*, 3rd edn. Elsevier, Edinburgh.

The unconscious child

Disease, injury, or intoxication may alter the conscious level in a child. Conscious level can vary from mild drowsiness to unconsciousness where the child is unrousable and unresponsive.

Causes of unconsciousness

- Hypoxic ischaemic brain injury
- Seizures
- Trauma
- Infection of the central nervous system
- Poisoning
- Metabolic disturbances
- Vascular lesions, including bleeding, arteriovenous malformations, and arterial or venous thrombosis
- Hypertension
- Obstructive hydrocephalus
- Space-occupying lesions

Approach to the unconscious child

- Primary assessment of ABC. If necessary, immediate support of ABC to prevent further deterioration secondary to ischaemia and/or hypoxia.
- Assess neurological function. Rapid measurement of consciousness using the AVPU scale:
     A   *Alert*
     V   responds to *Voice*
     P   responds to *Pain*
     U   *Unresponsive.*
- Assess and note pupil size and reaction.
- Note the child's posture.

Airway

The first requisite is to maintain a patent airway. If the AVPU score is P or less, the airway is at risk.

Breathing

Once the airway is protected, provide high-flow O_2 with a non-rebreathing mask.

Circulation

- Obtain IV or intra-osseous access
- Obtain blood
- Consider administration of IV antibiotics if infection is suspected

Nursing care

- It is often impossible in the first hour to ascertain a diagnosis; therefore the immediate aim is to maintain child's condition and
▶ *Treat the treatable.*
- Maintain the airway. If airway is not patent, open it with the airway manoeuvre and use an oropharyngeal airway. Summon medical help.

Fiona Smith, Royal Aberdeen Children's Hospital

- Assess respiratory effort.
- Monitor heart rate and SaO_2 continuously.
- Coma scale recordings (as described on p. 268). Perform every 15 min initially.
- Measure vital signs of temperature, heart rate, respiration, blood pressure, and SaO_2 hourly. Altered vital signs may indicate abnormal pathology or assist in identifying the cause of unconsciousness.
- Provide high-flow O_2 via non-rebreathing mask—regardless of SaO_2.
- Regular blood sugars and arterial blood gas monitoring, because abnormalities of these can cause coma in themselves.
- While primary assessment and resuscitation are being carried out, a detailed history of the child's health over the past 24 hours should be gained.
- Re-assess coma score, pupil responses, posture, and tone regularly.

Further reading

Williams, C., Asquith, J. (2000). *Paediatric intensive care nursing.* Churchill Livingstone, Edinburgh.

Epilepsy

The term 'epilepsy' is used for a group of neurological disorders resulting from uncontrolled electrical discharges from nerve cells in the cerebral cortex, characterized by recurrent episodes of convulsive seizures, sensory disturbances, abnormal behaviour, and/or loss of consciousness. There are different types of seizures, dependent upon which part of the brain is affected.

Generalized seizures

Both sides of the brain are involved together:
- absence (petit mal): brief loss of awareness
- myoclonic: shock-like contractions of different muscles
- atonic/astatic (drop fit): a sudden loss of muscle tone
- tonic: sudden stiffening of the limbs or whole body, causing a fall like a tree being felled
- clonic: jerks or twitches caused by repeated rhythmical contractions of muscles, limbs, or whole body
- tonic–clonic (grand mal): tonic stage followed by clonic stage.

Partial seizures

These occur when electrical activity starts in part of one lobe of one hemisphere. Partial seizures that spread to the majority of the brain are called secondary generalized seizures.
- Simple: level of consciousness not affected. Involves a change in sensation such as smell or taste, unexplained fear, feeling of déjà vu, or tingling and numbness of the face or arm.
- Complex: consciousness is affected. May look confused or dazed or behave in a strange way.

Diagnosis

- Take a history—a detailed description of events before, during, and after a seizure.
- Diagnosis is rarely made following one seizure; there are presentations in childhood and adolescence that may be mistaken for epilepsy, such as:
  - shuddering spells and jitteriness
  - benign myoclonus in infancy
  - tics and ritualistic movements
  - panic attacks, which can present with psychic and autonomic symptoms.

Investigations

- Blood tests to exclude other causes
- Electroencephalogram (EEG), to record electrical activity
- CT scan: shows abnormalities in the structure of the brain
- MRI scan: shows subtle cerebral malformations

Management

- Drug therapy: a balance between seizure control and side effects.

Angela Shead, Royal Devon and Exeter NHS Foundation Trust

- Ketogenic diet: myoclonic and atonic seizures respond best. Most frequently used in Lennox–Gastaut syndrome.
- Surgery: depends on the focus of epilepsy and poor control with drug therapy. Must be weighed against possible negative outcome.
- Vagal nerve stimulation (VNS): it remains to be determined which seizure type/epilepsy syndromes may benefit from VNS, and at what age children should have the procedure.

Further reading

Appleton, R., Gibbs, J. (2004). *Epilepsy in childhood and adolescence*, 3rd edn. Martin Dunitz, London.

Chappel, B., Crawford, P. (2001). *Epilepsy at your fingertips*, 2nd edn. Class Publishing, London.

National Society for Epilepsy website.www.e-epilepsy.org.uk

Head injury management

Head injury is the leading cause of death and disability in children and adolescents.

Two processes involved in brain damage after head injury are:
- primary brain injury: direct result of trauma, occurs immediately
- secondary brain injury: resulting from intracranial and extracranial complications of the initial injury, occurs later.

Primary brain injury
- Non-accidental injury: most severe head injuries in children under 1 year of age are the result of child abuse.
- Penetrating injury: injury to the brain is localized at the site of penetration; neurological signs reflect the focal nature of any brain damage, e.g. in penetration of the pre-central motor area, the child presents with limp paresis.
- Crush injury: the head becomes compressed between moving and stationary surfaces (e.g. mechanically operated door or falling masonry).
- Acceleration and deceleration injury (diffuse axonal injury): this is the most common form of trauma to the brain; occurs in the majority of road accidents, falls, and assaults.

Secondary brain injury
Arises when the brain is starved of O_2, which makes damage from the initial injury worse.

Causes
- Cerebral oedema
- Cerebral hypoxia (resulting from respiratory failure due to raised intracranial pressure (ICP) causing compression of the brainstem, or injury to the lungs)
- Cerebral ischaemia (due to raised ICP or systemic hypotension)
- Intracranial haematomas

Priorities for immediate management of head injury
- To restore blood pressure, blood O_2, and carbon dioxide (CO_2) levels to normal values as rapidly as possible, in order to minimize or prevent secondary brain injury.
- Subsequent resuscitation—the aim is to protect the brain by prevention of ischaemia due to intracranial haematomas, rising ICP, or the consequences of brain shift.

Management of head injury
- Airway: evaluation and management of airway.
- Breathing: continuous SaO_2 monitoring; assist with intubation and artificial ventilation if the child is in a coma.
- Circulation: administer prescribed IV fluids (monitor fluid input/ output).
- Disability: neurological examination and assessment.
  - monitor meticulously, using the GCS or modified GCS for young children, to assess the level of consciousness.

Gillian M. Robinson, Central Manchester and Manchester Children's University Hospitals NHS Trust

- observe and record pupil responses, focal neurological deficits, and other vital signs (TPR and blood pressure).
▶ Report any deviations in observations immediately.
- Evaluation and stabilization of other injuries.
- Seizure care and management as necessary.

▶ Despite technological advances, the most important aspect is skilled observation carried out by the nurse.

Significance of nursing care

- Assessment (acute, medium, and long-term)
- Observation and monitoring
- Administration of prescribed medication: observe and record effects
- Nutrition: may be NG/gastrostomy fed
- Rehabilitation (member of interdisciplinary team)
- Coordinate discharge planning
- Information and counselling:
  - head injury advice
  - child and family adjustment
  - access to resources and support mechanisms

Further reading

National Institute for Health and Clinical Excellence (2003). *Head injury: triage, assessment, investigation and early management of head injury in infants, children and adults.* Clinical Guideline 4. NICE, London. ▣ www.nice.org.uk
▣ Children's Brain injury Trust information. ▣ www.cbituk.org

Acquired brain injury

Acquired brain injury is an injury to the brain that is not hereditary, congenital, or degenerative.

Causes
- Traumatic brain injuries
- Aneurysms
- Infection, e.g. encephalitis or meningitis
- Hypoxic–ischaemic cerebral insult (caused by reduction of blood flow and supply of O_2 to brain)
  - stroke
  - near-drowning accidents
  - asphyxiation/suffocation (strangulation/smoke inhalation)
  - prolonged status epilepticus
  - during major surgical procedure, particularly cardiac surgery
- Toxins (e.g. drugs, salicylates, and CO_2 poisoning)
- Tumour
- Complications of metabolic or biochemical impairment (e.g. diabetes mellitus, due to hypoglycaemia and hyperglycaemia)

Priorities for immediate management of acquired brain injury
- Airway: evaluation and management of airway
- Breathing: SaO_2 monitoring; assist with intubation/ventilation if child in coma
- Circulation: administer prescribed IV fluids (monitor fluid input/output)
- Disability: neurological examination and assessment
  - monitor clinical signs of rising ICP (see below)
  - seizure management and care as necessary

Clinical signs of rising ICP
- Decrease in level of consciousness
- Fall in respiratory rate or change in respiratory pattern
- Decrease in heart rate
- Rise in blood pressure
- Pupil changes (dilate, become unequal, or non-reacting)

Significance of nursing care
- Assessment (acute, medium, and long-term)
- Observation and monitoring
- Administration of prescribed medication: observe and record effects
- Nutrition: may be NG/gastrostomy fed
- Prevent spread of infection: standard precautions
- Rehabilitation (member of interdisciplinary team)
- Coordinate discharge planning
- Information and counselling:
  - acquired brain injury advice
  - child and family adjustment
  - access to resources and support mechanisms

Gillian M. Robinson, Central Manchester and Manchester Children's University Hospitals NHS Trust

Support groups

Refer to the Contact a Family website for an extensive list of support groups at ⌨ www.cafamily.org.uk.

Further reading

Savage, R.C. (1999). *The child's brain: injury and development.* Lash and Associates Publishing/ Training, Wake Forest, NC.
Walker, S., Wicks, B. (2005). *Educating children with acquired brain injury.* David Fulton, London.

Cerebral palsy

A permanent, but not unchanging, disorder of movement and posture due to dysfunction of the brain.

Types of cerebral palsy

- Spasticity: due to damage in the cerebral cortex. Can affect both sides of the body or just one side, depending on which cells are damaged. It results in increased tension in the muscles, difficulty in relaxing, stiffness, and slowing of movement. This is the most common disorder and occurs in about 75% of cases.
- Hemiplegia: affects either the left-hand or right-hand side of the body, and involves one arm and one leg. Difficulty in movement is usually noticed in the arm first and may only manifest itself in the leg on weight bearing or walking.
- Diplegia: affects the legs only. Stiffness may be noticed at an early age when trying to separate the legs when changing a nappy. Walking is delayed and characterized by walking on the toes with knees bent.
- Quadriplegia: manifests itself in all four limbs and those affected usually have severe difficulties in all forms of movement: legs, arms, and trunk. It also interferes with sucking, chewing, swallowing, and speech.

Cerebral palsy affects approximately 1 in every 400 children. It usually occurs as a result of some hazard adversely affecting the brain some time after conception, around birth, or during early childhood. Some of the hazards are:
- Prenatal (conception to birth):
  - inefficient placenta
  - genetic disorders
  - infections
  - high blood pressure
  - premature birth
- Perinatal (during the birth):
  - birth trauma, i.e. prolonged labour
  - occasionally forceps delivery
  - lack of O_2
- Neonatal (0–28 days after birth):
  - breathing problems
  - hypoglycaemia
  - blood group incompatibility
  - convulsions
  - infections to the brain, which do not respond to treatment

Half of those born with cerebral palsy will have normal intelligence. The other half will have some kind of learning disability possibly due to other factors such as epilepsy, visual impairment, speech, etc.

Conditions associated with cerebral palsy

When caring for a child with cerebral palsy the following areas should be taken into consideration. Each child will have differing needs.

Barbara Southcombe, Royal Devon and Exeter NHS Foundation Trust

Mobility

- Non-ambulant children, especially those that are enterally fed, can suffer with osteopenia, causing bone fractures secondary to minor injuries.
- Ensure that mobility aids are used correctly to prevent/reduce further deterioration.

Visual impairment

One-third of children with cerebral palsy suffer with some kind of visual impairment, making it even more difficult to overcome their disability, undermining their motivation, and causing lack of self-esteem.

Nutrition

Many children with cerebral palsy have swallowing problems caused by poor tongue control. Feeding while sitting up, to extend the neck, reduces the risk of choking.

Communication

Because of poor tongue thrust, some may have difficulty with speech; this can lead to frustration, confusion, and depression.

Epilepsy

Occurs in one-third of those with cerebral palsy and usually manifests itself within the first 2 years.

Further reading

Bobath Children's Therapy Centre, Wales, (2004) information pack:
- www.bobathwales.org.
- www.associatedconditionsofcerebralpalsy.com
- www.caringforcerebralpalsy.com

The paralysed child

Paralysis results when an injury occurs to the spinal cord. The most common cause of serious spinal cord injury in children is a congenital defect, e.g. myelomeningocele. Other causes include:

- falls
- motor vehicle accidents
- quad bike accidents
- trampoline accidents.

Types of paralysis

- Quadriplegia—involves loss of movement and sensation in all four limbs, as well as the chest muscles, so respiratory support is required
- Paraplegia—involves loss of movement and sensation in the lower half of the body

Nursing care

The nursing care of the paralysed child is complex and challenging. The diagnosis of paralysis is devastating for the child and family, and it may be some time before the parents and child are ready to absorb any information. The level of paralysis will affect the amount of nursing intervention and the prevention of secondary complications is important. The nursing care includes the following.

- Maximizing potential for self-help and education.
- Respiratory (quadriplegia)—tracheostomy care and positioning.
- Skin—pressure relief and hygiene.
- Body alignment—support, splints, and passive exercises.
- Elimination—importance of bladder and bowel care.
- Remobilization—as active as possible to prevent muscle wasting, and contractures.
- Psychosocial—includes child and family needs. Important to set realistic goals and focus on maximizing capabilities with positive reinforcement.
- Sexuality—self-esteem problems and sexual health.
- Liaison with multidisciplinary team.
- Pre-operative and post-operative care if surgery indicated.
- Ongoing specialist support.
- Play.

Children work through their problems in play and it is vital that the child begins to play as soon as he/she is able. Boredom may be a problem, and imagination and creativity will be useful nursing skills to help the child adjust to his/her new situation.

Further reading

Spoltore, T., Mulcahey, M.J., Johnston, T., Kelly, K., Morales, V., Rebuck, C. (2000). Innovative programs for children and adolescents with spinal cord injury. *Orthopaedic Nursing*, **19**(3), 55–63.

Andrea Gibson, Queen's University Belfast

Meningitis

Meningitis is an acute inflammation of the lining around the brain and spinal cord. It occurs far more commonly in children than adults, with the peak age of incidence in children under 5 years of age. Signs and symptoms may present insidiously. The younger the child, the more difficult the diagnosis. Meningitis is usually bacterial or viral in origin.

Common pathogens

Bacterial

- Meningococcal (*Neisseria meningitidis*) infection accounts for most bacterial meningitis cases in the UK.
- Pneumococcal (*Streptococcus pneumoniae*) infection second most frequent cause and is associated with a higher fatality and neurological sequelae.
- Hib has become rare since the introduction of the Hib vaccine in UK in 1992.
- Group B streptococci (GBS) are the main cause of meningitis during the neonatal period. GBS with *Escherichia coli* and *Listeria* spp. are more uncommon causes.

Viral

- Mumps
- Enteroviruses
- Epstein–Barr virus
- Viral meningitis is almost never life threatening, with antibiotic administration not indicated.

Clinical features

- Early symptoms of meningitis are non-specific and may include fever, vomiting, irritability, and drowsiness.
- More specific signs in infants include a tense or bulging fontanelle and a high-pitched or moaning cry.
- In older children, headache, neck stiffness, and photophobia may be present.
- Kernig's sign (inability to extend the knee when the leg is flexed at the hip) and Brudzinski's sign (bending the head forwards results in flexion movements of the legs) may be positive.
- Seizures may also occur at any age.
- Meningococcal infection can present with a characteristic non-blanching purpuric rash if septicaemia is present (📖 *Meningococcal disease*).

Diagnosis

A lumbar puncture is the definitive diagnostic test but is contraindicated if there are signs of raised ICP. Blood cultures may also indicate the causative organism.

Treatment

Acute bacterial meningitis is a life-threatening condition that requires early recognition and prompt treatment with IV antibiotics.

Dawn Ritchie, University of Nottingham

Nursing management

Management includes treatment of the cause, prevention of secondary complications, and depends on the condition of the child.

* If the child is critically ill, support of ABC is essential.
* Closely monitor and assess the child's neurological and cardiorespiratory function to detect signs of deterioration in conscious level, rising ICP, and shock.
* Administer IV antibiotics for a minimum of 10 days.
* Give prophylactic antibiotic therapy to all family and close social contacts of meningococcal meningitis.
* Maintain optimal hydration through IV therapy or oral fluids. Measure accurately and record fluid balance, including urinary output.
* Isolation precautions.
* If at all possible, keep the child in a quiet room with reduced light and environmental stimuli.
* Support and reassure parents; give clear explanations of their child's progress and all treatments and procedures.
* All children will require a hearing assessment 6–8 weeks after discharge, or sooner if hearing loss is suspected.

Further reading

Meningitis Research Foundation. www.meningitis.org
Meningitis Trust. www.meningitistrust.org.uk

Meningococcal disease

Meningococcal meningitis and meningococcal septicaemia are together known as meningococcal disease and are systemic infections caused by the Gram-negative diplococcus *N. meningitidis*. This bacterium has many distinct serogroups: A, B, C, W135, and Y. Groups B and C are the most common in the UK, although the incidence of group C is declining since the advent of the MenC vaccine in 1999.

Incidence of meningococcal disease is highest in children under 5 years, with a peak in children under 1 year of age and a second smaller peak in young people aged 15–19 years.

- Transmission is via nasopharyngeal droplets.
- The incubation period is 2–10 days.
- Meningococci can be found naturally at the back of the throat or nose, with approximately 10% of the population being carriers, rising to 25% in young people aged 15–19 years.
- The reasons why invasive disease occurs are not fully understood.
- Increased incidence in winter.
- Overcrowding and smoking increase the risk of the disease.
- The majority of cases of meningococcal disease occur sporadically, with <5% of cases occurring in clusters.
- Travel to the Indian subcontinent, Middle East, and sub-Saharan Africa has in recent years increased the incidence of Group A and W135 cases in UK.

Children can present with meningitis alone, septicaemia alone, or both. Meningococcal septicaemia is the more serious. Meningococcal disease continues to have a significant mortality, about 10% cases overall, and morbidity. Early recognition and aggressive early treatment improve outcome.

Signs and symptoms

Frequently mild non-specific symptoms are followed by severe illness and, in >50% of cases, a rash.

Symptoms of septicaemia

- Rash: may be sparse or profuse, and may vary from tiny petechial spots to large purpuric lesions
- Fever
- Aches: children usually experience bad muscle and joint aches, making them feel restless and uncomfortable
- Myalgia and especially leg pain
- Weakness
- Gastrointestinal symptoms, including abdominal pain, vomiting, and diarrhoea.

Symptoms of meningitis

- Fever
- Headache
- Vomiting
- Irritability/drowsiness/confusion

Dawn Ritchie, University of Nottingham

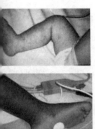
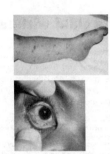

Meningococcal disease. From *Early Management of Meningococcal Disease in Children* ©
A.J. Pollard, S. Nadel, P. Habibi, S.N. Faust, I Maconochie, N. Metha, J. Britto, M. Levin.
Department of Paediatrics, Imperial College School of Medicine, St Mary's Hospital,
London W2. Reproduced with kind permission of Meningitis Research Foundation.

- Seizures
- Photophobia
- Neck stiffness
- Infants may also have a bulging fontanelle

Differential diagnosis

Meningococcus may be grown from aspirate of skin lesions, blood
cultures, CSF, or pharyngeal swab.

Nursing management

- Initial assessment includes patency of the airway, and adequacy of
  breathing and circulation. Resuscitation should start where indicated.
  Refer to early management of meningococcal disease algorithm.
- Assess circulation, including core–peripheral temperature, capillary refill,
  demarcation of circulatory insufficiency, and systolic blood pressure.
- Secure venous/intra-osseous access. The nurse's role in the administra-
  tion, monitoring, and evaluation of efficacy of fluid administration
  cannot be overstated.
- Monitor for early indications of raised ICP, GCS.
- Administer IV antibiotics for a minimum of 10 days.
- Isolate child for first 24 hours.
- Public health: meningococcal disease is notifiable.
- Prophylaxis for close contacts.
- Provide psychological support for the family; help them to cope with
  the very real possibility of the sudden death of their child.
- Long term: the child may need help to adjust to surviving a life-
  threatening illness, and there may also be concerns due to altered
  body image because necrosis due to meningococcal lesions may result
  in soft tissue losses and amputations.

Further reading

Pathan, N., Faust, S.N., Levin, M. (2003). Pathophysiology of meningococcal meningitis and
    septicaemia. *Arch. Dis. Child.*, **88**, 601–7.
Meningitis Research Foundation 🖳 www.meningitis.org
Meningitis Trust 🖳 www.meningitistrust.org.uk
🖳 www.isobel.org.uk

Care of a child with febrile convulsions

A febrile convulsion or febrile seizure (FS) is defined as an event in infancy or childhood that is associated with fever; an FS usually only occurs between 3 months and 5 years of age. They are further identified as events where there is no other cause for seizure, such as intracranial infection. FSs are brief, lasting <15 min, and generalized convulsive movements can be observed.

Signs and symptoms	Action
Child with previous symptoms of fever has generalized convulsive movements for <10–15 min	Place child in recovery position to maintain airway, observe all movements, and record timing of event
Child may feel hot	Keep child covered with light covering such as a sheet. Remove all tight or restrictive clothing
Body temperature significantly higher than normal	Administer antipyretic under prescription

General concerns	Response
Carer/parent very anxious and frightened, and worried that something may be very wrong	Reassure that this is a common event with incidence between 2% and 5% of all young children. Contact medical help to identify source of fever and eliminate serious infections. Reassure parent that child will receive appropriate care
Parents keen to know cause of FSs	Reassure that cause of fever will be investigated. 85–90% of FS events are caused by viral illness, otitis media, and tonsillitis. Urinary tract infections, gastroenteritis, upper respiratory tract infections, and meningitis account for the other 10–15%. The actual cause of FSs is still under debate
Parent very concerned that seizure may recur	FSs only recur in about 30% of children
Parent very concerned the possibility that FSs will occur in all fever episodes	Very difficult to predict when and if FSs will recur in individual children; 70% of children with FSs will have a recurrence within the first year, especially if first FS occurred at <15 months of age. Use of antipyretic medication to prevent the reoccurrence of FSs is ineffective

Maureen Harrison, University of Southampton

Contd.

Parents anxious to know what factors are likely to predict a recurrence.	Family history of FSs, epilepsy in first-degree relative, or attendance at pre-school nurseries (more febrile events in these children)
	If no risk factors, 10% risk of recurrence of FSs; if one risk factor, 25% risk; and if two risk factors, 50% risk
Parent very concerned that child will develop epilepsy following a FS	Risk of future epilepsy is only 1%, compared with 0.4% of epileptic children without a history of FSs
Concerns that fever might be harmful to child	Significant evidence that fever is not harmful. Evidence to support use of paracetamol in reducing fever is very weak, although some evidence for use of ibuprofen in reducing fever. Antipyretics do not prevent recurrence of febrile episodes
General worries about FSs and fever	Nurses need to be well informed in order to support and educate parents

Further reading

▪ www.prodigy.nhs.uk/guidance.asp?gt=febrile%20convulsion
▪ www.nhsdirect.nhs.uk/en.asp?TopicID=197

Space-occupying lesions

Paediatric brain tumours are the most common solid tumour found in children and the second most common neoplasm, representing approximately 20–25% of childhood cancers. Current treatment involves surgical resection where possible, usually followed by radiotherapy and/or chemotherapy. Although advances in treatment have been many, morbidity and mortality remain high in this group of children.

The aetiology of CNS tumours remains uncertain, although there are predisposing factors such as certain genetic factors, exposure to ionizing radiation, pesticides, and poliomaviruses.

Presentation

Variations depend on the following:
• compression or infiltration of specific cerebral tissue
• related cerebral oedema
• raised ICP.

Signs and symptoms will vary according to the child's age, development and cognition, and the location of the tumour. Early morning headache and vomiting are common features and should always be investigated. Secondary hydrocephalus often occurs, triggering an acute deterioration in the child with signs of raised ICP. Focal neurological signs in line with the location of the tumour may include visual changes, pituitary disturbance, hemiparesis, seizures, intellectual difficulties, ataxia, and cranial nerve involvement.

Investigation

CT and MRI scans remain the main diagnostic tools, with angiography occasionally being undertaken to define abnormal vascular pathology.

Treatment

The aim of surgery and the risks involved must be discussed in detail with the parents. Surgery should be undertaken in a dedicated specialist centre, where a paediatric neuro-anaesthetist, neurosurgeon, and specialist nurse are available.

Adjuvant therapy

Chemotherapy and/or radiotherapy are usually required following surgery, although a 'watch and wait' policy may occasionally be appropriate. Recent studies indicate that significant morbidity occurs following both treatments, and a skilled neuro-oncology nurse is essential in helping the family obtain necessary interventions and assistance.

Long-term concerns

• Neurological
• Endocrinological
• Cognitive and personality changes
• Change of body image
• Change of family dynamics
• Quality of life
• Long-term prognosis

Lindy May, Great Ormond Street Hospital for Children NHS Trust

Multicentre trials are essential to move treatment forward for this group of children, and molecular-targeted therapy may become the treatment of the future.

Further reading

May, L. (2001). *Paediatric neurosurgery—a handbook for the multidisciplinary team*. Whurr, London.
Walker, D., Perilongo, G., Punt, J., Taylor, R. (2004). *Brain and spinal tumours of childhood*. Arnold, London.

Benign intracranial hypertension

Benign intracranial hypertension (BIH) is increased pressure of CSF.

BIH is a headache syndrome. 'Benign' means not fatal; however, untreated BIH can permanently damage the child's eyesight. Headaches can be very debilitating.

Incidence
BIH is uncommon in children, 1–2 cases/year per large referring hospital. Children as young as 4 months can be affected. The sex distribution is equal.

Possible causes
- Unknown
- Some medicines have been associated with BIH, e.g. tetracycline, isotretinoin, and nitrofurantoin
- Oral contraceptives
- Corticosteroid withdrawal, including topical use for eczema
- Sinus disease and clots in veins around the brain have also been implicated

Signs and symptoms
- Lethargy and tiredness
- Dizziness, mood changes, and 'buzzing sounds inside my head'
- Young children may have a change in sleep pattern
- Nausea and vomiting
- Headaches, mostly frontal, become worse on lying down and may wake the child at night

Visual disturbances
Children describe a variety of visual disturbances:
- diplopia
- blurring of vision and intermittent loss of sight
- photophobia
- 'shimmering lights' with coloured centres

Clinical features
- Neurological examination: normal reflexes except for papilloedema, or sixth nerve palsy, when the eye cannot look outwards but can look inwards.
- Ophthalmic findings: BIH can occur with or without papilloedema in adults and children. To date there is no evidence that BIH *without* papilloedema is a threat to vision.

Diagnosis
- Normal MRI or CT.
- Lumbar puncture (LP) can be used to lower the CSF pressure.
- CSF can return to pre-tap concentrations within 2 hours.

Sarah Hayward, Royal Devon and Exeter NHS Foundation Trust

- Accepted 20 cmH$_2$O as an upper limit. Paediatric neurologists use 18 cmH$_2$O, with legs in a piked straight position.
- CSF pressure can be persistently raised for years after the initial episode of BIH, which implies that it is a chronic condition.

Management
- MRI, LP, and CSF pressure measurement in the sedated child (using a technique of tap manometry and/or a pressure transducer).
- If pressure of CSF >40 cmH$_2$O, fluid removed to obtain pressure of 30 cmH$_2$O.
- If CSF pressure <40 cmH$_2$O, fluid removed until pressure resembles normal 12–20 cmH$_2$O, or halved.
- LP may be repeated if:
  - papilloedema persists
  - headaches persist
  - minimal improvement.
- Visual fields and visual acuity are measured using a Snellen chart at presentation and followed up closely.

Treatments
The goals of treatment are symptom relief and preservation of vision:
- corticosteroids, acetazolamide, and furosemide
- repeated LPs
- optic nerve slits to the back of the eyes.

Complications
Acetazolamide is a carbonic anhydrase inhibitor and is the medication of choice. Continuous medication may result in low-pressure headaches, which become worse when moving from lying to standing. Because BIH can recur months or years after the first presentation, early recognition of symptoms could prevent any eyesight damage by BIH in the future.

Further reading
Soler, D., *et al.* (1998). Diagnosis and management of benign intracranial hypertension. *Archives of Disease in Childhood*, **78**, 89–94.

Francis, P., *et al.* (2003). Benign Intracranial hypertension in children following renal transplantation. *Paediatric Nephrology*, **18**(12), 1265–9.

Lumbar puncture

General principles
- Performed to obtain a specimen of CSF from the subarachnoid space, to aid diagnosis, remove excess fluid, or inject medication.
- CSF is normally a clear, colourless, and sterile liquid.
- Performed by an experienced doctor.

Action	Rationale
1. Undertake comprehensive nursing and medical assessment	Contraindicated when ICP is elevated: brain 'coning' may result
2. Explain procedure to child and carer. Obtain informed written consent	Gain cooperation and minimize distress and anxiety
3. Consider local anaesthetic cream, sedation, or general anaesthetic as appropriate for individual child and condition. Additional care as appropriate	Minimize distress and discomfort, and facilitate procedure
4. Gather and prepare all equipment: LP set LP needles (appropriate sizes) Local anaesthetic agent Sterile containers (according to local protocols) and specimen forms Sterile towels Sterile gloves Small adhesive plaster Antiseptic agent Suitable distraction aids, e.g. story book, tape, etc	Avoid unnecessary delay
5. Position child on their side, at edge of bed, and facing away from operator. Draw knees up to chest, flex neck. Craniospinal axis parallel to bed. Correct positioning is vital	Maximum widening of intravertebral spaces and easier access to subarachnoid space
6. Adopting aseptic technique, the doctor will:	
prepare skin with antiseptic	Minimizes risk of infection
towel up sterile field	
locally anaesthetize skin and between spinous process	Reduces pain and distress
undertake procedure	
7. Discard first few drops of CSF	Likely to be blood contamination from insertion trauma

Paula Dawson, Nottingham University Hospitals NHS Trust

Contd.

8. Allow 1–2 mL CSF to flow into each sterile container	Suitable quantity for analysis
Usually collected for:	
(1) glucose and protein	
(2) Gram stain and culture and sensitivity	
(3) cell count and differential	
Additional tests may be required	
9. Apply plaster to site. Leave *in situ* for 24 hours	Reduce risk of infection
10. Dispose of equipment appropriately	Reduce risk of cross-infection and/or wastage
11. Observe child post-procedure for :	
Headache—usually settles within 24–48 hours. Lay child flat. Give paracetamol. Encourage oral fluids	Caused by reduction in pressure around brain with CSF withdrawal
CSF leakage from site. Lay child flat	
Meningitis, 'coning', spinal epidural abscess, and haematoma possible. Observe vital signs and neurological status	

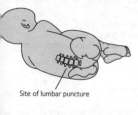

Site of lumbar puncture

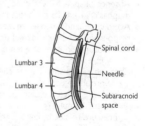

Spinal cord

Lumbar 3

Needle

Lumbar 4

Subarachnoid space

Lumbar puncture

Further reading

Blows, W.T. (2002). Diagnostic investigations Part 1: lumbar puncture. *Nursing Times*, **98**(36), 25–6.

Hickey, J.V. (1997). *The clinical practice of neurological and neurosurgical nursing.* Lippincott, Williams and Wilkins, Philadelphia, PA.

Coma scale

Failure to note deterioration in a child's level of consciousness or a lack of appreciation of its significance can lead to inappropriate management and could potentially cause irreversible brain damage or even death.

GCS

This takes three principal areas of behaviour and organizes them in an order of increasing dysfunction:
- eye opening
- verbal response
- best motor response

When the results from all three areas are combined, a measure of a patient's consciousness is obtained: maximum score 15, minimum score 3 (see table below).

Modified paediatric coma scale

The standard GCS is unsuitable for use in infants and young children. Modified paediatric scales have been adapted so the descriptors of verbal and motor response are relevant to children under 5 years of age. The paediatric coma scale has not been validated.

Remember

- Swollen or permanently closed eyes (e.g. after tarsorrhaphy) do not necessarily indicate decreasing level of consciousness.
- Absence of speech—the child may not speak English or may be deaf, dysphasic, or have a tracheostomy.
- Avoid commands such as 'squeeze my fingers/open eyes', because responses can be coincidental or a reflex grasp.
- Best motor response for a 6-month-old baby is flexion; localization not until 1 year.
- Only use painful stimuli if the child does not respond to age-appropriate commands:
  - trapezius pinch is easier and safer than supra-orbital pressure (central stimulus)
  - pressure to side of finger—third and fourth fingers are most sensitive (peripheral stimulus).

Further reading

Simpson, D.A., Cockington, R.A., Hanieh, A., Raftos, J., Reilly, P.L. (1991). Head injuries in infant and young children: the value of the Paediatric Coma Scale. Review of literature and report on a study. *Child Nervous System* **7**, 183–90.

Warren, A. (2000). Paediatric coma scoring researched and benchmarked. *Paediatric Nursing* **12**(3), 14–18.

Gillian M. Robinson, Central Manchester and Manchester Children's University Hospitals NHS Trust

Coma scales

Modified paediatric coma scale, <5 years		Glasgow coma scale, 5 years to adult	
Eye opening			
Spontaneous	4	Spontaneous	4
To speech	3	To speech	3
To pain	2	To pain	2
None	1	None	1
Eyes closed by swelling	C	Eyes closed by swelling	C
Best verbal response			
Alert, babbles, coos, words, or sentences to normal ability	5	Orientated	5
Less than usual ability or spontaneous irritable cry	4	Confused	4
Cries inappropriately	3	Inappropriate words	3
Occasionally whimpers and/or moans	2	Inappropriate sounds	2
None	1	None	1
Silent or mute	S	Silent or mute	S
Intubated	T	Intubated	T

Use grimace score if there is no audible verbal response, i.e. if silent (S) or intubated (T)

Grimace score	
Spontaneous normal facial/oro-motor activity	5
Less than usual spontaneous ability or only response to touch stimuli	4
Vigorous grimace to pain	3
Mild grimace to pain	2
No response to pain	1

Best motor response			
Normal spontaneous movements	6	Obeys commands	6
Localizes pain	5	Localizes pain	5
Withdraws to pain	4	Flexion to pain	4
Abnormal flexion (*decorticate* posture)	3	Abnormal flexion to pain	3
Extension to pain (*decerebrate* posture)	3	Extension	3
None	1	None	1

Neurological observations

Neurological observation relates to the integrity of an individual's nervous system. These observations are required to monitor and evaluate changes in the nervous system, by indicating trends and therefore aiding diagnosis and treatment, which in turn affect prognosis and rehabilitation.

The GCS assesses three modes of behaviour. It was designed for use in adults; the Adelaide Scale has been developed for use in children but is based on the GCS:

- eye opening
- verbal response
- motor response.

Both are scales of increasing dysfunction; each point is scored and a total level of consciousness is indicated. The maximum total score for GCS is 15, indicating a fully conscious state. A score <8 indicates that the patient is comatose. Altered consciousness indicates abnormalities within the brain.

States of consciousness

Consciousness is defined as 'a state of wakefulness, alertness, and awareness of one's self and one's environment'. The level of consciousness can vary from slight to severe changes, indicating the degree of brain malfunction:

- fully conscious—patient is aware of self and his environment
- lethargic—the patient is inactive and indifferent, responses are slower, and he might not respond verbally
- coma—there is a total absence of awareness.

Assessing the level of consciousness

- Eye opening: indicates that the arousal mechanism in the brain is active. Eye opening may be spontaneous or in response to speech, painful stimuli, or not at all. Arousal must be the first measurement taken during assessment; without this, cognition does not occur.
- Verbal response:
  - orientated—an individual is fully aware
  - confused—responses to simple questions are incorrect
  - incomprehensible—the patient moans and groans, but there are no recognized words
  - no verbal response at all.
- Motor response: to obey commands is the best motor response recordable. Ask the child to perform an action and record his/her best motor response. If not possible, use upper limbs to test the motor response, because lower limb responses can reflect spinal function. Response to painful stimuli may be:
  - localized, when the child moves his/her hand to the site of pain
  - flexor, which occurs when child flexes away from the pain
  - extensor, when child extends from the pain
  - no response when painful stimuli are applied.

Andrea Peters, Central Manchester and Manchester Children's University Hospitals NHS Trust

- Painful stimuli: implement this *only* if the child does not respond to firm and clear commands. When applying painful stimuli it is important to remember that the brain responds to central stimuli and the spine responds to peripheral stimuli. Central stimuli include trapezium squeeze, supra-orbital pressure, and sternal rub. The sternal rub can lead to severe bruising—do not use this for repeated assessment.

▶ It cannot be overemphasized that the methods of patient assessment should be carried out appropriately by *qualified health professionals*.

- Pupil activity: reaction of the pupils to light is an important part of neurological assessment. Note the size, shape, equality, reaction to light, and position of each eye. An impaired pupil response indicates that the midbrain may be suffering from an increase in pressure exerted by swelling in the brain.
- Motor function: damage to any part of the motor nervous system can affect the ability to move. Motor function assessment involves evaluation of muscle strength, muscle tone, and muscle coordination, and abnormal movements should also be documented.
  - Test muscle strength against your own muscle persistence and then against the pull of gravity.
  - Test muscle tone by flexing and extending the child's limbs on both sides and noting how much movement is resisted.
  - Test muscle coordination by rapidity and rhythm of alternating movements and point-to-point movements.
  - Abnormal movements: document seizures, tremors, tics, etc.
- Vital signs: include the recording of the child's temperature, pulse, respiration rate, and blood pressure. The respiratory pattern gives a clear indication of how the child's brain is functioning. Record the rate, pattern, and character of the respirations. A grossly fluctuating temperature in a child can indicate damage to the hypothalamus. A decrease in the pulse rate and increase in the blood pressure can indicate raised ICP.

It is essential to carry out an effective assessment of a child's conscious state when there is any indication that the child may suffer from impairment to this state, either at the present time or at any point in the near future during their admission to hospital.

Further reading

Frawley, P. (1990). Neurological observations. *Nursing Times*, **86**(35), 29–34.

Hofer, T. (1993). Glasgow Scale relationship in paediatric and adult patients. *Journal of Neuroscience Nursing*, **25**(4), 218–27.

Warren, A. (2000). Paediatric coma scoring researched and benchmarked. *Paediatric Nursing*, **12**(3),14–18.

Respiratory problems

Anatomy and physiology

- The respiratory tree can be divided into:
    - pre-acinus: conducting structures, developed by week 16 *in utero*
    - acinus: gaseous exchange structures, continue to develop throughout early childhood.
- Lungs continue to remodel until skeletal growth ceases.
- Features of the respiratory tree peculiar to the infant/young child are detailed in the table opposite.

Ventilation–perfusion ratio

Self-ventilating young children preferentially ventilate the non-dependent lung. Perfusion is less affected by the pressure gradient between the dependent and non-dependent lungs, but is affected by gravity. To maximize this ratio, lie the child on his/her side with the affected lung in the dependent position.

Further reading

Prasad, A., Hussey, J. (1995). Physiology of the cardiorespiratory system. In *Paediatric respiratory care: a guide for physiotherapists and health professionals*, pp. 13–24. Chapman & Hall, London.

Dave Morgan, Central Manchester and Manchester Children's University Hospitals NHS Trust

Respiratory tree of the infant/young child

Anatomical/physiological feature	Key point
Obligatory nasal breather	Upper respiratory tract infection can lead to significant respiratory distress
Relative macroglossia	Predisposes to airway occlusion
Proportionately large lymphoid tissue	Predisposes to airway occlusion during chronic infection
Epiglottis is floppy, attaching at an acute angle to the larynx	Predisposes to airway occlusion when level of consciousness decreased
Cricoid cartilage is the narrowest point of the airway	Risk of oedema
Short trachea with fewer cilia	Function as a filter, protecting the lungs, is reduced
Narrow airway diameter	Distal airways offer greater resistance to gas flow as a proportion of total airway resistance
Reduced smooth muscle within airway structure	Sensitivity to β_2 agonists (bronchodilators) decreased/absent
Absence of collateral ventilatory pathways	Predisposition to areas of lung collapse (atelectasis)
Cartilagenous rib cage	Decreased stability for muscle contraction, less resistance to elastic recoil of lungs, and more compressible
Horizontal ribs	Bucket-handle mechanism (antero-posterior diameter) unable to increase tidal volume
Lower percentage of type I muscle fibres (25% versus 50% in adult) in diaphragm	Prone to fatigue more rapidly when the work of breathing increases
High metabolic demand for O_2	In the presence of respiratory distress, failure ensues
Closing volume (volume at which distal airways collapse) is greater than functional residual capacity (volume in lung at end of expiration)	Degree of airway collapse always present
Rapid eye movement sleep inhibits intercostal muscle activity	Affects chest wall stability, causing paradoxical chest movement leading to a decrease in functional residual capacity

Apnoea

Definition

Apnoea is a disorder of respiratory control. There is no one clear definition, but it is widely accepted that apnoea is a cessation of breathing for 15–20 s, or less if it is associated with bradycardia and hypoxaemia.

Classification

Apnoeas can be classified as central, obstructive, or mixed:
- Central: respiratory effort is absent. These tend to last <20 s.
- Obstructive: obstructive air flow, but persistent chest wall movement. Usually observed in infants with upper airway abnormalities. Less common.
- Mixed: difficult to identify. Child appears to stop breathing, then makes respiratory effort but with ineffective gas exchange.

Presentation

Apnoeas generally present as apnoea of prematurity (AOP), apnoea of infancy (AOI), or obstructive sleep apnoea (OSA).

AOP

Apnoeas in pre-term infants are usually considered as a normal maturational process.

Causes
- Immaturity of the respiratory centre
- Infection
- Intraventricular haemorrhage
- Cardiovascular causes
- Upper airway collapse

Investigations/management
- Full septic screen.
- Gentle stimulation—▶ not shaking!
- Bag and mask ventilation if prolonged.
- Position prone, although re-iterate to parents that this is only while the baby is being monitored in hospital; at home he/she should be positioned supine.
- Medication, i.e. theophylline and caffeine.

AOI

These apnoeas generally occur in infants older than 37 weeks. The infants will often present with an apparent life-threatening event (APLE). This event is usually a combination of cessation of breathing, and colour change (usually cyanosis or pallor), often with marked hypotonia. The parents/carer will inevitably be stressed.

Causes
- Infection, e.g. meningitis and bronchiolitis
- Seizures
- Hypoglycaemia
- Metabolic disorders

Kelly L. Owens, Portsmouth Hospitals Trust

● Gastro-oesophageal reflux (GOR) has been cited as a cause of AOI; however, recent evidence suggests that episodes of apnoea were seldom associated with GOR. Furthermore, if there was a correlation between the events, the apnoea preceded the incidence of GOR.

Investigations/management
● Detailed history and physical examination.
● Infection screen.
● Monitor: at home if appropriate. Ensure that parents are CPR trained.

OSA

Apnoeas due to failure to maintain upper airway patency during sleep. Leads to impaired daytime performance and sometimes severe health complications, e.g. poor growth and developmental delay.

Causes
● Adenotonsillar hypertrophy
● Obesity

Investigations/management
● Polysomnography; recording of sleep state
● ECG
● SaO$_2$
● Adenotonsillectomy provides immediate relief.

Further reading

Arad-Cohen, N., Cohen, A., Tirosh, E. (2000). The relationship between gastroesophageal reflux and apnea in infants. *Journal of Pediatrics*, **137**(3), 321.

Asthma

Childhood asthma is one of the most common chronic diseases world-wide and should never be underestimated.

What is asthma?

Asthma is a condition that causes inflammation of the airways in response to an allergen. Common allergens in children are:

- viral infections
- cigarette smoke
- pollen
- animal dander
- house dust mite
- mould
- exercise
- emotion

When the airways come into contact with an allergen the muscles around the walls of the airways tighten, the lining of the airways swell, and mucus is produced.

Prevalence

Large-scale studies in the UK have estimated that between 12.5% and 15.5% of all children have asthma.

Mortality

In the UK, 25 children die from asthma each year.

Causes

The exact cause of asthma is unknown. Studies suggest that asthma runs in families and that exposure to cigarette smoke before and after birth increases the risk of a child developing asthma.

Clinical features

Accurate observations are imperative for assessment of the severity of a child's asthma and to enable prompt accurate treatment.

Signs and symptoms

- Coughing, particularly at night and after exercise
- Wheezing
- Breathlessness
- Noisy breathing

Differential diagnosis

Always consider other cause of wheeze and respiratory distress in young children:

- bronchiolitis
- virus-induced wheeze
- aspiration pneumonitis
- pneumonia
- congenital anomalies, tracheomalacia, and cystic fibrosis

Lisa Owen, North East Wales NHS Trust Wrexham

Normal airways

Asthma airways

Asthma can cause your airways to
become inflamed and swollen

In addition, the airway walls can become 'twitchy'
and thicker, making the airways narrower

Management

The aim of asthma management is to control symptoms, prevent exacerbations, and enable the child to lead a full and active life.

Treatment

Asthma treatments can be divided into:
- relievers (short-acting and long-acting β_2 agonists, and anticholinergics)
- preventers (inhaled steroids, oral steroids, and tablets (leukotriene receptor antagonists))
- combination therapies (long-acting β_2 agonists with inhaled steroids).

Follow-up

After a hospital admission, the child should see:
- specialist asthma nurse or respiratory paediatrician within 1 month
- GP or practice asthma nurse within 2 weeks.

Management of acute asthma in children (aged >2 years) in hospital

ASSESS ASTHMA SEVERITY

Moderate exacerbation
- SpO_2 ≥92%
- PEF ≥50% beat of predicted (>5 years)
- No clinical features of severe asthma

NB: If a child has signs and symptoms across categories, always treat according to their most severe features

Severe exacerbation
- SpO_2 <92%
- PEF <50% beat of predicted (>5 years)
- Heart rate
  - >130/min (2–5 years)
  - >120/min (>5years)
- Respiratory rate
  - >50/min (2–5 years)
  - >30/min (>5years)
- Use of accessory neck muscles

Life threatening asthma
- SpO_2 <92%
- PEF <33% beat of predicted (>5 years)
- Silent chest
- Poor respiratory effort
- Altered consciousness
- Cyanosis

Oxygen via face mask/nasal prongs to achieve normal saturations

- β_2 agonist 2–4 puffs via spacer ± facemask
- Increase β_2 agonist dose by 2 puffs every 2 minutes up to 10 puffs according to response
- Oral prednisolone
  - 20mg (2–5 years)
  - 30–40mg (>5 years)

Reassess within 1 hour

- β_2 agonist 10 puffs via spacer ± facemask or nebulised salbutamol (2–5 years: 2.5mg; >5 years: 5mg) or terbutaline (2–5 years: 5mg; >5 years: 10mg)
- Oral prednisolone (2–5 years: 20mg; >5 years: 30–40mg) or IV hydrocortisone 4mg/kg
- If poor response add 0.25mg nebulised ipratropium; repeat β_2 agonist and ipratropium up to every 20–30 minutes according to response

- Nebulised salbutamol (2–5 years: 2.5mg; >5 years: 5mg) or terbutaline (2–5 years: 5mg; >5 years: 10mg) plus ipratropium 0.25mg
- IV hydrocortisone 4mg/kg

Discuss with senior clinician, PICU team or paediatrician

- Repeat bronchodilators every 20–30 minutes

ASSESS RESPONSE TO TREATMENT
Record respiratory rate, heart rate and oxygen saturation every 1–4 hours

RESPONDING
- Continue bronchodilators 1–4 hours prn
- Discharge when stable on 4 hourly treatment
- Continue oral prednisolone for up to 3 days

At discharge
- Ensure stable on 4 hourly inhaled treatment
- Review the need for regular treatment and the use of inhaled steroids
- Review inhaler technique
- Provide a written asthma action plan for treating future attacks
- Arrange follow up according to local policy

NOT RESPONDING
- Continue 20–30 minute nebulisers and arrange HDU/PICU transfer

Consider:
- Chest X–ray and blood gases
- Bolus IV salbutamol 15μg/kg (over 10 minutes)
- Continuous IV salbutamol infusion 1–5μg/kg/min (200μg/ml solution)
- IV aminophylline 5mg/kg loading dose over 20 minutes (omit in those receiving oral theophllines) followed by continous infusion 1mg/kg/hour
- >5 years: Bolus IV infusion of magnesium sulphate 40mg/kg (max 2g) over 20 minutes

Thorax 2003; **58** (Suppl I) i1–i92

Management of acute asthma in children (aged >2 years) in hospital

DIAGNOSIS

A definitive diagnosis of asthma can be difficult to obtain in young children. Always consider other causes of wheeze and respiratory distress:
- bronchiolitis
- aspiration pneumonitis
- pneumonitis
- tracheomalacia
- complications of underlying conditions (congenital anomalies, cystic fibrosis)

ASSESS ASTHMA SEVERITY

Moderate exacerbation
- SpO_2 ≥92%
- Audible wheezing
- Use of accessory neck muscles
- Still feeding

NB: If a child has signs and symptoms across categories, always treat according to their most severe features

Severe exacerbation
- SpO_2 <92%
- Cyanosis
- Marked respiratory distress
- Too breathless to feed

Life threatening asthma
- SpO_2 <92%
- Cyanosis
- Apnoea
- Brandycardia
- Poor respiratory effort

Oxygen via facemask/nasal prongs to achieve normal saturations

Discuss with paediatrician or PICU team

Give trial of β_2 agonist: salbutamol up to 10 puffs via spacer and close fitting facemask Consider soluble prednisolone 10mg

Nebulised β_2 agonist: salbutamol 2.5mg or terbutaline 5mg Consider adding nebulised ipratropium bromide 0.25mg Give soluble prednisolone 10mg daily for up to 3 days

ASSESS RESPONSE TO TREATMENT
- Heart rate
- Pulse rate
- Pulse oxumetry
- Supportive nursing care with adequate hydration

RESPONDING
- Continue β_2 agonists
  - 1–4 hourly (moderate exacerbation)
  - 20–30 minutes (severe/life threatening exacerbation)
- Add or continue soluble prednisolone 10mg for up to 3 days

NOT RESPONDING
- Continue nebulisers bronchodilators
- Arrange HDU/PICU transfer
- Consider chest X-ray

Thorax 2003; **58** (Suppl I) i1–i92

Further reading

Levy, M.L., Pearce, L. (2004). *Asthma rapid reference*. Mosby, London.
www.brit-thoracic.org.uk

Recognition of respiratory distress

When a child presents with a breathing difficulty, it is important to assess the severity of the problem and to identify those children who require basic and advanced life support.

Signs of increased effort to breathe
- Increased respiratory rate
- Chest in-drawing
- Nasal flaring
- Tracheal tug
- Use of accessory muscles
- Grunting
- Too breathless to talk
- Too breathless to feed/eat

Signs of a child with a severe breathing difficulty
- Inappropriate drowsiness (difficult to rouse)
- Agitation
- Cyanosis

Pre-terminal signs of a child with breathing difficulty
- Exhaustion
- Bradycardia
- Silent chest
- Significant apnoea

▶ The child presenting with life-threatening or pre-terminal signs or severe breathing difficulty requires urgent attention.

Nursing management
- Ensure adequate oxygenation: measure and record SaO_2 and relevant clinical signs.

All children presenting to hospital with an acute breathing difficulty should have their SaO_2 measured. A combination of pulse oximetry and clinical signs can detect hypoxia in a child with respiratory distress.

Care must be taken to ensure that the device is correctly sized and the probe correctly positioned. An accurate measurement of saturation can only be obtained if there is a good pulse signal when the child is still and quiet.

- Administer O_2 via a face mask to maintain SaO_2 >92%. Use distraction to aid compliance if child not too exhausted to resist.
- Administer oral (or parenteral) steroids as prescribed. Explain clearly the reason for, and the side effects of, taking steroids.
- Administer adequate hydration (oral or parenteral) fluid as prescribed. Dehydration may occur because of poor fluid intake, sweating, and hyperventilation. Correct dehydration carefully because of potential risks of overhydrating children.

Gilli Lewis, Queen's University Belfast

- Re-assess frequently for worsening of condition. A child's condition can deteriorate very quickly. Close observation of a child in respiratory distress is required.
- Reduce anxiety:
  - explain clearly to child and family regarding any interventions/measurements/tests required
  - encourage rest and distraction by quiet play.
- Advise parents on feeding. If a child is able to eat or drink, encourage smaller, frequent feeds and guard against vomiting.

Further reading

ALSG (1997). *Advanced paediatric life support: the practical approach*. BMJ, London.

Bronchiolitis

This is the most common lower respiratory disease affecting children under 1 year old.

It is usually caused by RSV. The virus replicates in the epithelial cells of the bronchioles, causing necrosis and shedding of the cells. New epithelial cells are not ciliated. The lack of cilia and the increased secretions cause obstruction of the small airways. This, in turn, impairs gaseous exchange. The work of breathing and O_2 consumption increases. Impaired ventilation and ventilation–perfusion imbalance can result in hypoxaemia.

Diagnosis is made on clinical findings and the obtaining of a nasopharyngeal aspirate.

Characteristics

- Dry cough and wheeze
- Nasal discharge
- Pyrexia
- Anorexia
- Tachycardia
- Tachypnoea
- Recession
- Head bobbing
- Nasal flaring
- Grunting
- Hypoxia

Hazards

- Because of the highly infectious nature of the virus, avoid cross-infection by strict barrier nursing.
- The increased work of breathing may exhaust the infant, who will then need ventilatory support.
- Failure to observe any deterioration in the infant's condition may result in result in respiratory arrest.
- Inadequate fluid intake can result in dehydration.
- Constant handling of the infant may result in hypoxia and deterioration of the condition.

Treatment

- Supportive, with O_2 therapy and adequate fluid intake.
- The value of antiviral drugs is debatable.
- Prophylactic medication is usually only considered for 'at-risk' infants, such as premature infants and those with cardiac problems.

Nursing management

- Reduce anxiety:
  - handle the child minimally
  - give clear concise explanations to the parents.
- Maintain airway:
  - nurse with the head of the cot raised
  - consider nursing with the child prone.

Barbara Slee, Royal Devon and Exeter NHS Foundation Trust

- Maintain and monitor respiratory function:
  - monitor respiratory status
  - continuous monitoring of SaO_2 with pulse oximetry
  - use appropriate O_2 delivery system.
- Nutrition:
  - ensure adequate daily fluid intake
  - feed via the most appropriate route: orally, by NG tube, or IV.

Prevent the spread of infection
- Use standard precautions.

Prevention of further attacks
- Advise avoiding those with coryzal symptoms.
- Advise avoiding contact with cigarette smoke.

Further reading
McFarlane, K. (1994). Respiratory syncytial virus and bronchiolitis. *Paediatric Nursing*, **6**(8), 23–5.
Peter, S., Fazakerley, M. (2004). Clinical effectiveness of an integrated care pathway for infants with bronchiolitis. *Paediatric Nursing*, **16**(1), 30–5.
www.nlm.nih.gov/medlineplus/ency/article/000975.htm

Croup syndromes

Croup is a generic term applied to the sound made when a child has the characteristic 'barking' or 'brassy' (croupy) cough heard when the upper respiratory tract has degrees of swelling or obstruction associated with inflammation.

This inflammation is usually caused by a virus, but the trachea may become infected with *Staphylococcus aureus* and the epiglottis may be infected with *H. influenzae* bacteria. To some extent this can affect any number of the areas of the upper respiratory tract, larynx (laryngitis), epiglottis (epiglottitis), and larynx, trachea, and bronchi (laryngotracheo-bronchitis (LTB)). Infection of the larynx is usually the most significant, with the voice box and breathing being affected.

Characteristics of croup syndromes

• Stridor
• Brassy cough
• Hoarseness of voice resulting from inflammation of the voice box
• Dyspnoea
• Restlessness
• Irritability
• Low-grade to high-grade fever, depending upon where the infection is
• Drooling of secretions due to dysphagia
• Symptoms worse at night, particularly when supine
• Rapid pulse due to infective process and fright
• Suprasternal and substernal retractions may be seen in severe cases of croup

Hazards

• Most cases of croup and LTB are mild, but in some more severe cases, the child may struggle to inhale air past the obstruction and symptoms of hypoxia may occur.
• The child may progress to severe restlessness, anxiety, pallor, sweating, and rapid respirations.
• Occasionally the child may progress to life-threatening symptoms of cyanosis and cessation of breathing.

Treatment

• Most cases of croup can be treated at home with simple measures to relieve symptoms: paracetamol for pain, discomfort, and reduction of pyrexia may be the only treatment necessary.
• Encourage the child to rest and drink to reduce the discomfort of a dry and inflamed larynx and pharynx.
• Reassure the child that he/she will get better in time, and give gentle encouragement to drink and eat soft foods to build up energy. *

Further reading

Chandler, T. (2002). Croup. *Paediatric Nursing*, **14**(7) 41–7.
Grotjehann-Ernst, S. (2001). NHS National Electronic Library for Health. Clinical Guidelines for treatment of Croup. ▣ www.kidshealth.org

Martin Firth, University of Nottingham

Epiglottitis

Epiglottitis

- Children aged 2–5 years.
- Usually Hib.
- Condition becoming rare because of Hib immunization of infants.
- Inflammatory oedema of the supraglottic area, which includes the epiglottis and the pharyngeal structures.

Characteristics of epiglottitis

- Short history
- High fever
- Rapid pulse and respirations
- Stridor: frog-like croaking on inspiration
- Voice thick and muffled
- Dyspnoea: mild hypoxia → cyanosis
- Dysphagia and drooling
- Systemically unwell: pale, toxic, and lethargic
- Absence of spontaneous cough
- Child often adopts the characteristic posture of sitting upright, mouth open, with his/her chin thrust forward, tongue protruding
- Suprasternal and substernal retractions may be seen
- Extreme anxiety and agitation

Hazards

- If the condition is suspected, examination of the mouth is avoided as acute or total airway obstruction could result.
- The child should only be examined with an experienced anaesthetist ready to intubate if required. Do not lie the child down because this forces the epiglottis to fall backwards, leading to complete airway obstruction.
- Radiography of the neck is only justified if diagnosis is in doubt and should only take place if the child is stable. Radiography in lateral position may also precipitate respiratory arrest due to complete airway obstruction.
- It is also not advisable to perform any procedure that may increase the child's anxiety, e.g. taking a blood specimen, because this could precipitate airway spasm and cause death.
- Respiratory arrest can appear suddenly: progressive obstruction → hypoxia + hypercapnia + acidosis → decreased muscle tone + reduced level consciousness → death.

Treatment

- If epiglottitis is suspected, then emergency intubation should be performed to protect the airway.
- IV antibiotics are required immediately following intubation, usually cefotaxime, followed by 7–10 days oral therapy.
- Corticosteroids to reduce oedema in initial stages, also 24 hours before extubation.
- Recovery is usually rapid once the airway is established and antibiotic therapy given; child usually extubated on third day.

Gill McEwing, University of Plymouth

Nursing management

Reduce anxiety

- Epiglottitis is extremely frightening for child and parents; act quickly but calmly to provide support.
- Parent to hold/comfort child at all times to reduce anxiety, ensure child has security object.
- Reassure parents.
- Give clear explanations to child and parents before any procedure is carried out.
- Provide appropriate diversional activities.
- Provide a suitable environment to allow the child to rest.

Maintain airway

- Suction to remove secretions
- Assist child to expectorate sputum
- Chest physiotherapy
- Pain management
- Keep emergency equipment available

Maintain and monitor respiratory function

- Allow child to adopt the position that they find most comfortable
- Continuous monitoring of respiratory status
- Pulse oximetry to monitor SaO_2
- Use appropriate O_2 delivery system

Nutrition

- Nil by mouth to avoid aspiration
- IV infusion

Prevent spread of infection

- Use standard precautions

Prevention

Routine Hib vaccine

Pneumonia

Pneumonia is an inflammation of the pulmonary parenchyma that is common in childhood, especially in infancy. It may occur either as a primary disease or as a complication of another illness.

Usually classified by aetiological agent (i.e. viral, bacterial, mycoplasmal, or aspirational), it can be further categorized into three types:
- Lobar pneumonia: all, or a large segment, of one or more of the pulmonary lobes is involved. When both lungs are infected, it is known as double pneumonia.
- Bronchopneumonia: begins in the terminal bronchioles, which become clogged with mucopurulent exudates to form consolidated patches in nearby lobules. Also called lobular pneumonia.
- Interstitial pneumonia: the inflammatory process is confined within the alveolar walls (interstitium) and the peribronchicular and interlobular tissues.

Clinical features
- Neonates and infants: cough, fever, refusal of feeds, lethargy, tachypnoea, grunting, recession, cyanosis, and noisy breathing.
- Pre-school children: cough, post-tussive vomiting, fever, chest pain, and abdominal pain.
- Older children: fever, cough, chest pain, and dyspnoea.

Diagnosis
Based on clinical picture and investigations, including:
- full blood count and cultures
- chest X-ray
- nasopharyngeal aspirate
- pulse oximetry

Treatment
- O_2 therapy.
- Oral antibiotics or IV antibiotics in those unable to absorb orally (i.e. if vomiting) or those with severe signs and symptoms.
- Supportive measures, including oral and IV fluid and oral antipyretics.
- Regular respiratory and standard observations, including pulse oximetry, to monitor condition.
- Isolation may be necessary, depending on local policy.
- Physiotherapy is of little benefit.
- Consider moving to high-dependency with HDU or PICU if:
  - signs of shock
  - potential for deterioration needing advanced respiratory support
  - circulatory instability due to hypovolaemia
  - increasing respiratory and/or pulse rate due to respiratory distress/exhaustion.

Matthew Powell, St Mary's NHS Health Care Trust, Isle of Wight

Nursing management
- Administer antibiotic therapy as prescribed by doctors.
- Maintain oxygenation, monitoring pulse oximetry, and administering supplemental humidified O_2 to maintain saturations above 94%.
- Maintain adequate hydration, increasing oral intake and infusing IV maintenance fluids of 0.45% sodium chloride and 5% dextrose at the correct rate for body weight. Remember to calculate and factor in degree of dehydration. Observe strict fluid input and output.
- Monitor temperature, administering antipyretics where appropriate to decrease metabolic demands.
- Promote rest and sleep, planning nursing care around a normal routine and sleeping pattern.

Prognosis
The prognosis for pneumonia is generally good, with rapid recovery when treated early. Complications rarely occur because of early recognition, vigorous antibiotic, and supportive therapy. Some children, especially those who are immunosuppressed, may develop empyema, pneumothorax, or pleural effusion. Fine-needle aspiration, thoracentesis, and insertion of a chest drain may be indicated in these cases.

Further reading
www.brit-thoracic.org.uk/bts_guidelines_pneumonia_html
www.brit-thoracic.org.uk/pdf/paediatriccap.pdf

Respiratory syncytial virus

Epidemiology
- RSV is the single most important respiratory pathogen in childhood and occurs worldwide.
- In temperate zones, annual epidemics happen in winter or early spring.
- By 2 years, most infants have had RSV infection.
- Severe RSV-related bronchiolitis is associated with infants 2–6 months of age.
- Effective immunity is incomplete, and re-infection (less severe) can occur throughout life.
- The incidence of RSV infection has been linked to:
  - increased exposure to other children (urban environments, overcrowded accommodation, or attendance at day care centres)
  - bottle rather than breast feeding
  - exposure to tobacco smoke.

Clinical condition
RSV → bronchiolitis and pneumonia in infants and young children.

Symptoms
- Fever
- Dyspnoea
- Nasal congestion
- Tachypnoea
- Wheeze and cough
- Hyperinflation of the chest
- Apnoea

Pathophysiology
- Virus particles migrate to the epithelial cells lining the nasopharynx.
- Necrosis and sloughing of the epithelial cells, releasing quantities of virus.
- Immune response is evoked, airways become swollen and plugged with mucus.
- Virus particles spread to the lower respiratory tract.

Infection
Route of transmission
- Aerosol droplets from nasal and oral secretions; enter the host through mucous membranes of the eyes and nose.
- Virus can survive on inanimate surfaces (metals and plastics) for several hours, clothing for more than 2 hours, and unwashed hands for over 30 min, allowing spread of the virus through contact with people and the environment.

Incubation period
Incubation period of 5–8 days; this may be extended in immuno-compromised children.

Pamela Joannidis, Hospital for Sick Children Glasgow

Period of communicability
Communicable 1–2 days before the onset of symptoms and for as long as symptoms persist (usually 7–10 days).

Most at risk
- Premature babies <33 weeks' gestation.
- Immunocompromised children, i.e. those with leukaemia and organ transplant.
- Children with congenital heart disease.
- Children <2 years old, with no previous exposure.

Prevention and treatment
- There is no effective vaccine against RSV. Studies with RSV immune globulin may prevent severe bronchiolitis in premature infants (<32 weeks) with chronic lung disease.
- Treatment is supportive and may include:
  - gentle suction to remove mucus from upper airways
  - O_2 therapy
  - enteral feeding.

Precautions to reduce risk of nosocomial RSV
- Isolate or cohort patients suspected or known to have RSV.
- Early screening for RSV.
- Wear apron and gloves when in direct contact with infected child or environment.
- Hand hygiene before and after every direct patient contact and after removal of gloves.
- Do not share medical equipment between patients if possible. Decontaminate all equipment between patients with neutral detergent and water.
- Staff: educate in the most effective methods to reduce the risk of transmission.

Further reading
Hall, C.B. (2001). Respiratory syncytial virus. *New England Journal of Medicine*, **345**(15), 1132–3.

Macartney, K.K., Gorelick, M.H., Manning, M.L., Hodinka, R.L., Bell, L.M. (2000). Nosocomial respiratory syncytial virus infections: the cost-effectiveness and cost-benefit of infection control. *Pediatrics*, **106**(3), 520–6.

Madge, P., Paton, J.Y., McColl, J.H., Mackie, P.L. (1992). Prospective controlled study of four infection-control procedures to prevent nosocomial infection with respiratory syncytial virus. *Lancet*, **340**, 1079–83.

Pulse oximetry

The non-invasive peripheral monitoring of oxygen saturation (SpO_2) of haemoglobin in capillary blood. Expressed as a percentage, it provides an adjunct to the assessment and monitoring process and should be used in conjunction with direct observation of the child/young person and the monitoring of other parameters.

Principle

A sensor probe is placed on the finger, toe, foot, ear lobe, or occasionally the nose. Red and infrared-emitting diodes are on one side of the probe and a photodetector is sited on the other. Flashing sequentially, there is a slight pause when both are off in order to enable compensation for ambient light. A microprocessor analyses the changes in light absorption during the arterial pulsatile flow.

Estimation of oxygen saturation is based on the Beer–Lambert law, a combination of two laws describing the effect on light intensity made by an increasing concentration of a transparent substance and an increasing distance travelled through that substance. In effect, there is an inverse absorption relationship with haemoglobin saturation, i.e. very little red light is absorbed by highly saturated haemoglobin, whereas poorly saturated haemoglobin absorbs a larger amount.

Interpretation

Normal range:
• newborn: 85–90%
• thereafter: 95–99%.

Interpretation for assessment should be in conjunction with what is known to be normal for the individual child. There is a suggestion that children living at altitude have developed a physiological adaptation with a lower mean SaO_2.

Practical aspects

Site

Should be warm, with good capillary perfusion, and comfortable for the child. The choice of the sensor will be dependent upon the site as it is essential to ensure that photodetector is opposite the light source. Sensor may be of 'slip on' or 'wrap around' variety; ensure that sensor is not too tight or constrictive as perfusion will inevitably be affected and, consequently, give an aberrant result. Minimize movement of the sensor because this will cause motion artefact.

Care of site

Check site regularly (hourly) and document; sustained pressure will cause tissue compromise and may lead to necrosis. Site should be altered frequently, every 2 hours as a minimum but maybe more frequently depending upon assessment of the probe site.

Neil Bloxham, Plymouth Hospitals NHS Trust

Monitoring process

Signal adequacy is vital for accurate reliable assessment; monitors have signal indicators of either bar or wave form which demonstrate pulse strength at measurement.

Sources of inaccuracy

Cardiac arrhythmia presence as pulse is measured over several sustained beats.

False low readings

May result from:
- methaemoglobinaemia
- presence of dyes, e.g. methylene blue—used for some surgical procedures and in the management of methaemoglobinaemia.

False high readings

May result from carboxyhaemoglobinaemia—oximeter will overestimate saturation.

Further reading

Casey, G. (2001). Oxygen transport and the use of pulse oximetry. *Nursing Standard*, **15**(47), 46–53.
Chandler, T. (2000). Oxygen saturation monitoring. *Paediatric Nursing*, **12**(8), 37–42.
Medical Devices Agency (2001). *Tissue necrosis caused by pulse oximeter probes*. Medicines and Healthcare products Regulatory Agency, London

Nasopharyngeal aspirate

Although nasopharyngeal lavage/washout is the preferred method of obtaining a nasopharyngeal specimen, nasopharyngeal aspirate is seen as a suitable alternative in those children who are coryzal with a large amount of nasal secretion. Although used in the diagnosis of young babies with bronchiolitis, a routine specimen is no longer recommended other than in specific circumstances such as:

• infants under 6 weeks old
• cardiac patients
• chronic lung disease
• born at a gestational age of <32 weeks
• immunodeficiency
• neuromuscular disease
• very severe bronchiolitis.

The specimen should ideally be obtained prior to the infant/child being fed. Before undertaking the collection of a specimen, the nurse/doctor must ensure the room is prepared by ensuring the availability of emergency O_2 and suction at the bedside.

• The NPA collection device should be connected to the suction pack (similar to VYGOB534.10).
• Suction should be set at:
  • neonates: 60–80 mmHg
  • infants: 80–100 mmHg
  • children: 100–120 mmHg.
• The infant/child should be lying down on an examination couch or alternatively sat on a parent's knee with his/her head in an extended position 'sniffing the air'.
• The suction catheter should be passed up the nostril pathway to the pharyngeal space.
• Suction should be applied with the withdrawal of catheter.
• 0.5–1 ml of mucus should ideally be obtained, and this can be processed in up to 5 ml of normal saline through the sample tubing.
• The specimen should be chilled immediately and transported to the laboratory on melting ice; the laboratory should be informed it is on its way to them.

As in all procedures, the preparation of the child and parent is paramount.

Local and national guidelines and procedures should be adhered to in relation to the holding and restraint of babies, children, and young people.

Local and national infection control procedures should be adhered to for both protective garments, such as gloves and aprons, transportation, and labelling of specimens.

Nursing alert

Unlike the bronchiolitis specimen for RSV, a nasopharyngeal aspirate should not be misused in the diagnosis of *Bordetella pertussis*, where the preferred method of specimen collection should be a nasopharyngeal

Maureen Wiltshire and Penelope Aitken. Southampton University Hospitals NHS Trust

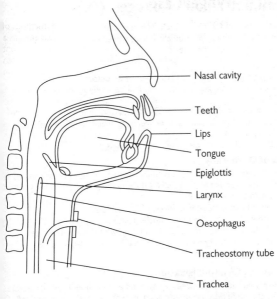

swab. The procedure differs slightly from the NPA in that it requires the insertion of a swab into the nostril parallel to the palate:

- leave the swab in place for a 2–3 s to absorb secretions
- remove and ideally repeat in the second nostril
- for best results, it should be plated and cultured at the bedside.

Further reading

Balfour-Lynn, I.M., Girdhar, D.R., Aitken, C. (1995). Diagnosing respiratory syncytial virus by nasal lavage. *Archives of Disease in Childhood*, **72**, 58–9.

White, H. (1997). Suctioning: a review. *Paediatric Nursing*, **9**(4), 18–20.

Administration of oxygen (O_2)

Administration of O_2 is a common effective practice in paediatric nursing. Uncorrected prolonged hypoxia can lead to cell death and may also lead to brain and/or heart damage.

Remember:
- O_2 is a drug and should be prescribed by a doctor.
- The amount of O_2 given is the fractional inspired O_2 concentration (FiO_2).
- There are risks associated with O_2 therapy and so the lowest possible concentration of O_2 should be delivered to maintain FiO_2 within normal parameters.
- O_2 therapy should be discontinued as soon as possible.

Risks of O_2 therapy
- In neonates it has been well documented that high O_2 concentrations can raise the partial pressure of O_2 (PO_2) above 15 kPa, resulting in retinopathy of prematurity.
- Prolonged exposure to high levels of O_2 in neonates can cause permanent lung damage (e.g. bronchopulmonary dysplasia).
- Too high a concentration of O_2 in children with chronic lung disease can cause respiratory failure. A lower SaO_2 is accepted in these children to prevent this.

Methods of O_2 administration
Different methods of O_2 delivery give different amounts of achievable FiO_2, so this should be taken into account when choosing the method of delivery.

Maximum achievable FiO_2 at 6 l/min of O_2

Method of delivery	Maximum FiO_2
Nasal prongs	50%
Simple mask without reservoir bag	50%
Mask without reservoir bag (partial rebreathing)	70%
Mask with reservoir bag (non-rebreathing)	90%
Head box	95%

Nasal cannula
These are fairly well tolerated by children. Extra humidification is not needed as the nasal passage is warm and moistens the O_2 as it passes through. The main disadvantage is that a flow >6 l/min is uncomfortable and dries the mucosa; however, a flow rate <1 l/min is possible.

Face masks
Not all children tolerate these for long periods. If O_2 is given this way for >4 hours, humidification should be added to prevent drying of the mucosa and to aid loosening of any secretions.

Denise Toplis, Royal Devon and Exeter NHS Foundation Trust

Head box

This method of delivery is only suitable for infants <8 months of age.
Head boxes give effective O_2 delivery, are non-invasive, and the FiO_2 is
monitored easily.

Disadvantages
- Carbon dioxide (CO_2) rebreathing occurs at low flow rates
  (<7 l/min).
- Removal of the box causes a drop in the FiO_2.
- A cold gas supply will cool the infant.
- Carers are unable to cuddle their baby because of the resultant drop
  in FiO_2.
- A warmed humidified O_2 supply is required.

Further reading

Foss, M.A. (1990). Oxygen therapy. *Professional Nurse*, 188–90.
Sims, J. (1996). Making sense of pulse oximetry—oxygen dissociation curve. *Nursing Times*, **92**(1),
    34–5.

Tracheostomy, changing tapes, and cleaning stoma site

Action	Rationale
1. Assess need for procedure	Skin care should be performed to prevent infection and skin breakdown and should be assessed on an individual day-by-day basis
2. Perform tracheostomy care before feeding or at least 2 hours after feeding	Risk of aspiration
3. Explain procedure as appropriate for the child's age and understanding, and parents if present	Enable self-regulatory behaviours. Promote partnership with the family
4. ⚠This should be performed by two people, one of whom should have previous experience	Maintain child's safety
5 Position infant supine, swaddled in a blanket with a small towel roll under the shoulders. Older children may prefer to sit up	Blanket roll → hyperextension → ease of access to site
6. Both wash hands	Prevent cross-infection
7. Prepare equipment: Lyofoam dressing (if required) Dressing pack (gauze and gallipot) Normasol/sterile water Gloves Scissors (if required) New tapes Apron and goggles	Prevent unnecessary delays/interruptions in procedure
8. Open dressing pack and don sterile gloves	Prevent cross-infection. Universal precautions
9. Person 1 holds trach. tube in place throughout procedure	Prevent accidental removal
10. Person 2 cuts old ties or releases Velcro tapes on one side and inserts one side of new tape	Facilitate cleansing of stoma

Marion Aylott, University of Southampton

Contd.

Action	Rationale
11. Divide stoma site visually into four. Work from the centre outwards using four swabs, one for each quarter turn around the stoma. Use gauze soaked in Normasol/sterile water to cleanse site, taking care not to allow any liquid to get under the tube. Apply the same technique with separate pieces of gauze to dry each quadrant	Maintain good skin integrity by removing old secretions while ↓ risk of aspiration. ↓ introducing contamination
12. Feed new tape around neck and secure new ties before removing old ties. Allow one finger space between the neck and ties	Hold tube securely. ↓ risk of pressure injury to skin
13. Monitor skin for signs of infection or skin breakdown	Instigate early treatment of complications. ▶ Remember to check skin under ties, especially back of neck
14. If there is drainage or inflammation, apply an appropriate dressing	Gauze is contraindicated → inhalation of small particles of gauze
15. Praise the child while assessing respiratory status	Trach. care can be emotionally difficult for some. Early detection of complications
16. Record procedure and observations made during and after tube change	Maintain accurate records and provide a point of reference in the event of any queries

Further reading

Wilson, M. (2005). Paediatric tracheostomy. *Paediatric Nursing*, **17**(3), 38–44.

Woodrow, P. (2002). Managing patients with a tracheostomy in acute care. *Nursing Standard*, **16**(44), 39–46.

⊞ www.tracheostomy.info/print.php?sid=9

Tracheostomy: suctioning a tracheostomy

Action	Rationale
1. Assess need for suctioning: to remove mucus, secretions, and to allow for easier breathing	Suctioning should be performed on an individually assessed basis *not* routine to ↓ risk of complications associated with the suctioning procedure
2. Explain procedure in a way appropriate for child's age and understanding, and to parents if present	Enables child self-regulatory behaviours. Promotes partnership with the family
3. Wash hands	↓ risk of cross-infection
4. Prepare equipment:	Prevent delays and interruptions in procedure, which might ↑ safety risks
Connect suction catheter to suction machine tubing (switch on and check it works)	Higher levels of negative pressure can cause mucosal damage. Maintain clean suction tubing
Catheters—correct size (catheter diameter half trach tube size)	
Turn on suction machine and check pressure setting (50–100 mmHg)	
Pour sterile water into suction bowl	
Nebulized 0.9% normal saline pre-suctioning if thick secretions are present	⚠ Saline instillation is never recommended. 0.9% saline nebulizers are preferred if secretions are thick and difficult to aspirate
Gloves	
Tissues	
Waste bag	
5. Don gloves. Remove catheter from paper sheath and hold without touching the part of catheter that is to be inserted.	Keep the catheter clean and ↓ risk of cross-infection
6. Pre–oxygenate as ordered	Extra O_2 may be given to prevent hypoxia
7. Gently insert catheter without applying suction. Suction only length of tube—premeasured suctioning	↓ risk of hypoxia; prevent damage to the tracheal mucosa and carina

Marion Aylott, University of Southampton

Contd.

Action	Rationale
8. Use finger-tip control to apply continuous suction while with drawing the catheter. ▶ Apply suction for as long as necessary to remove secretions without compromising cardiorespiratory safety	Remove secretions from the lumen of the tube; ↓ risk of hypoxia and discomfort
9. For cuffed trach. tubes, it may be necessary to deflate the cuff for suctioning	Prevent pooling of secretions above trach. cuff
10. ▶ Assess child's respiratory status during and following procedure	Early detection of complications; occluded airway and compromised respiration
11. Dispose of suction catheter by wrapping hand around catheter and pulling the glove over the catheter; discard appropriately	↓ risk of cross-infection
12. Draw water from bowl through suction tubing	Clean the tubing and ↓ risk of cross-infection
13. Allow rest and for vital signs and SaO₂ to return to normal. ▶ Repeat suction procedure as needed	Maintain a clear airway while ↓ the risk of hypoxia and discomfort from the suctioning procedure itself
14. ▶ Some children may need extra breaths with an Ambu bag (approximately 3–5 breaths)	For hyperoxygenation, hyperinflation, and hyperventilation of the lungs
15. Congratulate the child	Suctioning can be emotionally difficult for some
16. ▶ Record the colour, amount, consistency, and odour of the secretions	Maintain accurate records and provide a point of reference in the event of any queries

Further reading

Buglas, E. (1999). Tracheostomy care: tracheal suctioning and humidification. *British Journal of Nursing*, **8**(8), 500–4.
Hough, A. (2001). *Physiotherapy in respiratory care. An evidence-based approach to respiratory and cardiac management*, 3rd edn. Nelson Thornes, Cheltenham.
www.tracheostomy.info/print.php?sid=9

Changing a tracheostomy tube

Action	Rationale
1. Assess need to have the procedure	Tracheostomy tubes are changed weekly to monthly, according to manufacturer's instructions
	Prevent mucus build-up (maintain airway patency)
	Prevent infection
2. Change tube before or at least hours after feeding	↓ risk of aspiration
3. ⚠Tube change performed by two people, one of whom has recent previous experience	Maintain safety
4. Explain procedure to child and parents as appropriate	Enables self-regulatory behaviours. Promotes partnership with the family
5. Prepare equipment: Same size tube and tube a half size smaller Ties Towel roll K-Y- jelly Tracheal dilators Suction catheters and Yankeur sucker Scissors Gloves, apron, goggles	Prevent delays/interruptions in procedure; ↓ physiological and psycho-emotional risks
6. Position infant supine, swaddled with towel roll under shoulders. Older children may prefer to sit up	Towel roll → hyperextension → access to site
7. Wash hands. Don gloves, apron, and goggles	Prevent cross-infection. Universal precautions
8. Open dressing pack and set out equipment as for aseptic dressing technique	Prevent cross-infection
9. Inspect new tube for cracks and flexibility before use, especially if reusable. For cuff tubes, inflate cuff to check function. Avoid touching part of the tube that is inserted into the trachea	↓ risk of introducing infection and ↓ risk to child through faulty equipment
10. Thread new tie through one end of new tube	↓ risk of accidental dislodgement

Marion Aylott, University of Southampton

Contd.

Action	Rationale
11. Insert obturator into new tube (if required); ensure it slides in and out easily	Obturator helps to guide tube, and rounded tip adds protection to stoma during insertion
12. Suction tube prior to procedure	Clear airway and prevent obstruction of stoma as old tube is removed
13. One person cuts/removes old ties while one person holds tube in place	When ties are insecure, coughing can dislodge the tube
14. One person gently removes old tube following angle of the tube, an upward, outward arc, and immediately inserts the new tube in a smooth, curving motion, directing the tip of tube towards the back of the neck in a downward, inward arc	⚠ Never force tube.
If tube *does not* go in easily, extend neck, insert dilators, and attempt to re-pass tube	Gain ↑ access to stoma
If unsuccessful: attempt to pass tube a half size smaller	
If unsuccessful, provide respiratory support	Maintain respiratory stability until further assistance arrives
15. Once *in situ*, remove the obturator (if used) immediately while one other person holds tube securely	Child cannot breathe with obturator in place. Changing the tube will cause child to cough
16. Assess respiratory status	Early detection of complications → appropriate intervention
17. Allow child to sit up and congratulate	Procedure can be emotionally difficult for some
18. Record procedure and observations made	Maintain accurate records; provides a point of reference in the event of any queries

Further reading

Serra, A. (2000). Tracheostomy care. *Nursing Standard*, **14**(42), 45–55.

Wilson, M. (2005). Paediatric tracheostomy. *Paediatric Nursing*, **17**(3), 38–44.

Woodrow, P. (2002). Managing patients with a tracheostomy in acute care. *Nursing Standard*, **16**(44), 39–46.

Oropharyngeal and nasopharyngeal suctioning

Children and infants normally clear their airways by means of coughing, sneezing, and nose blowing. At times, due to infection or disease, overproduction of mucus and secretions occurs and these natural protective mechanisms may be ineffective. In some childhood conditions and following surgery (and/or anaesthesia), the coordination of the cough-and-gag reflex may be compromised; therefore suction may be required to maintain airway patency.

Oropharyngeal suction is the introduction of a fine catheter into the mouth, pharynx, and trachea via an airway adjunct and application of suction to remove secretions.

Nasopharyngeal suction is the introduction of a fine catheter into the nose, pharynx, and trachea, either directly through the nose or via an airway adjunct, and application of suction to remove secretions.

Indications

Suctioning may be required if the child demonstrates any of the following symptoms *and* their natural mechanisms are insufficient to maintain a clear airway:
- visible frothing or bubbling from the nose or mouth
- audible secretions—rattling or bubbling sounds can be heard with or without a stethoscope
- decreased SaO_2
- change in skin colour—redness, pallor, or cyanosis
- altered chest movements
- raised heart rate and raised respiration rate
- nasal flaring
- increased use of accessory muscles
- deteriorating arterial blood gases
- suspected aspiration.

Suction may be necessary if a specimen is required to aid diagnosis.

Contraindications

- Suction should *not* be performed on a child who is awake, alert, neurologically normal, over the age of 1 year, able to cough and swallow secretions, and not in severe respiratory distress.
- Contraindication for suctioning is normally with stridor and/or clotting disorders. Nasopharyngeal suctioning is normally contraindicated in children with CSF leakage, severe intranasal disease or trauma, and suspected or proven basal skull fracture.
- Caution is required in children with pulmonary oedema, severe bronchospasm, and/or recent lung, tracheal, or oesophageal surgery and raised ICP.

Pauline Donaldson and Louise Holliday, Royal Aberdeen Children's Hospital

Risks

When performing oropharyngeal/nasopharyngeal suctioning, potential risks include:
- trauma to the mucosa of the upper and lower airways
- atelectasis (collapse of the alveoli)
- vaso-vagal nerve stimulation (caused by the catheter touching the tracheal mucosa or hypoxia), which could lead to:
  - bradycardia
  - tachycardia
  - arrhythmias
  - hypotension
  - hypertension
  - cardiac arrest
- hypoxaemia
- laryngospasm caused by the larynx being touched
- infection.

Because of these, suctioning should not be performed routinely, but should only be performed when it is clinically indicated.

Documentation

In the hospital setting, document the procedure on a fluid-balance chart to comment on secretion type, volume, and colour

Codes	Secretions
1	Small
2	Moderate
3	Large
4	Copious
C	Clear
B	Bloody
W	White
G	Green

Further reading

Huband, S., Trigg, E. (2000). *Practices in children's nursing, Guidelines for hospital and community*, pp. 273–6. Churchill Livingstone, Edinburgh.

Macmillan, C. (1995). Nasopharyngeal suction study reveals knowledge deficit. *Nursing Times*, **91**(50), 28–30.

Moore, T. (2003). Suctioning techniques for the removal of respiratory secretions. *Nursing Standard*, **18**(9), 47–53.

Performing nasopharyngeal/ oropharyngeal suction in children

Equipment required	Suction unit and tubing
	O$_2$ unit, tubing, and mask (if required)
	Sterile suction catheters (size appropriate)
	Non-sterile disposable gloves (sterile if obtaining a laboratory specimen)
	Plastic apron
	Clean small plastic bowl with fresh tap water
	Goggles and face masks or visors (if there are copious secretions or risk of cross-infections)
	Stethoscope (if required)
Procedure	1. Wash your hands and put on an apron
	2. Explain procedure to parent/carer and child. Allow time for questions and ensure consent is obtained and documented. In an emergency situation, consent may not be obtainable
	3. Pre-oxygenation should be considered for children who are receiving O$_2$. If the child is able to cooperate, ask him/her to take a couple of deep breaths
	4. The appropriate catheter size must be determined. Sizes are suggested below:

Infant (0–2 years)	5–6 FG
Toddler (2–5 years)	6–8 FG
Younger child (5–10 years)	8 FG
Older children (over 10 years)	8–10 FG

5. Turn on suction machine and ensure that applied suction pressures are 60–120 mmHg/8–16 kPa. For infants, the pressure should be no higher than 100 mmHg/13 kPa

6. Position child on his/her side, or with his/her head to one side, to reduce the risk of aspiration. Unless complete patient cooperation can be assured, an assistant will be required. To prevent the infant wriggling, wrap him/her in a blanket or towel, to include both arms. Older children may prefer to sit in an upright position; use distraction or relaxation therapy

7. Wash your hands. Put on goggles and mask or visor, where appropriate. Put on non-sterile disposable gloves

8. If obtaining a specimen put on sterile gloves

9. Attach the suction tubing to the catheter

Pauline Donaldson and Louise Holliday, Royal Aberdeen Children's Hospital

Contd.

Equipment required	Suction unit and tubing
	10. For nasopharyngeal suctioning, premeasure the catheter from nose to suprasternal notch (top of the rib cage). For oropharyngeal suctioning, premeasure from mouth to suprasternal notch. Remove the catheter from its sleeve, keeping it uncontaminated
	11. Gently introduce the catheter into the child's mouth (via airway adjunct) or nose (this may or may not be via an airway adjunct), not yet applying suction. If resistance is met in the nose, withdraw the catheter and attempt a second pass. If resistance is still met, attempt the other nostril and/or consider trying a smaller catheter
	12. Once the catheter is passed to the premeasured length, apply suction pressure. Avoid rotating the catheter when withdrawing because this can cause trauma
	13. The time from the catheter entering the child's mouth or nose to its removal should be between 10 s and 15 s
	14. Observe the child's colour at all times during the procedure. In children who are being monitored, observe for a decrease in SaO_2 or heart rate
	15. Wrap the catheter around your gloved hand, and then pull the glove back over soiled catheter and discard in a clinical waste bin
	16. Re-assess the child's condition and recommence O_2 therapy if required
	17. If further suction is required, repeat the procedure with a new glove and catheter
	18. The patient should be allowed a period of rest before repeat suctioning
	19. Flush the suction tubing with tap water
	20. Dispose of all waste and wash hands
	21. Wash out bowl with multi-purpose detergent and water, and dry it
	22. Ensure emotional and physical comfort is provided for the child and family

Listening to chests

Auscultation is just one component of a respiratory assessment and i only useful when combined with a patient's history. It is important to be systematic, listening first for the types of breaths sounds and then for any added sounds. A comparison should always be made between the two sides of the chest, auscultating anteriorly and posteriorly where possible.

Anatomy

The right lung comprises three lobes, which are divided by two fissures. The horizontal/minor fissure:

- separates the upper lobe from middle lobe.
- runs horizontally from the fourth intercostal space at the sternal edge to the mid-axillary line.

The oblique/major fissure:

- separates the upper and middle lobes from the lower lobe.
- runs from the spinous process of the second thoracic vertebra around the chest to the sixth costochondral junction anteriorly.

The left lung comprises two lobes, which are divided by one fissure. The oblique/major fissure:

- separates the upper lobe (which incorporates the lingular region) from the lower lobe.
- runs from the spinous process of the second thoracic vertebra around the chest to the sixth costochondral junction anteriorly.

Further reading

Parker, S., Middleton, P.G. (1993). Assessment. In *Physiotherapy for respiratory and cardiac problems*, (ed. B.A. Webber and J.A. Pryor), pp. 17–19. Churchill Livingstone, Edinburgh.

Catherine Thornton, Central Manchester and Manchester Children's University Hospitals NHS Trust

Breath sounds

Sound	Description	Differential diagnosis
Vesicular/normal		
Normally heard over all lung regions	Soft, muffled, and continuous sound	*Quiet:* atelectasis, sputum retention, and hyperinflation
Quieter basally	Inspiration louder than expiration	*Absent:* pleural effusion, pneumothorax, severe asthma
	Expiration longer than inspiration	
Bronchial		
Normally heard over the trachea and larynx	Hollow, tubular sound	Consolidation indicated if heard over lung fields
	Equal intensity on inspiration and expiration	
	Pause between inspiration and expiration	

Added sounds

Sound	Description	Cause	Differential diagnosis
Fine crackles	High frequency, late inspiratory bubbling sound	Opening of alveoli/ respiratory bronchioles; airflow past sputum/fluid	Pulmonary oedema, atelectasis, sputum retention, and bronchiolitis
Coarse crackles	Low frequency, early inspiratory bubbling sound	Opening of bronchioles; airflow past sputum/fluid	Sputum retention, bronchitis
Monophonic wheeze	Single musical sound; pitch increases with narrowing	Single airway obstruction	Foreign body aspiration or tumour
Polyphonic wheeze	Multiple musical sounds; pitch increases with narrowing	Widespread airway obstructions	Bronchospasm, sputum retention, inflammation, or bronchiolitis
Pleural rub	Coarse rubbing/creaking	Infected/inflamed pleura	Pleuritis, tuberculosis, or chest rain
Stridor	High-pitched continuous wheeze	Airflow obstruction at tracheal level	Croup/epiglottitis or foreign body aspiration

Chest physiotherapy

Chest physiotherapy is performed following a thorough respiratory history and assessment performed by a physiotherapist. It can be useful for modification of an ineffective/altered pattern of breathing, to optimize ventilation–perfusion, and to facilitate removal of secretions.

Indications

Sputum retention and/or increased work of breathing due to:
- intubation and ventilation
- pneumonia (when in the productive phase)
- post-operative thoracic/abdominal surgery
- underlying chronic lung disease (e.g. cystic fibrosis, bronchiectasis, or primary ciliary dyskinesia)
- lobar/lung collapse (atelectasis) resulting from mucus plugging
- neuromuscular weakness

Precautions

A physiotherapist must assess whether treatment is indicated for:
- non-productive pneumonia
- pleural effusion
- asthma (when sputum retention, not bronchospasm, is the main problem)
- lung abscess
- tuberculosis
- empyema
- abnormal blood clotting values

Contraindications

- Pulmonary oedema (with absence of sputum retention)
- Severe bronchospasm
- Frank haemoptysis
- Reduced respiratory effort as a result of uncontrolled pain
- Undrained pneumothorax
- Bronchial tumour

Adjuncts

The use of humidification and mucolytics (where indicated) can also facilitate secretion clearance.

Further reading

Prasad, S.A., Hussey, J. (1994). Chest physiotherapy techniques and adjuncts to chest physiotherapy. In *Paediatric respiratory care—a guide for physiotherapists and health professionals* (ed. S.A. Prasad, I. Hussey), pp. 67–105. Chapman & Hall, London.

Hough, A. (1996). Physiotherapy for children and infants. In *Physiotherapy in respiratory care—a problem-solving approach to respiratory and cardiac management* (ed. A. Hough), pp. 286–302. Chapman & Hall, London.

Nicola Brogan, Central Manchester and Manchester Children's University Hospitals NHS Trust

Treatment techniques

Technique	Rationale
Positioning	To utilize gravity to ease work of breathing and optimize ventilation/perfusion
Postural drainage	To utilize gravity to aid drainage of secretions
Manual techniques (percussion, vibrations, and shakes)	To loosen and mobilize secretions
Breathing techniques (active cycle of breathing technique, autogenic drainage, blowing activities, e.g. bubbles and incentive spirometers)	To utilize collateral ventilation channels to mobilize secretions and encourage thoracic expansion
Positive-pressure techniques (intermittent positive pressure, breathing, manual hyperinflation, positive expiratory pressure, and oscillatory mucus clearance devices)	To utilize collateral ventilation channels to mobilize secretions and can facilitate thoracic expansion
Mechanical inexsufflation (cough machine)	To mobilize secretions and facilitate expectoration in those with an ineffective cough due to muscular weakness

Chest drain

General principle

Chest drains are inserted into the pleural cavity through an intercostal space under sedation, with a local or general anaesthetic, by an experienced surgical registrar or consultant.

- Chest X-ray confirms correct positioning.
- Treatment for thoracic trauma, surgery, and infection.
- Designed to remove air or fluid safely, preventing their reintroduction and facilitating lung expansion.

Care of chest drain *in situ*

Action	Rationale
The following equipment must always be at the bedside:	To take prompt action if pneumothorax develops and give routine care
Non-toothed clamps x 2	
Spare underwater seal chest drain bottle and tubing	
Sterile water	
Sterile gloves	
Alcohol swabs	
Sterile gauze swabs/small dressing pack	
Sterile clear occlusive dressing	
Sterile saline solution	
1. Explain procedures to child and carer	Gain cooperation and minimize distress
2. Maintain observation for signs/symptoms of pneumothorax; inform medical staff immediately of concerns	Early detection of complications
3. Observe entry site for redness, leakage, swelling, and bleeding. Observe tubing for visible side holes	To detect infection/haemorrhage. Call doctor immediately
4. Re-dress site aseptically with clear occlusive dressing	To minimize infection risk and allow wound observation
5. Tape drainage tube in line with patient's ribs	More comfortable
6. Ensure water level maintained above minimum level and that tube from patient is kept beneath water level	To maintain water seal
7. Maintain correct positioning. Bottle must remain lower than insertion site	Correct placement and patency indicated by bubbling of air, drainage of fluid, and swinging movement in drainage tubing

Paula Dawson, Nottingham University Hospitals NHS Trust

Contd.

Action	Rationale
	Fluid drawn away from pleural cavity by gravity; siphoning effect prevents back-flow into pleural cavity
	Fluid will stop swinging when lung is reinflated or tubing is blocked
8. If tubing disconnects or bottle breaks, apply clamps to tubing immediately. Reconnect tubing to new sterile bottle	To prevent air from entering pleural cavity and to reduce risk of infection
9. Tubing should be free from kinks	Dependent loops have negative effect on air and fluid drainage.
10. Position patient in semi-sitting position, towards chest-drain side	To promote drainage
11. Record amount and colour of drainage; mark drainage level on bottle with tape	To monitor drainage
12. Change bottle as necessary (no more than three-quarters full) using aseptic technique	To minimize infection risk; pressure will rise and affect drainage if bottle is too full
13. Suction pressure may be applied. Low flow meter or portable suction unit used. Pressure set according to written medical instructions	To assist removal of fluid/air from the pleural cavity
14. Encourage mobility; refer to physiotherapist	To promote optimum drainage and ventilation
15. Give regular analgesia	To minimize distress, discomfort, and any reluctance to breathe or mobilize

Removal of chest drain	
1. The drain may be clamped for a trial period to simulate removal	To aid decision to remove
2. Give prescribed analgesia	To alleviate discomfort
3. Position patient sitting up	To facilitate removal
4. Ask child (if able) to hold his breath while doctor removes the drain. Apply firm pressure, followed by sterile dressing	To prevent air re-entering pleural space before wound is sealed
5. Send tip of drain for culture and antibiotic sensitivity	To detect presence of pathogens

Further reading

Allibone, L. (2003). Nursing management of chest drains. *Nursing Standard*, **17**(22), 45–54.
Avery, S. (2000). Insertion and management of chest drains *NT Plus*, **96**(37), 3–6.

Using a humidifier

Why humidify?

Inhaled air is normally warmed and humidified by the nose and upper respiratory tract. Warming a gas increases its capacity to hold vapour.

Typical humidity values

	Medical gases	Typical room air	Lungs
Temperature	15°C	20°C	37°C
Relative humidity	2%	50%	100%
Absolute humidity (optimal environment)	0.3 mg/l	9 mg/l	44 mg/l

Effects of dry inhaled O_2

Reduced humidity in inspired air → heat and moisture being taken from mucociliary epithelium → mucosal drying → cilial dysfunction → accumulation of secretions → increased infection risk → retained secretions → blockage of small airways → atelectasis and reduced functional residual capacity → impaired gaseous exchange (ventilation–perfusion mismatch) → reduced oxygenation.

Humidity helps to maintain normal lung defence mechanisms by encouraging mucociliary transport.

Indications for humidification

- If more than 2 l (28%) O_2 is used for more than 5 hours
- Thick retained secretions
- When the upper respiratory tract is bypassed by an endotracheal tube or tracheostomy
- Babies with respiratory problems, because their immature respiratory system and smaller airways are functionally inefficient
- Dehydration
- Direct trauma to the respiratory system, e.g. burns or smoke inhalation
- Reduced mucociliary clearance, e.g. induced by anaesthetic or sedation

Types of humidification

- The heated passover humidifier is the most efficient, because the particle size/vapour is smaller than in cold systems and saline nebulizers. Increased particle size allows for more pathogens to be carried, therefore increasing infection risk.
- Cold humidity may be sufficient for those who are able maintain their body temperature; however, it cannot achieve atmospheric humidity. A quattro system (Venturi) should be used with bottled sodium chloride and elephant tubing; it should be avoided in patients who have hyper-reactive airways, e.g. asthmatics. There is no evidence for using bubble-through humidity with fine-bore tubing.

Rachael Hufton, Central Manchester and Manchester Children's University Hospitals NHS Trust

Setting up heated humidity

- Fit the chamber and secure the unit, placing it below the level of the bed.
- Hang the water bag 50 cm away from the chamber.
- Connect the circuit, temperature probes, and heater wire.
- Turn on the humidifier; ensure that the correct mode and temperature are used; allow 20–30 min to achieve temperature (check the humidifier manual).
- Ensure that the circuit is changed every 7 days.
- If there is condensation in the circuit, drain back to chamber.
- If the patient complains of the circuit being hot, increase the circuit length and check the temperature.
- If the patient is ventilated, switch off the humidifier on disconnection of tubing, to avoid overheating and potential burns.

Further reading

Williams, R., Rankin, N., Smith, T., Galler, D., Seakins, P. (1996). Relationship between humidity and temperature of inspired gas and the function of the airway mucosa. *Critical Care Medicine*, **24**(11), 1920–9.

Peak-flow monitoring (new EU device)

The device
Hand-held peak-expiratory-flow meters (PFMs) assess pulmonary function and aid self-management of asthma.

Normal range

Low range

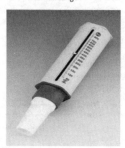
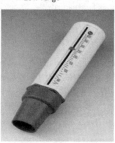

Monitoring peak flow
- Instruct the child to follow these steps:
  - make sure the device's arrow reads zero or is at base level
  - stand up (unless there is a physical disability)
  - take as deep a breath as possible
  - place the meter in your mouth, and close your lips around the mouthpiece
  - blow out as hard and as fast as possible (1–2 s)
  - do not cough or block the mouthpiece with your tongue.
- Write down the value obtained.
- Repeat the process twice more, and record the highest of the three values on a peak-flow chart.

New PFMs have been available from 1 September 2004. These new meters are manufactured to the new European standard (EN 13826) and may read differently from the traditional Wright PFMs that are being phased out.

Why use a new device?
- The Wright scale is non-linear and can over-read in the mid-range by up to 30%. PFMs with this scale have been used for the diagnosis and management of asthma in the UK and Europe since 1959.
- The new standard is based on absolute flow.
- The new device should produce peak-flow measurements similar to those obtained by conventional spirometry and a more accurate assessment of peak flow across the entire measurement range.

Gilli Lewis, Queen's University Belfast

When monitoring peak expiratory flow

- Remember this change may cause confusion in the interpretation of results by all users, particularly for patients who have their asthma treated solely on the basis of peak-flow measurement.
- Do not interchange Wright and EU PFM devices.
- Reassess patients' personal best peak flows and recalculate action levels for personalized asthma action plans when issuing a new EN 13826 PFM. Record EN 13826 on the action plan for reference.
- Note that current predictive values are based on the Wright scale and should not be used with the new EN 13826 PFMs. New revised predictions will become available.
- EN 13826 specifies one measurement range from 60 to 800 l/min, and is suitable for all users. However, low-range models are also available.
- PFMs do not need to be changed immediately; a gradual replacement programme over 12 months is recommended.
- New PFMs are labelled 'EN 13826' or 'EU scale'.

Further reading

British Thoracic Society (2004). *British Guideline on the Management of Asthma*, revised edn. www.brit-thoracic.org.uk/sign/index.htm

Miller, M.R. (2004). Peak expiratory flow meter scale changes; implications for patients and health professionals. *Airways Journal*, **2**(2), 80–2. www.airwaysextra.com

www.peakflow.com/top_nav/meter/index.html (accessed 2 August 2005).

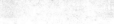

Cardiovascular problems

Anatomy and physiology of the circulatory system

The circulatory system is made up of a complex network of veins arteries, and capillaries:

- veins: thin-walled tubes carrying deoxygenated blood
- arteries: thick-walled, flexible tubes carrying oxygenated blood; the arteries divide into smaller branches known as capillaries.

At the core of the system is the heart. It is made up of three layers:

- myocardium: cardiac muscle that forms the wall of the heart
- endocardium: thin membrane that lines the chambers
- pericardium: the outer covering of the heart.

Within the heart there is a sophisticated mechanical structure that enables it to simultaneously collect and dispatch blood to all regions of the body. It consists of four chambers:

- the filling chambers—the atria
- the pumping chambers—the ventricles.

There are also four one-way valves:

- tricuspid valve, situated between the right atrium and right ventricle
- pulmonary valve, situated between the right ventricle and main pulmonary artery
- mitral valve, situated between the left atrium and left ventricle
- aortic valve, situated between the left ventricle and aorta.

A thick wall called the septum divides the left and right sides of the heart.

The right side of the heart has the job of collecting the deoxygenated blood from the body and delivering it to the lungs. Blood reaches the right atrium from the superior and inferior vena cavae. Once the tricuspid valve opens, the blood can flow into the right ventricle. When heart contraction occurs, the blood is ejected through the pulmonary valve into the main pulmonary artery. Once in the artery, the blood then flows into the lungs via the right and left pulmonary artery branches. Once it is in the lungs, the blood becomes oxygenated and flows back to the left side of the heart.

Blood reaches the left atrium via the pulmonary veins. Once in the atrium, the mitral valve opens, allowing it to pass into the left ventricle. At the point of contraction, the aortic valve opens, enabling the oxygenated blood to flow through the aorta to the rest of the body.

Further reading

Watson, R. (2000). *Anatomy and physiology for nurses.* Baillière Tindall, London.
☒ www.jdaross.cwc.net/heart.htm

Sarah Baker, Royal Devon and Exeter NHS Foundation Trust

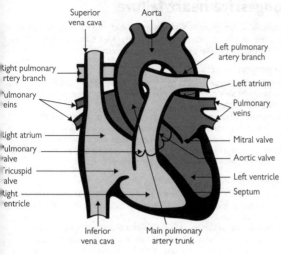

The normal heart

Congestive heart failure

Congestive heart failure is a condition in which the heart cannot effectively meet the metabolic demands of the body. Heart failure often occurs in children with congenital or acquired heart defects.

Congenital defects

- Various congenital defects result in blood being shunted from the left to the right side of the heart and then to the lungs again, instead of going out to the body.
- Increased pulmonary blood volume increases pressure and thus increases the work of the myocardium.
- The increased blood flow to the lungs gives rise to pulmonary arterial congestion, with subsequent pulmonary oedema and eventual systemic venous congestion and resulting generalized oedema.

Acquired defects

- Acquired heart conditions, e.g. valvular or endocardial damage caused by rheumatic fever or bacterial endocarditis, affect the pumping ability of the heart.
- If the left side of the heart fails to pump blood effectively into the arterial systemic system, there will be backlogging into the pulmonary venous system, which is eventually referred back to arterial system, again giving rise to pulmonary oedema and systemic venous congestion.

Signs and symptoms of congestive heart failure

- Feeding difficulties
- Sweating while feeding
- Breathless: tachypnoea
- Increased respiratory rate
- Increased respiratory effort: costal and subcostal recession
- Cough and congestion in lungs
- Hypoxaemia: SaO_2 decreased
- Increased heart rate
- Cyanosis of lips, nail beds, and around mouth
- Pallor
- Mottled/cold peripheries
- Limited activity
- Easily fatigued

Long-term effects

- Growth impairment
- Development delay
- Polycythaemia: as the body compensates to increase O_2-carrying capacity of blood

Confirmation of diagnosis

- History
- Assessment
- Clinical observations
- Clinical examination
- Chest X-ray
- Electrocardiogram (ECG)
- Echocardiogram
- Cardiac catheterization

Phil Morrow, Queen's University Belfast

Care of the child with congestive heart failure

Goals
- To improve cardiac output
- Decrease cardiac demands
- Improve respiratory function
- Maintain adequate nutritional status
- Reduce fluid excess
- Support and educate the child and family

Nursing care
- Continually assess and monitor the child's condition.
- Administer the following drugs safely, and monitor their effects and unwanted effects:
  - Digoxin—cardiac glycoside, slows and strengthens heart
  - ACE inhibitors—captopril, dilates blood vessels making it easier for the heart to pump blood forward
  - Sildenafil—vasodilation
  - Diuretics: furosemide, removes excess fluid from body, thus decreasing oedema and fluid retention; side effect is hypokalaemia
  - spironolactone—helps retain potassium.
- To improve respiratory function:
  - ensure availability of suction and O_2
  - assess degree of respiratory distress and monitor SaO_2
  - maintain the child's position to encourage lung expansion and rest
  - ensure the child wears loose clothing
  - provide periods of uninterrupted rest—cluster care.
- To maintain nutritional status:
  - the child has a high metabolic rate and therefore requires higher calorie intake
  - collaborate with dietitian and doctor to ascertain daily fluid intake and calorie requirements
  - give small frequent feeds and monitor intake
  - NG feeding may be necessary
  - monitor bladder and bowel function
  - monitor and record fluid intake and output.
- To maintain hygiene:
  - because of the high metabolic rate, the infant or child will be prone to sweating and will present with higher temperatures
  - attention to hygiene of skin and mucous membranes is vital to prevent breakdown of skin which will predispose the infant or child to infection
  - daily bed bath and inspection of skin folds and pressure areas
  - frequent oral hygiene
  - clean loose clothing.

Phil Morrow, Queen's University Belfast

Prevention of infection:
- all care interventions must adhere to the policy of infection control
- the child with a cardiac condition is prone to bacterial endocarditis—this requires attention to monitoring for signs of infection and response to antibiotic therapy; specific health education is necessary, particularly to situations that potentially predispose the infant or child to infection; this is reflected in information and advice given in relation to dental care

Family support:
- the care you give must reflect the ethos of family-centred care
- provide information about all care, treatment, or interventions, to obtain informed consent
- use visual aids to increase understanding of condition
- give information about support agencies, e.g. British Heart Foundation
- early planning for discharge, which requires ongoing teaching and education
- reference and referral to cardiac liaison nurse.

Further reading

Glasper, E.A., Richardson, J. (2005). *A textbook of chidren's nursing*. Elsevier, London.
British Heart Foundation. ⊞ www.bhf.org.uk

Shock

Shock results from an acute failure of circulatory function. Inadequate amounts of nutrients, especially O_2, are delivered to the body tissue and there is inadequate removal of tissue waste products. The most common causes of shock in the paediatric patient are hypovolaemia from any cause, septicaemia, and the effects of trauma.[1]

Shock can develop rapidly in children because the loss of relatively small amounts of fluid can compromise a high percentage of their intravascular volume.[2]

Shock may be described as either compensated or uncompensated:
- Compensated shock: vital organ function is maintained by intrinsic mechanisms, and the child's ability to compensate is effective.[1] Early signs are subtle and include:
  - irritability, agitation, or confusion
  - increased heart rate
  - decreased capillary return
  - normal blood pressure
  - narrowing pulse pressure
  - thirst
  - pallor
  - decreased urinary output.
- Uncompensated shock: the compensatory mechanisms start to fail and the circulatory system is no longer efficient.[1] The signs may include:
  - tachypnoea
  - tachycardia
  - falling blood pressure
  - moderate metabolic acidosis
  - oliguria
  - very slow capillary return
  - decreased skin turgor
  - decreased cerebral state.

There are many types of shock, four of which will be discussed here:
- cardiogenic shock
- septic shock
- hypovolaemic shock
- distributive shock.

Cardiogenic shock
Can be defined as shock resulting from a decline in cardiac output secondary to serious heart disease. Possible causes:
- arrhythmias
- cardiomyopathy
- heart failure
- myocardial infarction
- myocardial contusion
- valvular disease.

Stefan Cash, University of Central England Birmingham

Septic shock

Septic shock is associated with sepsis, which is associated with the presence of pathogenic organisms in the blood or tissue. Possible causes:
  septicaemia
  abdominal infection/pelvic infection following trauma or surgery.

Hypovolaemic shock

This is caused by a reduction in the volume of blood. Possible causes:
  haemorrhage
  dehydration
  vomiting
  diarrhoea
  ketoacidosis
  ascites
  pancreatitis
  intestinal obstruction
  burns
  peritonitis
  volvulus.

Distributive shock

A profound decrease in systemic vascular tone. The most common etiology of distributive shock is sepsis due to infection. Possible causes:
  anaphylaxis
  spinal chord injury/shock
  head injury
  early stages of sepsis
  drug intoxication.

Further reading

Advanced Life Support Group (2001). The child in shock. In *Advanced paediatric life support*, pp. 99–111. BMJ, London.
Morton, R. Phillips, B. (1994). Signs of early circulatory failure. In *Accidents and emergencies in children*, p. 37. Oxford University Press, Oxford.

Cardiovascular status

This is the clinical picture arising from assessment of the cardiovascular system. The assessment gives an indication of the current performance of the system, how efficiently the heart is working, and the effect that this is having on other major organs/systems, such as the respiratory system, the neurological system, and the renal system. The cardiovascular system includes the heart and blood vessels.

How is it assessed?

In order to assess the cardiovascular system, the practitioner needs to have a comprehensive understanding of the normal anatomy and physiology of the child and young person.

History

A complete history should be taken first, because this will enable the practitioner to undertake a more guided physical assessment. It should include questions about the mother's pregnancy, the birth, family history, current medications, and daily activities, including feeding.

Chief concerns emerging from the history include maternal infections during pregnancy, difficult resuscitation at birth, family history of congenital heart disease, fatigue, poor feeding, poor weight gain, failure to thrive, frequent respiratory infections, and cyanosis.

Physical assessment

General appearance
- Age-appropriate behaviour
- Immediate signs of cardiovascular insufficiency
  - lethargy
  - tachypnoea
  - abnormal posture
  - skin colour
  - small for age

Inspection
- Colour
  - polycythaemia
  - cyanosis
  - duskiness
- Clubbing
- Jugular venous pressure
- Precordial activity
  - prominence of left side of chest: indicating levocardia
  - flat chest: accentuating heart sounds

Palpation
- Peripheral and central pulses
  - grading of pulses
- Blood pressure in all four limbs to rule out aortic coarctation
- Capillary refill time, should be <2 s
- Liver edge, may be enlarged

Kerry Cook, Coventry University

Precordial activity
- palpable cardiac activity, particularly in flat chests

Auscultation
Heart sounds
Added sounds/murmurs
Bruits

Other investigations
ECG
Echocardiography
Radiography
MRI
CT
Exercise testing
Laboratory tests

Further reading

Archer, N., Burch, M. (1998). *Paediatric cardiology. An introduction.* Chapman & Hall, London.

Cook, K., Montgomery, H. (2005). Assessment. In *Practices in children's nursing*, 2nd edn, (ed. T. Mohammed, E. Trigg), Routledge, London .

Cardiac-related Diagnostic Methods. Physical Exam, Process, Questions, and Answers (revised October 2004). ▣ www.cincinnatichildrens.org/health/heart-encyclopedia/diagnostic/exam.htm

ECG traces

An ECG trace is a graphic representation of the electrical activity of the heart throughout the cardiac cycle. Electrodes are placed in standard positions on the surface of the skin and sense low-voltage electrical activity, which is then amplified by the ECG machine. The views may be three-lead (three electrode positions) or 12-lead (12 electrode positions); each electrode will depict a different part of the heart. The trace can be achieved either as a printed record or on a cardiac monitor screen. Although an ECG provides important information, the practitioner should always consider the clinical picture first.

The waveform

This refers to any movement away from a baseline (or straight line) and is represented either as a positive (above the baseline) or negative (below the baseline) deflection. One small square on ECG paper is equivalent to 0.04 s and one large square is equivalent to 0.20 s.

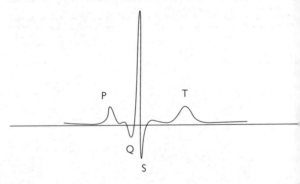

The normal PQRST complex. Reproduced with kind permission by cardioweb.co.uk

Kerry Cook, Coventry University

The PQRST wave represents a full cardiac cycle.

The P wave depicts the electrical impulse that has been fired by the sino-atrial node; this spreads out across the two atria. Here, depolarization of the left and right atria takes place, demonstrated by a positive deflection—a smooth curve above the baseline, which takes about 0.08 s in infants and 0.10 s in adults.

The PR interval is the time that it takes the electrical impulse to pass across both atria, through the internodal pathways towards the ventricles. This is actually the distance from the beginning of the P wave to the beginning of the QRS complex. The lower limits of normal start at 0.08 s in infants to 0.12 s in adults; the upper limit in adults is 0.20 s.

The QRS wave represents the conduction of the electrical impulse from the bundle of His through the ventricular muscle. The Q wave is a downward deflection, followed by the ventricular depolarization, which causes an upward deflection above the baseline (the R wave) and then another downward deflection (the S wave). The normal QRS complex ranges from 0.07 s in infants to <0.12 s in adults.

The ST segment depicts the beginning of ventricular repolarization; and is normally consistent with the baseline, although it may be altered in situations such as hyperkalaemia, digoxin administration, or myocardial damage in children.

The T wave is a positive deflection, signifying ventricular repolarization: at this point there is no associated ventricular muscle activity. This is the resting phase of the cardiac cycle.

Further reading

Gardner, J. (2005). *The ECG. What does it tell?* 2nd edn. Nelson Thornes, Cheltenham.
Mehta, C., Dhillon, R. (2004). Understanding paediatric ECGs. *Current Paediatrics*, **14**, 229–36.
www.cardioweb.co.uk/ecg/ecgpage54.asp

Gastrointestinal problems

Anatomy and physiology of the gastrointestinal system

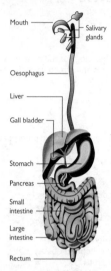

Functions of the gastrointestinal tract
- To provide the body with water, electrolytes, and nutrients.
- To secrete enzymes: exocrine and endocrine.
- To act as a barrier to organisms: forms part of the immunological system.

Structure
The gastrointestinal tract is fully formed by 24 weeks' gestation. The liver is immature at birth and continues to develop into adulthood.

Oesophagus
- Thin-walled tube joining pharynx to stomach.
- A sphincter at each end.
- Distal sphincter incompetent in some young babies, causing oesophageal reflux.

Stomach
- Reservoir for food.
- Approximate capacity of 30 ml at birth, increasing to 1500 ml in adulthood.
- Gastric secretions are regulated by two glands: the oxintric and pyloric glands.
- The oxintric gland secretes acid, mucus, pepsinogen, and intrinsic factor.

Andrea Macarthur, Central Manchester and Manchester Children's University Hospitals NHS Trust

The pyloric gland secretes gastrin, a hormone that stimulates histamine receptors to produce histamine.

The stomach mixes food to produce chyme and releases small amounts of it at 20 s intervals, via the pyloric sphincter, into the small intestine.

Clear fluids take 1–2 hours to be emptied from stomach. Milk feeds take longer. Total emptying after a meal takes 3–5 hours. Refer to Trust guidelines on fasting times prior to procedures.

Small intestine

- Approximately 275 cm long in neonates, increasing to 5–6 m in adults.
- Consists of duodenum, jejunum, ileum, and ileocaecal valve.
- Principal function is absorption of fats, amino acids, sugars, vitamins, and bile salts.
- Large surface area (multiple folds and villi). Immaturity and malnutrition compromise regeneration of villi.
- Peristalsis propels chyme through small intestine to the large intestine.

Pancreas

- Exocrine and endocrine gland.
- Exocrine portion secretes enzymes into the duodenum to digest and absorb fats, carbohydrates, and fats. Also secretes sodium bicarbonate.
- Endocrine portion secretes hormones from the islets of Langerhans. Alpha cells secrete glucagon, beta cells secrete insulin, and delta cells secrete somatostatin.

Large intestine

- Approximately 40 cm long in neonates and 150 cm long in adults.
- Consists of caecum, colon, rectum, and anal canal.
- Principal functions are absorption of water and electrolytes, and storage and expulsion of faecal matter.

Liver

- Largest gland in the body.
- Situated in the upper right part of the abdomen.
- Two lobes: one large right lobe and one small left lobe.
- Hepatic artery supplies oxygenated blood to liver.
- The hepatic portal vein transports products of digestion to the liver.
- The hepatic veins remove blood.

Gall bladder

- Pear-shaped sac located beneath the liver.
- Stores and concentrates bile.
- Empties bile into the duodenum as required.

Further reading

Williams, C., Asquith, J. (2000). *Paediatric intensive care nursing*, pp. 259–61. Churchill Livingstone, London.

The main functions and structure of the liver

Situated below the diaphragm, occupying most of the right hypochondrium and some of the epigastric region, the liver is the largest solid organ in the body.

The functional cell of the liver is the hepatocyte. The organ receives nutrients from branches of the lymphatic system and blood supply from the hepatic artery and portal vein. The liver is also unique in its ability to survive limited damage through regeneration.

The liver is metabolically active, accounting for an estimated 200 functions and as a result of these reactions produces heat as a by-product.

Functions
- Forms and destroys red blood cells.
- Produces lymph fluid.
- Synthesizes coagulation factors.
- Manufactures plasma proteins.
- Destroys bacteria, toxins, and worn out blood cells.
- Metabolizes carbohydrates, lipids, and proteins.
- Produces and secretes bile.
- Stores glycogen, vitamins, iron, and copper.
- Detoxifies drugs and waste products.

Immaturity of the liver may cause
- Deficient plasma protein formation and potential fluid shifts due to changes in oncotic pressures.
- Deficient gluconeogenesis (conversion of glycogen to glucose).
- Poor conjugation of bilirubin.
- A lack of clotting factors.
- A reduced ability to break down and excrete drugs.

Some of the liver's more important functions are described below.
- Carbohydrate metabolism: maintenance of plasma glucose levels is controlled by the conversion of proteins, fats, and other sugars to glucose (gluconeogenesis) in times of fast, and the conversion of glucose into glycogen and triglycerides for storage in times of plenty.
- Lipid metabolism: triglycerides transported to the hepatocytes by the lacteals are either hydrolysed to glycerol and fatty acids and used in the production of adenosine triphosphate (ATP) or bound to proteins (lipoproteins) and transported to adipose tissue for storage.
- Amino acid metabolism: the liver manufactures most of the plasma proteins and converts amino acids into glucose or triglycerides for metabolism or storage. This process of deamination produces ammonia, a toxic molecule that is further detoxified by the liver into urea, which is easily excreted by the kidneys.

Mark Broom, University of Glamorgan

Detoxification of drugs and hormones: the liver detoxifies alcohol and drugs and excretes them directly into bile. The liver can also alter or excrete hormones, such as thyroid hormone and the steroid hormones.

Recycling of haemoglobin: the haem molecule is split into iron and is re-used or stored. The remaining components are converted into bilirubin and are conjugated. This water-soluble compound is excreted via the bile ducts and ultimately into the intestines.

Synthesis of bile salts: bile salts are used to emulsify fats in the small intestine, reducing their size and, as a result, maximizing the effects of the digestive enzymes.

Storage: the liver stores glycogen and is the primary site for storage of vitamins A, B_{12}, D, E, and K.

Further reading

Martini, F.H. (2006). *Fundamentals of anatomy and physiology*, 7th edn. Benjamin Cummings, San Francisco.

Montague, S.E., Watson, R., Herbert, R.A. (ed.) (2005). *Physiology for nursing practice*, 3rd edn. Elsevier, Edinburgh.

Appendicitis

Refers to an acute inflammation of the appendix which is a narrow 'worm-like' sack attached to the caecum and no longer has any useful physiological function in humans.

Can occur at any age, although is more common during adolescence.

Occurs more frequently in boys and is one of the most common forms of emergency requiring operation. The cause is unknown; however obstruction by a foreign object or faeces can lead to a blockage and subsequent swelling and inflammation, which, in turn, can lead to serious complications unless treated promptly.

Clinical features

- Vague abdominal pain around the umbilicus, gradually becoming sharper and more intense
- Pain moves to right iliac fossa region of the abdomen and becomes more constant
- Any movement or coughing intensifies the pain; the child will tend to lie still and quiet, although finding it difficult to sleep
- Drawing the legs up to the fetal position to alleviate pain
- Positive Rovsing's sign (rebound pain in the right iliac fossa when pressure is applied to the left side of the abdomen)
- Rapid pulse
- Fever, flushed face
- Loss of appetite or vomiting
- Decrease in urine output
- Diarrhoea
- Bad breath, furred tongue

Complications

- Peritonitis: occurs when the appendix 'bursts' and infected material from it circulates freely in the peritoneal cavity, leading to widespread infection.
- Abscess: infected material remains contained within the appendix but swells to form a lump, which if untreated, can 'burst' and cause widespread infection.

Treatment

- The standard treatment for appendicitis is surgical removal—an appendicectomy.
- If the appendix has 'burst', the infection will be washed out of the abdominal cavity using a saline solution and antibiotics prescribed to prevent further infection.

Nursing intervention
Post-operative care
- Maintain airway
- Make regular observations of temperature, pulse, respirations, and blood pressure
- Assess and manage pain—regular analgesia

Denise Owens, University of Salford

Fluid balance: input and output—may require IV fluids
Medications: antibiotics/anti-emetics
Wound care and management: may have wound drain; suture type
Reduce child and parent anxiety: comfort/support/reassurance/
encouragement
Enable rest/sleep
Provide distraction and play
Nutrition: as advised by medical staff
Mobility: encourage movement around bed and early mobilization

Further reading

www.sugical-tutor.org.uk

Peritonitis

Acute inflammation of the membrane lining the abdominal, cavity. Affect both sexes and all age groups.

History

Arises as a result of trauma or surgery to the abdomen.

Physical signs

- Pain: acute and localized, spreading across the abdomen, and becoming severe and generalized; may have shoulder pain
- Pyrexia
- Nausea and vomiting
- Tachycardia
- Rigid tender abdomen
- Hypotension
- Dehydration
- Malaise

Causes

Foreign material in the abdominal cavity: bacteria, blood, faecal matter gastrointestinal fluids, and undigested food.

Investigations

- Physical examination
- X-ray
- CT scan
- Blood for and U&Es, and culture

Treatment

- Surgery: laparotomy
- Antibiotics
- IV fluids
- NBM until bowel sound heard
- NG aspiration
- Antipyretics
- Analgesia

Complications

Multiple organ failure

Nursing intervention: post-operative care

- Maintain airway
- Regular observations of pulse, respiratory rate, blood pressure, and temperature
- Observe for abdominal distension
- Antipyretics
- Pain assessment and management
- Fluid balance: input and output
- Wound care and management
- Nutrition when bowel sounds heard
- Rest and sleep
- Parental support

Further reading

🖳 www.surgical–tutor.org.uk

Denise Owens, University of Salford

Pyloric stenosis

Also known as infantile hypertrophic pyloric stenosis, this is the mo[st]
common cause of intestinal obstruction in infancy. Usual age of presentation is 3–12 weeks and it is more prevalent in boys. Occurs secondary t[o]
hypertrophy and hyperplasia of the muscular layers of the pylorus.

History
• Progressive vomiting or regurgitation, which may become projectile
• Vomiting is intermittent, usually occurring after feeding
• Hungry baby—crying, not satisfied with pacifier or dummy
• Weight loss
• Dehydration
• Lethargy
• Decrease in urinary output and bowel movements

Physical signs
• Epigastric distension
• Visible peristaltic action across abdomen
• Depressed fontanelles, dry mucous membranes
• Poor skin turgor, pallor
• Lethargy
• Signs of shock

Causes
• Unknown
• Possible links to inheritance

Investigations
• Blood for electrolytes, pH, creatinine
• Abdominal X-ray and/or ultrasound
• Physical examination
• Barium feed
• Test feed

Treatment
• IV fluids
• NBM
• Surgery: pyloromyotomy

Complications
• Bowel obstruction due to adhesions or perforation
• Persistent vomiting (usually underlying cause, e.g. obstruction)

Denise Owens, University of Salford

ursing intervention

ost-operative care

Maintain airway

Make regular observations of temperature, pulse, respiratory rate, and blood pressure

Observe for abdominal distension

Assess and manage pain

Fluid balance: measure input/output, note vomiting, and bowel movements

Wound care and management

Nutrition: re-introduce feeds

Enable rest and sleep

Provide parental support

urther reading

www.surgical-tutor.org.uk

Mesenteric adenitis

Mesenteric adenitis is inflammation of the lymph nodes in the right lower quadrant of the abdomen. Difficult to diagnose, often confused with appendicitis; however, on examination the pain is usually more diffuse and the site of pain can shift when the patient changes position, whereas appendicitis is more localized.

More prevalent in children under 15 years and diagnosed when all other causes of abdominal pain eliminated, i.e. gynaecological, gastrointestinal disorders, appendicitis, and urinary tract infections. It is the large lymph nodes that cause the pain; peritonism and guarding never occur in mesenteric adenitis.

Cause

It is most frequently caused by a viral infection, although a previous infection, such as an upper respiratory tract infection, chest, or gastrointestinal infection, can often be the cause, and signs may still be present.

Symptoms
- Pyrexia
- Abdominal pain in the right lower quadrant
- Nausea/vomiting
- Occasionally diarrhoea

Treatment
- It is a diagnosis of exclusion: a laparotomy may be performed to rule out appendicitis.
- Surgery if abscess formation, signs of peritonitis.
- Antibiotics used if evidence of bacterial infection.
- Hydration and electrolyte balance.
- Analgesia and antipyretics.

Nursing care
- When unclear diagnosis, admit for observation. Reassure the child and parents that the disease is benign.
- Mesenteric adenitis is a self-limiting inflammatory illness that can take several weeks to clear.

Complications
- Volume depletion/electrolyte imbalance with protracted vomiting
- Abscess formation
- Peritonitis (rare)
- Sepsis (relates to aetiological agents such as *Streptococcus pneumoniae* and *Yersinia* spp.)

Prognosis
Prognosis—good. Complete recovery without specific treatment.

Jody Nevile, Royal Cornwall Hospital Trust

urther reading

dolph, M.C.J., Levene, M.I. (1999). *Paediatrics and child health*. Blackwell Science, London.
www.gpnotebook.co.uk/cache/2013659143.htm
www.emedicine.com/radio/topic444.htm

Gastroenteritis

Gastroenteritis is characterized by a sudden onset of vomiting and/or diarrhoea. Poor appetite, fever, and abdominal pain can also occur. The severity of this illness can vary from being a minor condition to a life threatening state. Gastroenteritis affects the absorption process in the gastrointestinal tract. This results in fluid loss. Infants and young children are particularly susceptible. This is because they have a higher proportion of water in their body weight, have an increased metabolic rate, and also an immature renal system.

Causes
Viral, bacterial, and protozoal.

Assessment
Vomiting and diarrhoea can also occur in other childhood conditions, and these need to be excluded.
- An assessment of the level of dehydration is required. It can be categorized broadly into:
  - severe dehydration (>10%)
  - moderate dehydration (5–10%)
  - mild dehydration (<5%).

The level of dehydration can change rapidly, children do not necessarily move through each stage.

- A stool specimen is usually obtained for M, C&S.
- A urine specimen for M, C&S maybe required.
- A blood test for U+Es is often required.

Care management
- Infection control measures must be in place to prevent cross-infection
- IV fluids are required if it is severe dehydration. For mild and moderate dehydration, oral rehydration therapy is generally sufficient.
- Breastfeeding is not normally stopped and is used in conjunction with the supplements.
- Once rehydration has taken place, a normal feeding pattern is introduced. The traditional practice of regrading is not generally recommended with most children able to tolerate their usual diet.
- Prior to discharge, give verbal and written advice and make appropriate liaison with the community services.
- Undertake notification of the infection if required; tell the parents that this has been done.

Further reading
Armon, K., Stephenson, T., MacFaul, R., Eccleston, P., Werneke, U. (2001). An evidence and consensus based guideline for acute diarrhoea management. *Archives of Diseases in Childhood* **85**, 132–42.
McVerry, M., Collin, J. (1999). Managing the child with gastroenteritis. *Nursing Standard*, **13**(37), 49–53.
 hcd2.bupa.co.uk/fact_sheets/html/gastroenteritis_children.html

Theresa Pengelly, University of Worcester

Coeliac disease (gluten-sensitive enteropathy)

Coeliac disease is a condition of the small intestine, which is usual diagnosed in the first year of life when cereals are introduced to a child diet.

Gluten, a protein substance found in wheat, barley, rye, and oats, provokes a damaging immunological response to the mucosa of the small intestine, which results in the atrophy of the villi. Villi provide a large surface area for the absorption of nutrients from food. When damaged the surface area for absorption of nutrients is reduced, resulting in diarrhoea and malnutrition.

In adults the disease often presents in atypical form, in that they may not have the bowel symptoms. They approach their doctor with symptoms of tiredness, psychological problems, or a skin rash (dermatitis herpetiformis).

Incidence
- 1 in 300 in the UK.
- 1 in 100 on the west coast of Ireland.

Clinical features
- Developmental delay
- Weight loss
- Poor muscle tone
- Abdominal distension
- Growth delay
- Decreased appetite
- Iron deficiency anaemia
- Folate deficiency
- Chronic diarrhoea/steatorrhoea
- Vitamin and mineral deficiencies

Diagnosis
- History of weight loss, failure to thrive, and poor feeding.
- Abnormal blood tests: coeliac screening blood tests measure antibodies in the blood to gluten or gliaden in the diet and the damaged endomysial muscle in the bowel.
- Delayed growth.
- Endoscopy, intestinal biopsy: confirms the presence of coeliac disease.

Management
- Gluten-free diet for life. Safe to eat maize, corn, or rice.
- Involve dietician.
- Calcium supplements.
- Folic acid and vitamin supplements.
- Prognosis good and improvements rapid when commenced on gluten-free diet.

Lorna Liggett, Queen's University Belfast

Provide health education regarding diet and dental care.
Provide psychological support for the child and family.

Complications

arely:
infertility in women
autoimmune diseases
osteoporosis.

here is also a slight increased risk of developing bowel cancer.

Further reading

ullivan, A. (1999). Coeliac disease. *Nursing Standard*, **14**(11), 48–52.
eighery, C. (1999). Coeliac disease. *British Medical Journal*, **319**, 236–9.
www.coeliac.co.uk

Constipation

Constipation is defined as the painful passage of hard infrequent stools. is a common problem and diagnosis is made on clinical history and phys cal examination. When parents initially report the problem, commo issues identified include number of stools passed per week, stool volume difficulty in passing stools, a sensation of abdominal fullness, abdomina distension, and overflow incontinence.

The causes of constipation are complex, but often constipation is only temporary problem, resolved with a diet high in fibre and fluids. Unfortu nately, many children have protracted constipation. The causes fall int three categories, which are often interlinked and some of which have been identified: social, psychological, and physical.

Children with protracted constipation or functional faecal retention ofte have encopresis, which is the repeated expulsion of faeces, whethe involuntary or intentional, in inappropriate places (e.g. clothing or th floor) in a child of at least 4 years of age (or equivalent developmenta level). These children often lack the sensation, which normally leads to expulsion. This results in retention of a large bulk of stool, and liqui stool leaks on to underclothes.

Nursing management of intractable functional constipation

The standard treatments include the following:
- Initial disimpaction with stool softeners and stimulants.
- Education of child and parent about diet (fibre and fluid, and possible removal of cows' milk or wheat).
- General exercise, which helps stimulate peristalsis.
- Toilet training, including regular, timed toilet sitting and toilet posture training; stool charts.
- Training regarding coordination of relaxation of sphincters with effective contraction of diaphragm (biofeedback training).
- Information regarding laxatives.
  - stool softeners (e.g. lactulose and docusate sodium) and stimulants
  - stimulants (senna, bisacodyl, and sodium picosulphate).
- Psychological referral: counselling, cognitive and family therapies, and psychotherapy.

Unfortunately, the response to treatment is often poor owing to the complex interaction of psychosocial influences and the pathophysiological effects of prolonged faecal retention.

It is considered that at least 50% of children who have unsuccessful therapy regimens, have slow-transit constipation (STC). These children cannot be considered as having a behavioural disorder, even though the symptom of the disorder causes considerable anxiety. Knowing that there is a physical cause should reduce the psychological stress of the child and parents. In the future, some treatment regimens for STC may change; e.g. high-fibre diets, rather than aiding bowel movements, will tend to block up the bowel. Low-fibre diets would reduce the stool

Maureen Harrison, University of Southampton

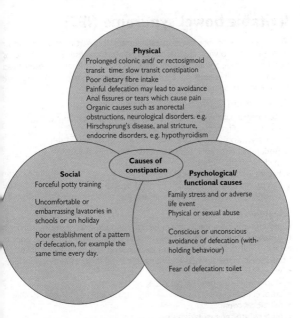

Physical
Prolonged colonic and/ or rectosigmoid
transit time: slow transit constipation
Poor dietary fibre intake
Painful defecation may lead to avoidance
Anal fissures or tears which cause pain
Organic causes such as anorectal
obstructions, neurological disorders. e.g.
Hirschsprung's disease, anal stricture,
endocrine disorders, e.g. hypothyroidism

**Causes of
constipation**

Social
Forceful potty training

Uncomfortable or
embarrassing lavatories in
schools or on holiday

Poor establishment of a pattern
of defecation, for example the
same time every day.

**Psychological/
functional causes**
Family stress and or adverse
life event
Physical or sexual abuse

Conscious or unconscious
avoidance of defecation (withholding behaviour)

Fear of defecation: toilet

content and be more easily propelled, in combination with therapies to
stimulate intestinal peristalsis.

Further reading

Brazzelli, M., Griffiths, P. (2001). Behavioural and cognitive interventions with or without other
    treatments for defaecation disorders in children. *Cochrane Database of Systematic Reviews*,
    Issue 4.

Price, K.J., Elliott, T.M. (2001). Stimulant laxatives for constipation and soiling in children. *Cochrane
    Database of Systematic Reviews*, Issue 3.

Irritable bowel syndrome (IBS)

IBS is a disorder of the lower intestinal tract. It is part of a broader group of disorders known as functional gastrointestinal disorders. It is recognized in children, and many adult sufferers can trace their symptoms back to childhood. It seems to be more common among 11–17-year-olds. Both sexes are affected equally in children.

Presentation
- Abdominal pain, which may be colicky, dull, or sharp in nature.
- Diarrhoea alternating with constipation.
- Mucusy stools.
- Abdominal distension (although less commonly reported in children than adults).
- Feeling of incomplete defecation.
- Symptoms may be preceded by psychosocial issues, such as schooling problems, eating disorders, etc.

Diagnosis
Children with IBS appear active, healthy, and experience normal growth. It is important to rule out other medical conditions with similar appearances. A full medical history and examination are undertaken. Investigations should be performed according to clinical features and may include
- urine culture
- stool studies for ova and parasites
- stool cultures
- full blood count
- erythrocyte sedimentation rate.

Some paediatric areas have adopted the Rome II criteria to make positive diagnosis of IBS. These criteria can be applied to children who are old enough to provide an accurate pain history.

Cause
There is no identifiable cause for IBS, although there may be a positive family history.

Prognosis
IBS is a chronic condition but is not life threatening. Most children have mild symptoms and continue with a normal life. However, some children may have moderate to severe symptoms that interfere with schooling and activities of daily living. IBS may persist into adulthood.

Treatment
IBS is a chronic condition and there is no cure. The aim of treatment is to establish regular bowel action and relieve symptoms:
- high-fibre diet
- peppermint oil may be of some benefit in relieving the symptoms of abdominal pain
- support and reassurance that although the symptoms may be difficult to treat, the condition is not a threat to the child's health

Yvonne Riley, Chorley and South Ribble District General Hospital Lancashire

psychological care: referral to psychologist if symptoms are
exacerbated by psychosocial issues.

urther reading

ine, R., Kline, J., Di Palma, J., Barbero, G. (2001). Enteric-coated, pH dependent peppermint oil
capsules for the treatment of irritable bowel syndrome in children. *Journal of Pediatrics*, **138**(1),
125–8.

ewart, M., Stewart, A. (1997). *No more IBS!* Vermilion, London.
www.about-irritable-bowel-syndrome.co.uk/

Crohn's disease

This is a chronic inflammatory bowel disease that, as yet, has no confirmed origin. It also has no cure and is a lifelong condition characterized by periods of exacerbation and remission. It affects all the layers of the bowel wall and can occur in any part of the gastrointestinal tract, from mouth to anus.

Characteristics of Crohn's disease
- Abdominal pain, often in the lower right region
- Diarrhoea
- Rectal bleeding, which may be serious and persistent, leading to anaemia
- Weight loss
- Fatigue
- Fever (may occur)
- Children with Crohn's disease may suffer delayed development and stunted growth

Complications
- One of the most common complications is a blockage of the intestine because the disease tends to thicken the intestinal wall with swelling and scar tissue. This then causes narrowing of the passage.
- Can cause sores and ulcers that tunnel (fistulas) through the affected area into surrounding tissue.
- Nutritional imbalances due to poor absorption, inadequate diet, and intestinal loss of protein.
- May have inflammation of eye, joints, skin, or liver. Possibly the result of altered immune function.

Treatment
Treatment for Crohn's disease depends on how severe it is and where it is. The objectives are to:
- control the inflammation
- maintain nutritional status
- alleviate symptoms such as the diarrhoea and pain.

Treatment may include the following:
- A combination of drugs:
  - 5-aminosalicylic acid (5-ASA) derivatives are prescribed frequently to reduce inflammation
  - in severe attacks corticosteroids and sometimes immunosuppressive agents are used
  - supplements of iron, calcium, and vitamins D and B_{12} may be needed due to poor absorption
  - analgesic, antidiarrhoeal, and antispasmodic drugs may be prescribed.
- Surgery may be indicated if the patient is unresponsive to medical therapy or has severe peri-anal infection, intestinal stricture, intestinal perforation, bleeding obstruction, fistulae, or abscesses.

Julia Edge, South Devon Health Care NHS Trust

Nursing management

Reduce anxiety

Ensure emotional and educational support is given, taking into account possible feelings of isolation and depression.

Empower patients.

Inform patients/carers of all nursing and medical interventions.

Access to toilets

It is important for patients to have easy access to a toilet, preferably an en-suite room, because sufferers have increased urgency, diarrhoea, and rectal bleeding. To have a commode on the ward behind a curtain is unpleasant because bowel motions are often explosive, noisy, and foul-smelling.

Nutrition

It is important to provide a nutritional and balanced diet but to take into account that patients may not fully absorb all the nutrients from their food. Children may associate eating with pain and diarrhoea, and thus may not want to eat, or eat less. Some patients may find that dairy products or a high-fibre diet may aggravate symptoms, so it is often constructive to refer to a dietician.

Further reading

Nightingale, A. (2004). An overview of the diagnosis and management of Crohn's disease. *Gastrointestinal Nursing*, **2**, 31–9.

NACC (2002). IBD: a guide for general nurses. 🖵 www.naccc.org.uk

Ulcerative colitis

Ulcerative colitis is a chronic lifelong illness with periods of exacerbation and remission. It represents >50% of the 20 000–25 000 new cases of inflammatory bowel disease each year. It is characterized by acute, non infectious inflammation of the colorectal mucosa. It can begin early in childhood, although the peak age for onset in young people is between 15 years and 25 years. Together with Crohn's disease, and because of their similar symptoms and treatments, it is known as inflammatory bowel disease (IBD). The usual area affected is the gastrointestinal tract but it is, in fact, a systemic disease. Because of its debilitating and protracted effects, this disease can have potentially serious consequences for the child's normal growth and development, and a young person would be faced with problems such as biological, psychological, and social changes, as well as role changes related to family and peers.

Although the aetiology of the disease is not known, diet, lifestyle, and infection, as well as a genetic influence, are thought to be relevant.

Signs and symptoms
Include:
- abdominal pain
- frequent bloody diarrhoea
- gastrointestinal bleeding
- fever
- tachycardia
- peritoneal irritation
- electrolyte imbalance
- malnutrition.

In children with ulcerative colitis, approximately one-quarter present with proctitis, one-third have left-sided colitis, and in almost half of children the disease extends to the transverse colon or beyond.

One-third of patients with IBD have other systemic symptoms, such as arthritis, osteoporosis, and mouth lesions.

Diagnosis
- Routine laboratory tests, including full blood count, would indicate anaemia, inflammation (elevated erythrocyte sedimentation rate and C-reactive protein), and malnutrition.
- Faeces may be positive for red and white blood cells.
- A plain X-ray would reveal if any abdominal organs were involved in disease activity.
- The disease is confirmed by biopsy following endoscopy, which would demonstrate evidence of chronic inflammation. This inflammation is usually presented as continuous uniform areas.

Treatment
The aim of treatment is to eliminate symptoms, optimize nutrition status, promote normal growth and development, and be aware of, and

Mair Sinfield, University of Glamorgan

prevent, psychological problems associated with a chronic debilitating disease.

Medical treatment

- Includes sulfasalazine and aminosalicylates, used for mild disease, with acute steroid therapy reserved for moderate to severe disease.
- Close monitoring is required because of the adverse side effects.

Surgical treatment

- Curative for intestinal symptoms but not extra-intestinal symptoms.
- Procedure involves partial or complete removal of the colon, usually with subsequent ilio-anal anastomis. The avoidance of a permanent colostomy is not always possible.
- General principles of gastrointestinal post-operative care apply.
- Provide support following surgery, and as the young person learns to cope with the disease.

Further reading

Glasper, A., Richardson, J. (ed.) (2006). *A textbook of children's and young people's nursing*. Churchill Livingstone, London.

Wong, D. (2003). *Nursing care of infants and children*. Mosby, St Louis.

📖 www.aboutkidsgi.org/ulcerative colititis.html

Hirschsprung's disease

Definition

Hirschsprung's disease is a rare genetic disease, affecting 1 in 5000, and is associated with Down syndrome. It is a functional intestinal obstruction, which results from the congenital absence of parasympathetic ganglion cells (aganglionosis) in the mesenteric plexus of the distal bowel. These cells are responsible for the peristaltic movement of the bowel, and when they are absent constipation results.

It affects the rectum and sigmoid, but can also involve the colon and extend into the large bowel. A functional obstruction of the bowel, with dilation of the proximal colon and hypertrophy of the muscle, occurs as a result of the disease. It is also known as megacolon.

Clinical features

Although symptoms usually begin within the first few days after birth, some people do not develop symptoms until later childhood, or even adulthood.

In infants, the main symptom is not passing meconium within the first 24–48 hours of life. Other symptoms include:
- abdominal distension and vomiting
- chronic constipation
- enterocolitis (inflammation of the small intestine and colon)
- pyrexia.

Symptoms in older children include:
- passing small, watery stools
- diarrhoea
- poor appetite.

Diagnosis

Good history taking and close assessment are essential. Hirschsprung's disease is confirmed by a combination of barium enema and rectal biopsy, where a small piece of bowel is removed and examined for the presence of nerve cells.

Treatment

- Hirschsprung's disease requires surgery to remove or bypass the affected bowel:
  - traditionally—temporary colostomy with definitive reconstruction planned for later
  - recently—single-stage repair or even a transanal 'incisionless' approach, requiring shorter hospital stays, less pain, and less scarring.
- General principles of gastrointestinal pre-operative and post-operative care apply.

Long-term problems

May include persistent constipation, incontinence, inflammation, and occasionally the need for a permanent colostomy.

Mair Sinfield, University of Glamorgan

The family can receive advice and support from the specialist centre treating their child. Psychological care may also be required.

Further reading

Rinhheanu, M., Markowitz, J. (2002). Inflammatory bowel disease in children. *Current Treatment Options in Gastroenterology*, **5**(3),181–96.

Rogers, J. (2004). Paediatric bowel problems. *Gastrointestinal Nursing* **2**(4), 31–9.

www.aboutkidsgi.org/hirschsprungs.html

Hernia

A hernia is a protrusion of a portion of an organ or organs through an abdominal opening. Usually treated with simple surgery, but the danger from herniation arises when there is constriction, which may impair the circulation, or when the protrusion interferes with the function or development of other structures.

Types of hernia

- Congenital diaphragmatic: allows abdominal contents to herniate up into the chest area. This is a serious condition that is treated surgically as soon as the baby's condition allows, and, although improving, mortality can be high. Hopefully the condition will have been detected antenatally by ultrasound scan, when plans will have been made to deliver the baby at a regional centre with paediatric surgical expertise. At birth, the paediatrician electively intubates and ventilates the baby to reduce the risk of air entry into the gastrointestinal tract. A thorough assessment and stabilization take place before surgery to repair the defect. The severity and involvement of other organs will determine the outcome and speed of recovery.
- Inguinal: the prolapse of a portion of the intestine into the inguinal ring above the scrotal sac, usually caused by a congenital weakness or failure of closure. Most common type of childhood hernia, especially in boys and is often bilateral. The incidence is greatest during infancy.
- Umbilical: common in infants, especially in African-American children because of the use of 'home remedies' such as 'belly binders'. Umbilical hernias normally protrude and expand when the child coughs, cries, or strains.
- Femoral: more common in girls and felt as a small mass on the anterior surface of the thigh just below the inguinal ligament in the femoral canal.

Hernias are indicated by the presence of a swelling in the relevant area, which may be accompanied by pain and restricted movement.

Treatment

A simple hernia will be repaired surgically, usually as a day case with follow-up as appropriate.

Oesophageal atresia

This is a congenital malformation of the oesophagus, which ends in a blind pouch. Occurring commonly with a tracheo-oesophageal fistula, it can present with other anomalies (see VACTERL association). There is no known cause.

Incidence
- Occurs in 1 in 3500 live births, equally in boys and girls
- Usually a lower than average birth weight
- 10–20% mortality in premature babies or those with other anomalies

Diagnosis
- Antenatal polyhydramnios in 50% of cases
- Noisy breathing and frothy saliva soon after birth
- Choking, coughing, and cyanotic episodes, particularly on feeding
- Pulmonary problems if fed prior to diagnosis
- A size 10 FG or 12 FG NG tube has resistance at 9–11 cm
- Chest and abdominal X-ray shows NG tube usually at T2–T4 level

Management
- Maintain airway: suction using Replogle double-lumen tube on free drainage with frequent aspiration
- NBM
- IV fluids
- Surgery: end-to-end anastomosis is performed. If there is a long gap, surgery is delayed until the ends have grown. If the two ends are too far apart, colon interposition, gastric tube, or gastric interposition surgery is performed
- Gastrostomy and/or cervical oesophagostomy may be performed until the oesophagus is complete and functioning
- Provide parental support to promote attachment and reduce anxiety
- 'Sham' feeds: feeds that exit via the oesophagostomy may be commenced
- Gastrostomy feeding
- Pacifiers to encourage sucking
- Upright position with oral feeds
- Stoma care of oesophagostomy and/or gastrostomy

Complications
- GOR can be resolved by practical measures, and prescribed medication
- Strictures: these may need to be stretched under anaesthetic
- Normal feeding programmes will take longer to achieve
- Peristalsis is less coordinated
- Dysphagia
- Lodging of food in the oesophagus
- Anastomotic leaks

Ruth Davies, Royal Devon and Exeter NHS Foundation Trust

Prognosis

This is related to the birth weight, associated anomalies, and time of diagnosis.

• Feeding and difficulties are common in the first 2 years.
• Normal life expectancy and abilities notwithstanding other anomalies.

Further reading

Huband, S., Trigg, E. (ed.) (2000). *Practices in children's nursing: guidelines for hospital and community*. Harcourt, London.

Wong, D. (1997). *Whaley and Wong's Essentials of pediatric nursing*, 5th edn. Mosby, St Louis.

🖳 www.tofs.org.uk/info_vacterl.htm

Biliary atresia

- Biliary atresia is a progressive disease, usually present at birth, which leads to cholestasis, hepatic fibrosis, and cirrhosis.
- The most common cause of neonatal jaundice.
- Late diagnosis may result in irreversible liver damage and a need for liver transplantation in the first year of life.
- Frequency is 1 per 16 000 live births.
- Usually no family history.
- Slight female preponderance.
- Aetiology is unknown.
- 10% have extra-hepatic abnormalities (polysplenia, situs inversus, interrupted inferior vena cava, preduodenal portal vein, and cardiac defects); biliary atresia splenic malformation syndrome.
- Neonatal screening using dry blood spots is unreliable.
- All infants who have conjugated jaundice after 14 days of age should be investigated to exclude biliary atresia.
- Referral to specialist centres is mandatory for suspected cases in order to facilitate early surgery.

Clinical features and history

- Conjugated hyperbilirubinaemia
- Dark urine
- Pale acholic stools
- Hepatomegaly
- Birth weight and gestation usually normal
- Feed and thrive appropriately at first
- Lack of fat-soluble vitamin K absorption may result in coagulopathy, rarely with a bleed which may be intracranial
- Older infants may have ascites and splenomegaly

Diagnosis is by excluding medical causes (α_1-antitrypsin deficiency) and identifying the characteristic histological appearance of a percutaneous liver biopsy. Abdominal ultrasound will exclude other surgical causes such as choledochol cyst and inspissated bile syndrome. An absent or contracted gall bladder after fasting is suggestive. Radionuclide hepatobiliary imaging fails to show bile excretion into the bowel within 24 hours. Infants with a high suspicion are recommended for surgery.

Surgery

- Right-sided transverse incision across the midline
- Operative cholangiogram to confirm diagnosis
- Exposure of porta hepatitis
- A complete resection of the extrahepatic biliary tree
- Continuity restored with a Roux loop as a portoenterostomy after the technique of Professor Kasai
- Bile drainage is achieved in 60% of infants.

Graham Gordon, Birmingham Children's Hospital NHS Trust

Post-operative care
- IV antibiotics followed by oral prophylactic antibiotics
- IV fluids with early return to feeding with medium-chain triglyceride-based feed
- Epidural analgesia
- Steroids for 2 weeks
- Discharge often by 7 days
- Choleretics (phenobarbitone or ursodeoxycholic acids)
- Fat-soluble vitamins (A, D, E, and K) for up to 1 year
- Normal vaccination times, including Prevenar®, Pneumovax®, and influenza

Main complications
- Nutritional consequences of cholestasis
- Ascending bacterial cholangitis
- Cirrhosis and portal hypertension

Any of these may lead to liver transplant in infancy or childhood. Most common indication for paediatric liver transplant (up to 50%).

Further reading

Stringer, M.D., Howard, E.R. (2003). Surgical disorders of the liver and bile ducts and portal hypertension. In *Diseases of the liver and biliary system in children* (ed. D.A. Kelly). Blackwell, Oxford.

www.childliverdisease.org/jaudine/baby

Childhood obesity

The number of overweight and obese children in the UK has risen steadily during the past 20 years. Obesity is a condition where weight gain poses a serious threat to health.

Measurement

- Child's weight, obese: body weight >25% fat in boys and >32% in girls.
- Body mass index (BMI), as determined by calculations of weight and height, can overestimate weight status because it does not account for increased fat-free mass, e.g. muscle.
  - BMI does not account for changing adiposity, fat distribution, and muscle mass with age difficult to apply to children.
  - BMI percentile uses different cut-off points to define overweight and obese children, depending on age and gender. Best tool available for screening obesity in children.

Prevalence

- Childhood obesity reflects trend of adult population in the UK and other countries.
- The National Audit Office (NAO) has projected that by 2010, 1 in 4 adults will be obese and the total cost to the NHS and wider economy will be £3.6 billion.
- 8.5% of 6-year-olds and 15% of 15-year-olds are obese in England.

Causes

- Obesity occurs when intake of energy is greater than that expended.
- Children more likely to be overweight if their parents are obese.
- Genetic factors are less significant than eating and activity habits.

Causes of childhood obesity

Diet	Physical activity
High-calorie foods, such as fast foods and confectionery, are abundant, relatively cheap, and heavily promoted, specifically at children	Sedentary lifestyles: 40–69% of children over the age of 6 years spend less than 1 hour/day doing physical activity of moderate intensity
Large portion sizes	A decline in the number of young people playing sport at school
High proportion of food prepared outside the home	A decline in the proportion of children walking or cycling to school
Increased eating frequency	A possible rise in sedentary pastimes such as watching television, playing computer games, or accessing the Internet
Heavy marketing of fast foods and high intakes of sugar-sweetened drinks	An Independent Television Commission survey shows that the average 4–15-year-old watches ~2.5 hours of television per day
Alcohol	

Gill McEwing, University of Plymouth

Effects

- Overweight child has a 70% chance of becoming an overweight adult.
- Higher risk of developing serious health problems in later life, including heart attack and stroke, type 2 diabetes, bowel cancer, osteoarthritis, and high blood pressure.
- Overweight child → psychological distress → stigmatization, prejudice, low self-confidence, isolation, and depression.
- Type 2 diabetes mellitus is occurring in school-age children.

Further reading

Joint WHO/FAO Expert Consultation (2002). *Diet, nutrition and the prevention of chronic diseases.* WHO, Geneva.

Management of childhood obesity

- Overweight children should not be encouraged to actually lose weight.
- Advise children to maintain their weight, and gradually 'grow into it' as they get taller.
- Never put child on a weight-loss diet without medical advice, because this can affect their growth.
- Unregulated dieting—particularly in teenage girls—can to lead to the development of eating disorders, e.g. anorexia nervosa and bulimia nervosa.
- No drug treatment has proven effective in the treatment of weight problems in children.
- Helping children to achieve and maintain a healthy weight involves:
  - a healthy well-balanced diet.
  - changes to eating habits.
  - increasing physical activity.

National initiatives

National initiatives are being developed.
- HealthyStart: means for disadvantaged families to buy foods such as fruit.
- SureStart: for families and children up to the age of 4 years living in the most deprived areas; provides family support, advice on nurturing, etc.
- Compulsory nutrition standards for school lunches.
- National school fruit scheme: all 4–6-year-olds to have a free piece of fruit each day.
- Food labelling: the Food Standards Agency (FSA) is developing a range of resources (with the DfES) for use in schools to explain how to use food labels effectively.
- PE is a compulsory part of the national curriculum up to the age of 16 years.
- Healthy travel to school: a school travel advisory group publishes guidance for local authorities to encourage children to walk or cycle to school.

Management of childhood obesity

Eating habits	Diet	Physical activity
Set a good example with your own eating habits	Starchy foods, which are rich in 'complex carbohydrates', are bulky relative to the amount of calories they contain. This makes them filling and nutritious. Sources such as bread, potatoes, pasta, rice, and chapattis should provide half the energy in a child's diet.	Encourage walking to places such as school and the shops, rather than always jumping in the car
Provide meals and snacks at regular times to prevent 'grazing'	Reduce/remove high-fat foods such as chocolate, biscuits, cakes, and crisps;	Suggest going to the park for a kick around with a

Gill McEwing, University of Plymouth

Contd.

Eating habits	Diet	Physical activity
	try healthier alternatives such as fresh fruit, crusty bread, or crackers	football or a game of rounders, cricket, or frisbee
Do not allow your children to eat while watching television or doing homework	Try to grill or bake foods instead of frying	Visit a local leisure centre to investigate sports and team activities to get involved in
Make mealtimes an occasion by eating as a family group as often as possible	Avoid fizzy drinks that are high in sugar. Substitute them with fresh juices diluted with water or sugar-free alternatives	Make exercise a treat by taking special trips to an adventure play park or an ice-skating rink, or suggest whole-family bike rides, swimming, and in-line skating
Encourage children to eat when they are hungry rather than out of habit	A healthy breakfast of a low-sugar cereal (e.g. wholemeal wheat biscuits) with milk plus a piece of fruit is a good start to the day	When it is safe to do so, teach your child to ride a bicycle
Teach children to chew food more slowly and savour the food. They will feel fuller more quickly and be less likely to overeat at mealtimes	Instead of sweets, offer dried fruit or tinned fruit in natural juice	Reducing physical inactivity pastimes such as watching television or playing computer games. These should be reduced to no more than 2 hours a day or an average of 14 hours a week
Do not keep lots of high-fat, high-sugar snack foods in the house		Do not use food to comfort a child—give attention, listening, and hugs instead
Do not make outings for fast foods part of the weekly routine		Avoid using food as a reward, instead buy a gift, go to the cinema, or have a friend to stay overnight
Try to get children involved in preparing food as this will make them more aware of what they are eating		
Keep a food diary		

Further reading

Food Standards Agency. ◪ www.foodstandards.gov.uk/healthiereating
Parliamentary Office of Science and Technology, 7 Millbank, London SW1P 3JA. Tel: 020 7219 2840. ◪ www.parliament.uk/post

ABC of viral hepatitis

Viral hepatitis is the most common cause of liver disease. The main viruses are hepatitis A, B, and C. They infect the liver cells, leading to acute or chronic infection, ranging from mild inflammation to cirrhosis (irreversible liver damage) and/or hepatocellular carcinoma.

Acute viral hepatitis

Infection can be asymptomatic, present with mild to moderate symptoms dependent on the immune response of the host, or may lead to acute liver failure, which may require liver transplant.

Signs and symptoms

Usually experienced in hepatitis A and B and rarely in hepatitis C.

- Tiredness
- Nausea
- Loss of appetite
- Vomiting
- Dark urine
- Pale stools
- Right upper quadrant and epigastric pain
- Jaundice
- Raised liver transaminases
- Raised serum bilirubin
- Hepatomegaly

Acute viral hepatitis is a notifiable disease.

Management

- Hepatitis A needs source isolation.
- No isolation required for hepatitis B or C.
- Handling blood and bodily fluids → infection-control policies.
- Supportive medical treatment, with rest analgesia, and hydration.
- Prevent stigmatization: education and awareness.
- Usually patients recover with rest; some need hospitalization.
- Symptomatic patients usually seroconvert, clear the virus, and become immune. They are at no further risk of infection and do not require vaccination.
- Acute hepatitis A resolves spontaneously, followed by lifelong immunity.
- If patients with acute hepatitis B and C do not clear the virus and viraemia continues for >6 months, chronic infection (carriers) develops. Children/young people are mostly asymptomatic and unaware of the infection until tested for it.

Acknowledgements

Professor Dierdre Kelly, Dr Elizabeth Boxall, and Julie Taylor.

Further reading

Kelly, D.A. (2004). *Diseases of the liver and biliary system in children*, 2nd edn. Blackwell, Oxford.
🔲 www.doh.gov.uk/chidrenbbvs

Jaswant Sira, Birmingham Children's Hospital NHS Trust

Hepatitis A virus (HAV)

Hepatitis A is the most infectious, self-limiting, and common form of acute viral hepatitis in developing countries. In the UK the incidence shows a cyclical pattern; while the majority of cases are sporadic, outbreaks do occur.

HAV
A single-stranded RNA virus—picornaviridae family.

Incubation period
14–40 days.

Transmission
- Infectious during incubation period and for the following 30 days.
- Oral–faecal route.
- Source:
  - contaminated food and drinking water
  - poor hygiene.

Diagnosis
Confirmed by a blood test.

HAV markers
- HAV antibody immunoglobin (Ig) M positive
  - indicative of recent infection, present for 4–6 months.
- HAV antibody IgG
  - persists lifelong, conferring protection.

Management
Acute viral hepatitis
- Usually asymptomatic in children and severity tends to increase with age.
- 1% of children develop fulminant hepatitis → intensive clinical care and probable transplant. Most recover, cholestasis or relapse may persist for 2–3 months, no chronic liver disease.

Prevention
- Good hygiene
- Improve sanitation
- Follow universal precautions
- Health education and awareness
- Vaccination of those at risk, i.e.
  - travellers to high-risk areas
  - immunocompromised
  - routine vaccination of care workers not indicated.

Vaccination
First dose provides 1 year of immunity; booster dose, 6–12 months after primary dose, provides up to 10 years of immunity.

Hepatitis B virus (HBV)

- If virus persists longer than 6 months → chronic infection. The WHO estimates that about 350 million people may have chronic infection.
- Higher prevalence (8–20%) in Eastern Europe, Asia, and Africa, whereas in Western Europe and USA it is <2%.
- It is one of the top 10 causes of death worldwide.

HBV
- A double-stranded DNA virus belonging to the hepadnavirus family. It is 100 times more infectious than HIV.
- Virus may remain active for 10 days, even in a dry blood spot.

Incubation period
15–180 days.

Diagnosis
Confirmed by a blood test.

Natural history

HBV-positive markers
- Hepatitis B surface antigen (HBsAg): infection, first marker hepatitis B surface antibody (HBsAb); fully immune, the last marker to appear, or immune response to vaccination
- Hepatitis B core antibody (HBcAb) IgM: acute infection, usually present up to 6 months
- HBcAb IgG: contacted infection, usually present after 6 months
- Hepatitis B e antigen (HBeAg): viral replication, high risk of liver damage and transmission
- Hepatitis B e antibody (HBeAb): partial immunity, low risk of liver damage and transmission

HBV NATURAL HISTORY

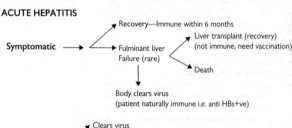

Hepatitis B Virus

Jaswant Sira, Birmingham Children's Hospital NHS Trust

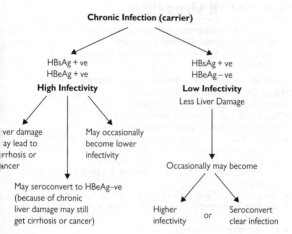

Chronic Infection (carrier)

HBsAg + ve
HBeAg + ve
High Infectivity

HBsAg + ve
HBeAg − ve
Low Infectivity
Less Liver Damage

...ver damage
...ay lead to
...rrhosis or
...ncer

May occasionally
become lower
infectivity

May seroconvert to HBeAg−ve
(because of chronic
liver damage may still
get cirrhosis or cancer)

Occasionally may become

Higher   or   Seroconvert
infectivity   clear infection

Risk factors

Infected mother to baby during childbirth—90% of babies born to
antigen-positive mothers develop chronic infection.
Sharing contaminated needles/equipment for drug abuse.
Non-sterile equipment—tattoos, body piercing, or acupuncture.
Contaminated needlestick injury of care workers.
Unprotected sex with an infected partner.
Sharing tooth brushes, razors, combs, or nail clippers.
Recipients of blood or blood products in countries with no screening
programme (all blood and blood products in the UK have been
screened since 1969).

Management

Acute hepatitis B
As acute viral hepatitis.

Chronic hepatitis B
Although asymptomatic, patients are at risk of serious liver disease and
hepatocellular carcinoma in adulthood. Regular monitoring of patients'
liver function and marker for liver tumour is required.
No effective treatment, but antiviral treatments such as interferon,
lamivudine, and adefovir are used by some specialists.
Information, counselling, and psychological support by specialists.
Alcohol within normal limits.
Career advice.
Advice about insurances/mortgages.

Prevention of hepatitis B
- All pregnant women should be offered counselling and screening.
- Delay in the vaccination course may result in the baby becoming infected, sometimes with fatal consequences that could have been prevented. Inform parents of this risk, advise them not to miss or delay appointments.

Accelerated vaccination programme for the newborn of a mother with hepatitis B
- Initial dose at birth (within 48 hours).
- Second dose at 4 weeks } must be given.
- Third dose at 8 weeks } as scheduled.
- Booster dose at 12 months and a blood test to check for response (HBsAb) to the vaccination course:
  - responders: HbsAb >100 miu/mL; protected
  - non-responders: <10 miu/mL; may need a booster dose or repeat vaccination.
- The babies of HBeAg-positive or HBeAb-negative mothers will also require immunoglobulin, with the first dose of vaccine for immediate protection.
- Breastfeeding is encouraged.

Vaccination of at-risk population
- Healthcare workers, families of infected people, travellers to high-risk areas, recipients of multiple blood products, those in institutions, and adopted and immunocompromised patients.

Preventative measures
- Wear disposable gloves, aprons, and, if necessary, goggles to prevent direct contact with blood or body fluids.
- Waterproof dressings for cuts/broken skin.
- Injecting drug users should be informed of the risk and the need to use sterile needles/syringes. Encourage accessing needle exchange programmes.
- Never share toothbrushes, razors, combs, or nail clippers.
- Sterile equipment for body piercing or tattoos at registered premises.
- Blood spillage or body fluids (see your Trust infection-control policy). At home use bleach diluted in a 1:10 ratio with water.
- Wash bloodstained clothing in cold and then hot water.
- Health education and awareness to reduce transmission and stigmatization.

Acknowledgements
Professor Dierdre Kelly, Dr Elizabeth Boxall, and Julie Taylor

Hepatitis C virus (HCV)

Chronic HCV infection is an increasing health problem worldwide, with 170 million people infected. In England 200 000 people may be chronically infected, of which 1% are children. Many remain unaware of their infection.

HCV
- Single-stranded RNA virus belonging to the flavivirus family. Ten times more infectious than HIV.
- The virus remains active for 2–3 days following blood spillage.

Incubation period
14–70 days.

Diagnosis
Confirmed with blood tests

HCV markers
- HCV antibody positive:
  - contact with the virus, present or past infection
  - need further tests to confirm infectivity, as below.
- HCV RNA PCR positive—indicates infection.
- HCV antibody positive and HCV RNA PCR negative: marker of past infection, not infectious. Antibodies may remain for life.

Further testing
- HCV genotypes (groups): most common in UK are 1a, 1b, 2a, 2b, 3a, and 3b.
- Genotypes are significant in response to treatment, but no difference is known in liver pathology.

Transmission
- Similar to hepatitis B, higher risk—contaminated equipment for illicit drug use.
- 6% risk infected mother to baby at birth; increases to 10% if co-infected with HIV.
- Risk is low via sexual intercourse with infected partner without a condom, but increases with multiple partners.
- Blood transfusions, blood products, or invasive treatment in countries with no blood screening programme. All blood and blood products have been screened for HCV in the UK since 1991.

Signs and symptoms
- Usually asymptomatic, but risk of serious liver disease and hepatocellular carcinoma in later adulthood.
- Occasionally tiredness, abdominal pain, or headaches.
- Psychological problems—stigmatization and discrimination.

Jaswant Sira, Birmingham Children's Hospital NHS Trust

Management of HCV

MANAGEMENT OF HIGH-RISK INFANTS/CHILDREN AND YOUNG PEOPLE

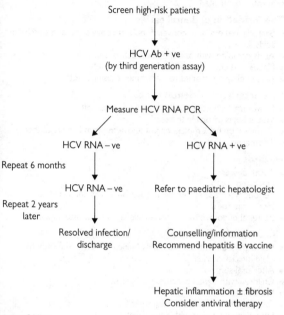

Screen high-risk patients

↓

HCV Ab + ve
(by third generation assay)

↓

Measure HCV RNA PCR

HCV RNA – ve | HCV RNA + ve

Repeat 6 months

HCV RNA – ve | Refer to paediatric hepatologist

Repeat 2 years later

Resolved infection/discharge | Counselling/information Recommend hepatitis B vaccine

↓

Hepatic inflammation ± fibrosis Consider antiviral therapy

Hepatitis C Virus

Monitor patients regularly for liver function and liver tumour, and give advice.

Antiviral treatment

Interferon and ribavirin treatment: excellent response to genotypes 2 and 3, but is less effective for genotype 1.

Patients/families need to live a normal healthy life, including a balanced diet.

Need specialist advice about:
• transmission, careers, insurances, and mortgages.

Prevention

Vaccination is not yet available.

Elective caesarean section is not proven to prevent the infection, but avoid lengthy premature rupture of membranes or invasive fetal monitoring.

Breastfeeding does not pose a risk to the baby unless there is broken skin or mother is co-infected with HIV.

Follow universal precautions.

Dental caries

Dental caries, tooth decay, or cavities are holes that damage the structure of the tooth. Dental caries is common and could be successfull prevented/controlled.

The formation of dental caries
- Bacteria in the mouth convert food (especially sugar and starch) into acids.
- Acids combine with bacteria, food debris, and saliva to form plaque.
- Plaque, a sticky substance, adheres to the teeth.
- Acid in plaque dissolves tooth enamel, causing a hole.

Characteristics of dental caries
- Brown marks on the teeth that will not brush off
- Visible holes or pits in the teeth
- Common on back molars or just above the gum line on all teeth
- Toothache

Hazards
- Tooth abscess
- Fractured tooth
- Periodontal disease, causing alveolar bone loss and eventual loss of the tooth
- Bacterial endocarditis for those children with cardiac conditions

Children at risk
- Some children with special needs (difficult to clean their teeth)
- Maxillofacial injuries
- After oral surgery
- Children with dental prosthesis or braces
- No dentist
- Families with poor health awareness
- Low-income families with a poor diet
- Prolonged bottle feeding

Treatment
- Analgesia
- The decay is drilled out and the tooth filled or the tooth extracted

Nursing management
- Recognition and referral:
  - oral assessment
  - child's dental history; those at risk of poor oral hygiene
  - complaints of a painful mouth or toothache
  - refusal of the child to eat
  - liaise with paediatricians and oral surgeons
- Support and education of the parents and child:
  - how to clean the child's teeth and mouth effectively
  - the importance of a reduced sugar diet and healthy snacks
  - the dangers of prolonged bottle feeding and sugary drinks at night

Sue Mason, Royal Devon and Exeter NHS Foundation Trust

- the importance of regular dental checkups
- a list of dentists if they are not registered
- liaise with appropriate health professionals

Nutrition:
- analgesia to control discomfort
- good sugar-free oral intake
- encourage regular healthy meals
- sweet treats only after meals to help prevent snacking

Oral hygiene:
- keep mouth clean and moist to prevent the build-up of plaque
- correct brushing at 45° to ensure maximum plaque removal and minimal trauma to gums

Prevention

Health promotion and education
Fluoride toothpaste
Access to NHS dentist
Dental sealants

Further reading

Huband, S., Trigg, E. (2000). Assessment. In *Practices in children's nursing: guidelines for hospital and community*. Churchill Livingstone, London.
Xavier, G. (2000). The importance of mouth care in preventing infection. *Nursing Standard*, **14** (8), 47–52.
www.nlm.gov/medlineplus/ency/article/001055.htm (accessed 25 April 2005).

Posseting

Definition: posset
- Small quantities of undigested milk are regurgitated repeatedly into the mouth soon after feeding.
- Many babies have problems with regurgitation (posseting) during their first year of life; in the majority of infants this resolves by 12–18 months of age or when solid feeds commence.
- Regurgitation is generally due to the gastro-oesophageal sphincter not yet being fully mature in babies; it takes approximately 12–18 months to function correctly.

Signs and symptoms
These start within the first few months of life and present as regurgitation of small volumes of undigested milk soon after a feed.
Severe signs and symptoms that would cause concern and need further investigation are:
- vomiting (large volume)
- repeated chest infections
- weight loss
- failure to thrive
- pain (heartburn)
- irritability with feeding
- anaemia or signs of blood in the vomit
- arching of the back and crying
- poor sleep pattern
- chronic cough.

Prevention
Simple changes can often help:
- smaller more frequent meals
- feeding the baby in a more upright position
- not laying the baby flat after feeding
- using a feed thickener
- change of milk or diet
- slightly elevating the head of the cot when lying the baby down.

Posseting is usually self-limiting and resolves with time over the first 12–18 months of life, without signifying any serious underlying disease.

Hazards
More severe forms of regurgitation are found when infants do not respond to simple lifestyle changes and possets become larger (vomits). The infant should then be assessed for GOR. GOR refers to the inappropriate opening of the gastro-oesophageal sphincter, releasing gastric contents into the oesophagus, which may cause harm, such as coughing, wheezing, painful swallowing, oesophagitis, failure to thrive, or respiratory problems.

Nicola J. Gibbons, Nottingham University Hospital NHS Trust

Treatment and nursing management

Initially, use feed thickeners These naturally inhibit the regurgitation of food into the oesophagus.

Do not give the baby too much milk or allow him/her to swallow a lot of air with feeds. Air swallowing occurs when the bottle is horizontal and both milk and air are drawn into the mouth when sucking. Promote regular 'winding'.

Although the prone sleeping position is favoured for infants with GOR, this conflicts with the 'back-to-sleep advice' which aims to reduce the risk of cot death. Lying the baby on the left side or slightly elevating the head of the cot/bed may be an alternative.

Infants with continuous possets should be assessed for GOR by their GP, who may recommend antacid treatment with prokinetic agents and histamine (H_2) receptor blockers, in addition to feed thickeners. The GP may refer the infant to a paediatrician or paediatric gastroenterologist for further investigations.

Further reading

British Society of Gastroenterology (2002). *A study guide in GI physiology.* Association of GI Physiologists, London.

Fleisher, D. (1994). Functional vomiting disorders in infancy: innocent vomiting, nervous vomiting, and infant rumination syndrome. *Journal of Pediatrics,* **125**, S84–94.

(2000). *Practices in children's nursing: guidelines for hospital and community.* Feeding—part 1: Breast, bottle, and weaning. Churchill Livingstone, Edinburgh.

Infantile colic

Colic is a commonly used but ill-defined term that refers to problemat excessive crying in infancy (mostly within the first 4 months), with a rang of variable associated signs in an intermittently distressed baby. Estimate of prevalence vary greatly, but one in six families consult a GP or heal visitor for help.

Causes

Many potential causes.
- Physiological disturbance:
  - cow's milk protein allergy or other gut pathology
  - transient autonomic nervous system anomaly affecting the respons to normal stimuli
  - transition from one neurobehavioural developmental state to another.
- Infant temperament and maternal response predisposing to behaviour or responses.
- Deficient, inadequate, or unresponsive parental care.

Why is excessive crying or colic a problem?

- Lasting effects from excessive crying are uncommon.
- Distressed behaviour is found in later childhood in a small subset.
- Effects are felt mostly by the family: exhaustion, strained relationships, social isolation, and feelings of guilt.
- Risk of non-accidental injury may be increased.
- Significant workload for GPs and health visitors.

Solutions and interventions

Intervention depends on the perceived cause. A detailed history and period of listening to the parents' story are essential.
- Medical screening to exclude physical illness.
- Sensitive observation of parenting for obvious problems, such as poor feeding technique or inappropriate handling.
- Drug treatment (drops) has a poor record of effectiveness. In confirmed lactose intolerance, lactase drops can be effective for breast-fee babies, but otherwise lactose-free formulae are more appropriate.
- Replacement of standard milk formula with soya or hydrogenated formulae has limited success.
- Behaviour modification to emphasize diurnal rhythm can improve sleeping patterns and reduce crying in some babies.
- Support for parents, emphasizing the absence of blame, offering moral support, and taking time to listen can enhance the parents' ability to cope. Support groups are available, notably BM Cry-Sis.[1]
- Usually resolves gradually and spontaneously within the first 4 months, with a gradual return to normal life.

Further reading

Long, T. (2004). *Excessive crying in infancy*. Whurr Publishers.

1 www.crysis.com

Tony Long, University of Salford

Rickets

This childhood condition occurs more in boys than girls and befor
fusion of the epiphyses. It can be inherited, a nutrient deficiency, or sec
ondary to a disorder. Adult rickets is known as osteomalacia.

Characteristics
- Bowing of the legs
- Pigeon chest deformity
- Curvature of the spine
- Flattening and squaring of the skull
- Fracture risk
- Teeth: slower to appear and enamel softer
- Low levels of calcium and phosphate
- X-rays show lowered amounts of minerals and bones

Types
- Rickets
- Vitamin-D-resistant rickets

Rickets
Causes
- Calcium deficiency due to a vitamin D (calciferol) deficiency or abnor-
  mality of metabolism (coeliac disease)
- Dietary calcium deficiency
- Lack of sunlight
- Phosphate deficiency due to decreased gut absorption or increased
  renal losses
- Neurofibromatosis
- Fluorosis—adverse effects of fluoride

Treatment
Ongoing vitamin D supplements, high-calcium foods, such as milk, and
adequate exposure to sunlight. When rickets occurs as a result of a
underlying condition, e.g. kidney disease, the treatment will be dependen
on the cause.

Vitamin-D-resistant rickets
Causes
- The most common inherited form of rickets is X-linked hypophos-
  phataemic rickets, which can also appear sporadically. Mothers pass
  the defective gene to either son or daughter, but a father only passes
  the defective gene to daughters. The renal tubules cannot reabsorb
  phosphorus and often have a defect in phosphate transport in the
  proximal tubule, producing hypophosphataemia—decreased level
  of phosphates in the blood and high levels of phosphate in the urine.
- This form resembles rickets but does not respond to vitamin D and
  affects approximately 1 in 20 000 people.

Sonya Clarke, Queen's University Belfast

Treatment

Large doses of phosphate medication plus active vitamin D hormones given by mouth, e.g. calcitriol. Rare hereditary types may need other family members to take small doses of vitamin D.

Complications of rickets

Too much vitamin D can cause kidney damage, and arthritis may result from bone distortion.

Further reading

Berg, E. (2004). Rickets. *Orthopaedic Nursing*, **23**(1), 53–5.
Wharton, B., Bishop, N. (2003). Rickets (Overview of causes and development in children, especially vitamin D deficiency). *Lancet*, **362**, 1389–1400.

Intestinal obstruction

Obstruction occurs when the passage of contents is stopped, either by narrowed or blocked lumen. In general, intestinal obstruction is characterized by abdominal pain, nausea and/or vomiting, abdominal distension and a change in bowel habits. The progression and combination of symptoms can vary considerably. In many conditions complications, such as dehydration and necrosis, can occur soon after the onset of symptoms.

Congenital causes

- Imperforate anus: the normal opening is closed; usually detected at birth.
- Meckel's diverticulum: a remnant of fetal development, this is a pouch of tissue (usually gastric) which is in the intestine. This is often asymptomatic but can cause intestinal obstruction in childhood. It is more likely to occur in children under 10 years of age.
- Hirschsprung's disease: the absence of ganglion cells in sections of the intestine, usually the colon. The affected section cannot relax, resulting in the non-passage of faeces. If this is severe, obstruction can occur within 48 hours of birth.
- Volvulus: during fetal development the intestine fails to become fixed in the correct position. This means that twisting can occur, resulting in partial or total occlusion. It is more likely to occur in the first year of life.
- Meconium ileus: meconium is waste material that is normally expelled from the intestine shortly after birth. Failure to do this will result in obstruction. It can be associated with cystic fibrosis.

Acquired causes

- Intussusception: a proximal section of intestine telescopes into a more distal section. It generally presents with a sudden onset of acute abdominal pain. The leaking of blood and mucus can cause 'redcurrant jelly' stools.
- Post-operative adhesions and tumours: can also cause obstruction to occur.

Care management

There should be an initial assessment of vital signs, including hydration status; dehydration and subsequent electrolyte imbalance can quickly occur. A pain assessment and a record of all fluid intake and output must be maintained. Sudden onset is common and parents may be feeling shocked. This should be reflected in the care management.

Further reading

Hockenberry, M., Wilson, D., Winklestein, M., Kline, N. (2003). *Wong's Nursing care of infants and children*, 7th edn. Mosby, St Louis.
Rodgers, J. (2004). Paediatric bowel problems. *Gastrointestinal Nursing*, **2**(10), 33–9.

Theresa Pengelly, University of Worcester

Nutritional management: calculating infant feeds and energy requirements

Sufficient nutrition is required to support the infant's normal growth an development. In addition, the premature or ill infant may requir increased levels of nutrition to support the disease process.

Calculating the amount of infant feed required

Infants should ideally be given milk according to their expected weigh rather than their actual weight, although the infant's feed requiremer can be calculated on their actual weight.

The amount per kilogram body weight used to calculate feeds increase in the first week of life and decreases as the baby is introduced to weaning diet.

Amount of feed (average requirement/kg body weight/day)

Newborn	30 ml
2 days	60 ml
3 days	90 ml
4 days	120 ml
5 days	150 ml
6 days to 9 months	150 ml
>9 months	120 ml

A single feed requirement is calculated using the following equation:

Weight (kg) × Amount of feed required per kg body weight (from the table)

In practice

The precise amounts can vary between neonatal and children's practitic ners and between wards. It is vitally important, if you are concerne about the infant's ability to take or absorb the nutrition offered, to involve the local paediatric dietician and ask for a specific assessment c the infant or child's current nutritional and energy needs.

Estimating energy requirements

Measuring, monitoring, and calculating energy requirements require specific methods: calorimetry or 'doubly labelled' water. Ensuring suffi cient energy is generally assessed on the degree of weight gain an growth in response to the amount and type of feed given.

When estimating specific requirements you need to consider:
• basal metabolic rate
• thermal environment—energy is required to maintain warmth
• rate of growth

Gill Langmack, University of Nottingham

- exercise/sleep
- faecal and urinary losses.

As measurement techniques improve, estimation of the actual energy expenditure, and therefore requirements, are being refined. Currently these are:

- breast-fed infants: 56–152 kcal/kg body weight/day
- full-term infants up to 6 months old: 110–120 kcal/kg body weight/day
- by 1 year: 95–100 kcal/kg body weight/day
- premature infants: 114–180 kcal/kg body weight/day.

Further reading

Bayes, R., Campoy, C., Molina-Font, J.A. (1998). Some current controversies on nutritional requirements of full-term and pre-term newborn infants. *Early Human Development*, **53**(suppl.), S3–13.

Huband, S., Trigg, E. (ed.) (2000). *Practices in children's nursing*. Churchill Livingstone, Edinburgh.

World Health Organization Child and Adolescent health. ☒ www.who.int/child-adolescent-health/nut.htm

Gastrostomy care

Percutaneous endoscopic gastrostomy

- After insertion, clean the stoma site daily with sterile water and gauze for 1 week.
- For the next 2 weeks, clean it with cooled boiled water and gauze.
- Once the stoma site has completely healed, it can be cleaned in the bath.
- The stoma site should not be soaked in water for the first 10 days. If the child is incontinent a very shallow bath is permitted.
- Once the stoma site has healed and the fixation palate can be opened, check with manufacturer's guidelines, because early opening of the fixation device can cause peritonitis. The gastrostomy should then be rotated in a full circle and moved in and out of the stoma site by 1–2 cm on a daily basis. Once the stoma is well established this can be done on a weekly basis, to ensure the tract is kept open, and that buried bumper syndrome cannot occur.

Mic-Key button

- The button will require changing every 3–6 months. The button is kept in place by a water-filled balloon, and the water needs to be changed on a weekly basis. As the child develops, the button size will need changing.
- Children with respiratory conditions may require a shaft length of 0.5 cm longer than measured; this will aid movement when the child is coughing and prevent the balloon splitting.

Tube blockages

- Using a 50 ml syringe, draw back (aspirate) any excess fluid.
- Flush the tube with warm water, leave for 30 min, and flush again.
- Try a carbonated drink or pineapple juice. Using a 50 ml syringe, syringe the drink into the gastrostomy. Close the clamp and leave for 30 min, during which move the gastrostomy between your fingers, which will aid enzymic breakdown of the blockage. Then flush using cooled boiled water.
- If this fails, try pancreatic enzyme solution.

Overgranulation

- Use Terra-Cortril with Lyofoam. Place a pea-sized amount of Terra-Cortril on a small keyhole dressing of Lyofoam and around the base of the gastrostomy tube.
- The last resort is silver nitrate.

Infection

- Take a swab.
- If the stoma site is sticky and oozing, use Sofradex ointment; apply to the area once daily for 7 days. This line of treatment can be started before the swab results are returned.
- If the area appears generally sore, use Cavillon spray or sticks. This acts as a barrier, enabling the skin to heal.

Jayne Deaves, South Devon Healthcare NHS Trust

Candida/thrush
- Treat with a course of nystatin, both orally and topically.
- A sample of stomach aspirate should be sent for analysis.
- Once treatment is completed, change the gastrostomy if possible.

Further reading

Arrowsmith, H. (1996). Nursing management of patients receiving gastrostomy feeding. *British Journal of Nursing*, **5**, 2688.

Klein, S. *et al.* (1990). The burried bumper syndrome: a complication of percutaneous endoscopic gastrostomy. *American Journal of Gastroenterology*, **85**(4), 448–51.

Passing a short-term (PVC) NG tube

Action	Rationale

1. Assess need
 	
    Inability to achieve adequate oral intake
 	
    Gastric decompression
	Passing a NG tube is not benign. Associated complications: apnoea, bradycardia, obstructed nasal passage, tissue trauma, and infection

2. Gather supplies and wash hands
 	
    NG tube ~50% diameter of nostril
 	
    Water (lubricate tube)
 	
    Tape to secure
 	
    50 ml syringe
 	
    pH paper
 	
    Cup of water (drinking during passage may be helpful)
	Minimize risk of cross-infection; avoid unnecessary interruption in procedure

3. Explain procedure as appropriate for child's age and understanding, and parents if present	Enable self-regulatory behaviours; promote partnership with family
4. Select nostril using child preference (if appropriate) and skin integrity as a guide	Often inserted in alternating nostrils, ↓ risk of nasal trauma

5. Position appropriately
 	
    Swaddle infant ☞
 	
    Choice
 	
    Upright; if drinking
	Promote comfort

6. Measure insertion length from the end of nose to top of ear lobe to half way between the xiphisternum and naval	Pass correct tube length
7. Dip tip of NG tube in water to lubricate ●	Ease passage. ⚠ Never use oil-based lubricants
8. Insert NG tube into nostril smoothly, guiding it towards the oropharynx; ask child to slightly extend neck (if able)	Promote accurate passage through oropharynx; Never force, remove and start again
9. Once through the oropharynx (ask child to flex head) ▶▶ pass NG tube to premeasured length at nostril. Encourage child to drink or infants to suck on a pacifier to: aid passage of tube; distraction	Coughing or colour change indicates tracheal placement. ⚠ If cough or colour change: *stop* and *remove* tube immediately

Marion Aylott, University of Southampton

Contd.

10. Secure tubing. Confirm gastric placement by gently aspirating ~0.5 ml stomach contents; use 50 ml syringe	Large syringe (50 ml) creates smaller negative suction, less likely to damage mucosa
11. Test aspirate using pH paper. pH of 0–4 indicates stomach aspirate ∴ correctly positioned	pH is 86% reliable. Factors that elevate pH, e.g. histamine and antagonists H_2-receptor, antacids
If no aspirate; reposition child on left side; re-aspirate	Tube and stomach contents will pool in fundus
If no aspirate; inject a small volume of air ~3–5 ml; re-aspirate	Blows tube away from stomach lining → freeing ports → aspiration of fluid
If no aspirate; withdraw or insert NG tube a small distance (1–2 cm); re-aspirate	May not be optimally placed
If still no aspirate, report to medical staff	Doctor will consider use of chest X-ray to confirm placement. *Never* inject air and auscultate: unreliable, and associated with untoward incidents
12. Document: size, date, time of insertion, nostril used, complications, and action taken	After ~10 days PVC tubes harden → potential perforated gut
13. Always reconfirm position: before use and following coughing or vomiting	Detect displacement into oesophagus or lung

Further reading

Christensen, M. (2001). Bedside methods of determining nasogastric tube placement: a literature review. *Nursing in Critical Care*, **6**(4), 192–9.

Medicines and Healthcare Products Regulatory Agency (2004). *Enteral feeding tubes (nasogastric)* Ref. MDA/2004/026. 🖳 www.mhra.gov.uk

NHS Quality Improvement Scotland (2003). *Nasogastric and gastrostomy tube feeding for children being cared for in the community. Best Practice Statement.* NHS QIS, Edinburgh. 🖳 www.nhshealthquality.org

Enteral feeding tubes

Enteral feeding tubes enable babies/children to be fed via a tube.

NG tube

The NG tube is passed though the nostrils, down the back of the throat and via the oesophagus into the stomach. This short-term tube is made from PVC plastic and should be changed every 5–7 days. Its biggest advantages are that no surgery is required and it can be used straight away.

Disadvantages of using the NG tube:
- can cause irritation to both the nose and oesophagus
- increases mucus secretion and partially block the nasal airways
- in some babies it may decrease their sucking reflex
- it is possible to pass the tube into the trachea, delivering fluid into the lungs; this could be fatal.

Appropriate training must be given to staff and parents or carers of these children. They need to know where to get appropriate help after discharge from hospital.

Gastrostomy tube

Long-term tube made from very soft plastic which requires changing every 2–3 months. New tube should be replaced quickly to avoid stoma closing. Tube inserted surgically. The most popular choice of long-term tube is held in place by a balloon inflated by 5 ml of sterile water, which needs to be changed on a regular basis.

Caring for a child with an NG tube *in situ*

- Provide psychological support
- Maintain skin integrity
- Always wash hands before handling the tube
- Make sure the tube is securely fixed
- Flush the tube before each feed and medications
- Always check tube is correctly positioned before instilling anything in it
- Stop feed immediately if there is any sign of breathing difficulty
- Prevent bacterial contamination of feed
- Do aspirate and flush NG tube every 4 hours to check position and maintain patency

Maintaining tube patency

Small tubes are prone to obstruction. Common causes: large molecule feeds, partially digested gastric residue, and instilling crushed or hydrophilic medications.
- Flush tube before and after feeding with water.
- Flush every 4 hours if continuously fed.

Sarah Wiggins, Royal Devon and Exeter NHS Foundation Trust

Further reading

Huband, S., Trigg, E. (2002). *Practices in children's nursing, guidelines for hospital and community*. Churchill Livingstone, Edinburgh.

imby, B. (2005). Fundamental nursing skills and concepts, 8th edn. Lippincott Williams & Wilkins, Philadelphia.

www.dietetics.co.uk/article_enteral_feeding2.asp

Feeding via an NG tube

A child with an NG tube will be having close input from a dietician and a planned feeding regime.

If possible, feed the child at mealtimes, with the family so he/she gets used to it being associated with a mealtime. If appropriate, give the child some finger food or soft food that he/she can touch and taste, to help with the transition to oral feeding. Children who have NG tubes can become poor feeders, so encouragement, where possible, is important.

Equipment

- pH paper
- Disposable latex gloves
- Boiled cooled water for flushing tube
- 2 sterile gali pots
- Plastic apron

- Fluid balance chart
- 2 syringes 5–10 ml for PVC tube or 50–60 ml for polyurethane tube
- Feed at room temperature

Method

- Wash hands and put on gloves.
- Reassure child and parent, and explain what you are going to do.
- Ensure the child is in a comfortable position; head higher than stomach, preferably sitting or at 30°. Neonates—prone or on right side.
- Using the appropriate syringe, aspirate fluid from the stomach and test it using pH paper: should read <5.5 (some medications can alter the pH).
- Flush the tube to ensure patency and prime the tube.
- Apply clamp to tube.
- Attach syringe and fill barrel with feed.
- Slowly release clamp to allow feed to slowly enter the stomach.
- The higher the syringe is held above the stomach, the greater the hydrostatic pressure and the faster the liquid will flow. Administer the feed at a rate similar to the time taken to have the feed orally (15–30 min).
- Top up the barrel of the syringe as it empties, avoiding the entry of air into the system.
- When feed is complete, flush tube with water and cap off the feeding tube.
- Make the child comfortable.
- Complete the fluid balance chart.

Further reading

Huband, S., Trigg, E. (2002). *Practices in children's nursing, guidelines for hospital and community.* Churchill Livingstone, Edinburgh.

Goff, K. (1998). Enteral and parenteral nutrition—transitioning from hospital to home. *Nursing Care Management,* **3**(2), 67–74.

Mensforth, A., Spalding, D. (1998). Discharge and planning for home enteral tube feeding. *Clinical Nutrition Update,* **3**(2), 8–10.

Sarah Wiggins, Royal Devon and Exeter NHS Foundation Trust

How to change a stoma bag

What is a stoma?

- Stoma comes from the Greek word *stomoun* meaning 'opening or mouth'.
- There are various types: colostomy, ileostomy, vesicostomy[*], urostomy, and jejunostomy.
- These stomas may be created for a number of different reasons, e.g. congenital abnormality, inflammatory bowel disease, trauma, and cancer, and all usually require some form of appliance to collect the stomal waste.

Equipment required

- New appliance (stoma bag)
- Gauze/soft wipes
- Warm tap water
- Scissors
- Tie or clip if not part of the appliance
- Appropriate disposal bag or nappy sack

Further reading

Collett, K. (2002). Practical aspects of stoma management. *Nursing Standard*, **17**(8), 45–52, 54–5.
Trainor, B. *et al.* (2003). Changing an appliance. *Nursing Standard*, **18**(13), 41–2.
▣ www.convatec.com

---

[*] In an infant with a vesicostomy an appliance may not be used, because drainage directly into the nappy may be an alternative option.

Marc Crocker, Birmingham Children's Hospital

Clinical skills: procedure for changing a bag

Action	Rationale
1. Prepare all equipment prior to removal of old appliance	To ensure that a safe and efficient procedure is carried out, minimizing the child's anxiety
2. Empty contents of the bag prior to removal	To prevent spillage of contents onto child's peristomal skin
3. Peel flange away from skin, applying gentle pressure to underlying skin	To minimize trauma to the child
Optional use of non-alcohol adhesive remover wipes or spray	Aids removal of flange from peristomal skin
4. Using warm tap water clean around peristomal skin and stoma	To remove excess stomal content from skin and stoma, thus reducing risk of peristomal contact dermatitis. Removal of residue from previous flange base
5. Dry area using patting technique	Minimize skin trauma. To ensure flange adherence to skin
6. Cut flange to appropriate size to incorporate stoma. Use of stoma measuring guide will help with sizing	To ensure snug fit, protecting peristomal skin but ensuring sufficient size to minimize entrapment of stoma, causing stoma stricture
7. Apply new bag, starting at bottom edge of stoma and working in an upwards direction	Aids visualization of position of bag over stoma
8. Apply gentle pressure to flange	Maximize flange adherence to skin
9. For drainable appliances, secure bottom of bag using tie, clip, or in-built sealing device	Prevent leakage of contents
10. Retain template (backing of new bag flange)	Used as stoma-measuring guide for subsequent bag changes

Genito-urinary problems

Anatomy and physiology of the renal system

The renal system is fully developed by 36 weeks' gestation.

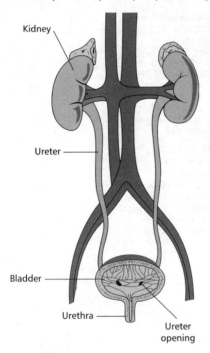

Kidney

Ureter

Bladder

Urethra

Ureter opening

The kidneys
- Consist of an outer cortex and an inner medulla.
- Urine is drained into the renal pelvis and out through the ureter into the bladder.

Andrea Macarthur, Central Manchester and Manchester Children's University Hospitals NHS Trust

Nephron
- The nephron is the functional unit of the kidney.
- 1–1.5 million nephrons are present at birth.
- Each nephron is made up of a renal corpuscle, where fluid is filtered, and a renal tubule, into which filtered fluid is passed.
- The renal corpuscle consists of a glomerulus, which is surrounded by the Bowman's capsule.
- Blood enters the glomerulus through the afferent arteriole and leaves through the efferent arteriole.
- Water and solutes filter from the blood into the renal tubule.
- The renal tubule consists of three sections: proximal convoluted tubule, loop of Henle, and distal convoluted tubule.
- Pressure is higher in the glomerular capillaries than in the renal tubules, resulting in constant filtration.
- Water and solutes are re-absorbed in the renal tubules.

Functions of the kidneys
- Excretion of waste product of metabolism, including urea, creatinine, and ammonia.
- Regulation of solutes, including sodium, potassium, chloride, calcium, phosphate, and magnesium.
- Regulation of plasma pH through hydrogen ion secretion and bicarbonate re-absorption and production.
- Regulation of blood pressure by secreting renin.
- Activation of vitamin D, which influences calcium and phosphate balance.
- Production of erythropoietin, which stimulates red blood cell production from the bone marrow.

Further reading
Bissinger, R.L. (1995). Renal physiology. Part 1: Structure and function. *Neonatal Network*, **14**, 9–19.

Nephrotic syndrome

Definition

Two types: steroid-sensitive nephrotic syndrome (SSNS), and steroid-resistant nephrotic syndrome (SRNS). SRNS cases should be referred to a paediatric nephrology centre.

Incidence

2–4 per 100 000 children aged under 16 years. 80% (SSNS) present by the age of 6 years, and boys predominate in this period (ratio, boys: girls = 3:2).

History

Peri-orbital oedema (morning) and swollen legs (evening); increasing weight gain; and 'frothy' urine.

Clinical features

- Oedema
- Proteinuria
- Hypoalbuminaemia
- Lethargy, poor appetite, and abdominal pain
- Hypovolaemia
- Transient hypertension

Investigations

- Plasma U+Es creatinine, and albumin
- Full blood count and haematocrit
- Lipid profile: cholesterol and triglycerides
- Urine for M, C&S and early morning protein: creatinine ratio

Treatment

- 20% albumin plus diuretics mid-transfusion (if clinically hypovolaemic)
- Prednisolone (tailored dose when remission induced)
- Penicillin (until oedema resolves)
- Diuretics
- No added salt in diet

Complications

- Relapses
- Medication side effects
- Arterial and venous thrombosis
- Increased infection risk (immunological dysfunction)
- Hyperlipidaemia
- Striaie (SRNS)

Outcome

- SSNS: relapses become more infrequent and the disease generally 'burns out' by 20 years of age.
- SRNS: children remain under the care of a paediatric nephrologist for treatment, which may include dialysis and transplantation.

1 Barratt, T.M. *et al.* (1994). Consensus statement on management and audit potential for steroid responsive nephrotic syndrome. *Archives of Disease in Childhood*, **70**, 151–7.
2 Hodson, E.M. *et al.* (2005). Corticosteroid therapy for nephrotic syndrome in children. *Cochrane Database of Systematic Reviews*, Issue 1.

Maggie Randall, Southampton University Hospitals NHS Trust

Chronic renal failure

Definition

Chronic renal failure is a continuous irreversible process, extending from mild renal impairment to end-stage disease, which requires renal replacement therapy.

It is represented by a glomerular filtration rate of <75 ml/min/1.73 m compared with <10 ml/min/1.73 m^2 in end-stage renal failure.

Incidence

It affects 53 per million of the child population.

Causes

- Congenital abnormalities:
  - renal dysplasia
  - reflux nephropathy
  - obstructive uropathy
- Hereditary conditions:
  - congenital nephrotic syndrome
  - polycystic kidney disease—autosommal recessive
  - cystinosis
- Glomerulonephritis:
  - focal segmental glomerulosclerosis
- Systemic disease:
  - lupus erythematosus
  - Henoch–Schönlein purpura
  - haemolytic uraemic syndrome
- Miscellaneous:
  - renal vascular disease
  - kidney tumour

Clinical features

Children present in a number of ways relating to the primary disease or as a consequence of deteriorating function. These features include:

- anorexia and lethargy
- poor growth
- hypertension
- peripheral oedema
- renal osteodystrophy
- haematuria
- urinary tract infection

Management

Good management is achieved via a multidisciplinary team approach aiming to:

- prevent symptoms, i.e. nausea and vomiting
- promote normal growth and development
- preserve residual renal function
- prepare family unit for renal-replacement therapy, i.e. dialysis and transplantation

Ruth Underhill, Southampton University Hospitals NHS Trust

Key management points for nursing awareness

Nutrition
Calorific supplementation is necessary to meet the child's estimated average requirements for age, i.e. glucose polymers and/or fat emulsifiers via oral, NG, or gastrostomy route. Regular dietetic review is required to monitor progress.

Anaemia
Inadequate erythropoietin production leads to renal anaemia. Regular subcutaneous injections of recombinant human erythropoietin can be administered in conjunction with iron and folate supplements to improve child's haemoglobin levels.

Fluid and electrolyte balance
Some children pass large urine volumes secondary to high urinary sodium losses. Salt supplementation, as well as extra water intake to control thirst, is a necessary measure.

Acid–base balance
Metabolic acidosis can be a problem when bicarbonate ions are no longer regenerated in renal failure. Sodium bicarbonate is a suitable replacement therapy.

Renal osteodystrophy
Good dietetic control of phosphate and adequate patient adherence to phosphate binders and vitamin D supplements help keep renal bone disease at bay.

Hypertension
Administration of antihypertensives and diuretics in combination with reduced dietary salt intake lead to better blood pressure control.

Infection
Antibiotic prophylaxis is necessary for renal tract abnormalities.

Education and preparation
Renal failure requires an ongoing programme of education for children and their families to best prepare them for renal-replacement therapy in whatever form it may take.

Psychosocial support
Chronic illness disrupts normal family living. Support comes in many guises. Renal social workers and psychologists are essential members of the multidisciplinary team.

Further reading
Ramage, I.J. et al. (2003). Principles of management in chronic renal failure. *Current Paediatrics*, **13**, 496–501.

Shaw, V. (1999). Nutritional management of renal disease. *Paediatric Nursing*, **11**(4), 37–43.

Acute renal failure

Acute renal failure is a sudden decline in kidney function, which results a build up of nitrogenous waste products in the blood and an inability t regulate fluid, electrolyte, and acid–base balance. It is potentially reve sible and can present with or without oliguria.

Incidence

It is estimated that each year 7.5 cases per million children are diagnose in the UK.

Causes

Pre-renal failure (reduced blood flow to kidney)

Hypovolaemia:	dehydration
	gastrointestinal losses
	burns
	haemorrhage
Third-space losses:	sepsis
	nephrotic syndrome
Circulatory failure:	congestive cardiac failure
	cardiac tamponade

Intrinsic renal failure (structural damage to glomeruli, vessels, and/or tubules)

Tubular:	acute tubular necrosis
	drug/toxin injury
Interstitial:	interstitial nephritis
	drug-induced
Vascular:	haemolytic uraemic syndrome
	vasculitis
	renal artery stenosis
Glomerulonephritis:	systemic lupus erythematosus

Post-renal failure (obstruction to urine flow)

- Obstruction of solitary kidney
- Bilateral ureteric obstuction
- Urethral obstruction, i.e. clot or stones
- Posterior urethral valves

Extensive patient assessment is required to determine the severity and cause of renal failure

- History: onset of complaint, drug history, past medical history, and family history
- Physical examination:
  - cardiovascular, respiratory, and neurological assessment
  - height and weight recording
  - hydration status

Ruth Underhill, Southampton University Hospitals NHS Trust

- presence of rashes or swollen joints
- physical evidence of palpable kidneys, bladder, or any masses

Blood picture: biochemistry, haematology, coagulation, immunology, and microbiology profiles

Urine investigations: urinalysis, urinary electrolytes, and microscopy

Other diagnostic tests: chest X-ray, renal ultrasound, ECG, echocardiogram, and renal biopsy

Treatment

Close attention to fluid balance, monitoring electrolytes, and blood pressure.

Dietetic involvement is crucial because patients are catabolic.

Some patients managed conservatively, i.e. without dialysis; hence there is greater emphasis on strict fluid balance.

Renal-replacement therapy in the form of peritoneal dialysis, haemodialysis, or haemofiltration. Indications for dialysis:

- hyperkalaemia.
- fluid overload.
- metabolic disturbances.
- remove nephrotoxic poisons.
- facilitate space for nutrition.

Surgical intervention may be necessary if the renal failure is post-renal in nature.

Nursing management

Continuous monitoring of cardiovascular, respiratory status, and peripheral perfusion

Monitor neurological function (if indicated); neurological assessment recorded on age-appropriate GCS.

Fluid balance:

- accurately record all fluid input and output
- support and education in adherence to fluid allowance
- weigh daily.

Nutrition:

- care of parenteral or enteral nutrition
- provide educational support regarding dietary restrictions.

Prevention of infection:

- care of dialysis access, post-operative wounds or drains
- monitor for signs of sepsis
- antibiotic administration (if indicated).

Reduce anxiety. Provide:

- educational support to child and family
- clear explanations of procedures to be performed
- appropriate environment for child to rest.

Further reading

Philips, A.S. (1999). Management of acute renal failure. In *Paediatric nephrology*, 4th edn, (ed. T.M. Barratt et al.), pp. 1119–33. Lippincott, Williams & Wilkins, Baltimore.

Proesmans, W. (2002). Acute renal failure in childhood. *ETDNA ERCA Journal*, suppl 2, 26–9.

Vesico-ureteral reflux (VUR)

Introduction

VUR is defined as the back-flow of urine from the bladder up the ureter to the kidney. The back-flow of urine is caused by a structural defect in the ureter, which is not long enough and allows urine to flow back towards the kidney every time the bladder contracts. It is a risk factor for progressive renal damage associated with persistent and repeated urinary tract infections (UTIs). VUR affects 1% of infants and up to one-third of children who have repeated UTIs. It is usually diagnosed between 2 years and 3 years of age. VUR is a genetic disorder and familial VUR is common.

Clinical manifestations

The child may present with any of the following:
- persistent and repeated UTIs
- enuresis
- flank pain
- abdominal pain.

Investigations

Young children and infants warrant intensive investigation of UTI because younger children are at a higher risk of developing renal damage in later years. Both child and family require constant information and explanations regarding the necessity for the investigations and the subsequent results obtained. These investigations include:
- abdominal X-ray
- DMSA scan
- micturating cysto-urethogram (MCU)
- renal ultrasound.

Treatment

There are two pathways: (1) medical, which focuses on the prevention of UTIs and renal damage, with the administration of prophylactic anti-biotics, and (2) surgical, which may be considered the last option and involves re-implantation or reconstruction of the ureters so that they are of sufficient length to prevent the reflux from occurring.

Nursing management

The use of prophylactic antibiotics may continue for years, and nursing management involves education and support of the child and family. Educational points should include:
- monitoring the child for signs of UTI, e.g. foul smelling and concentrated urine, ↑ temperature, and abdominal pain
- administration, dosage, and duration of antibiotics and the importance of compliance
- maintaining adequate fluid intake
- administration of anticholinergics (if appropriate) to decrease bladder pressure

Susie Barnes, Queen's University Belfast

how to collect a urine sample to ensure prompt attention if UTI presents

where and when to ring for sensitivities of a urine culture and how to ask whether the child is on the appropriate antibiotic

what investigations are planned and what follow-up care may be required.

Information and education of families is of the utmost importance, because they need to feel secure in looking after their child. It is important to encourage compliance with their child's medication and management.

Further reading

Potts, N.L., and Mandleco, B.L. (ed.) (2002). *Paediatric nursing. Caring for children and their families.* Delmar Thomson Learning, Clifton Park, NY.

www.kidney.org

Acute glomerulonephritis (AGN)

Introduction

AGN is an acute or sudden inflammation of the glomeruli in the kidney leading to deterioration in renal function, resulting in sodium and water retention. The cause is usually an infectious agent, bacterial or viral (the most common organism is streptococcus). This initiates an immune response within the child. This antibody–antigen reaction leads to the laying down of immune complexes within the renal glomeruli, resulting in gross inflammation. The inflammatory process alters the permeability of the glomerular basement membrane (GBM) or the 'sieving part' of the glomerulus, resulting in protein 'leaking' into the urine.

Clinical manifestations

The child may present with some of the following.

- Haematuria (glomeruli inflamed and red blood cells leak into the urine); urine is described as being 'tea-like' in colour or smoky.
- Proteinuria (glomeruli inflamed and protein leaks into the urine).
- Dependent and peri-orbital oedema (retention of sodium = retention of water).
- Decreased urinary output as renal damage progresses and glomerular filtration rate falls.
- Fatigue.
- Hypertension (not all cases).
- Disturbed electrolyte levels: increased serum sodium, increased serum potassium, and increased creatinine; dependent on the level of renal damage.

Susie Barnes, Queen's University Belfast

Investigations

- White blood cell count, including differential
- Serum complement (C3)
- Streptozyme assay (positive if that infection is present)
- Culture (throat)

- Urinalysis (protein and/or red blood cells)
- Renal function (GFR/U&Es)
- Quantify proteinuria
- Auto-antibody screen

Treatment

Focuses on:
- identifying infectious agent
- ↓ oedema (maintain fluid balance status)
- maintain electrolyte levels
- maintain blood pressure.

This is a stressful time; the nurse has a vital role in terms of providing continuous relevant information to both child and family regarding the various investigations, results, and subsequent management.

Nursing management

Fluid overload	Hypertension	Electrolyte imbalances
Daily weight (same time)	Monitor blood pressure regularly	Monitor U&Es
Assess for dependent oedema and peri-orbital oedema	Administer antihypertensives if appropriate	Restrict sodium/potassium diet if appropriate
Input–output balance		
Assess skin integrity/meticulous hygiene		
Careful positioning/elevation of legs		

The child and family will need continuing health education on issues such as signs of oedema, skin integrity, and the need for cleanliness, to encourage empowerment. A multiprofessional approach is important, with the play specialist having a key role. The nurse can assist the play specialist in developing periods of distraction and play activities interspersed with rest, because the child will tire easily.

Further reading

Potts, N.L., Mandleco, B.L. (ed.) (2002). Paediatric nursing. Caring for children and their families. Delmar Thomson Learning, Clifton Park, NY.

www.gosh.nhs.uk/factsheets/families (look under 'K' for 'kidney')

Haemolytic uraemic syndrome (HUS)

Epidemiology

HUS is the most common cause of acute renal failure in infants and children in Britain, with an average annual incidence of 0.71 per 100 000. It occurs mostly in children under 5 years of age, with female predominance and peak occurrence in spring and summer.

Referral to a paediatric nephrology centre is appropriate.

There are two subgroups: epidemic and sporadic

Epidemic/typical	Sporadic/atypical
Younger children	Very young or older children
Preceded by gastric illness	Preceded by upper respiratory tract infection
Good prognosis	Poorer outcome, frequent relapses

Causes

- Undercooked meat, dairy products, and visits to livestock farms
- E.coli 157: H7, *Shigella* spp, and *S. pneumoniae*

History

- Bloody diarrhoeal illness (90% of cases) for 1–15 days, with abdominal pain, cramping, vomiting, and pyrexia
- Haematuria
- Lethargy, pallor, and irritability
- Oliguria (lasting >1 week in 60% of cases)

Clinical features

A multisystem disease characterized by a classical triad of symptoms:
- haemolytic anaemia
- thrombocytopaenia
- acute renal failure.

CNS involvement (30% of cases): altered consciousness, tone and movement, and seizures.

Investigations

- Plasma U+Es, creatinine, bone profile, and liver function
- Full blood count, blood film, and clotting studies
- Blood cultures
- Urine for M, C&S
- Stool for M, C&S and virology
- Ultrasound scan for kidney size and gastric involvement
- CT scan and EEG if cerebral oedema/infarctions suspected

Diagnosis

- E. coli 157: H7 stool culture
- Burr-shaped red cells on microscopy film

Maggie Randall, Southampton University Hospitals NHS Trust

Treatment

Supportive
Blood and platelet transfusions
Fluid balance
Electrolyte monitoring
Dietary/total parenteral nutrition (catabolic state)
Early dialysis (improved outcome)

Outcome

5% acute mortality
5% end-stage renal failure
10% residual hypertension (renal scarring)
Recurrence rare
Severe acute disease and prolonged anuria associated with
worse prognosis

Follow-up

Annual blood pressure, urinalysis, and plasma creatinine need to be
reviewed for 5 years by a paediatric nephrologist.

Further reading

ynn, R.M. et al. (2005). Childhood hemolytic uremic syndrome, United Kingdom and Ireland. *Emerging Infectious Diseases*, **11**(4), 590–6.

egler, R. et al. (2005). Hemolytic uremic syndrome: pathogenesis, treatment and outcome. *Current Opinion in Pediatrics*, **17**(2), 200–4.

Circumcision

A circumcision is an operation to remove the foreskin of the penis. Th
involves tearing the foreskin away from the glans (head) of the penis, ar
cutting the foreskin off, leaving the end behind. The amount of foreski
remaining can vary.

A circumcision would be carried out for religious or medical reasons, th
latter being chronic phimosis, posthitis, paraphimosis, or balanitis xerotic
obliterans.

- Chronic phimosis: the opening of the foreskin narrows so that it
  cannot be retracted. This may result from scarring and thickening by
  repeated attacks of posthitis. It is also a normal condition in young
  children, as the foreskin may not completely separate from the glans
  until the child is 4 years old or more. If it persists, it can be difficult for
  the child to pass urine. The foreskin may seem to balloon out when
  the child urinates, and infection may occur.
- Posthitis: inflammation of the foreskin and the glans. It is usually mild
  and self-limiting, but with repeated attacks the foreskin becomes
  narrowed and scarred, leading to impossible retraction. Caused by
  thrush, streptococci, herpes, human papilloma virus, Chlamydia, and
  other harmful organisms.
- Paraphimosis: this occurs when a tight foreskin is retracted behind the
  head of the penis but then cannot be replaced.
- Balanitis xerotica obliterans: irritation, discomfort, and eventually
  shrinkage of the tissues. Adhesions form between the foreskin and the
  glans. The condition arises in both childhood and adult life, and is
  completely cured by circumcision.

Aftercare

- Give regular pain relief and encourage the child to take fluids.
- He will be able to go home once he has passed urine, which may be
  uncomfortable and frightening at first.
- The penis will be sore, bruised, and inflamed for a few days.
- The child can have a bath 24–48 hours after circumcision.
- The dissolvable stitches will take up to 3 weeks to dissolve and the
  penis will take up to 6 weeks to heal fully.
- The child will need to wear loose clothing.
- He should remain off school until comfortable.

Problems that may occur at home

- Bleeding, requiring 20 min firm pressure to stop. Contact GP
  if it continues.
- Swelling and crusting, requiring regular baths.
- Infection, requires the attention of the GP.
- Penile adhesion: requires regular retraction for 2 weeks after
  the operation.

Layla Price, Royal Devon and Exeter NHS Foundation Trust

urther reading

ofVander, Y. (2002). Circumcision in boys. *World Hospitals and Health Services*, **38**, 215–17.
Caffey, M. (2002). Circumcision: Is a local anesthetic appropriate? *Nursing*, **32**, 24.
Great Ormond Street. www.aoswers.com/circumcision
Circumcision information and resource pages. www.ciro.org

Renal transplantation in children

Renal transplantation is the treatment of choice for children with faili
kidney function. Ideally this should be performed before the child reach
end-stage renal failure, avoiding the need for dialysis. Organs for rer
transplantation in children are usually retrieved from either cadaveric
living related kidney donors. The advances in laparoscopic surgery hav
revolutionized the living related donor (LRD) transplant programme
significantly reducing the donor's potential for complications and lengt
of stay in hospital.

Cause of renal dysfunction

Renal insufficiency in children is often associated with a congenit
malformation or associated syndrome:

- Malformations: aplastic, hypoplastic, and dysplastic kidneys
- obstructive uropathy/PUV/reflux
- polycystic kidney disease
- Alport's syndrome
- Prune belly syndrome and Vater's syndrome
- Wilms' tumour
- congenital nephrotic syndrome
- focal segmental glomerulosclerosis.

Transplantation in children is both technically and physiological
challenging. The prevention of a major physiological disturbance relate
to fluid and electrolyte imbalance is paramount. A strict fluid
replacement protocol should be followed.

A child receiving an adult kidney may excrete a volume of urine ever
hour that approximates the total blood volume; a small error i
replacement therapy may create a potentially lethal imbalance. If kidney
are lost within a few weeks of transplantation, this is usually due to vas
cular events or recurrence of the original disease.

Post-renal transplant fluids

	Fluid	Rate
Maintenance	0.45% sodium chloride/2.5% glucose (insensible losses at 400 ml/m² /24 hours)	Insensible losses + previous hour's urine output
Bolus fluids: if CVP falls below 7 mmHg and poor perfusion	4.5% albumin 5–10 ml/kg body weight	ml over 30 min
Bolus fluids: if CVP falls below 7 mmHg	0.9% sodium chloride 5–10 ml/kg body weight	ml over 30 min

The age of the recipient is a significant prognostic factor for both LRD
and cadaveric donor grafts. The 1 year graft survival rates for LRD
recipients improve with age.

Eileen Brennan, Great Ormond Street Hospital for Children NHS Trust

Age	Cadaveric	LRD
0–1	49%	77%
2–5	65%	83%
>6	70%	86%

Estimated transplant survival in years		
Years	Cadaveric	LRD
1	86%	95%
5	76%	81%
10	56%	58%

Selection of immunosuppressive therapy

Cyclosporin/prednisolone/azathioprine
Tacrolimus/prednisolone/azathioprine
Tacrolimus/prednisolone/mycophenolate
± Basiliximab
± Serolimus

The long-term risks of immunosuppression medication are cytomegalovirus and Epstein–Barr virus which are associated with lymphoproliferative disease and other malignancies. After transplant, one of the most serious problems, especially in the adolescent age group, is non-compliance. This may result in graft loss or dysfunction; this age group often express concern about their outer appearance, e.g. facial oedema, obesity, acne, and short stature.

Further reading

Webb, N.J., Johnson, R., Postlewaite, R.J. (2003). Renal transplantation. *Archives of Disease in Childhood*, **88**, 844–7.
Royal College of Physicians (2002). *Fourth Annual Report of the UK Renal Registry*. Royal College of Physicians, London.
www.nelh.nhs.uk/nsf
www.nice.org.uk

Ethical issues in the live donation of organs/tissue by children

- Beneficence
- Non-maleficence
- Fidelity (trust)
- Justice
- Veracity (truth)
- Confidentiality
- Autonomy

In the sphere of organ donation, the principles of beneficence, non maleficence, justice, and autonomy are the overriding themes.

There are two types of organ/tissue donation: cadaver (dead) and living.

The legalities of live donation

In British law, no person is deemed capable of consenting to being killed or seriously injured. Donation by living donors is therefore effectively restricted to the donation of kidneys, liver segments, lung lobes, blood and bone marrow. Because it is possible to assess the risks and benefits of a given procedure, the common law legality of live *adult* organ donation is settled; consent to a surgical procedure that is, in itself, non therapeutic will be valid so long as the consequent infliction of injury can be shown not to be against the public interest.

With regard to children, any medical intervention must be believed to be in the child's best interests.

The function of ethics

There is a controversy over whether the function of ethics in the sphere of paediatrics is to assure children of their right to participate in activities or protect them against the risks of doing so.

Relevant ethical principles

Beneficence

The beneficence requirement may or may not discount live donation by minors, depending on one's accepted definition of 'benefit'. In some instances, the good of society may be considered sufficient, providing the second principle of non-maleficence is applied.

Autonomy

Autonomy in children may automatically be compromised by virtue of their limited understanding and societal status. However, mature minors are allowed to make decisions regarding other aspects of treatment, and a decision not to allow children to provide organs and tissue may conflict with the principle of justice.

Justice

As the long-term physical effects of live donation are unknown and the psychological effects difficult to quantify, it may appear logical to prevent minors from donating any form of organ or tissue until they reach the

Paula Flint, Central Manchester and Manchester Children's University Hospitals NHS Trust chronological age of majority. However, preventing children from donating underestimates the sense of achievement they may feel in the future, and perhaps children should not be deprived of the right to contribute to the good of others.

Obligations and altruism

The Law Commission (1995) confirms that courts have created a more expansive concept of the best-interests test to include social interests. Children are part of larger communities and have some limited obligations to be altruistic to their community. However, if societal interests are allowed to take precedence, a risk–benefit approach here could place the minor donor in jeopardy in the face of the recipient's need.

Conclusion

- Whether the harvesting of organs and tissue from minors is ethically acceptable depends on the accepted overriding ethical principle.
- Whether non-maleficence equals 'zero' or 'minimal' physical risk is not clear, yet this is of paramount importance to the ethics of a procedure which does not intend physical benefit to the donor.

Further reading

Kopelman, L.M. (1989). When is the risk minimal enough for children to be research subjects? In *Children and Healthcare* (ed. L.M. Kopelman and J.C. Moskop), p. 221. Kluwer Academic, Dordrecht.

Mason, J.K., McCall Smith, R.A., and Laurie, G.T. (2003). *Law and medical ethics*, p. 428. LexisNexis, London.

Veatch, R. (2000). *Transplantation ethics*. Georgetown University Press, Washington, DC.

Suprapubic urinalysis

Action	Rationale
1. Assess need: clean urine to ascertain infection	Taking a suprapubic urine specimen is not benign. Associated complications: pain, risk of infection, and tissue trauma. Performed when a urine sample is required to identify infection quickly, prior to starting antibiotics
	When the baby has thrush, vulvovaginitis urethritis, or balanitis and a specimen would be contaminated if taken from a bag or pad
2. Gather supplies and wash hands Sterile dressing pack 5 ml syringe 23 FG (blue) needle Skin preparation for disinfection Sterile urine container Spot plaster	Prevent cross-infection. Avoid unnecessary interruption in procedure
3. Explain procedure to parents, and obtain verbal consent. Explain risks and the need to obtain a clean urine specimen	Enable self-regulatory behaviours. Promote partnership with family
4. Clean the area of skin around the midline of the pubic bone	To prevent infecting the urine with flora and fauna from the skin
5. Position appropriately, swaddle infant, holding the legs firmly out straight so that the pelvis does not move	Promote comfort. Reduce the risk of trauma and to prevent needlestick injury
6. The doctor's needle should pass through the abdominal wall at a point that is about 0.5–1 cm above the pubic bone. The blue needle is connected to the 5 ml syringe and is aspirated as it is advanced to a depth of around 5 mm. A flash of urine will indicate the entry to the bladder. If no urine is aspirated at this depth the needle should be withdrawn while still aspirating. Apply a plaster after removal of the needle	NB: If an assistant gets ready with a sterile pot the stimuli of cleaning the skin often precipitates micturition and a clean catch may become available!
7. Document amount, date, time of procedure, and action taken	Observe child's urine after the procedure for evidence of trauma. Microscopic haematuria is frequent. Macroscopic haematuria soon resolves

Sarah Hayward, Royal Devon and Exeter Hospital NHS Foundation Trust

Further reading

Huband, S., (ed) Trigg, E. (2000). *Practices in children's nursing: guidelines for hospital and community.* Churchill Livingstone, Edinburgh.

Clean catch urine

Action	Rationale
1. Assess need: clean urine to ascertain infection	Taking a urine specimen is benign
2. Gather supplies and wash hands Sterile collecting vessel Syringe 5 ml or 10 ml Skin cleanser: usually 0.9% saline with cotton wool wipes Sterile urine container	Prevent cross-infection. Avoid unnecessary interruption in procedure
3. Explain procedure to parents and child. Explain the need to obtain a clean urine specimen. Explain the need to collect the urine as a mid-stream, i.e. not the first flow of urine becasue this will contain flora and fauna from the urethral passage	Enable self-regulatory behaviours. Promote partnership with family
4. Clean the area of skin around the urethral opening. Explain to the child how to clean his or her own body, or explain to parents how to help	To prevent infecting the urine with flora and fauna from the skin
5. Ensure privacy and assistance where required	Promote comfort and dignity
6. Transfer the urine specimen aseptically to the urine container, using the sterile syringe. Ensure the specimen is labelled correctly and sent to the laboratory with the correct form	To ensure accuracy of specimen. To ensure the specimen gets to the laboratory to be analysed
7. Document: amount, date, time of procedure, and action taken	

Further reading

Glasper, A,. Richardson, J. (2005). *A textbook of children's and young people's nursing.* Elsevier, Edinburgh.

Sarah Hayward, Royal Devon and Exeter Hospital NHS Foundation Trust

Clean catch urine from a baby

Action	Rationale
1. Assess need: clean urine to ascertain infection	Taking a urine specimen is benign
2. Gather supplies and wash hands Sterile collecting vessel Syringe 5 mL or 10 mL Skin cleanser: usually 0.9% saline with cotton wool wipes Sterile urine container	Prevent cross-infection. Avoid unnecessary interruption in procedure
3. Explain procedure to parents. Explain the need to obtain a clean urine specimen. Explain the need to collect the urine as a mid-stream, i.e. not the first flow of urine because this will contain flora and fauna from the urethral passage	Enable self-regulatory behaviours. Promote partnership with family.
4. Clean the area of skin around the urethral opening or explain to parents how to help	To prevent infecting the urine with flora and fauna from the skin
5. Ensure privacy and assistance where required	Promote comfort and dignity
6. Parents can often keep a vigil with an open sterile container and catch a specimen as the child is in mid-flow	
7. A urine bag may be used on cleansed skin	
8. Also wipe the base of the bag prior to aspirating with aseptic technique, using a needle to obtain the urine and place in a sterile urine collection pot	
9. Alternatively a collection pad placed inside a nappy will collect urine which can then be aspirated from the pad (using a sterile syringe and no needle) and placed into a sterile urine pot	
10. Transfer the urine specimen aseptically to the urine container using the sterile syringe. Ensure the specimen is labelled correctly and sent to the laboratory with the correct form and details of how it was obtained	To ensure accuracy of specimen. To ensure the specimen gets to the laboratory to be analysed
11. Document amount, date, time of procedure, and action taken	

Sarah Hayward, Royal Devon and Exeter Hospital NHS Foundation Trust

Further reading

Whaley, L.F., Wong, D.L., Hockenberry, M.J. (2005). *Wong's Nursing care of infants and children.* Mosby, London.

Normal composition of urine

Substance	Normal value in urine	Presence may indicate	Appearance
Urine	96% water, 2% urea, 2% uric acid, creatinine, phosphates, sulphates, oxalates, and chlorides		Urine is amber coloured, and is acid in reaction. A healthy well-hydrated child should pass between 1 and 2 ml of urine/kg of body weight
pH	pH 4–8. The wide range reflects diet and the role of the kidney in acid–base balance	Alkaline urine may indicate an infection. Some bacteria contain the enzyme urease, which causes urea molecules in urine to split, releasing ammonia. This causes a nasty smell and an alkaline pH	
Blood/ erythrocytes	Not normally present in urine (on dipstick)	Haematuria may be due to trauma or impact, renal stones, post-catheterization, inflammation of the mucosal lining. Some chemotherapy irritates the bladder mucosa	Colour ranges between a pink tinge and dark red
Haemoglobin	Not normally present in urine (on dipstick)	Haematuria may be the result of severe burns, haemolytic uraemic syndrome, transfusion reactions, Henoch's purpura	Dusky tea-coloured, Coca Cola coloured
Protein	Not normally present in urine (on dipstick)	May indicate urinary tract infection, or a protein-losing condition, e.g. nephrotic syndrome, glomerular nephritis, heart failure, severe hypertension, pregnancy, or high protein diets	Frothy
Leucocytes	Not normally present in urine on dipstick	May indicate pyuria or infection	

Sarah Hayward, Royal Devon and Exeter Hospital NHS Foundation Trust

Contd.

Glucose	Not normally present on dipstick (not normally more than 0.28 mmol/l)	May indicate stress, diabetes mellitus, steroid therapy, renal problems	
Mucus	Not normally present in urine	May indicate a previous bladder augmentation or infection	Stringy egg-white strands mixed in the urine, sometimes cloudy
Crystals or deposits	Not normally present in urine	May indicate infection or renal disease. Chemical analysis needed to define problem	
Nitrites	Not normally present in urine (on dipstick)	May indicate infection	
Bilirubin	Not normally present in urine	May indicate liver disease or jaundice	May be dark-orange colour
Colour other than straw coloured	Urine normally straw coloured	May indicate the use of some medicines	Rifampicin colours urine orange; methyl blue colours urine blue
Specific gravity	Normal range between 1020 and 1030	Variations will indicate overall hydration of the child	Pale water-like urine indicates dilute urine. More concentrated urine appears darker in colour

Normal blood values

Electrolyte	Chemical sign	Normal value in venous blood	Potential problem if too high	Potential problem if too low	Source/excretion
Creatinine (Cr)		0–60 mmol/l African–Caribbean and very muscular children have higher values. Creatinine is a product of metabolism. Creatinine can be mathematically estimated using the patient's height	Creatinine is usually seen as a marker of renal function. A creatinine of 1200 mmol/l would not be a problem in a child. However, with a raised creatinine level the child would usually have other electrolyte imbalances, and these will be physiologically significant	No problem	Creatinine is derived from the breakdown of creatinine phosphate in muscle, by catabolism. It is excreted by the kidneys
Phosphate	PO_4	0.8–1.4 mmol/l Phosphate is important for healthy bones and teeth. A feedback mechanism governed by the parathyroid hormone prevents demineralization of bone			PO_4 is ingested in diet, e.g. dairy foods. Milk, cheese, yogurt, and chocolate are high in PO_4. Excreted by the kidney or ingested, if eaten with PO_4 binders, e.g. aluminium hydroxide or calcium carbonate, will bind with the phosphate and be passed out of the gut, in stool
Sodium	Na^+	135–145 mmol/l Na^+ is an essential requirement for the 'Na⁺–K⁺' pump which is a mechanism providing energy for cell and brain development. Na^+ blood levels have an impact on the extracellular fluid in the body. Angiotensin–renin mechanism allows Na^+ to be re-absorbed in the kidneys in order to maintain blood pressure	Hypernatraemia may indicate dehydration and hypovolaemia	Hyponatraemia may indicate a hypervolaemic or waterlogged over-loaded child	Ingested. Excreted by the kidneys. Lost in sweat

Sarah Hayward, Royal Devon and Exeter Hospital NHS Foundation Trust

Potassium K⁺	3.5–4.5 mmol/l. K⁺ is essential for muscle contraction	Hyperkalaemia is dangerous. Arrhythmias may occur and cardiac arrest	Ingested in food. Bananas strawberries, chips, and chocolate are high in K. Excreted by kidneys. Also is lost through diarrhoea, stoma losses, and vomiting. Iatrogenic causes of low K are IV fluid supplements, without K additives. Excessive use of diuretics. Insulin infusions: insulin causes cells to increase their uptake of K into cells. Hyperkalaemia occurs with insulin deficiency, e.g. DKA, burns, and any condition where there is cell damage, e.g. tumour lysis
		Hypokalaemia can cause dysrhythmias	
Urea	2.5–4.5 mmol/l End product of metabolism, produced by the liver	Hyperuraemia will indicate the child has begun to metabolize his/her own body reserves due to poor nutritional intake or reflect renal failure. High urea levels may give the child nausea, vomiting, anorexia, lethargy, confusion, and itchiness. Very high levels will result in siezures, clotting deficiencies, and coma	Excreted by the kidneys
		Hypouraemia has little or no significance to the child	

Principles of haemodialysis

Haemodialysis is indicated when the child's renal function can no longer regulate electrolytes and/or fluid levels. It is a treatment that is carried out at least three times weekly in hospital, thus disrupting both the child's and family's daily living. Chronic illness will affect the physical, psychosocial, and cognitive development of the child, and this cannot be underestimated. Both child and family will need continuous guidance and support.

Definition

Haemodialysis is a term used to describe the removal of solutes and water from the blood across a semipermeable membrane (dialyser). It involves the use of three transport mechanisms.

- Diffusion: the movement of solutes from an area of higher solute concentration to an area of lower solute concentration through a semipermeable membrane. Here, a concentration gradient is essential, and is provided by the dialysate. This is a fluid delivered to the dialyser on the opposite side to the blood. It contains essential solutes in similar concentrations to normal blood and no waste products.
- Osmosis: the movement of water from an area of higher water concentration to an area of lower water concentration through a semipermeable membrane. Excess water is also removed by a process called ultrafiltration, which is controlled and set on the haemodialysis machine.
- Convection: the movement of solutes with water flow, also known as 'solvent drag'.

Susie Barnes, Queen's University Belfast

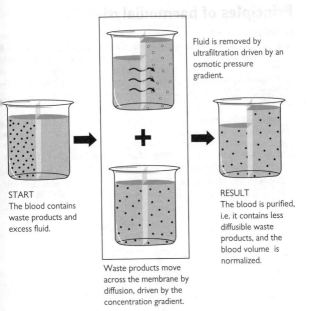

Fluid is removed by ultrafiltration driven by an osmotic pressure gradient.

START
The blood contains waste products and excess fluid.

RESULT
The blood is purified, i.e. it contains less diffusible waste products, and the blood volume is normalized.

Waste products move across the membrane by diffusion, driven by the concentration gradient.

Principles of peritoneal dialysis

Definition

Peritoneal dialysis involves the transport of solutes and water across a semipermeable membrane (in this case, it is the child's peritoneum) which separates two fluid-containing compartments: blood in the peritoneal capillaries and dialysate. The same transport mechanisms that are employed in haemodialysis are used here, i.e. diffusion, osmosis, and convection.

The child instils dialysate solution via a catheter, which is placed in the peritoneum. It remains there for approximately 4 hours, the glucose drawing in excess water and the electrolytes diffusing from the child's capillary system into the dialysate. After 4 hours, the child drains the 'dirty' dialysate into the toilet and begins the process over again.

Exchange times tend to be 8 a.m., 12 p.m. midday, 6 p.m. and just before night-time, although they can be altered to fit in with the child's daily routine.

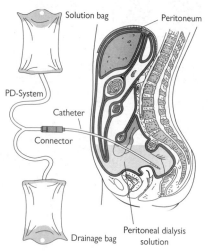

Principle of peritoneal dialysis

Susie Barnes, Queen's University Belfast

Reproductive problems

Male reproductive system

The male has reproductive structures both inside and outside the pelvis.

The external genitalia consist of the scrotum, which encloses the testes and the penis, an erectile organ through which the distal portion of the urethra passes.

The internal genitalia consist of the testes, which produce the reproductive cells, the spermatozoa. These leave the testes and travel within the epididymis, the ductus deferens, the ejaculatory duct, and the urethra before leaving the body. The seminal vesicles, the prostate gland, and the bulbourethral glands secrete into the ejaculatory ducts and the urethra.

Function

To produce and release semen into the female reproductive system and also produce sex hormones that will eventually result in puberty, maturity, and libido.

Conditions related to the male reproductive system

- Testicular trauma: results in acute pain, e.g. when torsion takes place and a testicle twists around.
- Varicocele: varicose vein in the network of veins that run from the testicle; commonly develops boys in at puberty. Not usually harmful but may result in reduced sperm production.
- Testicular cancer: most common cancer in men under 40 years of age. Can spread to other parts of the body but the cure rate is excellent with early detection.
- Epididymitis: inflammation of the epididymis usually caused by infection
- Hydrocoele: collection of fluid in the membranes around the testis. Although this causes swelling, it is usually painless.
- Inguinal hernia: a portion of the intestines pushes through the abdominal wall at a weak point and into the groin or scrotum.

Disorders of the penis

- Inflammation: redness, itching, swelling, and pain.
- Balanitis: swelling of the glans.
- Prosthitis: inflammation of the foreskin. Bacterial or yeast infections.
- Hypospadias: urethra opens on the underside of the penis not the tip.
- Phimosis: tightness of the foreskin.
- Paraphimosis: penis retracted, blood flow to the penis impaired. The child may experience pain and swelling.
- Micropenis: penis has normal form but is well below average size.
- Ambiguous genitalia: not clearly male or female. In boys, very small penis but testicles present.

Further reading

🔲 www.patient.co.uk/showdoc21692440

John Bastin, University of Plymouth

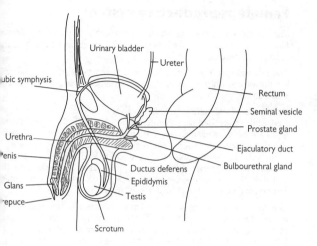

Urinary bladder

Ureter

ubic symphysis

Rectum

Seminal vesicle

Prostate gland

Urethra

Ejaculatory duct

enis

Bulbourethral gland

Glans

Ductus deferens

Epididymis

epuce

Testis

Scrotum

Female reproductive system

The female reproductive system is entirely located within the pelvis; it functions are to produce sex hormones and gametes, and to protect an support the developing embryo.

The external part, the vulva, is located between the legs. The vulva covers the vagina, which leads to the internal organs: the uterus, Fallopia tubes, and ovaries.

At the top of the vulva is a fleshy area called the mons pubis and two pairs of skin flaps filled with adipose tissue called the labia majora. Within these are the labia minora, which are flaps covered with smooth hairless skin that surround the vaginal opening. The clitoris is located at the front of the vulva where the labia join at the top, behind this lies the urethra opening and then the vaginal opening. The vagina connects with the uterus at the cervix. The cervix has strong thick muscular walls which relax during child birth to allow the baby to pass through.

The uterus is shaped like an inverted pear and, again, is very muscular. A its external upper corners are the Fallopian tubes, which form a pathway to the ovaries. At ovulation, eggs enter the funnel-shaped end of the tubes and are wafted away towards the uterus by the action of cilia.

At puberty, the reproductive system becomes cyclic—the menstrual cycle—driven by oestrogen and progesterone.

Conditions related to the vulva/vagina

- Vulvovaginitis: inflammation of the vulva and vagina, which can be caused by soap, bubble baths, bacteria, or fungal agents.
- Non-menstrual bleeding: caused perhaps by the presence of a foreign body in the vagina, a urethral prolapse, trauma from sexual abuse.
- Labial adhesions: in infants and young girls, sticking together of the labia in the midline. Increased risk of infection.

Conditions related to the ovaries, Fallopian tubes, and uterus

- Ovarian tumours: although rare, can occur in young girls.
- Ovarian cysts: non-cancerous sacs filled with fluid, may push on surrounding organs.
- Polycystic ovary syndrome: may appear in the teens; too much testosterone causes ovaries to swell and develop cysts.
- Ovarian torsion: twisting of the ovary; leads to restricted blood flow and atrophy.

Further reading

www.mic.ki.se/Diseases/C13html

John Bastin, University of Plymouth

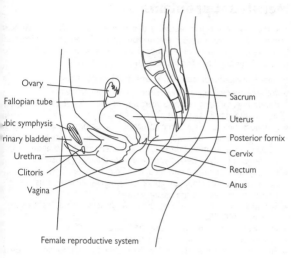

Female reproductive system

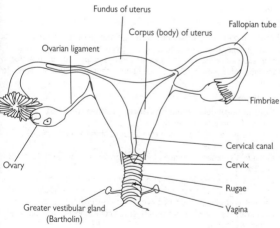

Menstrual problems

The main gynaecological problems that present to the GP or healthcare professional are related to menstruation, either the absence or irregularity of periods or heavy or painful periods. Girls who have had a period have a uterus and have had some oestrogen production.

Possible characteristics of menstrual problems

- Puberty: average age 12.8 years (precocious puberty when girl has developmental signs before 8 years and possibly delayed when no signs of puberty at 14 years).
- Amenorrhoea: absence of menstruation, can be primary of secondary.
- Primary amenorrhoea (with no secondary sexual characteristics): could be due to constitutional delay, chronic systemic illness, ovarian failure/gonadal dysgenesis, hypothalamus/pituitary dysfunction.
- Primary amenorrhoea (with secondary sex characteristics): due to Müllerian duct development abnormalities or Rokitansky–Kuster–Hauser syndrome (no uterus and vagina).
- Secondary amenorrhoea: pregnancy, weight loss, or polycystic ovarian syndrome (PCOS).
- Heavy or irregular periods: heavy >80 ml/cycle.
- Dysmenorrhoea: painful menstruation.
- Endometriosis: tissue identical to the endometrium is found outside the uterus.

Consideration

Because adolescence is a time of change and developing self-awareness and self-image, due care needs to be given to the need for vaginal o rectal examinations. Clinical examination is important in practice bu diagnostic information can be sought by other methods, such as ultra sound.

Treatment

- Constitutional delay: often familial, no treatment required (unless issues of worry or concern).
- Chronic systemic illness: due to infection, physical, endocrine, or emotional disorders.
- Gonadal dysgenesis: streaked ovaries, most common form Turner's syndrome.
- Müllerian duct development abnormalities: imperforate or absent vagina; surgical correction if there is a uterus present. Adolescent presents with haematocolpos, which may need only incision of the membrane or, if higher in the vagina, vaginal reconstructive surgery or hysterectomy.
- Absent vagina: reconstructive surgery (vaginoplasty) of dilatation from a vaginal dimple.
- PCOS: girls should be encouraged to lose weight, as little as 5% can be associated with improvements in menstrual cycle, hirsutism, rates of ovulation, and pregnancy. Most girls with PCOS have normal levels of oestrogen, but as they are not ovulating they are not producing

Caroline Saunders, Royal Liverpool Children's Hospital NHS Trust

progesterone. Unopposed oestrogen increases the long-term risk
of endometrial carcinoma; therefore treatment with the combined
oral contraceptive is suggested.

Heavy periods: pharmacological treatments (non-hormonal and limited
hormonal treatments because of longer-term data on possible later
breast cancer if combined pill used for >4 years when <20 years old).

Dysmenorrhoea: painful menstruation is caused by the contractions of
the myometrium associated with excessive prostaglandin production.

Endometriosis: treatment is to manage pain and preserve later fertility.

urther reading

arden, A.S. (1998). *Paediatric and adolescent gynaecology. Arnold. Oxford University Press.*

uint, E.H., Smith, Y.R.J. (2003). Abnormal uterine bleeding in adolescents. *Midwifery Womens Health*,; **48**(3), 186–91.

ap, G.B. (2003). Menstrual disorders in adolescence *Best. Pract. Res. Clin. Obstet. Gynaecol.*, **17**(1), 75–92.

Delayed puberty

The absence of secondary sexual characteristics or the slow appearance of normal secondary sexual characteristics in girls over 13 years or boys over 14 years of age.

Incidence
- A higher incidence in boys than girls.
- Usually constitutional delay of growth and puberty (CDGP) in boys.
- High incidence of pathology in girls.

Cause associated with low gonadatrophins
- Constitutional delay, usually familial
- Chronic disease, e.g. asthma or Crohn's disease
- Poor nutrition/anorexia nervosa
- Multiple pituitary hormone deficiency
- Tumours, e.g. craniopharyngioma or optic glioma
- Trauma, head injury, and surgery
- Cranial irradiation
- Hypothyroidism

Cause associated with high gonadatrophins
- Gonadal dysgenesis, e.g. Turner syndrome or Klinefelter syndrome
- Primary gonadal failure, e.g. testicular torsion, anorchia
- Abdominal irradiation
- Chemotherapy
- Intersex disorder

Investigations
- Bone age: to assess skeletal maturity
- Endomyseal antibodies, T_4/thyroid stimulating hormone (TSH)
- Chromosomes
- Pelvic ultrasound
- Human chorionic gonadotrophin test
- MRI scan

In CDGP only investigation required is bone age.

Treatment

If constitutional delay:
- reassure and monitor
- if the child is distressed and/or bullied, testosterone therapy can be used for boys and oestrogen for girls (see below)
- continue to monitor until puberty is completed.

If due to chronic disease:
- treat cause or improve nutritional status
- replace sex hormones:
    - boys: testosterone tablets, injections, patches, or gel
    - girls: oestrogen tablets or patches.
- support and provide counselling about future fertility.

Amanda Stoner, University of Leeds

ong-term outcome

May have reduced final height
May have reduced bone mass, potential for higher incidence of
fractures
Infertility
Inability to carry foetus after abdominal irradiation

urther reading

ook, C.G.D., Hindmarsh, P.C. (2001). Disorders of puberty. In *Clinical paediatric endocrinology*,
4th edn. Blackwell Science, Oxford.
rfar, J.O., Arneil, G.C. (2004). Endocrine and growth disorders. In *Textbook of paediatrics*, 6th
edn. Churchill Livingstone, Edinburgh.

Precocious puberty

Definition

Puberty is the development of secondary sexual characteristics and th preparation of the individual for reproductive capability, together wit the accompanying psychological changes.

Normal puberty follows a set sequence of hormonal events and can la from 18 months to 3 years.

It is centrally initiated by a pulsatile release of gonadatrophin-releasir hormone (GnRH) from the hypothalamus, which acts on the anterio pituitary to produce luteinizing hormone (LH) and follicle-stimulatir hormone (FSH). LH and FSH stimulate oestrogen and testosterone pro duction in women and men, respectively, which, assisted by adren steroids, stimulates the development of physical sex characteristics.

Physical changes at puberty

Puberty is staged using the Tanner method.

Girls

- The first change is breast budding.
- Peak height velocity occurs at breast stage 3 before menarche (approximately age 12 years).
- Periods start at breast stage 4 (approximately age 13 years).
- Menarche is the last event of puberty.
- After menarche has been achieved, very little growth occurs.

Boys

- The first sign of puberty is enlargement of the testes.
- Peak height velocity occurs mid-puberty (approximately age 14 years).
- Voice 'breaks'.
- Facial hair growth is one of the final stages.

Central precocious puberty

The early activation of the hypothalamic–pituitary–gonadal axis befor the age of 8 years in girls and 9 years in boys. The endocrine and physica changes are the same as in normal puberty, i.e. following the same order

Incidence

- Higher incidence in girls (ratio of girls:boys is 23:1)
- Female: 80% of cases are idiopathic
- Male: high incidence of pathology

Cause

- Idiopathic
- CNS lesions: tumours, hamartoma of hypothalamus, infection, trauma, hydrocephalus, irradiation, or surgery
- Hypothyroidism
- Congenital adrenal hypoplasia
- McCune–Albright syndrome: usually affects girls
- Testotoxicosis

Amanda Stoner, University of Leeds

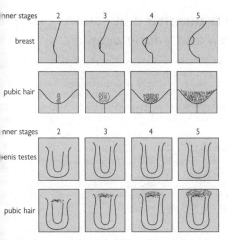

nner stages   2   3   4   5

breast

pubic hair

nner stages   2   3   4   5

enis testes

pubic hair

vestigations

ot all of these will be necessary.

GnRH test
Thyroid function test
Adrenal androgens
Bone age X-ray
Cranial MRI
Pelvic ultrasound scan
Synacthen test
Adrenal scan

reatment

Idiopathic:
- GnRH analogues
- cyproterone acetate
- ketoconazole
- family support

Non-idiopathic:
- treat underlying cause

ong-term outcome

Precocious puberty does not lead to early menopause
Normal reproductive function
No significant psychological consequences
No impairment in bone density

urther reading

ook, C.G.D., Hindmarsh, P.C. (2001). Disorders of puberty. In *Clinical paediatric endocrinology*, 4th edn. Blackwell Science, Oxford.

rfar, J.O., Arneil, G.C. (2004). Endocrine and growth disorders. In *Textbook of paediatrics*, 6th edn. Churchill Livingstone, Edinburgh.

Sexually transmitted infections (STIs) in children and young people

It is important that all adolescents are given accurate information regardi positive sexual health. Risks are explained and reinforced in a sensiti manner appropriate to age and level of understanding. There should access to services that can provide advice about, test for, and treat ST confidentially. The presence of an STI in an adolescent who denies volu tary sexual activity may be secondary to abuse/possibly rape—seek appr priate interventions.

More common STIs
- Gonorrhoea: often goes unnoticed but can cause vulvar itching, discharge, and urethritis.
- Chlamydia: majority asymptomatic; high risk of developing pelvic inflammatory disease, inter-menstrual bleeding, post-coital bleeding, and occasionally an increase in vaginal secretions.
- Syphilis.
- Genital warts: sexually transmitted (human papilomavirus (HPV)).
- Herpes: mild itching and then appearance of vesicles.
- Vaginal infections: most common are *Trichomonas vaginalis* (offensive malodorous vaginal discharge with vulvar soreness and irritation) candidiasis (not sexually transmitted but partner may develop symptoms—vulvitis and cottage-cheese-like discharge), and bacterial vaginosis (possibly due to a retained tampon).
- Foreign bodies.
- HIV.

Hazards
Asymptomatic infection is common and there is often coexistence several STIs; therefore thorough screening is necessary. Health surve lance is suggested as a follow-up; on, to trace partners where possible.

Treatment
- Examination and history of sexual activity
- Screening for STI/culture swabs/blood tests/microbiology and possibl immediate microscopy/antigen testing
- Pharmacology
- Treatment of sexual partner(s)
- Education and minimizing risk
- Psychological interventions for those who have self-harming behaviou
- Treatment for HIV, both medical and psychological counselling

Caroline Saunders, Royal Liverpool Children's Hospital NHS Trust

urther reading

estle, C.E., Halpern, C.T., Miller, W.C., Ford, C.A. (2005). Young age at first sexual intercourse and sexually transmitted infections in adolescents and young adults. *American Journal of Epidemiology*, **161**(8), 774–80.

ηton, K.A., Mercer, C.H., McManus, S., *et al.* (2005). Ethnic variations in sexual behaviour in Great Britain and risk of sexually transmitted infections: a probability survey. *Lancet*, **365**, 1246–55.

pp, J. and Viner, R. (2005). Sexual health, contraception, and teenage pregnancy. *British Medical Journal* **330**, 590–3.

Contraception

Contraception is an area of concern for many adolescents and young people. The range of contraceptives available is extensive; however adolescents often have concerns about their side effects.

Clinicians are required to assess a young person's competence to consent to treatment and document that such an assessment has been carried out. National guidelines exist to assist in the assessment; however, young people can be provided with contraceptive advice/treatment without parental knowledge.

Contraception is available from GPs, sexual health clinics, family planning clinics, and pharmacies. The table below identifies various methods, effectiveness when used properly, and some associated problems.[1]

Method	Effectiveness	Problems
Progestogen-only pill	99%	Irregular periods, no protection against STIs, acne, breast tenderness, weight gain, headaches, cysts on ovaries, ectopic pregnancy, and small risk of breast cancer
Combined pill	99%	Headaches, nausea, breast tenderness, mood changes, increased blood pressure, venous/arterial thrombosis, and small risk of developing breast, cervical, or liver cancer
Contraceptive patch	99%	May be seen, skin irritation, no protection against STIs, headaches, nausea, breast tenderness, mood changes, weight loss/gain, venous/arterial thrombosis, and small risk of breast cancer
Intra-uterine device	99%	Heavier, longer, and painful periods; no protection against STIs; pelvic infection, perforate womb/cervix, and ectopic pregnancy
Male and female condoms	99% and 95%, respectively	Interrupt sex, slip off/split; allergy to latex
Diaphragms and caps	92–96%	Interrupt sex, time consuming, cystitis, and allergy to latex
Emergency contraception	95%	Nausea, headaches, tiredness, breast tenderness, abdominal pain, and vomiting

1 🖳 www.fpa.org.uk

Jackie Johnston, Napier University Edinburgh

STIs

The rate of STIs among young people is very high and concern exists that in the long term the rate of infertility is set to rise. In order to prevent STIs, young people are encouraged to use condoms, in addition to other contraceptive methods.

Pregnancy

The UK has one of the highest rates of teenage pregnancy in the developed world. Pregnancy can occur because of lack of knowledge, failed contraception, and, in some instances, as a result of rape. Teenage pregnancy has implications for both mother and baby.

The mother can experience socio-economic deprivation and negative public attitudes, she may not be able to complete her education, and she has an increased risk of mental health problems and premature death.

There is an increased risk of low birth weight, congenital malformation, and perinatal death of the baby, childhood accidents and hospital admissions, developmental delay, and learning difficulties.

Further reading

Burtney, E., Fullerton, D., Hosie, A. (2004). Policy developments in the United Kingdom. In *Young people and sexual health* (ed. E. Burtney and M. Duffy), pp. 47–57. Palgrave Macmillan, New York.

Faculty of Family Planning and Reproductive Health Care Clinical Effectiveness Unit (2004). Contraceptive choices for young people. *Journal of Family Planning and Reproductive Health Care*, **30**, 237–51.

www.fpa.org.uk

Effect of chemotherapy on fertility

Childhood cancer

Chemotherapy, as well as radiotherapy, is an important treatment f‍ cancer in children. After treatment for cancer, most children will n have any serious long-term problems; however, certain treatments f‍ childhood cancers can have an impact on puberty and fertility.

Treatments

Treatments that may affect puberty and fertility include chemothera‍ drugs. Some drugs are implicated more than others and the cumulat‍ dose is also important. Fertility is particularly affected in high-d‍ therapies, such as in bone-marrow transplantation. In general, boys a‍ more liable to infertility after a given therapy than girls.

Radiotherapy to the brain and to the sex organs will also affect fertili‍ Surgery to the genital tract may also result in infertility.

Infertility

Fertility is the ability to become pregnant or father a child. Fertility pre‍ ervation is difficult in younger children, although reassurance should offered that the issue will be followed up in a late-effects clinic. In pub‍ tal males sperm banking can be offered prior to starting treatment. E‍ cryopreservation is not proven in females, and does not yet form part regular practice.

Nursing care

Prior to commencing any chemotherapy, parents should be made awa‍ of all the side effects, including late effects. In teenage girls, the patie‍ and families may need to be warned of amenorrhoea and early men‍ pause. Adolescent males should have sperm harvested prior to start‍ any treatment, and healthcare professionals should reassure the‍ patients that changes have no impotent effect. In both sexes, nursing st‍ should emphasize the need for contraception because sterility is no‍ certainty.

Further reading

CancerBACUP (2004). *Sexuality and cancer*. CancerBACUP, London.
Davis, C. (2003). The impact of treatment on male fertility. *Cancer Nursing Practice*, **2**(4), 25–31

Lynne Barnes, Central Manchester and Manchester Children's University Hospitals NHS Trus‍

Sexual assault

Sexual assault is unlawful and non-consensual sexual behaviour perpetrated against children or adults. In most countries sexual assault is a criminal offence and a breach of human rights. Across the UK the legal definition of sexual assault differs; however, it generally refers to a range of behaviours that are sexual in intent and are undertaken without consent or with a child under the age of sexual consent.

Rape
- Penetration of the vagina, mouth, or anus by a penis
- Perpetrators are male
- Victim can be either male or female

Assault by penetration
- Penetration of the vagina or anus by an object or part of the body
- Perpetrators and victims can be either male or female

Indecent assault
- Sexual touching by either male or female
- The degree of touching can be minimal or severe, but the intent is sexual
- Touching can be with objects or parts of the body
- Victim can be either male or female

Causing or inciting an individual to engage in sexual activity
- Where an individual makes another perform or receive sexual acts
- The victim might be forced to perform an act on themselves
- Both perpetrators and victims can be either male or female

Legislation also refers to sexual assaults resulting from prostitution, trafficking, and enforced marriages. For children and young people, the following tends to apply:
- age of consent to any sexual activity is usually 16 years for both males and females
- there is an age below which consent is not deemed to be possible, often 13 years.

If children are the victims of sexual assault, this is termed child sexual abuse, and requires specific child protection procedures to be implemented in addition to criminal proceedings. The child protection procedures are instigated to ensure that the child who has been assaulted, and any other victims, are immediately protected from harm and any future risks eliminated.

Criminal proceedings are also instigated to bring the perpetrators to justice and ensure that any risk they pose to children is managed.

Further reading

Corby, B. (2000). *Child abuse—toward a knowledge base*. Open University Press, Buckingham.
Family Planning Association (2004). The law on sex. 🖥 www.fpa.org.uk/about/PDFs/Law.pdf

Hydrocoele

Definition

During its passage from the peritoneal cavity into the scrotum, the testis is preceded by a sac-like extension of peritoneum called the process vaginalis. After the testicle has descended, the process vaginalis normally closes and the scrotum loses its connection with the abdomen. However, in cases where the process vaginalis remains patent, peritoneal fluid can enter the potential space, creating a swelling in the inguinal region or scrotum. This swelling is known as a hydrocoele. A hydrocoele may also develop if the testis becomes inflamed or damaged, e.g. due to trauma or tumour.

Characteristics and indications for treatment

- Hydrocoeles are not usually painful and have a bluish appearance.
- They transilluminate brightly if a pen-torch is used.
- Parents may report a variation in the size of the swelling.
- The condition is more common at birth, but most cases resolve spontaneously before the child is 1 year old.
- Surgery is recommended if the hydrocoele fails to resolve by the time the child is 2 years old or if the swelling becomes painful or enlarged.
- The important point in diagnosing this condition is to differentiate it from an inguinal hernia.

Hydrocoelectomy

- The hydrocoele is removed in an operation called a hydrocoelectomy.
- The surgery requires a small inguinal incision. The fluid is removed and the process vaginalis is closed. The incision is closed with dissolvable sutures.
- Complication rates are low. As with all surgery, there is a small risk of bleeding during or after the procedure. Haematomas, wound infection, and damage to the scrotum and surrounding tissues may also occur.
- Damage to the testicle is rare but may occur.

Post-operative care

Hydrocoele repair is usually done a day-case basis. Once the child has fully recovered from anaesthesia he may be allowed home and advised to take regular analgesia for 48 hours. Loose clothing is advised for comfort during this time. The child should be advised to avoid straddle positions, e.g. riding a bicycle, for at least 2 weeks after surgery.

Further reading

Burnard, G.B., Young, A.E. (ed.) (1998). *The new Aird's companion in surgical studies.* Churchill Livingstone, London.

Gill, F.T. (1998). Umbilical hernia, inguinal hernias, and hydroceles in children: diagnostic clues for optimal patient management. *Journal of Pediatric Health Care*, **12**(5), 31–5.

🔲 http://www.emedicine.com/emerg/topic256.htm

Claire Ferguson, Royal Liverpool Children's Hospital NHS Trust

Undescended testicle (cryptorchidism)

Definition

Testes develop high up in the abdomen, close to the kidneys, and gradually descend through the inguinal canal into the scrotum shortly before birth. Occasionally one or both of the testes fail to descend fully and remain in the abdomen or inguinal canal. The descent may be completed after birth and both testicles should have descended into the scrotum by the age of 1 year. The incidence of an undescended testis is much higher in premature infants than in full-term babies.

Examination and indications for treatment

- Examination will usually determine whether or not the testicle is fully descended.
- Sometimes a testicle that has not fully descended may be palpable outside of the scrotum.
- Usually a testicle that is impalpable will be present in the abdominal cavity, as complete absence of a testicle is very rare.
- Undescended testes are corrected by an operation called an orchidopexy.
- The main indications for performing an orchidopexy are to achieve optimal development of the testes and improve sperm production. The production of sperm is temperature dependent and because the temperature of the scrotum is lower than that of the abdominal cavity, production is improved.
- Other indications are cosmetic, psychological, and to reduce the risk of torsion, trauma, and possible malignancy.
- Ideally, an elective orchidopexy should be carried out by the age of 3 years.

Orchidopexy

- An orchidopexy involves a small incision in the groin.
- The testicle is mobilized and brought down into the scrotum.
- Occasionally it is difficult to bring the testicle down easily into the scrotum because the vessels supplying it are too short. If this is the case, the testicle is brought down as far as possible and the child will require a further operation in 6 months. This is known as a staged orchidopexy.
- If the testicle appears grossly abnormal at the time of operation and is unlikely to provide any useful function, it may be removed at this time (an orchidectomy).
- As with all surgery, there is a risk of bleeding and infection, and occasionally there may be bruising to the area.

Post-operative care

In the post-operative period the child should be given regular analgesia. Exercise and activity should be minimized for 2 weeks until the pain and swelling have reduced. The child should not use the straddle position (e.g. riding a bicycle) for 1 month. The surgeon will normally request to see the child in clinic approximately 1 month after surgery.

Claire Ferguson, Royal Liverpool Children's Hospital NHS Trust

Further reading

Barthold, J.S., Gonzalez, R. (2003). The epidemiology of congenital cryptorchidism, testicular ascent and orchidopexy. *Journal of Urology*, **170**, 2396–401.

Burnard, G.B., Young, A.E. (ed.) (1998). *The new Aird's companion in surgical studies*. Churchill Livingstone, London.

http://www.aafp.org/afp/20001101/2037.html

Hypospadias

Definition

Hypospadias is a common congenital defect in which the urethral meatus opens at any point along the shaft of the penis from the glans to the perineum. Hypospadias is also frequently associated with a downward bending of the penis (chordee) and malformation of the foreskin.

Hypospadias may prevent a child from passing urine when standing up. The chordee might also make sexual relationships difficult when the boy is older.

Hypospadias repair

The treatment of hypospadias is surgical correction with the following aims:

• to reconstruct the urethra and glans
• to reconstruct the foreskin
• to correct the chordee.

The type of repair will depend on the severity of the defect. Surgery is usually performed between 6 months and 18 months of age, before the child starts school.

Post-operative care

• A large foam dressing may cover the penis.
• A catheter will be inserted during surgery to drain urine from the bladder while the repair heals.
• The child should avoid activity while the dressing is in place. Walking may damage the repair.
• Laxatives may be given to help prevent the child straining during bowel evacuation.
• The surgeon may request that prophylactic antibiotics be given.
• Bladder spasms are a common occurrence while the catheter is in place. Regular analgesia and an anticholinergic medication can help prevent spasms and keep the child comfortable.
• It may be possible for the parents to take the child home with the catheter in place if they have received appropriate training, equipment and discharge advice. Good community nursing support must be available. The family should have access to transport in case there is a problem with the catheter and the child needs to return to hospital quickly.

The dressing and catheter are usually removed in hospital after 1 week. The swelling and bruising takes approximately 2 weeks to subside. Possible complications include fistula and/or stricture. These may require further operation. After hypospadias repair, children are followed up in clinic by their surgeon.

Claire Ferguson, Royal Liverpool Children's Hospital NHS Trust

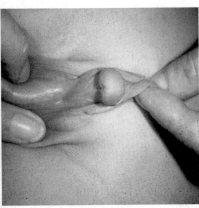

Reproduced with kind permission of Mr David Burge

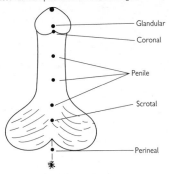

- Glandular
- Coronal
- Penile
- Scrotal
- Perineal

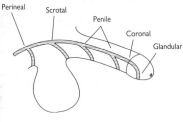

Perineal   Scrotal   Penile   Coronal   Glandular

Further reading

Burnard, G.B. Young, A.E. (ed.) (1998). *The new Aird's companion in surgical studies*. Churchill Livingstone, London.

Manzoni, G., Bracka, A., Palminteri, E., Marrocco, G. (2004). Hypospadias surgery: when, what and by whom? *BJU International* **94**(8) 1188–95.

www.pennhealth.com/health_info/Surgery/hypospadiasrepair_1.html

Examination of external female genitalia

As a routine assessment and not when there are causes for concern with respect to child protection issues.

Action	Rationale
1. Assess child's need to have the procedure undertaken; have knowledge of anatomy and physiology of the area	Establish the underlying physical need to examine the external genitalia. Be aware of the possible causes ofnormal and abnormal genitalia for your area of practice
2. Do not undertake assessment if issues of child protection have been raised or are known from medical records	The child should not be placed at further emotional or physical risk
3. Do not undertake this alone unless there is a clear indication/request from an older child	Both child and staff need to consider issues of protection. If an older child refuses to have a chaperone, this needs to be given consideration and documented in the notes
4. Ensure the environment is safe and fit for the purpose. Examination couch available. Explain the procedure to the child if an appropriate age and developmental level	Environment must ensure and maintain privacy, and the couch should be of a height that allows the procedure to be undertaken in comfort for the patient and the staff
5. Should the child refuse to cooperate with the request, then stop and reassure the child. The child/parent has to give verbal consent (where possible)	Refusal is just that, and the examination cannot go ahead if the child refuses. Should the child agree after reassurance, then staff could continue. If at any point there are worrying issues or concern, the examination be halted and advice sought
6. Ask the child to undress (where necessary from the waist/remove underwear). Ask child to lie on the examination couch; ensure lighting adequate	Maintain privacy by keep child covered as much as possible, removing child's trousers if necessary to be able to visualize the area to be examined
7. Ensure hygiene needs met. Any hygiene needs of the child should be addressed prior to inspection of the genital area and can be done by a parent. Handwashing and use of disposable gloves by the practitioner	Minimizing cross-infection

Caroline Saunders, Royal Liverpool Children's Hospital NHS Trust

Contd.

8. Always talk through what you doing. Ask the child to bend knees and move legs towards the body and relax legs to allow visualization of the area. Examine the perineal area for physiological problems and signs of disease, including the labia, clitoris, labia minora, urethra and vaginal opening, and anus where possible. Touch should be minimal, and visualization by opening the labia allows for inspection

Should the child wish to help in the examination, this can be encouraged after handwashing. It is important to identify any abnormalities and note these in the medical notes; give advice and reassurance to parents along with any medical treatment that is necessary (e.g. hormone cream for labial adhesions)

9. When the examination is complete, encourage child to dress and attend to hygiene needs. Give positive feedback to the child and thank her for her cooperation

Maintain privacy and dignity at all times. Record any finding in the child's notes and attend to any needs following examination

Examination of external male genitalia

As a routine assessment and not when there are causes for concern with respect to child protection issues.

Action	Rationale
1. Assess child's need to have the procedure undertaken; have knowledge of anatomy and physiology of the area	Establish the underlying physical need to examine the external genitalia. Be aware of the possible causes of normal and abnormal genitalia for your area of practice
2. Do not undertake assessment if issues of child protection have been raised or are known from medical records	The child should not be placed at further emotional or physical risk
3. Do not undertake this alone unless there is a clear indication/request from an older child	Both child and staff need to consider issues of protection. If an older child refuses to have a chaperone, this needs to be given consideration and documented in the notes
4. Ensure that the environment is safe and fit for the purpose. Examination couch available. Explain the procedure to the child if an appropriate age and developmental level	Environment must ensure and maintain privacy, and the couch should be of a height that allows the procedure to be undertaken in comfort for the patient and the staff
5. Should the child refuse to cooperate with the request, then stop and reassure the child. The child/parent has to give verbal consent (where possible)	Refusal is just that, and the examination cannot go ahead if the child refuses. Should the child agree after reassurance, then staff could continue. If at any point there are worrying issues or concern, the examination should be halted and advice sought
6. Ask the child to undress (where necessary from the waist/remove underwear). Ask him to lie on the examination couch ensure lighting is adequate	Maintain privacy by keeping the child covered as much as possible, removing the child's trousers if necessary to be able to visualize the area for examination
7. Ensure hygiene needs met. Any hygiene needs of the child should be addressed prior to inspection of the genital area and can be done by parents. Handwashing and use of disposable gloves by the practitioner	Minimizing cross–infection

Caroline Saunders, Royal Liverpool Children's Hospital NHS Trust

Contd.

8. Always talk through what you doing. Examine the groin area and also the perineal area; inspect the penis, foreskin, and scrotum for any physiological problems or signs of disease	Should the child wish to help in the examination, this can be encouraged after handwashing. It is important to identify any abnormalities and note these in the medical notes; give advice and reassurance to parents, along with any medical treatment that is necessary (e.g. problems with foreskin, glans, scrotum, testis, etc)
9. Once the examination is complete encourage the child to dress and attend to hygiene needs. Give positive feedback to the child and thank him for his cooperation	Maintain privacy and dignity at all times. Record any finding in the child's notes and attend to any needs following examination

Further reading

artley, E. (1998). *Children and sexuality: perspectives in health care*, (ed. T. Harrison). Baillière Tindall, London.

Musculoskeletal problems

Related skills

Bone

- One of the body's connective tissues, with a solid matrix of calcium phosphate and calcium carbonate
- Bones are strong but surprisingly light
- Two bone types: spongy and compact
- Bones contain cavities filled with bone marrow, which can be yellow or red

Generalized structure

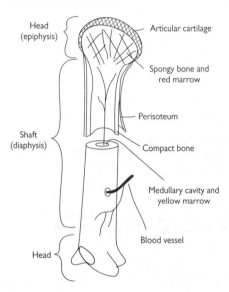

Head (epiphysis) — Articular cartilage

Spongy bone and red marrow

Perisoteum

Shaft (diaphysis) — Compact bone

Medullary cavity and yellow marrow

Blood vessel

Head

Compact bone

- Hard and dense, with a complex structure of parallel cylindrical structures called osteons.
- The matrix is composed of concentric layers in which osteocytes are found nestling in lacunae. A network of canals and vessels that provide nutrients and to the osteocytes are also found in the matrix.

Spongy bone

Made from a network of beams called trabeculae, which align along lines of stress to reinforce the bone. Trabeculae can be remodelled if the stress planes alter because of changes in activity.

Bone cells

Mature bone cells are called osteocytes and fall into three categories:
- osteoblasts—make bone

John Bastin, University of Plymouth

osteoclasts—break down matrix
osteogenic cells (progenitors)—can do both.

All osteocytes act dynamically to constantly remodel and maintain the strength of bone. These cells also come under the influence of testosterone and oestrogen throughout the life cycle.

Bone remodelling

Occurs all the time but is considerable after the repair of a fracture. In periods of immobility or inactivity, bone-matrix loss can be quite high and can result in fracture if bones are suddenly put under high stress. Remodelling counteracts changes in bone stress but also allows calcium homeostasis to be maintained.

Bone shape

Long bones: found in limbs
Short bones: movement areas
Flat bones: skull
Irregular bones: vertebrae

Bone growth

Growth of long bones is generated from epiphyseal plates at the end of the bone shaft. These plates originate in fetal development and continue to lay down bone until puberty, when androgen activity causes them to close. This tends to happen more quickly in girls than boys.

Achondroplasia—a genetic condition resulting in restricted growth—is caused by the epiphyseal plates not laying down new bone at the normal rate.

Epiphyseal plates can also be damaged by trauma, resulting in premature closure and loss of growth in the damaged bone.

Skeletal muscle

Relationship between bone and muscle:
- bone and muscle joined by tendons
- skeletal muscles move bones
- only one end of a muscle moves; the other end is fixed
- the prime mover is called the *agonist*
- the controlling opposing muscle is the *antagonist*
- stability results from the action of *synergistic muscles*
- skeletal muscle uses levers

Skeletal muscle
- Lies directly beneath the skin—the flesh.
- Each muscle is covered with dense connective tissue—the deep fascia.
- Muscles are arranged in bundles or fascicles.
- Muscles have a belly and are attached at both ends.

Muscle fibres
- Fascicles are complex bundles of muscle fibres.
- Muscle fibres are specialized cells: T tubules and sarcoplasmic reticulum.
- The inner core of the muscle fibre is made of myofibrils.
- Myofibrils are composed of contractile myofilaments.

Muscle fibre contraction
- Muscle contraction is an interaction between myofilaments in a subunit known as a sarcomere.
- There are two types of myofilaments: thick filaments of myosin and thin filaments of actin.
- Chemical interaction in the presence of ATP causes distortion of the two proteins, which results in contraction of the sarcomere. This, repeated throughout the entire fascicle, causes movement.
- ATP is released following nerve impulse activity in the region of the motor end-plate.
- At the same time there is an influx of calcium, which is recycled at the end of the contraction.

Muscle defects
- Birth defects can occur in muscle (and bone), although they usually occur in the face, hips, legs, and feet.
- Muscles may develop incompletely and may result in an abnormal appearance and function.

Further reading
www.leeds.ac.uk/cbh/lectures/anatomy5.html

John Bastin, University of Plymouth

Classification of fractures

A fracture is quite simply a break in the continuity of the bone. A number of classification systems have been developed, often concerned with specific bony areas, and largely used in diagnosis of adult fractures. Fractures in children are usually described and the following words are most commonly used:

- undisplaced: fracture/fragments in good position
- displaced: fracture/fragments in poor position; further described as axially displaced, angulated, or rotated
- open (compound) fracture: bone punctured through skin surface
- closed fracture: skin surface not broken
- intra-articular: fracture involves the joint surface

	A transverse fracture lies across the shaft of the bone
	An oblique fracture lies obliquely across the shaft of bone.
	A spiral fracture spirals around the shaft of bone
	A comminuted fracture is where the bone is broken into more than two segments
	A greenstick fracture only occurs in children where the bone is more elastic. A direct blow will cause the bone to bend but not completely break.

Salter–Harris classification of epiphyseal fractures

In children, a fracture through the epiphyseal (growth) plate may result in interference with, or complete cessation of, bone growth of the respective long bone, which will produce a limb-length discrepancy. These fractures are known as *epiphyseal fractures*. Salter and Harris classified these fractures into five types.

Brian Silverwood, Healthcare Commission

	Type I: Injuries occur when the fracture line is along the plane of the growth plate. Pain on weight bearing will be the main symptom
	Type II: Injuries occur when the fracture is along the plane of the growth plate but extends into the metaphysis (the growing portion of a long bone) on one side
	Type III: Injuries occur when the fracture line is along the plane of the growth plate, but extends into the epiphysis (bone end) on one side
	Type IV: Injuries occur where the fracture extends from the epiphysis through the growth plate into the metaphysis
	Type V: Injures involve a crush injury to the growth plate. This may not be obvious on X-ray but the clinical signs will suggest a serious injury

Open fractures

Classified by the following system:

Type I	An open fracture with a wound <1 cm long and clean
Type II	An open fracture with a laceration >1 cm long without excessive soft tissue damage, flaps, or avulsions
Type III	Massive soft tissue damage, compromised vascularity, severe wound contamination, and marked fracture instability
Type IIIA	Adequate soft tissue coverage of a fractured bone, despite extensive soft tissue laceration, flaps, or high-energy trauma irrespective of the size of the wound
Type IIIB	Extensive soft tissue injury loss with periosteal stripping and bone exposure; usually associated with massive contamination
Type IIIC	Open fracture associated with arterial injury requiring repair

Further reading

Bell, M.J. (2002). Polytrauma in children. In *Children's orthopaedics and fractures*, 2nd edn (ed. M.K.D. Benson *et al.*), pp. 579–86. Churchill Livingstone, London.

Danby, D.J., Edwards, D.J. (2001). *Essential orthopaedics and trauma*, 3rd edn. Churchill Livingstone, London.

McRae, R., Esser, M. (2002). *Practical fracture treatment*, 4th edn. Churchill Livingstone, London.

University of Bridgeport (2005). *Salter–Harris Classification*. 🖥 www.bridgeport. edu/~gwl/salter-harrisclassification.htm (accessed 18 August 2005).

Treatment of fractures

There are five main aims of fracture treatment and management. These are commonly summarized as the 'five Rs'.

Resuscitation
- A child should rarely need fluid resuscitation.
- However, be aware of signs and treatment for shock.
- Shock may be related to pain and blood loss.

Reduction
- Describes the realignment of fractured bone ends.
- Best achieved under general anaesthesia so that the surgeon can utilize an image intensifier and the child is protected from pain, discomfort, and psychological trauma.
- For greenstick fractures, alignment may be achievable under sedation and/or Entonox in the accident and emergency department.

Restriction
- Following reduction, the fracture needs holding in place until bony union occurs (around 6–8 weeks in children).
- Methods used depend on the bone affected and nature of injury, and may include:
  - plaster casts
  - traction
  - internal fixation
  - external fixation.
- The aim of restriction is to prevent bony deformity and allow bone growth to proceed normally.

Restoration
- There is a risk of muscles and joints stiffening and losing some function when a limb is immobilized.
- The child should be encouraged to exercise all joints and muscles except those directly affected by the injury, e.g. a child with a fractured arm can be encouraged to move all digits regularly, which keeps the fingers nimble, encourages muscle to move within the cast, and promotes venous return.

Rehabilitation
- When the immobilization method is removed, the child should be encouraged to exercise.
- Physiotherapist/exercise plan.

The child must receive adequate pain control during the period of resuscitation, reduction, and restriction, through adequate analgesia and diversional therapies. Pain usually subsides once reduction is achieved; however, the child may suffer from muscle spasms until swelling subsides.

Achievement of the five Rs will also be determined by the many potential complications of fractures, including:
- infection
- malunion

Brian Silverwood, Healthcare Commission

delayed union
non-union
avascular necrosis
fat embolism
damage to structures
compartment syndrome.

Further reading

pley, A.G., Solomon, L. (2001). *Concise system of orthopaedics and fractures*, 2nd edn. Edward Arnold, London.

enson, M.K.D. et al. (2002). *Children's orthopaedics and fractures*, 2nd edn. Churchill Livingstone, London.

agdin, J. (1996). The musculoskeletal system. In *Children's nursing*, (ed. L. McQuaid et al.). Churchill Livingstone, London.

Management of a child with a fractured femur

Femoral-shaft fractures are a common injury in children. Accidental trauma is the main cause, although consideration should be given to other pathological factors, i.e. osteogenesis imperfecta, or the possibility of non-accidental injury. In children <5 years of age, falls are the main cause of injury, whereas high-impact incidents, e.g. road traffic accidents are the more usual cause in older children.

Treatment

The aims of treatment are to relieve pain, achieve fracture alignment, and promote healing and optimal functional outcome.

Treatment options are based on:

- age
- position and type of fracture
- associated injuries
- general health.

Treatment options	Rationale
Pavlik harness	Child under 3 months of age.
Gallows traction	Child 3–18 months of age, under 16 kg weight
Hip spica plaster	Child 2–10 years, social circumstances
Thomas splint traction	Child ≥18 months. Long-term or initial management only. When femoral swelling reduced, then hip spica or surgical correction as decided by consultant
Surgical correction: internal fixation	Fracture reduction is necessary and pathological fractures. Allows early mobilization
Surgical correction: external fixation	Comminuted fractures and/or soft tissue injuries

Pavlik harness

The harness is used to splint the fractured femur with some additional padding. In a child in this age group, the fracture will heal in approximately 3 weeks. The family receives specific instructions about caring for a child in a harness.

Gallows traction

The traction apparatus is applied and the traction cords are tied to the top of the cot. It relieves pain by reducing muscle spasm and maintains fracture alignment. The child's buttocks are elevated off the bed and the child's body weight provides the counter-traction. In this age group, fractured femur will heal in approximately 4–6 weeks.

Elizabeth Wright, Southampton University Hospitals NHS Trust

Hip spica plaster

This moulded body cast supports and maintains the fracture alignment. It is worn for 6–8 weeks. Following family consultation and with provision of support services, the child can be cared for at home.

Thomas splint traction

Fixed traction which relieves pain by reducing muscle spasm and maintains fracture alignment. Duration of traction depends on age and fracture healing, but treatment can last up to 12 weeks.

Internal fixation

Flexible medullary nails are usually used in the 6–14-year age group. The flexible long wires are inserted into the medulla of the femur to stabilize and reduce the fracture. There is minimal scarring and the child can mobilize early. The nails can be removed 9 months after insertion if symptomatic.

External fixation

Fixation can be with either a monolateral or a circular frame. Wires pass through the bone and soft tissues, proximal and distal to the fracture. The wires are then attached the external fixator. This allows the fractured bone ends or fragments to be securely supported and the fracture alignment can be controlled. Early mobilization is possible.

Further reading

Davis, P., Barr, L. (1999). Principles of traction. *Journal of Orthopaedic Nursing*, **3**(4), 222–7.

Judd, J., Wright, E. (2005). Joint and limb problems in children and adolescents. In *Orthopaedic and trauma nursing* (ed. J. Kneale and P. Davis), pp. 244–64. Churchill Livingstone, London.

Parsch, K. (2002). Femoral shaft fractures. In *Children's orthopaedics and fractures*, 2nd edn (ed. M. Benson, J. Fixsen, M. Macnicol, and K. Parsch), pp. 640–5. Churchill Livingstone, London.

Fractured tibia and fibula

A fractured tibia (shinbone) is a relatively common injury sustained by children of all ages. For example, a toddler may fracture a shinbone by simply tripping over a toy, and twisting injuries may cause a spiral fracture. In older children/adolescents, a blunt blow often causes a severe fractured tibia/fibula, e.g through a sporting injury, fall, or road traffic accident.[1]

Symptoms
- Pain
- Swelling of soft tissue
- Tenderness
- Deformity
- Reduced movement
- Numbness and coolness below fracture site towards the foot

Investigation and treatment options
- Careful X-ray examination is required to ensure growth plate is intact if the fracture is towards the end of the bone.
- Simple undisplaced fractures (usually in toddlers) require immobilization through plaster cast application.

Surgical intervention is now commonly performed on fractured tibias/fibulas. A number of internal and external fixation devices are available and what is used will depend on the nature and location of the fracture and the amount of soft tissue damage.[2] It may also be down to the surgeon's preference and experience.

Internal fixation
- Screws
- Screws and plates
- Intramedullary nails or rods
- Nancy nails

External fixation
- Transfixing screws above/below the fracture and held by a fixed external sliding bar (Orthofix).
- External ring frame (Ilizarov) using a combination of transfixing screws and wires.
- Hybrid frame (a combination of a sliding bar system and ring frame) may be used for injuries around the knee area.

Nursing considerations

Conservative management
- Analgesia for pain control
- Neurovascular observations
- Plaster of Paris care
- Mobilization: non-weight-bearing with crutches
- Reassurance

Brian Silverwood, Healthcare Commission

nternal fixation

- Analgesia
- Neurovascular observations
- Routine pre-operative/post-operative care
- Care of wound/incision site
- 1–2 days bed rest required prior to mobilization
- A plaster cast may still be applied prior to a cast brace (a plaster cast with hinges to allow knee exercise) after a few weeks
- Physiotherapy

External fixation

- Similar to above
- Pin-site care
- Early exercise with continual passive movement (CPM) machine
- Anti-spasmodics for muscle spasm
- Psychological support

1 American Society of Orthopaedic Surgeons (2005). *Shinbone fractures.* orthoinfo.aaos.org/ (accessed 18 August 2005).
2 Apley, A.G., Solomon, L. (2001). *Concise system of orthopaedics and fractures*, 2nd edn. Edward Arnold, London.

Supracondylar fracture of humerus

This is the most common of all elbow fractures in children and is usually the result of a fall. It occurs in the distal end of the humerus, above the humeral condyles.

Important consideration

The brachial artery transverses the distal humerus. With a supracondylar fracture, there is a high risk of neurovascular compromise or even a Volkmann ischaemic contracture—a permanent hand contracture. Children with a supracondylar fracture of the humerus are usually admitted into hospital for 24-hour neurovascular observation. The radial pulse should be monitored to see if there is any pressure on the brachial artery. A weaker radial pulse compared with that on the opposite side demands emergency attention to save the circulation of the forearm. Continuous pulse oximetry can be applied to make an objective measurement of perfusion. Regular assessment for any evidence of injury to the median nerve must also be performed.

Treatment options

Treatment depends on the fracture classification, stability, and neurovascular status.
- Immobilization in plaster.
- Closed reduction/manipulation under general anaesthetic.
- Closed reduction/manipulation under general anaesthetic with Kirshner wire fixation. The Kirshner wires are removed at 4 weeks.
- Open reduction and internal fixation.

In all cases of displaced fracture, it is important to monitor children closely post-operatively for signs of compartment syndrome and vascular compromise. It is imperative that non-narcotic analgesics be given because narcotic analgesics can mask the early symptoms of vascular compromise. Active movements of the fingers are insisted upon to prevent oedema of the hand. A check radiograph is taken to confirm satisfactory reduction.

Ongoing care

The child is discharged home with the elbow immobilized in plaster. Plaster is maintained for 4–6 weeks. The child and family are given advice about caring for the plaster and observing for neurovascular impairment (📖 Care of plaster).

Removal of Kirshner wire

If a Kirshner wire was inserted, it needs to be removed 4 weeks after insertion. For younger children, this is done under a general anaesthetic, and for older children, the wire is removed in clinic. The arm is then placed in plaster again for the remaining 2 weeks.

Removal of plaster

After the plaster has been removed, it is not unusual for the elbow to have a restricted range of movement. The child is advised to use the arm

Elizabeth Wright, Southampton University Hospitals NHS Trust

or normal activities of living, to gradually regain the range of movement.
This is helped by a warm bath. However, sporting activity is restricted for
another 6 weeks to allow the fracture to consolidate fully.

Further reading

De Pablos, J., Tejero, A. (2002). Fractures of the shoulder, upper limb and hand. In *Children's
orthopaedics and fractures*, 2nd edn (ed. M. Benson, J. Fixsen, M. Macnicol, and K. Parsch).
Churchill Livingstone, London.
www.bonetumour.org/book/APTEXT/index.html

Fractured radius and ulna

Definition
- Commonly known as forearm fractures.
- The fracture can occur at the distal (farthest), middle, or proximal (top) end of the radius and ulna.
- Fractures may or may not be displaced.

Incidence
Forearm fractures account for 40–50% of all childhood fractures.

Causes
Falling on to an outstretched arm or as a result of a direct injury.

History and examination
- Ascertain cause and mechanism of injury.
- Be aware of non-accidental injury.
- Note deformity of arm, point of tenderness, and sensation in each finger.
- Ask child to flex (bend) and extend (straighten) each finger.

Risk factors
If pulses are absent and the hand is pale and cold, and has altered sensation, a neurovascular complication is indicated and immediate surgical treatment is needed.

Signs and symptoms
- Acute pain
- Deformity of arm
- Swelling
- Bruising
- Reduced function of arm
- Altered sensation in fingers

Diagnosis
An X-ray identifies the fracture and the degree of any displacement.

Treatment
- Analgesia.
- Immobilization of the arm by application of a backslab to allow for further swelling. Once swelling has settled, the plaster can be completed.
- Elevate.
- If the fracture is displaced, it will need manipulating under a general anaesthetic.
- If a closed manipulation is unstable, the fracture may need to be fixed by surgical intervention, such as screws or nails.
- The arm will need to be in a cast for 4–6 weeks, with regular check X-rays to monitor the position and new callus formation.

Louise Mould, Royal Devon and Exeter NHS Foundation Trust

Nursing management

- Reassure the child and family.
- Give explanations about treatment and procedures.
- Pain management.
- Application and care of the cast.
- Elevate the arm.
- Neurovascular observations.
- Prepare for theatre, both physically and emotionally, if surgery is required.
- Refer to physiotherapist to teach shoulder/finger exercises.
- Provide written advice on plaster care and signs to look out for.

Complications

- Neurovascular impairment: the cast may need to be split.
- Compartment syndrome: surgical intervention is required.
- Nerve damage may cause altered sensation of fingers, which may last for several weeks until the nerves repair themselves.
- Displacement of the fracture can recur after the swelling has subsided.

Further reading

Holt, L. (2000). Skeletal injuries. In *Accident and emergency. Theory into practice* (ed. B. Dolan and L. Holt). Ballière Tindall/Royal College of Nursing, London.

Larson, D. (2000). Assessment and management of hand and wrist fractures. *Nursing Standard*, **16**, 36, 45–53.

www.orthoinfo.aaos.org

Fractures of metacarpals and metatarsals

Definition
The metacarpals are the five bones that form the hand, and the metatarsals are the five bones that make up the forefoot.

Causes
• Fractures of the shaft of the metacarpals are caused by either a direct blow or a crush injury.
• Fractures of the metatarsals are usually caused by a crush injury.

History and examination
• Ascertain cause and mechanism of injury.
• Note pain, swelling, reduction in movement, and neurovascular status.
• In fractures of the metatarsals, the child may be partially able or unable to bear weight.

Risk factors
If metatarsal fractures develop severe swelling, with pain on movement of the toes, compartment syndrome must be considered.

Signs and symptoms
• Pain
• Swelling
• Bruising
• Reduction in movement
• Unable to totally weight bear (metatarsal fractures)

Diagnosis
An X-ray is taken to determine the position of the fracture and whether it is displaced or dislocated.

Treatment
• Metacarpal fractures are normally treated conservatively by neighbour or 'buddy' strapping.
• Elevation.
• If there is a wound, antibiotics may be given to prevent infection.
• If the fracture is displaced or dislocated, surgical intervention is required.
• Metatarsal fractures are also treated conservatively, depending upon severity of pain and swelling.
• If there is minimal swelling, rest, elevation, and application of ice is advised.
• More extensive swelling and pain may indicate compartment syndrome.

Nursing management
• Reassure child and family.
• Give explanations about treatment and procedures.

Louise Mould, Royal Devon and Exeter NHS Foundation Trust

Pain management.
Neurovascular status.
Strapping of fingers or toes.
Elevation of limb.
Application of ice.
Prepare child and family, both physically and emotionally, if theatre is required.
▶ Refer to a physiotherapist if crutches are needed to enable mobilization.

Further reading

arson, D. (2002). Assessment and management of foot and ankle fractures. *Nursing Standard*, **17**(6), 37–46.

Wilson, G. et al. (1997). *Emergency management of hand injuries*. Oxford University Press, Oxford.
🔲 www. emedicine.com

External fixation

External fixation devices have become a versatile and highly useful method of dealing with a range of orthopaedic conditions. Examples where external fixation devices may be used include:

- leg lengthening for children in whom growth-plate damage has occurred or for children with dwarfism syndromes
- severe congenital talipes (clubfoot)
- congenital abnormality of the lower arm and wrist
- realignment/repair of complex comminuted fractures
- fractures with severe soft tissue, nerve, or blood vessel damage
- infected fracture sites where internal fixation would be unwise.

Types of device

- Transfixing screws held together by a sliding bar (Orthofix). Most commonly used for straightforward leg lengthening and fixation of mid-shaft uncomplicated fractures.
- Circular frame (Ilizarov) held to the bone by a combination of transfixing screws and/or wires. Most commonly used for correction of deformities, repair of a fragmented fracture, and repair of small bone areas such as the foot.
- Hybrid frames are a combination of a sliding bar fixed to a circular frame, occasionally used for injuries around the knee area.

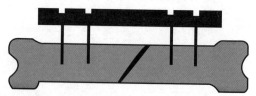

Sliding bar external fixator

Complications

- Pin-site infection common
- Occasionally delayed bony union
- Stress fractures following removal of the screws
- Overgranulation of skin around pin-sites
- Scarring of skin

Nursing considerations

- Following application, this treatment is painful until swelling subsides. Muscle spasms may occur due to position of screws/wires:
  - give regular analgesia and antispasmodic as required
  - find a comfortable position
  - play therapy.
- Psychological impact. Many children and parents find the frame difficult to accept:

Brian Silverwood, Healthcare Commission

- prepare before operation (detailed explanation, including examples of frames and photographs)
- show sensitivity during the early post-operative period; allow the child to cover with a pillowcase, etc.
- involve specialist limb reconstruction and pain team.
- Pin-site care (📖 see local procedure p.508).
- Help child to exercise:
  - CPM machine
  - child usually mobilized from post-operative day 2
  - close working partnership with physiotherapist.
- The device may be in place for 3–6 months before removal.
  - Older children can remove their own screws by utilizing Entonox in the out-patient department.
  - A hinged cast brace may be applied following removal, to prevent stress fractures and allow full mobilization.

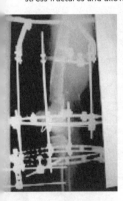 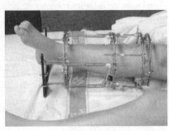

Examples of circular frames. From Glasper A, Richardson E. (Eds.). *A textbook of Children's and Young People's Nursing* (2006), Elsevier, (London); Brian Silverwood, Chapter 35 Caring for Children with Orthopaedic Disorders Fig 35.10 External fixation (Ilizarov frame) p.569, © 2006, with permission from Elsevier.

Further reading

Apley, A.G., Solomon, L. (2001). *Concise system of orthopaedics and fractures*, 2nd edn. Edward Arnold, London.

Pickup, S., Pagdin, J. (2000). Procedural pain: Entonox can help. *Paediatric Nursing*, **12**(10), 33–6.

Acute osteomyelitis

Definition
Acute osteomyelitis is a bacterial infection which, in children, most frequently affects the metaphyseal region of the long bones (near the growing epiphyhsis and therefore close to the joint). Pus collects in the medullary cavity of the bone and tracks through the cortex to form a subperiosteal collection, lifting the periosteum away from the bone. If left untreated, bone necrosis results and a sinus forms, with the infection tracking to the skin. The infection is usually accompanied by a systemic illness and requires prompt diagnosis and early treatment to prevent long-term implications for the child's growing bones.

Incidence
- 2 per 100 000 population.
- The incidence is higher in boys than girls.

Causes
The most common causative organism in children is *S. aureus*. In the neonate it is *H. influenzae*. The bacteria reach the site of infection either by haematogenous spread (via the bloodstream) from another infected part of the body or through a surgical or traumatic open wound.

Risk factors
- Open fracture
- Bone surgery

Suspected bone infection

Clinical features	Investigations
• Pain and non-use of affected limb	• Full blood count (white cell count elevated)
• Reduced movement of neighbouring joint	• CRP (elevated)
• Localized swelling, warmth, and redness	• Erythrocyte sedimentation rate (elevated)
• Pyrexia	• Blood cultures (to determine organism before commencing IV antibiotics)
• General malaise and nausea	• Bone scan or MRI (to confirm bone infection)
• History of recent infection, e.g. upper respiratory infection	• X-ray (not confirmatory, changes are insidious, 7–10 days, useful for follow-up)
• Sepsis	

Differential diagnosis
- Irritable hip (transient synovitis)
- Septic arthritis (infection in the joint requiring urgent drainage of pus)

[4]. Southampton University Hospitals NHS Trust

Treatment

- IV antibiotics, commenced immediately after blood cultures taken.
- The antibiotic is determined by:
  - organism (change appropriately with results of blood cultures)
  - age of child.
- Effective drug choices are benzylpenicillin and flucloxacillin, with oral Fucidin®; continue until repeat blood test results indicate a trend of improvement in the blood parameters and there is clinical improvement in the child's symptoms.
  - ▶ For infants who have not had the Hib vaccine, a cephalosporin is the drug of choice.
- Oral antibiotics are continued for a total of 6 weeks.
- Occasionally surgery is necessary to drain the abscess (ultrasound is helpful in determining soft tissue collection).

Nursing management

- 4-hourly monitoring of body temperature
- Pain relief
- Rest and immobilization of affected limb (consider use of a plaster backslab)

Complications

- Septic arthritis
- Chronic osteomyelitis (rare in children)
- Growth-plate arrest, resulting in limb-length discrepancy or deformity
- Fracture non-union
- Septicaemia

Follow-up

Children are seen in the clinic 2 weeks after discharge from hospital. The blood test is repeated and an X-ray performed to measure the response to treatment.

Further reading

Judd, J., Wright, L. (2005). Joint and limb problems in children and adolescents. In *Orthopaedic and trauma nursing* (ed. J. Kneale and P. Davis), 2nd edn, pp. 244–64. Churchill Livingstone, London.

Saxton, V.J. *et al.* (1997). Bone and joint infection. In *A textbook of paediatric orthopaedics* (ed. N.S. Broughton), pp. 149–64. WB Saunders, London.

▣ Osteomyelitis. www.orthoseek.com/articles/osteomyelitis.html

Scoliosis

Definition
A deformity of the spine with lateral curvature and vertebral rotation.

Causes
- Neuromuscular: neuropathic or neurogenic
- Congenital: failure of formation or segmentation
- Idiopathic: no known cause

80% of all scoliosis cases are idiopathic and are classified by age at onset:
- early onset (infantile) occurs before the age of 5 years and is predominant in boys
- late onset (adolescent) occurs between the ages of 12 years and 16 years and is predominant in girls.

Signs
- Uneven hem line
- One shoulder higher than the other
- One hip more prominent than the other
- Girls may complain that one breast appears less prominent than the other

Often detected by school personnel, such as school nurse, gym teacher, or dance teacher.

Diagnosis
By clinical examination and spinal X-rays. When the subject bends forwards, one side of the chest or loin appears more prominent if scoliosis is present (Adams test). X-rays are taken with the spine erect. Measurements are taken and the degree of curvature determined.

Treatment
Aims
- Prevent curve progression and any resulting compromise of respiratory function
- Preserve good appearance
- Preserve function

Types
- Observation: spinal X-rays are taken at 3–6-monthly intervals with the spine erect. Each X-ray is compared with the previous one to determine curve progression.
- Bracing: sometimes used when the child is growing rapidly. The aim is to control the curve until the child is a more ideal age for surgery.
- Surgery: generally performed when it is thought the spinal curvature at skeletal maturity will be greater than 50°. The type and size of the curve and age of the child determine surgical procedure. Consists of correcting the spinal curvature and performing a bony fusion. The spine is then held in place with metal rods, hooks, and screws.

Pauline Heaton, Central Manchester and Manchester Children's University Hospitals NHS Trust

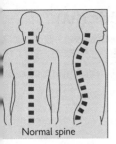 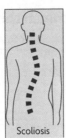 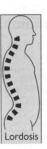 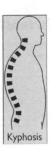

| Normal spine | Scoliosis | Lordosis | Kyphosis |

- Definitive: older children, either posterior or anterior approach.
- Combined: young children and those with severe curves may require both anterior and posterior surgery.
- Growing rods: young children where bracing fails to control the curve.

Scoliosis in infants

- Congenital: most common form in babies. Early surgery in patients with a poor prognosis generally gives rise to a satisfactory outcome.
- Postural moulding syndrome: a generally benign condition that resolves spontaneously.
- Early onset (infantile) idiopathic: well-recognized radiological markers separate this from the previous condition. Development can be arrested and regression induced by aggressive conservative treatment. The results are good if treatment is started early.

Further reading

De Wald, R.L. et al. (2003). *Spinal deformities the comprehensive text.* Thieme, New York.
Leatherman, K.D., Dickson, R.A. (1988). *The management of spinal deformities.* Wright, London.
🔲 www.srs.org

Juvenile idiopathic arthritis (JIA)

JIA: umbrella term for a variety of arthritic conditions which occur before age of 16 years (formerly known as Still's disease and subsequently juvenile chronic arthritis (JCA)).

- 1 in a 1000 children in the UK are affected by arthritis (incidence equal to diabetes mellitus).
- Aetiology unknown.

Characteristics of JIA

- Swelling: one or more joints >6 weeks
- Tender painful joints
- Joint stiffness (typically mornings)
- Restriction of movement
- Warmth in joints
- Joint deformity due to late diagnosis/treatment failure
- Poor growth due to late diagnosis/treatment failure

Systemic JIA subgroup

- Daily spiking pyrexia for 2 weeks (quotidian for at least 3 days)
- Rashes
- Multi-organ involvement—hepato-splenomegaly, serositis, and lymphadenopathy

Aims of treatment

- Reduction of joint inflammation.
- Maintain function and independence, to achieve full potential as individuals.
- Prevention of deformity.

Treatment modalities

- Non-steroidal anti-inflammatory drugs (NSAIDs), e.g. ibuprofen, naproxen, and diclofenac (often given in higher than normal dosages).
- Intra-articular steroid injections.
- Steroids pulsed, orally or IV, to effect disease remission.
- Disease-modifying anti-rheumatic drugs (DMARDs), e.g. methotrexate.
- Biological therapies, e.g. etanercept, Humira, or infliximab.
- Children and young people with more than oligo-arthritis should be referred to and supported by tertiary paediatric rheumatology centres, with shared-care arrangements initiated.
- Nurses caring for these children need to be trained and competent in the management of cytotoxic and biological therapies.

Therapeutic interventions

- Physiotherapy (and hydrotherapy): maintenance of normal function, posture, pacing, and exercise.
- Occupational therapy: functional assessment, aids, and splinting of joints as appropriate.
- Orthotics.
- Psychology.

Liz Hutchinson, Nottingham Children and Young People's Rheumatology Service
Helen Strike, Southmead Hospital Bristol

Opthalmology: children and young people with JIA should be referred for slit-lamp examination of the eyes because inflammatory eye disease (uveitis) can be a feature of arthritis and may be asymptomatic.

ursing management

Work as part of an interdisciplinary team, ideally including all of the following: paediatric rheumatologist, physiotherapist, occupational therapist, pharmacist, school teacher, social worker, psychologist, youth worker/hospital play specialist, complementary therapist, and dietician.

Provide holistic disease education/management for child, family, parents, carers, and others involved in care and consequences of the disease and its management.

Know how to care for patients who are immunosuppressed.

Provide psychosocial support for child and family/carers.

Know about treatment modalities and monitoring requirements (NICE guidance).

Assess disease activity (use of core outcome variables, e.g. childhood health assessment questionnaire) and response to treatment.

Liaise, as appropriate, with primary and secondary care teams, education, social services, and voluntary agencies.

Facilitate effective transition to adult care/life.

urther reading

nberg, D.A., Miller, P.J., Woo, P., Breedveld, F.C. (2004). *Oxford textbook of rheumatology*, 3rd edn. Oxford University Press, Oxford.

ediatric Rheumatology International Trials Organization (PRINTO). ▣ www.printo.it

yal College of Nursing (2004). *Subcutaneous methotrexate in inflammatory arthritis*. RCN, London. ▣ www.rcn.org.uk

Developmental dysplasia of the hip (DDH)

Can present at birth or as a dislocated hip or limp after 6 months of age
- DDH covers a variety of conditions, including dislocation, displacement of ball and socket, subluxation (the hip is not deep enough in the socket), and socket too shallow.
- DDH occurs in approximately 2 in 1000 births; generally more girls than boys are affected.

Diagnosis
- Diagnosed at birth with Ortolani and Barlow tests
- Lie baby on his/her back and gently move hips out sideways
- If hips do not move well, further investigation is required
- Ultrasound scan to confirm diagnosis

All babies' hips are rechecked at 6–8 weeks and 6–8 months as standard practice, because late diagnosis can occur.

Treatment
Conservative treatment
If DDH is diagnosed early, treatment is usually with a splint or harness which is worn for 6–12 weeks. This will flex the baby's hips out. This position is most satisfactory for the hip to develop.

Surgical treatment
Occasionally the baby will need to be put into a plaster cast to hold the joints more firmly in place. There may be surgery involving the release of tendons and, if still unstable, an osteotomy may be performed.

After surgery, the correction is maintained in plaster that extends from the waist down to the feet (📖 p.516, Caring for Children in hip spicas).

Nursing management
- Provide support for child and family.
- A diagnosis of DDH is often upsetting for parents. Diagnosis is often made at birth or in the few weeks thereafter when parents are already tired and emotional, and so easily overwhelmed. Therefore support and clear information are essential.
- The family is managed predominately in the out-patient department, but may require hospital admission for surgery.

Pre-operative and post-operative care
- Standard pre-operative and post-operative care for the child and family, depending on the child's needs.
- Advice on the management of a hip spica.

Further reading
Contact-a-Family Congenital dislocation and developmental dysplasia of the hip 🖳 www.cafamily.org.uk/Direct/c63.html
Knighton, J. (1998). Developmental dysplasia of the hip. *Fracture Magazine International*, **20**, 9–13.

Janina Chell, Royal Cornwall Hospital Trust

Congenital talipes equinovarus (CTEV) or talipes

Definition

- Congenital
- Talipes: the Latin word for 'foot and ankle'
- Equino: horselike, because the foot is in plantar flexion
- Varus: medical word for 'turned in'

CTEV is the most common congenital abnormality of the foot. One o both feet can be affected, and in cases of bilateral involvement one foo is usually worse than the other.

CTEV remains the most difficult foot abnormality to treat successfull because treatment includes treating several joints at the same time, an also treating joints that constantly change under the influence of growth.

CTEV is diagnosed either antenatally or immediately after birth, althoug a traumatic birth may cause talipes that can be easily resolved with sim ple exercises.

Characteristics

- The heel is drawn up
- The foot is inverted (twisted inwards)
- The hind foot is abducted
- Creases in the skin

Treatment

There are two types of treatment: conservative and surgical.

Conservative treatment

Performed in the first 3 months, and concentrates on the forefoot. This i achieved by using:

- below-knee plaster backslabs
- strapping
- above-knee plaster backslab.

Surgical treatment

This is necessary if the foot remains undercorrected. This will be decided at 3 months. The foot's response to the conservative treatment wil dictate how much surgery is required.

Surgery could consist of:

- soft tissue release, with or without tendon transfers
- osteotomies
- correction and lengthening of soft tissue structures

After surgery, the correction is maintained by an above-knee plaster. Treatment continues with the supply of special footwear, night splints, and stretching exercises.

Surgery may lead to a good result, but as the child grows, the soft tissue may tighten, occasionally leading to further surgery.

Janina Chell, Royal Cornwall Hospital Trust

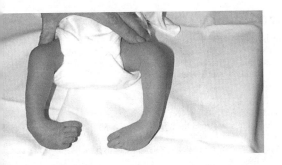

Nursing management

Support for child and family: a diagnosis of CTEV is often upsetting for parents, and because diagnosis is often made at birth, parents are already tired and emotional, and so easily overwhelmed. Therefore support and clear information is essential.

Parents often become quite upset about the constant exercises they have to undertake, causing pain and discomfort to their child. The family is predominately managed in the out-patient department.

Pre-operative and post-operative care: standard pre-operative and post-operative care for the child and family, depending on the child's needs.

Further reading

Dandy, J.P., Nugent, I.M., Ross, A.C. (1995). *Key topics in orthopaedic surgery*. Bios Scientific Publishers, Oxford.

Lorimer, L.D. (1993). *Neale's common foot disorders—diagnosis and management, a general clinical guide*, 4th edn. Churchill Livingstone, London.

Irritable hip (transient synovitis)

Irritable hip is a condition in which the synovial lining of the hips become inflamed. This usually causes the child to have pain and difficulty walkin. Irritable hip occurs in children (between 2 years and 10 years) and more common in boys than girls.

Causes

Unknown, but triggers may include:
- viral infection
- infection elsewhere in the body
- trauma may precede in a small number of cases
- post-vaccine or other drug-related reactions have been cited as possible causes.

Clinical signs

- Usually no temperature, but may have low-grade pyrexia
- Pain, causing crying at night
- The child can usually still walk, but with pain, and may limp
- Hip site may be tender
- Affected leg may be held in a position that causes the child the least amount of pain
- A small-to-moderate decrease in the range of hip movement
- May be a decrease in the range of knee movement
- History of a recent infection

Differential diagnosis

Following physical examination, investigation in hospital will include h. X-ray and ultrasound, and blood tests may be requested to rule ou conditions that present a similar clinical picture, such as Perthes disease.

Treatment

Mild cases
- Bed rest in a position of comfort (flexed if tolerated) for 7–10 days
- Regular analgesia
- NSAIDs
- Physiotherapy

More severe cases
- Bilateral or unilateral simple skin traction
- Aspiration of any hip effusion under general anaesthesia

In most cases, a full recovery is achieved. There is usually an X-ray an follow-up at around 6 months after easing of symptoms, to ensure the condition has completely cleared and no other hip conditions have developed.

Nursing considerations

Nursing care will depend on the choice of treatment. Should the chil require a period of traction, consider the following.
- Pain
  - regular analgesia
  - position of comfort

Brian Silverwood, Healthcare Commission

Boredom
- play specialist
- activities
- computer games and videos

Position, assist with:
- eating
- drinking
- washing
- elimination
- learning

Traction
- look for sensitive reactions of adhesive skin extensions
- check weights secure/hanging freely
- bed tilt to counterbalance weight
- prevent complications of bed rest

Further reading

enson, M.K.D. *et al.* (2002). *Children's orthopaedics and fractures*, 2nd edn. Churchill Livingstone, London.

Whitelaw, C.C. (2004). *Transient synovitis.* www.emedicine.com/ped/topic1676.htm (accessed 24 July 2005).

Perthes disease

Perthes disease is characterized by a loss of circulation to the head of the femur in a child, resulting in avascular necrosis (bone cell death in head of femur). This is followed by a period of revascularization lasting 18 months to 2 years. During this period, the bone is soft and at risk of fracture, usually resulting in the head either collapsing or moulding into an abnormal or non-spherical shape, leading to stiffness and pain.

Characterisics of Perthes disease

- Cause unknown
- More common in boys than girls
- Symptoms depend upon the stage of the disease

May present with:
- very painful hip (due to inflammation of hip lining)
- and/or a painful limp that has developed acutely over a few hours.

Or more frequently:
- presents with a fracture of the head of femur
- or a painful limp that occurred over days or weeks.

Not unusually:
- the child may go through the whole process of the disease without symptoms
- presents at his/her doctor as a young adult with hip pain due to degenerative arthritis of the hip caused by Perthes disease.

Treatment

- The condition is usually diagnosed by X-ray, following other investigations to rule out conditions that may cause similar symptoms.
- Traditionally, the child was placed on prolonged periods of bed rest and non-weight bearing, because it was thought this might stop the head of the femur collapsing.
- Treatment now centres on maintaining the head within the acetabulum. This may be achieved conservatively through casting or bracing, or surgically by a femoral rotational osteotomy or similar surgical hip procedure
- If the hip presents with stiffness, the child may already have a degree of flattening of the head, and this will be treated by a period of traction and physiotherapy, followed by surgical hip-adductor releases.

Nursing considerations

Nursing care will depend on whether the child is to receive conservative or surgical management. However, the following should be considered irrespective of the orthopaedic management:
- boredom: play specialist
- pain: regular analgesia, diversion therapy
- assistance with activities of daily living: if on bed rest or hip spica cast
- care of hip spica cast: trimming, strenghening, and waterproofing
- parental anxiety: explanation and information

Brian Silverwood, Healthcare Commission

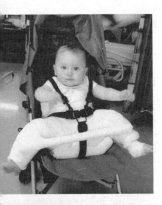

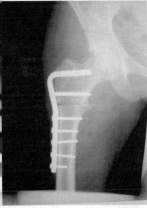

Example of rotational osteotomy with blade plate and screw fixation. Figures from Glasper A, Richardson E. (Eds.), A textbook of Children's and Young People's Nursing (2006), Elsevier (London); Brian Silverwood Chapter 35, Caring for Children with Orthopaedic Disorders, Fig 35.9 Internal fixation p.568, © 2006, with permission from Elsevier.

Further reading

Benson, M.K.D. et al. (2002). *Children's orthopaedics and fractures*, 2nd edn. Churchill Livingstone, London.

Orthoseek (2005). (Legg–Calve) Perthes Disease. 🖳 www.orthoseek.com/articles/perthes.html (accessed 8 August 2005).

Staheli, L.L. (2003). *Fundamentals of pediatric orthopedics*, 3rd edn. Lippincott Williams & Wilkins, Philadelphia.

Skin traction: application and care (principles)

Traction is a pulling force, which requires counter-traction (the child's body acting against gravity) in order to function effectively. When skin traction is used, the pull is not only applied directly to the child's skin, but also applied indirectly to underlying structures, such as bones, joints, and muscles. Normally a continuous pull applied to the leg(s) may be used on arm (e.g. Dunlop traction). Can be used alone (e.g. Gallows traction) or as part of more complex system (e.g. Thomas splint traction).

Action	Rationale
Assess child's need for traction	Other treatment options are available. Potential complications include pressure sores, skin damage, muscle wasting, constipation, and boredom
Reduction/treatment of fracture	
Relief of pain, contracture, or muscle spasm	
Pre-operative positioning	
Select and prepare equipment	Save time and promote efficiency
Skin traction kit—adhesive/non-adhesive strapping, bandages	Ensure correct size and type of kit
Balkan beams, connectors, pulleys, and weight(s)	Ensure compatibility and accessibility of equipment
Prepare child and parents	
Explain the procedure appropriately for child's age/level of understanding	Promote cooperation and family-centred care
Relieve pain/sedate child	Movement during application may cause pain
Select suitable bed or cot	Ensure compatibility of apparatus
Check integrity of child's skin	Adhesive strapping may cause allergic reaction or exacerbate existing problem
Measure strapping against limb, leaving a small gap between foot and spreader bar. Trim excess length	Ensure correct length; allow for ankle movement
Apply to medial and lateral aspects of limb, starting above malleoli	
Remove backing slowly to allow smooth application; ensure strapping is kept straight and malleoli are covered by foam padding	Prevent wrinkles in strapping because of potential skin damage; prevent unequal pull to medial or lateral aspect of limb; protect bony prominences from excess pressure
Bandage firmly but not tightly over strapping, starting just above malleoli; omit the knee(s)	Secure strapping; prevent excess pressure

Maggie Doman, University of Plymouth

Contd.

Action	Rationale
Adjust and secure cord(s) at spreader, pass through pulleys, and attach securely to weight(s); suspend weight(s)	Apply traction
Apply counter-traction:	Balanced system—pulling force maintained if child moves in bed
Elevate end of bed	
Check child's position	
Check colour, sensation, movement, pulse, and temperature of extremities; continue observations regularly; and adjust bandages or position as necessary	Excessive traction force or tight bandages may compromise neurovascular status
Ongoing care:	Promote and maintain comfort
Check pressure areas for skin integrity—remove bandages and check skin daily	Prevent soreness, especially of heels, sacrum, and elbow, and damage to skin under bandages
Diet and fluids	Promote healing
Elimination—regular nappy changes or slipper bedpan	Prevent constipation and soreness
Maintain privacy and dignity	
Play/other activities/family-centred care	Prevent boredom and promote normality
Check equipment daily and after alterations to system, e.g. following X-ray or movement of bed/cot	Maintain safety of child; ensure effectiveness of traction

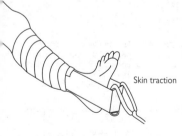

Skin traction

Further reading

Davis, P., Barr, L. (1999). Principles of traction. *Journal of Orthopaedic Nursing*, **3**(4), 222–7.
Bolcik, M.A., Carini-Garcia, G., Birmingham, J.J. (1994). *Traction: assessment and management*. Mosby, St Louis.
Styrcula, L. (1994). Traction basics. Part II: Traction equipment. *Orthopaedic Nursing*, **13**(13), 55–9.

Gallows traction: application and care (principles)

This involves the application of skin traction to both legs for children under about 18 months of age, up to a maximum weight of 12–14 kg (skin traction).

Action	Rationale
Assess child's need for traction	Other treatment options are available. Potential complications include pressure sores, skin damage, and muscle wasting
Reduction/treatment of fractured femur	
Positioning prior to hip surgery	
Select and prepare equipment	Save time and promote efficiency
Skin traction kits × 2	Ensure correct size and type of kit
Beams, connectors, pulleys, and weights	Ensure compatibility and accessibility of equipment
Prepare child and parents	
Explain procedure	Promote cooperation and family-centred care
Relieve pain	Movement during application may cause pain
Prepare suitable cot	Ensure compatibility of apparatus
Check integrity of child's skin	Adhesive strapping may cause allergic reaction or exacerbate existing problem
Measure strapping against legs, leaving a small gap between the foot and spreader bar. Trim excess length	Ensure correct length; allow for ankle movement
Apply strapping to medial and lateral aspects of legs, starting above malleoli	
Remove backing slowly to allow smooth application; ensure strapping is kept straight; and malleoli are covered by foam padding	Prevent wrinkles in strapping; potential skin damage; prevent unequal pull to medial or lateral aspect of limb; protect bony prominences from excess pressure
Bandage in place, starting just above malleoli	Secure strapping; prevent excess pressure
Suspend child's legs at right angles to his body	Apply traction (balanced)
Adjust and secure cords at spreader bar	

Maggie Doman, University of Plymouth

Contd.

Action	Rationale
Pass cords through pulleys attached to beams above cot Attach cords securely to weights at head or foot of cot Cords may be tied to beam (fixed traction)	
Check counter-traction by ensuring buttocks clear of mattress, using flat of hand	If buttocks on mattress, insufficient traction; if too high, excessive traction force and risk of damage to hips
Check colour, sensation, movement, pulse, and temperature of feet; continue observations regularly; and adjust bandages as necessary	Child's position, excessive traction force, or tight bandages may compromise neurovascular status
Ongoing care	Promote and maintain comfort
Check pressure areas for skin integrity, especially sacrum, shoulder blades, occiput, and under bandages Hygiene	Skin may become sore due to position and restricted mobility
Diet and fluids	
Elimination	
Maintain privacy and dignity	
Play and family-centred care	
Check equipment daily—all apparatus, cords, pulleys, etc	Maintain child's safety; ensure effectiveness of traction

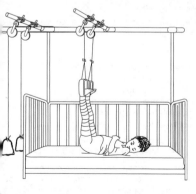

Further reading

Huband, S., Trigg, E. (ed.) (2000). *Practices in children's nursing*, pp. 293–301. Churchill Livingstone, Edinburgh.

www.steps-charity.org.uk.

Pin-site care

Definition

Pins or wires are used in conjunction with external fixators, such as the ilizarov frame, to secure a fracture, lengthen a limb, or correct a deformity.

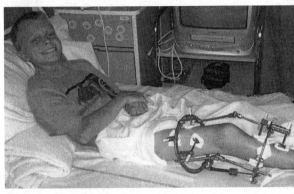

Ilizarov frame for correction of fixed knee contracture

Skeletal pins are in effect a foreign body and therefore have the potential to become infected. The rationale behind pin-site cleaning is to prevent bone infection (i.e. osteomyelitis).

Nursing management of pin-sites

The management of skeletal pins remains a source of constant debate (see below), although the principles are universal:

- evidence-based
- clean technique
- removal of crusts (to allow free drainage of serous fluid)
- avoid transfer of cleaning swabs between pins
- check pin-sites daily for signs of infection
- treat developing pin-site infection promptly with broad-spectrum antibiotic (after sending a swab to the laboratory)
- educate the parent/carer and child.

The ultimate aim is to prevent complications of severe infection that would lead to the pin(s) being removed, thereby compromising patient treatment.

External fixators may be in place for as little as 2 months or up to 12 months, depending on the child's underlying condition. Nursing intervention is aimed at assisting the parents, carers, and child to feel confident in pin-site cleaning, with knowledge of who and when to contact if in doubt about a developing pin-site infection.

Julia Judd, Southampton University Hospitals NHS Trust

Suggested pin-site cleaning regimens in current practice

Method 1	Method 2
Pin-sites covered with dry dressings after operation	After operation cover pin-sites with alcohol-moistened dressings
Theatre dressings left in place for 48 hours	Clean pin-sites daily for 3 days after operation using 70% alcohol, and cover with alcohol-moistened dressings
Pin-sites cleaned daily with normal saline using cotton buds	On day 4, clean and leave occlusive dressing in place
Crusts are removed	Clean pins and re-dress every 7 days using the same method

Clinical features of pin-site infection
- Redness around the pin-site
- Tenderness and pain at the pin-site
- Swelling
- Increased oozing from the pin-site or presence of pus
- Odour from the pin-site
- Pin loosening

Investigations for potential pin-site infection
- Pin-site swab
- Bloods: full blood count, eythrocyte sedimentation rate, CPK

Treatment of pin-site infection
An infected pin-site is painful or inflamed, with a discharge that is positive for bacterial culture or responds to antibiotic therapy.
- Preventive antibiotics are commenced at the first signs of pin-site infection.
- Admit for IV antibiotics if the infection is not controlled with oral therapy.

Complications
The most severe complication of pin-site infection is osteomyelitis; the infection tracks along the pin directly to the bone. Treatment:
- the external fixator is removed
- IV antibiotic therapy is administered.

Further reading
Davies, R., Nayagam, S., Holt, N. (2005). The care of pin sites with external fixation. *Journal of Bone and Joint Surgery, British Volume*, **87**(5), 716–19.

FROG pin-site care project. ▣ www.man.ac.uk/rcn/ukwide/frogpinsite.htm

Judd, J., Wright, L. (2005). Joint and limb problems in children and adolescents. In *Orthopaedic and Trauma Nursing* (ed. J. Kneale and P. Davis), 2nd edn, pp. 244–264. Churchill Livingstone, London.

Lee-Smith, J., Santy, J., Davis, P. (2001). Pin site management. Towards a consensus: part 1. *Journal of Orthopaedic Nursing*, **5**(1), 37–42.

Care of a child in plaster

Plaster or resin-based casts are commonly used to immobilize limbs following orthopaedic (bone or joint) trauma or surgery.

Why a cast?
- To maintain bone alignment for fracture healing
- To maintain surgical correction until healed
- To provide pain relief by resting the affected limb or joint
- To correct deformities, by plaster wedging or serial casting

Care of the child while applying plaster
- Explain the procedure fully to the child and parent/carer first.
- The plaster room environment is clinical and noisy. Try to make the environment more welcoming by the provision of familiar toys and comforters.
- Casts should only be applied by a qualified plaster technician.
- The limb is prepared with stockinet and/or wool padding.
- The cast bandage is soaked in water and then bandaged on to the limb.
- Initially the cast will feel warm.
- Plaster of Paris will take 24–48 hours to dry. Resin-based casts dry in 20–30 min.

Care of the child after cast application
- Handle the wet cast with the palm of your hand to prevent denting.
- The cast should be exposed to the air to facilitate drying. Do not use a hairdryer because plaster conducts heat and the patient could experience a burn.
- Elevate the limb with a cast on pillows covered with a towel. A towel will absorb excess moisture and aid drying. The softness of the pillow will prevent dents forming in the cast. Elevation will assist with reducing/discouraging oedema.
- Children in large body casts should be turned every 2 hours to facilitate drying of the plaster.
- Observe the cast regularly for dents, cracks, or skin rubbing.

Advice given on discharge
- Keep the cast dry.
- Allow the cast to dry naturally.
- Do not cover the cast with plastic for showering or bathing. Condensation can form under the plastic and make the cast wet.
- Do not put anything down the cast. Small objects may not be retrieved and will cause pressure sores.
- Do not use objects to scratch the skin under the cast, e.g. knitting needles. This may cause a skin laceration or traumatize the skin, making it more susceptible to sores.
- Avoid beaches and sandpits. Sand under a plaster can cause skin abrasions.
- Keep the limb elevated for the first 2 days. This reduces/prevents swelling.

Elizabeth Wright. Southampton University Hospitals NHS Trust

Follow specific advice, e.g. do not bear weight on a plastered limb.
➤ Seek medical advice if:
- the toes or fingers become blue, swollen, and painful to move
- the limb becomes more painful
- if the cast feels uncomfortable or rubbing is noticed
- if an unpleasant smell is noticed from the cast and/or a discharge is seen on the plaster

Further reading

ucus, B., Davis, P. (2005). Why restricting movement is important. In *Orthopaedic and Trauma Nursing* (ed. J. Kneale and P. Davis). Churchill Livingstone, London.
rior, M., Miles, S. (1999). Principles of casting. *Journal of Orthopaedic Nursing*, **3**(3), 162–70.
www.bettercare.vic.gov.au.bhcu2/bhcarticles.nsf/pages/Plaster_Care?OpenDocument

Observing for neurovascular impairment and compartment syndrome

Neurovascular impairment is the interruption, either partial or complete, of the nerve or blood supply to a limb. It may occur as a result of injury or from treatment of the injury or orthopaedic condition. If left untreated, it may precede compartment syndrome.

Compartment syndrome is defined as 'high pressure within the muscle compartment'. Muscle fascia which cannot expand encloses the muscle and so increased pressure 'reduces capillary blood flow below a level necessary for tissue viability'. If left untreated, muscle necrosis can occur, possibly resulting in limb amputation or death from renal failure.

Signs and symptoms

The signs and symptoms of compartment syndrome are listed as the 'five Ps': pain, pallor, paraesthesia, paralysis, and pulselessness. An additional indicator is coldness.

Signs and symptoms	Nursing observations
Increasing pain, out of proportion to the injury or surgical intervention. The first most reliable sign	Regular pain assessments using an age-appropriate pain tool. Give all patients prescribed analgesia
Pallor	Observe perfusion of digits on the affected limb. Capillary refill time should be <1 s
Paraesthesia	Ask if the child can feel 'pins and needles' in the digits. Lightly touch all digits, asking the child to confirm that he/she can feel the touch and that the feeling is normal or the same as in the non-affected limb
Paralysis	Ask the child to move the affected digits. The child may be reluctant to move the digits because of pain, but should be able to do so
Pulselessness. The final sign. If pulselessness occurs, then compartment syndrome is well established and amputation is likely	Record the pulse distal to the site of injury. It may be necessary to make a hole in the plaster to access the pulse
Coldness	Feel the digits for warmth and compare with the other limb

Nursing observations for neurovascular impairment should occur at least hourly, and more frequently if there is clinical concern.

Further reading

Dykes, P.C. (1993). Minding the five P's of neurovascular assessment. *American Journal of Nursing*, **93**(6), 38–39.

MedlinePlus medical encyclopaedia: compartment syndrome. 🖥 www.nlm.gov/medlineplus/emcy/article/001224.htm

Swain, R., and Ross, D. (1999). Lower extremity compartment syndrome: when to suspect acute or chronic pressure build up. *Postgraduate Medicine*, **105**(3), 159–68.

Elizabeth Wright, Southampton University Hospitals NHS Trust

Thomas splint traction

Thomas splint traction can be used as balanced or fixed traction for the management of children with a fractured femur. It consists of a proximal ring that fits around the upper leg and to which two long rigid slender steel rods are attached. These extend down to another smaller ring distal to the foot.

History

This was designed in 1857 by Hugh Owen Thomas, an orthopaedic surgeon and was used initially in the management of patients with tuberculosis. During the First and Second World Wars his nephew, Sir Robert Jones, introduced his uncle's ideas and the traction method was adapted to enable wounded soldiers to be safely transported from the battlefield. The mortality of compound fractures of the femur fell from 80% in 1916 to <8% in 1918. The Thomas splint remained the main treatment for fractured femur until the advent of modern surgical techniques.

Today, the Thomas splint is used primarily as the initial management for patients with a fractured femur. Once the patient's condition has been stabilized and the thigh swelling has reduced, other treatments are often selected.

Definition of traction

Traction is 'the application of a steady pull on an injured limb by weights and pulleys'.

Applying Thomas splint traction

- Ensure the child has received effective analgesia, ideally a femoral nerve block, plus morphine or ketamine.
- Explain the procedure to the child and family.
- Measure the non-injured limb. When fully pushed in, the splint must have 30 cm projecting beyond the foot.
- Prepare equipment:
  - adjust Thomas splint to correct size, and make up
  - place traction frame on bed
  - have weight hangers and weights available
  - additional equipment—bandages, scissors, tape, and traction cord.
- The Thomas splint is usually applied in the accident and emergency department. Its assembly requires two healthcare professionals.
- One nurse applies manual traction to the injured limb. This manipulates the fracture and may result in neurovascular compromise. It is essential that neurovascular assessments are made before and after. Manual traction is maintained until another nurse has applied and secured the splint.
- Adhesive skin traction is applied, taking care not to compress the peroneal nerve that transverses the back of the knee because this may cause foot drop. The leg is rested in the Thomas splint.
- The skin traction is tied to the splint and tightened using a windlass. This creates the fixed traction.

Elizabeth Wright, Southampton University Hospitals NHS Trust

An X-ray is taken to confirm the position of the fracture.
The child is transferred to a hospital bed in the ward area. Additional traction cords and weights are attached to support the Thomas splint. This allows the child greater mobility in the bed.

mportant considerations

Maintain neurovascular assessments of the affected limb at least hourly.
Assess effectiveness of analgesia.
Assess skin integrity daily. Ask the patient if the skin/traction feels comfortable.
Check the traction apparatus daily.
Take preventive action regarding possible complications of bed rest: pressure sores, constipation, chest infection, etc.

urther reading

acus, B., Davis, P. (2005). Why restricting movement is important. In *Orthopaedic and trauma nursing* (ed. J. Kneale and P. Davis), pp. 105–39. Churchill Livingstone, London.
oyal College of Nursing: Society of Trauma and Orthopaedic Nursing (2002). *A traction manual*, pp. 49–56. RCN Publishing, Harrow-on-the-Hill, Middlesex.
www.bonetumour.org/book/APTEXT/index.html

Caring for children in hip spicas

Definition

Hip spicas are a form of splintage usually constructed out of plaster of Paris. They are commonly used to immobilize the hip(s) following surgery (e.g. for developmental dysplasia of the hips) or in the treatment of fractured femur in the young child.

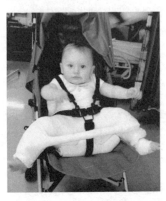

The spica is positioned with the hip(s) in flexion and abduction. It starts at mid-chest level, covers the hips, leaving an opening for toileting, and extends down the leg to the ankle (or foot if immobilizing a fractured femur). A spica can be single (extending down the affected limb only), double (both legs), or one-and-a-half (affected limb and to the knee of unaffected leg). The type depends on the underlying treatment and stability of the hip.

Nursing management

It is imperative that parents are supported in the care of their child in spica, and that they are provided with verbal and written information and practical guidance. There are three key areas of caring for a child in a hip spica: skin (and cast) care, mobility, and psychosocial needs.

Skin care

The cast and child's skin need to be kept dry and clean to prevent skin ulceration.

- Place pillows under the head of the mattress to prop the child in a semi-reclining position. This aids drainage of urine down into the nappy and prevents it seeping back up into the cast. It has the added benefit of positioning the child for play and activities.
- Prevent pressure sores: keep heels off the mattress (place a rolled-up towel under ankles), turn child regularly to reposition, and check elbows and back of head.

Julia Judd, Southampton University Hospitals NHS Trust

Tuck nappies up inside the cast. Check them every 1–2 hours during the day and last thing at night. Change if damp/wet. Use sanitary towels inside the nappy for extra protection. The older child can use a bedpan for toileting. Place thin strips of plastic inside the front and back of the cast and direct them into the bedpan. For girls, use toilet tissue as a wick to direct the flow of urine into the pan.

Wash exposed areas with soap and water. Dry carefully.

Inspect the skin daily for irritation and sore areas.

Inspect the cast regularly for indentations, cracks, and weak areas.

Teach parents how to check for normal circulation in their child's lower limbs: normal sensation, colour, and movement.

Mobility

Assist parents with safe lifting and turning their child in the spica. Liaise with the occupational therapy team regarding provision of necessary equipment to assist manual handling and mobility at home, e.g. hoist, buggy, car seat, and reclining wheelchair.

NB: The spica is not a walking cast and the child should not be allowed to stand or bear weight.

Psychosocial needs

Schooling and peer interaction for the older child: investigate whether the older child in a spica can return to school (may depend on assistance for toileting and wheelchair access).

Aim to provide normality as much as possible in the form of playtime, sleep time, and interaction with siblings and family.

Caring for a child in a hip spica is a daunting prospect for parents. They should feel supported by the hospital and community team and know who to contact for advice and when.

Further reading

Dodd, J., Wright, L. (2005). Joint and limb problems in children and adolescents. In *Orthopaedic and trauma nursing* (ed. J. Kneale and P. Davis), 2nd edn, pp. 244–64. Churchill Livingstone, London.

Smith, J. (2004). A literature review of the care of babies and young children in hip spicas. *Journal of Orthopaedic Nursing*, **8**(2), 83–90.

Sparks, L., Rush Ortman, M., Aubuchon, P. (2004). Care of the child in a body cast. *Journal of Orthopaedic Nursing*, **8**(4), 231–5.

Welcome to steps. 🖥 www.steps-charity.org.uk/links

Removing skeletal wires, pins, or screws

Definition

Skeletal wires or screws are used to fix external fixators to bones to treat fractures or in limb reconstruction treatments. There are many types of external fixators, but all rely the on the use of skeletal wires or screws. Skeletal wires or pins are also used to hold bony breaks together until the bone has healed through natural callus formation and regeneration. These bony breaks can follow either a traumatic event, e.g. fractured radius and ulna after a fall, or orthopaedic surgery, in which surgeon surgically breaks a bone to realign it and uses the skeletal wires or pins to hold the 'break' together until it heals.

Insertion of skeletal wires, pins, or screws

- Skeletal wires and screws are inserted during surgery under a general anaesthetic.
- If screws and wires are used to affix external fixators in limb reconstruction treatments, prepare children and their carers adequately pre-operatively.
- If screws or wires are used in the treatment of stabilizing fractures, it is unlikely the child will have been prepared thoroughly pre-operatively. Therefore care must be taken to counsel and support the child and his/her family post-operatively.
- Often, if skeletal wires or pins are used to stabilize breaks (whether traumatic or surgical), they are incorporated into a plaster of Paris cast.

Clinical features of infection

- Redness around the wire-site (may not be visible if a cast is in place).
- Tenderness and pain at the wire-site.
- Visible oozing at the wire-site through the cast.
- Odour from the cast.
- The child may develop pyrexia.
- The child may become systemically unwell.

Pin-site care (📖 p.508)

- When skeletal screws, pins, and wires are used under a plaster of Paris cast, the patient's carers must be made aware of the signs of potential infection.
- Encourage the family to contact the hospital if they suspect infection.

Removal of skeletal screws, wires, and pins

- Skeletal screws, wires, or pins are removed when the orthopaedic surgeon is content that the affected bone has healed.
- In many cases it may be decided to remove the screws, wires, or pins under a general anaesthetic and therefore the child will be admitted to hospital.

Jonathan Pagdin, Sheffield Children's Hospital

However, in certain circumstances it may be appropriate to remove the skeletal screws, wires, or pins in the out-patient setting, especially where they can be removed simply.

Many children, particularly those who have undergone repeated limb-reconstruction treatments, may readily volunteer to have skeletal screws, wires, or pins removed without a general anaesthetic, which they find unpleasant.

Removing skeletal screws, wires, and pins in the out-patient department also means that there is no requirement to admit the child, and this frees anaesthetic time for other cases. When removal takes place in the out-patient department, the child will be allowed home within approximately an hour of the procedure being performed.

Principles of skeletal screw, wire, and pin removal

Ensure consent given by the patient and/or parent/guardian.

Careful explanation of the procedure to the child and parent/guardian.

The procedure should be carried out in an appropriate setting, e.g. a treatment room.

Preparation of equipment prior to the procedure, e.g. use of dressing packs, cleansing and dressing materials, and the equipment to remove the screws, wires, and pins.

Ensure the child is comfortable prior to the procedure.

Encourage support from parents, nursing staff, or play specialists.

Use of distraction whenever possible, e.g. video games, taped music, books, etc.

Use of adequate analgesia, where appropriate use Entonox®.

Removal of skeletal screw, wire, or pin using the appropriate tool for removal.

Adequate cleansing and dressing of the wound site, e.g. the exit holes of the screw, wire, or pin.

Reinforcement of the signs of infection to the child's parents/guardians.

Using Entonox® for screw, wire, and pin removal can reduce patient and parent anxiety immensely and lead to successful removals in the out-patient setting, thereby reducing the need for admission to hospital and reducing the risks posed by a general anaesthetic.

Further reading

Pickup, S., Pagdin, G.J. (2001). Procedural pain: Entonox can help. *Paediatric Nursing*, **12**(10), 33–6.

Dealing with an orthopaedic emergency

An orthopaedic/trauma team should deal with any orthopaedic emergency. Nursing and medical intervention should be holistic, supportive to the child or adolescent, and yet family centred. All documented nursing care should narrate the nursing process (assess, plan, implement, and evaluate) and use an appropriate model of nursing.

Life- and limb-threatening injuries
- Vascular injuries proximal to the knee or elbow, with or without fractures.
- Crush injuries of the abdomen and pelvis.
- Compartment syndromes: traumatic amputations—complete or incomplete.
- Dislocations of the knee or hip.
- Fractures, with or without dislocations, about the knee or elbow.
- Major pelvic fracture and fractures with vascular or nerve injury.
- Open fractures with ragged, dirty wounds.

Injury assessment
The nurse should obtain a history that includes mechanism of injury and first-response findings.

Extremities should be assessed for:
- colour and perfusion (pulse, capillary refill, and warmth)
- deformities such as angulation or shortening, muscle spasm, and crepitation
- swelling, discoloration and bruising, and tenderness
- wounds, bleeding, or haematoma
- vascular impairment (sensation and pain)

Major emergencies
- Pelvic fractures: usually severe trauma, which may accompany visceral injuries to the abdomen; anticipate shock.
- Open fractures: remove gross contaminates; assist medical officer to align with proper splinting techniques; any obvious or suspected fracture near a wound should be assumed to be an open fracture and blood loss should be estimated.
- Amputations: potential for massive haemorrhage. An amputated part should be cleaned of any gross contaminant, wrapped in a sterile towel moistened with sterile saline, placed in a sealed plastic bag, and transported in a chest with crushed ice and water if available. Do not allow the limb to freeze; do not use dry ice.

General principles
- Pain management: regular pain assessment (valid and reliable tool) and adequate analgesia; WHO pain ladder.
- Cover wounds with damp or dry sterile dressing—depends on injury.
- Bleeding should be controlled with direct pressure.

Sonya Clarke, Queen's University Belfast

Tourniquet (applied by medical officer) should be used only as a last resort; if used, it should be loosened and re-applied every 40 min.
Check neurovascular status of limb before and after splinting and inform medical officer of any changes.
IV fluids protocols.
Hypovolaemic shock management.

Sensory problems

Anatomy and physiology of the ear

The ears have an important role in both hearing and balance. The convert the pressure changes generated by sound waves into electric potentials, which are then transmitted to the auditory areas of the brain. The ears also provide information about the position an movements of the head and initiate reflex postural adjustments th maintain balance. The ear is split into three parts: the outer ear, th middle ear, and the inner ear.

The outer ear

The pinna is a cartilagenous structure that has a relatively poor bloc supply. When a sound is made, the sound waves are 'collected' by th pinna and transmitted along the external auditory canal to the tympan membrane, through the middle ear via the ossicles, to the inner ear. Th cochlea in the inner ear converts the sound waves into electrical signa that are then passed to the brain via the auditory nerve. The presence a pinna on both sides of the head allows localization of sound.

External auditory canal

The cartilagenous portion of external auditory canal is lined by sk (keratinized squamous epithelium) which, in addition to having hair follicle has specialized wax (cerumen)-secreting glands in its outer one-third. A elsewhere, the skin sheds squames, but to prevent these building up the canal, the squamous epithelium gradually migrates from the tympan membrane out the canal. Wax is shed along with the squames. The bo portion of the external auditory canal is surrounded by the masto bone, occupies the inner one-third of the canal, and is very tender.

The tympanic membrane

The tympanic membrane has three layers. The outer layer is continuo with the skin of the external auditory canal. It is a shallow concave di divided into the pars tensa and the pars flaccida. The pars tensa is th larger inferior part of the eardrum and the pars flaccida is thus in th superior part of the middle ear, or the attic. The tympanic membrane is continually growing structure, which allows it to close if it is perforated.

Looking at the tympanic membrane should follow this process: th handle of the malleus should be identified first and followed up to th short lateral process. The pars flaccida is above this and the pars tensa below; the lateral process of the malleus is the key to examining th eardrum.

The middle ear

The middle ear is an air-containing space connected to the nasophary via the Eustachian tube. The middle ear space, including the mastoid cells, is closely related to the temporal lobe, cerebellum, jugular bu and the labyrinth of the inner ear. The space contains three bones (t malleus, incus, and stapes), which are collectively known as the ossic and are connected by synovial joints.

Jo Williams, Birmingham Children's Hospital NHS Trust

The ossicles

The malleus is the most lateral of the three ossicles. The long process of the malleus is attached to the inner layer of the tympanic membrane. The incus is attached to the malleus. The long process of the incus is attached to the head of the stapes. The stapes has a footplate which is seated in the oval window, which separates the middle ear from the perilymph of the inner ear.

When sound waves pass via the outer ear to the tympanic membrane, the tympanic membrane vibrates, which in turn causes the ossicles to vibrate, transmitting the vibration to the inner ear.

The inner ear

The inner ear is a dense bony capsule containing a membranous labyrinth, which forms the cochlea, vestibule, and semicircular canals. The cochlea contains the organ of hearing, which is connected to the auditory nerve by the brainstem. The vestibule and semicircular canals form the peripheral balance organ.

The cochlea

A snail-shaped structure that is the sensory organ of hearing. The vibrations that are intiated by the stapes footplate initiate a travelling-wave pattern within the cochlea. This wave-like pattern causes a shearing of the cilia of the outer and inner hair cells. This shearing causes hair-cell depolarization, resulting in neural impulses that the brain interprets as sound.

The vestibular labyrinth

The vestibular labyrinth is composed of the saccule and utricle (sense organs of balance), which inform the brain of the body's linear position in space. The horizontal, anterior, and posterior semicircular canals are also part of the vestibular labyrinth and inform the brain of rotational movements.

Further reading

Bluestone, C., Stool, S., Cuneyt, A., Arjmand, E., Casselbrandt, M., Donar, J., Yellon, R. (2003). *Pediatric otolaryngology*, 4th edn. W. B. Saunders, Philadelphia.
www.medicdirect.co.uk

Anatomy and physiology of the nose

The two functions of the nose are breathing and smelling. The nose divided into the external nose and the nasal cavity, including the na septum.

The external nose

The upper one-third of the nose is bony. The inferior two-thirds of t nose are cartilaginous (the upper and lower ala cartilages). The tip of t nose is pliable fibrocartilage.

The nasal cavity

Inside each nostril is a vestibule lined with skin, which contains sebacec and sweat glands. Also in the vestibule are coarse hairs which act filters and help to prevent the entry of foreign bodies. The nasal cavity divided by the osteocartilagenous septum. The lateral walls of the na cavity support a series of ridges called the turbinates. The maxilla frontal, ethmoid, and sphenoid sinuses drain into the nasal cavity. Ea nasal cavity leads to the nasopharynx through the posterior choanae.

Air entering the lungs should be moist, clean, and warm. The turbinates the nasal cavity are lined with columnar epithelium and contain erect tissue. Goblet cells and submucous glands secrete sticky mucus onto t surface of the epithelium. This mucus moistens inhaled air. The air is a warmed because the mucous membrane has a very rich blood supply.

The nose humidifies and filters the inhaled air. If a particle, such as poll enters the nose, it is trapped in the nasal vestibule which has a tac surface. It is transported posteriorly by the beating action of the na cilia. Once it reaches the posterior choanae, it is swallowed.

Nasal airflow varies from one side to the other and a cycle of fluctuati nasal blockage can be demonstrated in almost everyone at rest.

In the uppermost part of each nasal cavity lies the olfactory muco which contains the nerve cells sensitive to the presence of inha chemicals. Olfactory receptors are stimulated by airborne chemica Action potentials are transmitted to the olfactory areas of the bra Complete olfactory loss can occur following an acute viral infection o head injury.

Further reading

Bluestone, C., Stool, S., Cuneyt, A., Arjmand, E., Casselbrandt, M., Donar, J., Yellon, R. (20 *Pediatric otolaryngology*, 4th edn. W. B. Saunders, Philadelphia.
Drake-Lee, A. (1996). *Clinical otorhinolaryngology*. Churchill Livingstone, Edinburgh.
🖳 www.medicdirect.co.uk

Jo Williams, Birmingham Children's Hospital NHS Trust

Anatomy and physiology of the throat

The throat is composed of the oral cavity, pharynx, and larynx.

The oral cavity

The oral cavity is composed of the tongue, lips, hard palate, teeth, an mandible. The tongue is covered with squamous epithelium. The organ of taste (the taste buds) are found in the epithelial coverings of the tongue, soft palate, posterior wall of the pharynx, and epiglottis. The taste buds contain chemoreceptors that respond to chemicals in the die and generate patterns of impulses, which are transmitted to the gustator cortex in the parietal lobes of the cerebral cortex. It is here that the sensation of taste is perceived. Reflex stimulation of salivary and gastri secretion is mediated by neural pathways in the brainstem.

The pharynx

The pharynx is split into three parts: the nasopharynx, oropharynx, an hypopharynx. Food is masticated in the oral cavity by chewing, whic involves the teeth, mandible, hard palate, and tongue. The food bolu is then propelled voluntarily into the oropharynx. When a bolus o food hits the posterior wall of the oral cavity, the soft palate occlude the nasopharynx, the larynx is raised, and the epiglottis falls back. Th food bolus then passes into the oesophagus, where it is propelled b peristalsis into the stomach.

The larynx

The larynx is a rigid skeleton consisting of several cartilagenous stru tures, the most prominent being the thyroid cartilage. The epiglotti attached to the thyroid and occludes the laryngeal inlet when swallowin The larynx lies in the front of the neck, immediately above the trachea.

The larynx has three functions: it is a respiratory channel, it acts as sphincter protecting the lower airway, and it is an organ of communica tion. Communication is obviously a vital function of the larynx, bu protection of the trachea and the lower airway from aspiration of foo and secretions, especially during swallowing, is essential.

Further reading

Daya, H., Crittenden, G. (1998). *Inside ENT*. Pale Green Press, London.
Wetmore, R., Muntx, H., McGill, T., Potsic, W., Healy, G., Lusk, R. (2000). *Pediatric otolaryngolog* Thieme.
🖳 www.medicdirect.co.uk

Jo Williams, Birmingham Children's Hospital NHS Trust

The main structures of the eye

At birth the eye is three-quarters of the adult size of 2.5 cm, which is reached at the age of 14 years. Visual acuity at birth is poor, but gradually reaches adult acuity at 3 years.

External structures include the following.
- Lacrimal gland: responsible for producing tears that drain from the eye into the nasolacrimal duct. Lacrimal fluid contains salts, proteins, and oils, and an enzyme, lysozyme, that has a mild bactericidal action.
- Conjunctiva: a thin transparent tissue covering the visible part of the sclera and the inside of the eyelids, which starts the process of light refraction. Nourished by tiny blood vessels that also assist in the lubrication the eye.

The interior of the eye is divided into the aqueous and vitreous chambers.
- The aqueous chamber contains the iris (the coloured portion of the eye) which is suspended by cilia processes between the cornea and the lens, and secretes aqueous humour. Derived from plasma, aqueous humour supplies O_2 and nutrients to the lens and exerts pressure which influences the shape of the eye. Smooth and circular muscles form a disc that expands and contracts leaving an aperture (pupil). The amount of light that enters the eye is regulated by the parasympathetic nervous system. The lens is a transparent flexible biconcave structure which converges light onto the retina by the process of accommodation.
- The vitreous chamber contains a gel-like substance called vitreous humour, which maintains the shape of the eye and supports the delicate structures.

The retina is made up of five layers.
- Photoreceptor layer: light images are converted into electrochemical signals inside the photoreceptors and transmitted to the optic nerve. Cones situated at the centre of the retina give clarity and colour recognition to the image. The fovea centralis contains the highest density of cones and this is situated lateral to the optic disc, where the optic nerve leaves the eye. The rods offer peripheral vision and allow sight in situations of dim light.
- Retinal pigment epithelium (RPE): under the photoreceptors is a dark layer that absorbs excess light and transports O_2, nutrients, and cellular waste between the photoreceptors and the choroid.
- Bruch's membrane: separates the blood vessels of the choroid from the RPE
- The choroid: a layer of blood vessels that supplies O_2 and nutrients to the outer layers of the retina.
- The sclera: the fibrous white outer protective covering of the eye.

Further reading

Martini, F.H. (2006). *Fundamentals of anatomy and physiology*, 7th edn. Benjamin Cummings, San Francisco.

Montague, S.E., Watson, R., Herbert, R.A. (ed.) (2005). *Physiology for nursing practice*, 3rd edn. Elsevier, Edinburgh.

Mark Broom, University of Glamorgan

Acute otitis media

- Otitis media: short-term inflammation of the middle ear:
  - acute otitis media
  - otitis media with effusion (glue ear)
  - chronic suppurative otitis media.
- Common in children, because the Eustachian tube is relatively short, s it is easy for infection, such as the common cold, to spread from the nose and throat
- In the UK about 30% of children visit their GP with acute otitis media each year

Incidence

- More common in white children than black children
- More common in boys than girls
- Children with craniofacial abnormalities or Down syndrome are at greater risk
- Increased risk in children from lower socio-economic groups
- Increased risk in children who have enlarged tonsils and adenoids
- Lower incidence among breast-fed children
- Recurrent episodes of acute otitis media or chronic otitis media in young children increases the risk of hearing impairment

Signs and symptoms

- Rapid onset, often associated with a common cold.
- Presents with fever, irritability, crying, and sometimes vomiting and diarrhoea.
- The child may pull at the ears, showing signs of otalgia, and the tympanic membrane will be red and inflamed.
- The pain is acute, severe, and deep in the ear.
- There is often an effusion behind the tympanic membrane. If the effusion persists beyond 3 months, it is known as otitis media with effusion.

Diagnosis

Based on changes in the tympanic membrane with regard to colour opacity, contour, the light reflex, and mobility (if tested). Radial bloo vessels are a sign of an effusion in the middle ear.

Causes

The most common bacterial causes of acute otitis media are:

- *Streptococcus pneumoniae*
- *Haemophilus influenzae*
- *Moraxella catarrhalis*

Differential diagnosis

- Ear pain with discharge could be signs of a foreign body *in situ*.
- Eustachian tube dysfunction can cause transient ear pain, but the tympanic membrane is normal.
- Ear pain can be confused with dental pain.

Jo Williams, Birmingham Children's Hospital NHS Trust

Treatment

80% of cases resolve in about 3 days without antibiotic treatment.
Do not give antibiotics routinely. Exceptions:

- if the child is younger than 2 years old
- if the child has bilateral acute otitis media
- if the child has systemic symptoms, such as a temperature of above 38.5°C.

Give analgesia.

Some children will have a persistent effusion, which needs to be monitored on a 3-monthly basis. If this does not resolve and is affecting the child's hearing and development, insertion of grommets may be indicated.

Complications

Complications are rare, but they include hearing loss and acute mastoiditis, which may lead to meningitis and/or cerebral abscess. In this case cortical mastoidectomy and drainage of pus would be indicated.

Further reading

Barnes, K. (2003). *Paediatrics: a clinical guide for nurse practitioners*. Elselvier, Oxford.
Drake-Lee, A. (1996). *Clinical otorhinolaryngology*. Churchill Livingstone, Edinburgh.
www.nice.org.uk
www.prodigy.nhs.uk

Chronic otitis media

Chronic otitis media can be subdivided into tubotympanic and tympano-mastoid chronic suppurative otitis media.

- Tubotympanic otitis media arises from bacterial suppuration and perforation of the pars tensa of the tympanic membrane, following recurrent middle-ear infection.
- Tympanomastoid disease usually follows long-standing non-suppurative disease, often with chronic Eustachian tube dysfunction, resulting in retraction of the tympanic membrane in the attic of the eardrum. Skin can collect in this retraction. This skin, called a cholesteatoma, can expand, become infected, and erode the eardrum and the bones in the middle ear.

Signs and symptoms

- Deafness is the first symptom of chronic otitis media. This can range in severity according to which structures have been involved in the disease.
- Otorrhoea: the discharge depends on the type of disease present. If it is tubotympanic disease, discharge is often profuse, mucoid, and tends not to be offensive. Otorrhoea associated with tympanomastoid disease is often scanty and offensive.

Management

- Aural toilet: it is essential that this is performed by an experienced practitioner.
- Topical antimicrobial therapy.
- Surgical treatment will depend on the type of disease:
  - if it is tubotympanic, a myringoplasty can be performed once the ear is dry
  - if a cholesteatoma is present or suspected, an examination under anaesthetic should be performed and disease removed.

Complications

Complications of untreated or undetected middle-ear disease.

- Extracranial complications: ossicular discontinuity, middle-ear adhesions, tympanosclerosis, and lower motor facial palsy.
- Intracranial complications: extradural abscess, subdural abscess, meningitis, brain abscess, venous sinus thrombosis, and otitic hydrocephalus.

Further reading

Daya,.H., Crittenden, G. (1998). *Inside ENT*. Pale Green Press, London.
Drake-Lee, A. (1996). *Clinical otorhinolaryngology*. Churchill Livingstone, Edinburgh.
🖳 www.sign.ac.uk

Jo Williams, Birmingham Children's Hospital NHS Trust

Grommet insertion

A grommet is a plastic tube that is inserted into the tympanic membrane to allow ventilation of the middle ear.
• Grommets are inserted under a general anaesthetic.
• An incision is made in the tympanic membrane, the glue is aspirated, and a grommet is inserted into the incision.
• This is usually as a day-case procedure.
• Grommets fall out by themselves, usually after 9–12 months, and are carried out of the ear by the epithelial migration process.
• Longer-term grommets, such as T-tubes or permanent tubes, can stay in place for up to 5 years.

Indications
• Glue ear (otitis media with effusion) with hearing loss.
• Recurrent ear infections (recurrent acute otitis media).
• Retraction pocket within the tympanic membrane.

Complications
• Discharge: about 25% of children will have one ear infection while the grommet is in place. Infection is due to water entering the middle ear. Treatment consists of topical antibiotics.
• Residual perforation after the grommet comes out. Rare, occurs in 2% of patients with standard grommets but is more frequent after T-tubes.

Nursing management
General pre-operative care
• A hearing test prior to surgery may be required to ensure that grommets are still necessary.

Post-operative care
• There may be some discomfort that responds to simple analgesia.
• There may be some discharge from the ear, which may be blood-stained but should settle within a few days.
• Topical antibiotic drops are sometimes prescribed to prevent the grommet from becoming blocked with glue or blood.

Education
The ears need to be protected from entry of water into the middle ear:
• when washing hair, plug the ear with cotton wool smeared with vaseline.
• advise children that they can go swimming but should avoid swimming under water and diving.

Further reading
www.entnursing.com

Sarah Hill, Royal Cornwall Hospital Trust

Tonsillitis and tonsillectomy

- The tonsils are lymphoid organs that sit on either side of the base of the tongue.
- Tonsillitis can occur at any age but is most frequent in children under 9 years of age.
- It is spread by droplet infection.

Characteristics of tonsillitis

- Sore throat
- Difficulty in swallowing
- Pyrexia
- General malaise
- Halitosis
- Lymphadenopathy
- Exudative inflammation
- Enlargement of the tonsils
- Earache, as a result of referred otalgia

Tonsillitis is mainly caused by bacterial infection. Other conditions ca cause similar symptoms, including glandular fever and scarlet fever.

Treatment

- Rest.
- Simple analgesia.
- Encourage oral fluids to prevent dehydration. If the patient is unable to maintain adequate oral intake, IV fluids may be required.
- In severe cases, antibiotics may be required.
- Abscesses can occur if the infection has spread to the tissues lateral to the tonsils. Treatment consists of aspirating or incising the abscess. This gives instant symptomatic relief and the condition resolves quickly with antibiotics.

Indications for tonsillectomy

- Recurrent attacks of acute tonsillitis
- Tonsillar and adenoidal hypertrophy, causing airway obstruction
- Following quinsy
- Carriers of haemolytic streptococci or diphtheria
- Biopsy in suspected malignancy

Nursing management

General pre-operative care

- It is important that the child does not have tonsillitis at the time of surgery.
- Any suspicion of bleeding must be investigated fully.

Post-operative care

- Observe the child regularly.
- Record pulse, respiration, temperature, and blood pressure.
- Observe the child for signs of bleeding, excessive swallowing, or drooling, which may indicate that there is reactionary haemorrhage.

Sarah Hill, Royal Cornwall Hospital Trust

Post-operative bleeding must be stopped urgently. ▶ Delay may be fatal. This may require a return to theatre.

A secondary haemorrhage may occur 5–10 days after the operation, usually caused by infection. Hospital admission is required for treatment.

Encourage the child to eat and drink as normal; this is believed to promote a speedy recovery and helps prevent post-operative infection. Regular analgesia is required to keep the child comfortable and also helps the child to eat well.

urther reading

www.entnursing.com

Adenoidectomy

- Adenoidectomy is the removal of the adenoid tissue under general anaesthetic.
- The adenoids are lymphoid tissues, which are situated on the posterior wall of the nasopharynx and occupy much of that cavity in younger children. However, by the age of 6–7 years the adenoids begin to shrink, and by the age of 15 years, little or no adenoid tissue remains.
- In some children the adenoids undergo hypertrophy, which can cause problems, and therefore they need to be removed.

Indications

- Snoring
- Purulent nasal discharge
- Nasal blockage and mouth breathing
- Obstructive sleep apnoea
- Glue ear: large adenoids are thought to compromise the function of the Eustachian tube, resulting in secretory otitis media

Diagnosis

- The diagnosis is usually identified by history and clinical indications.
- The adenoids are difficult to examine because most children will not tolerate mirror examination or nasal endoscopy.
- The diagnosis can be confirmed when the adenoids are palpated under general anaesthetic.

Nursing management

Post-operative care

- Observe closely.
- Take pulse, respiration, blood pressure, and temperature measurements regularly.
- Reactionary haemorrhage: bleeding can occur at the time of surgery or shortly afterwards. ▶ Prompt action is required. If severe, the child may need to return to theatre to have the post-nasal space packed.
- Secondary haemorrhage: bleeding can also occur 5–10 days after surgery. This requires admission to hospital, but usually resolves with bed rest, observation, and antibiotics.
- Nasal obstruction may still be present after surgery but usually improves after a few days, once the oedema following surgery has settled.
- Simple analgesia for pain management.
- Advise children to remain off school for 2 weeks.

Further reading

🔲 www.entnursing.com

Sarah Hill, Royal Cornwall Hospital Trust

Strabismus

Definition

A squint (strabismus) occurs when one eye looks in a different direction from the other. A squint can be constant or intermittent and may affect only one eye or alternate from one eye to the other.

Characteristics

- Esotropia: eye turns inwards
- Exotropia: eye turns outwards
- Hypertropia: eye turns upwards
- Hypotropia: eye turns downwards

Causes

There are several, including:
- long or short sight
- a problem with brain control of eye position
  - associated with genes
  - associated with prematurity or developmental delay
- faulty eye muscles.

Clinical features

When a child has a strabismus, the eye turning (squinting) may be ignored. The child's vision then stops developing and may deteriorate the eye becomes lazy (amblyopic).

Risk factors

If treatment is not given, the child may lose most or all of the sight in the affected eye.

Treatment

- Varies in each child and is dependent on type of squint, level of vision, child's age, and whether glasses are needed.
- Should be started as soon as possible.
- Can start as young as 4–6 months old. Squints are not grown out of (over the age of 4 months).
- Can be successful in older children, even as old as 13 years (in general it is harder to treat amblyopia associated with squints over the age of 7 years). If intermittent, the child may learn to control the squint, but it often persists.
- First, deteriorating vision should be treated, which may involve glasses and/or patching.

Glasses

- Used to correct long or short sight or astigmatism (uneven curvature) of the eye.
- Can sometimes partially or totally correct the squint when worn. The squint may still be seen without the glasses.
- Often the corrective glasses may not be sufficient to improve the lazy eye. Patching may then be required to restore lost vision.

Julie Kitchen, Royal Devon and Exeter NHS Foundation Trust

Patching

The good or 'non-squinting' eye is patched to force the weaker eye to work. This treatment needs to be monitored carefully.

Atropine eye drops are sometimes administered by parents in the good eye as a patching alternative, because they blur near vision and the child will then use the lazy eye for close work.

Once vision has improved and has been maintained at an optimal level, the following treatments may be used if squint persists:

- change glasses
- specialized glasses, e.g. bifocals or prismatic lens
- brief patching for 30–60 min/day.

Surgery may be necessary for reconstructive reasons or if it is hoped that the two eyes will be used together to give binocular vision. Left untreated a squint can be disfiguring and cause teasing/social isolation for the child.

Surgery is *not* a substitute for patching. The patching restores and develops vision.

The 'good eye' is not adversely affected by patching, unless patching is almost full-time and the 'weak' eye reaches normal vision.

Further reading

Pediatric Eye Disease Investigator Group (2005). Two-year follow-up of a 6-month randomized trial of atropine versus patching for treatment of moderate amblyopia in children. *Archives of Ophthalmology*, **123**(2), 149–57.

www.orbis.org/strabminute

Surgical management of strabismus

Why is squint surgery performed?

Surgery may be necessary if the strabismus (squint) is cosmetically unsightly or if there is hope that the two eyes may be used together again (binocular vision). Squint surgery can be performed at any age.

Most squints (not corrected by spectacles) are due to a lack of ability by the brain to keep the two eyes lined up properly. Because the brain cannot be operated on, the eye muscles are operated on instead to try to compensate for the neurological problem by altering the muscle forces on the eye.

How is squint surgery performed?

Usually the operation is on the eye that squints all or most of the time but sometimes it is on both eyes.

Under general anaesthetic, the muscles around the eye are repositioned; this strengthens or weakens the appropriate muscles, helping to straighten the eye.

- Dissolvable stitches are used to place the eye muscles in new positions on the surface of the eyeball. The eye is never removed from the socket and lasers are not used.
- In older children/adolescents, surgery can be done using adjustable sutures. Instead of firmly tying the muscle stitches at the end of the operation (as usual), they are left tied in a bow-tie knot.
- When the patient has recovered from the anaesthetic and is alert, the eye surgeon can measure the position of the eye and change the muscle positions if the eye is not straight.
- Anaesthetic eye drops are instilled prior to, and at the time of, the muscle adjustment, to relieve discomfort.

Further reading

Callery, P. (2005). Preparing children for surgery. *Paediatric Nursing*, **17**(3), 12.

Editorial (2001). Adjustable suture strabismus surgery: continuing progress. *British Journal of Ophthalmology*, **85**, 2–3.

🖳 www.viscotland.org.uk

🖳 www.visionconnection.org

Julie Kitchen, Royal Devon and Exeter NHS Foundation Trust

Post-operative care following strabismus surgery

Squint surgery is normally performed as a day case. If the child makes satisfactory recovery, he/she can go home the same day as the surgery is performed.

Problem	Action/rationale
1. Following squint surgery children/ adolescents may return to the ward with an eye pad on the last eye operated on	To prevent injury when local anaesthetic is still effective. The pad could be removed if it causes any distress
2. White mucus may be discharged from the eye	Remove mucus with clean gauze and sterile water
Mucus discharge may be present in the morning on waking and periodically during the day	If the discharge increases and/or becomes markedly yellow or green in colour, the patient should be seen by an ophthalmic specialist
3. After surgery, the surface of the eye will be red and slightly swollen over the muscles that have been operated on	Most of the redness or 'bloodshot' appearance will disappear within the first 1–2 weeks, but can take up to 6 weeks
	Any redness of the eye(s) that spreads to involve the entire front surface of the eye, not just over the muscle(s) operated on, requires review by an ophthalmic specialist
	If there is markedly increased swelling or redness of the eyelids, this should also be reviewed by an ophthalmic specialist
4. The eye(s) may be sore	Give regular pain relief, as prescribed. Soreness over the operated muscle(s) can be aggravated by eye movement but should subside over the first few days after surgery
	If there is increasing pain, review by an ophthalmic specialist is required
5. There may be a sensation of something in the eye(s)	This is due to the incisions in the conjunctiva and sutures and will gradually go away within the first week or two
	The sutures are dissolvable
6. There may be tear production	Due to minor irritation from the sutures

Julie Kitchen, Royal Devon and Exeter NHS Foundation Trust

Contd.

Problem	Action/rationale
7. There may be some double vision	This can be common, but it usually goes away during the first days or weeks after surgery
	Some children/adolescents already have double vision before the operation
8. Prescribed eye medication should be administered according to prescription	To help prevent infection and promote healing

Follow-up care

The child/adolescent will be reviewed by their orthoptist or ophthalmic consultant, according to local policy.

Potential complications

- After surgery, the eye/s may become sore, red, and watery.
- Swimming in chlorinated pools should be avoided for approximately 3 weeks post-operatively, because the eyes can become very irritated.
- Dusty dirty environments or areas where there are irritating vapours or chemicals, should be avoided for at least 2 weeks because of risk of infection.
- The child/adolescent can return to work or school at their discretion, as long as they avoid the environments stated above. It may be advisable to take a few days off initially to aid recovery.

Further reading

Cropper, J., Hutchison, L., Llewellyn, N. (2003). Post-operative retention of urine in children. *Paediatric Nursing*, **15**(7), 15–18.

Higson, J., Bolland, R. (2000/2001). Telephone follow-up after paediatric day surgery. *Paediatric Nursing*, **12**(10), 30–2.

Conjunctivitis

Commonly known as 'pinkeye', conjunctivitis is an infection of the conjunctiva—the clear membrane that covers the white part of the eye.

There are three major types of conjunctivitis:
- infected
- allergic
- caused by an irritant.

Infected conjunctivitis

Manifests as a viral or bacterial infection.
- The bacterial infection causes copious amounts of purulent discharge, giving the sensation of a foreign body present in the eye. The child may be in considerable pain with intra-ocular pressure and sensitivity to light.
- The viral infection has a much clearer discharge and is often found in conjunction with S. pneumoniae, H. influenzae, and S. aureus.
- Both types of infection are highly contagious, passing through direct contact, coughing, and sneezing.
- They should be treated with mild corticosteroid/antibiotic drops or ointment, coupled with analgesics, cold compresses, and lubricants, or as much as the child can take.

Allergic conjunctivitis

Arises mainly at specific times of the year, e.g. triggered by dust mites or hay fever.
- Stringy mucoid discharge follows unbearable itching of the eyes and swelling of the eyelids.
- This condition is treated with mild vasoconstrictor decongestant drops and is known to be non-contagious.

Conjunctivitis caused by an irritant [1]

Could be caused by something as simple as a household soap, chlorine, fumes, or smoke.
- Intense itching and a clear thin discharge, with swollen eyelids, will be apparent.
- Treated simply with a prescription antibiotic drop or ointment.

Both allergic and irritant conjunctivitis have an incubation period of 3–4 days and can last for up to 2 weeks.

All conjunctivitis requires treatment, especially in the child, in order to avoid long-term eye damage.

Further reading

McMillan, A., De Angelis, B., Felgin, W., Warshaw, S. (1990). *Oski's paediatrics: principles and practice.* Lippincott Williams & Wilkins, London.
Whaley, L.F., Wong, D.L. (1991). *Nursing care of infants and children,* 4th edn. Mosby, London.
📖 www.patient.co.uk/showdoc/23068712

Anna Chick, Royal Cornwall Hospital Trust

Deafness

There are two types of deafness, conductive and sensorineural.
- Conductive deafness: if occurs there is a breakdown in the passage of sound from the external ear, through the middle ear, to the cochlea.
- Sensorineural hearing loss: occurs in the cochlea of the inner ear, involving either cochlear or auditory nerves.

Deafness may be in one or both ears. Profound hearing loss is usually obvious, but lesser degrees of hearing loss may present at any time. The parent usually notices hearing loss in children; however, school teachers often question a child's hearing, particularly if he/she exhibits lack of concentration and learning difficulties. Children may present with absent or delayed speech, which is sometimes due to a hearing deficit. Currently, a system of neonatal hearing screening is being established in the UK.

Sudden deafness in children
- Wax in the external ear can present as sudden deafness, which may be unilateral or bilateral. Advise removal of the wax by an experienced practitioner.
- Sudden deafness can present after a traumatic incident, such as a fracture to the skull. The trauma may have caused a perforation to the eardrum or disruption of the ossicular chain in the middle ear, causing a malfunction of the conduction of sound to the inner ear.
- Sudden irreversible sensorineural deafness can occur spontaneously following a cerebral incident or after meningitis or mumps.
- If a child presents in a clinic with a sudden hearing loss and there is no history of the above, a scan should be performed to rule out neoplasm.

Progressive deafness
- Glue ear is a common childhood condition which usually presents with mild continuous deafness. The glue in the middle ear prevents the eardrum and the ossicles from moving, and therefore a hearing loss may be present.
- If a child has chronic otitis media, scarring of the eardrum is likely to occur. This prevents the eardrum from moving adequately, so a conductive hearing loss may be present.
- Otosclerosis can occur in children. The ossicles in the ear become stiff or fixed and therefore are less able to pass on vibrations when sound enters the ear.

Systemic diseases, syndromes, and deafness
Deafness can be associated with:
- syndromes, such as Down and Treacher-Collins syndromes
- systemic diseases, such as renal and autoimmune diseases

Jo Williams, Birmingham Children's Hospital NHS Trust

Further reading

Drake-Lee, A. (1996). *Clinical otorhinolaryngology*. Churchill Livingstone, Edinburgh.
www.medicdirect.co.uk
www.ndcs.org.uk

Epistaxis

Epistaxis in children is quite common, and most children will suffer bleed from the nose at one time or another for various reasons. In children, the site of the bleeding is usually the anterior septum (Little's area), and the reason for the bleed is a break in a blood vessel within the nose It can be unilateral or bilateral.

Causes of epistaxis

Epistaxis may be due to:
- an injury to the nose
- blowing the nose too hard or too frequently
- picking the nose
- putting a foreign body in the nose
- local disease within the nasal cavity
- systemic disease, such as leukaemia
- anticoagulant therapy

Questions to ask
- How long have symptoms been present?
- Which side does the bleeding come from?
- How frequently does the child have nosebleeds?

Treatment
- Sit the child down, either by him/herself on the parent's/carer's knee.
- Reassure both child and parent/carer.
- Pinch the soft part of the nose between the thumb and finger for at least 10 min. Squeeze firmly and do not let go until 10 min has elapsed.
- Apply crushed ice, or a bag of frozen peas wrapped in a towel, to the bridge of the nose. This will cause the blood vessels in the nose to constrict and will help slow the bleeding.
- If the child's nose bleeds for >20 min, take him/her to the nearest accident and emergency department.
- Sometimes it may be necessary to pack the nose to stop bleeding. This must been done by an experienced practitioner.
- A child who has regular nosebleeds should see a doctor so that investigations can be performed. It may be necessary to cauterize some of the blood vessels at the front of the nose that give rise to bleeding.

Advice
- To avoid swallowing blood, do not tilt the child's head backwards.
- Do not put cotton wool up the nostrils.
- Advise avoiding hot drinks for the next 24 hours.
- Advise not to blow the nose for the next 24 hours.
- Apply Vaseline just inside each nostril to keep the skin of the nose moist and to prevent the formation of scabs.

Jo Williams, Birmingham Children's Hospital NHS Trust

Further reading

Barnes, K. (2003). *Paediatrics: a clinical guide for nurse practitioners*. Elsevier Science, Edinburgh.
www.medicdirect.co.uk

Assisting in the examination of the eye

Action	Rationale
1. Assess need for assistance in the examination Child is uncooperative Eye examination is necessary	Eye examination is vital in order to eliminate eye disease or sight-threatening condition
2. Introduce yourself to child and family. Explain procedure to child and parents	Reassurance of child and parents and promoting partnership with the family
3. Assess physical resources required in assisting in the safe examination	To ensure safe examination is performed
4. Offer parents opportunity to be present during the procedure	To ensure child's emotional needs are met. It can be emotionally disturbing for parents. Nurse to hold the child but ensure parents are offered opportunity to stay during procedure

In infant or child under 1 year old

Wrap infant in a blanket with arms at his/her side. Hold the infant's head still, to ensure equipment can be safely applied to eye(s)

If child is 1–5 years old

Try to distract child by using imaginary play, such as pretending the slit lamp is a motorbike and that the eye drops are magic raindrops. Utilize toys and resources available, such as hand puppets, to help focus the child's eyes

Explain the procedure to the child and family. If the child needs to be motionless, ask a parent/carer to sit child on his/her lap, then wrap one arm across the child's body with the child's arms underneath. With the other hand, keep the child's head still by placing a hand on his forehead

Ensure that the parent/carer is happy to participate; if not, explain rationale for restraint method and the nurse should hold the child

If child is over 5 years old:

Employ distraction technique as mentioned above. Reassure at all times

Julie Kitchen, Royal Devon and Exeter NHS Foundation Trust

Contd.

Action	Rationale
5. At the end of the procedure congratulate the child. Give reward, such as stickers/certificates	Procedure can be emotionally difficult for some children and parents/carers
6. If unable to examine eye, an examination under anaesthesia (EUA) may be necessary	To eliminate eye disease or sight-threatening condition

Further reading

RCN (2003). Restraining, holding still and containing children and young people. *Guidance for Nursing Staff*. RCN, London.
Valler-Jones, T., Shinnick, A. (2005). Holding children for invasive procedures: preparing student nurses. Paediatric Nursing, **17**(5), 20–2.

Examination of the ear

Before physical examination of the ear, listen to the patient, elicit symptoms, and take a careful history. The questions that you will need to ask will depend on what the child has presented with. Explain each step of any examination procedure and ensure that the patient and parent/carer understand and give consent.

It is important to ascertain the child's level of hearing. If the child is old enough, you could ask the child questions such as whether he/she has problems hearing at home or whether he/she can hear his/her teacher at school. You can ask the parent or carer what he/she thinks about the child's hearing. It is often useful to ask the parent or carer how the child is performing in school, because teachers often identify a hearing deficit.

Is there any discharge from the ear canal?
- Does the discharge affect both ears?
- What is its quantity?
- What is its colour?
- Is it mucoid?
- Is it painful or painless?
- Is it wax?

Is there any pain?
- Where is it localized?
- Is it bilateral or unilateral?
- Is there itching?
- Is there discharge? If so:
  - Did it come with the pain?
  - Was the pain relieved by the discharge?
- Is the pain referred?
- Is there pain and/or swelling behind the pinna?

Examination
- Once you have taken a detailed history, a careful physical examination of the ear can be performed. Ensure that the patient is sitting comfortably and you maintain privacy. It is also vital that you are positioned comfortably—remember your back!
- First examine the pinna, outer meatus, and adjacent scalp by direct light and check for scars from previous surgery. Examine both pinnae. Look at the size, shape, and position of each pinna. A pinna that is small, unusual in shape, or unusually low down on the face could be a variation of the normal structure, but may indicate a syndrome.
  - Is the ear red and inflamed? Are there signs of trauma or possible infection?
  - Is it deformed due to previous trauma?
  - Is there any damage to the ear lobes from earrings or studs?
  - Is there any scaling or cracking of the skin, associated with scaling of the scalp or eyebrow region—possibly seborrhoeic eczema?

Jo Williams, Birmingham Children's Hospital NHS Trust

- Gently pull the pinna upwards and backwards (in infants downwards and backwards) to straighten the meatus. Any localized infection or inflammation will cause this procedure to be quite painful. Common causes of pain might be a boil (furuncle) or a fungal infection in the meatus.
- Remember that the skin lining the meatus is very delicate and sensitive.
- Holding the otoscope as you would a pen, with your little finger resting against the patient's face, insert the specula gently into the meatus. Use the largest sized specula that will fit comfortably in the ear.
- Can you see the eardrum or is it obscured by wax? Earwax is a normal physiological substance that protects the ear canal. The quantity produced varies between individuals. If the earwax obscures the view of the tympanic membrane, It should be removed by an experienced practitioner.
- Carefully check the ear canal and the eardrum. The normal eardrum has a pearly grey appearance and you should be able to see the handle of the malleus in the middle ear through the drum. It is often possible to make out the long process of the incus. In a normal drum there is a reflection of light, called a cone of light, extending from the handle to the lower part of the drum—the pars tensa.
- The ear cannot be judged to be completely normal until the entire eardrum has been seen. To see into the roof of the meatus (pars flaccida and pars tensa) you may need to ask the patient to move his/her head. The normal appearance of the membrane varies and can only be learned by practice, which will lead to recognition of abnormalities.
- Methodically inspect all parts of the meatus and eardrum by varying the angle of the speculum. Carefully check the condition of the external auditory meatus as you withdraw the otoscope.
- If you are assisting with the examination of the child, it is vital that an explanation is given to both child and parent/carer. Encourage the child to sit on his/her parent's/carer's knee for the examination, but if that is not possible, you can assist. The best position for the examination is if the child sits sideways on the parent's knee with the ear facing the examiner. The parent/carer should then be advised to place one of his/her hands gently on the top of the child's head and the other hand on the child's shoulder. This position is comfortable for all concerned and reassuring for the child.

Further reading

Wormald, P., Browning, G. (1996). *Otoscopy: a structured approach.* Arnold, London.
www.bris.ac.uk/Depts/ENT/otoscopy_tutorial

Examination of the throat

Before physical examination of the throat, listen to the child, elicit symptoms, and take a careful history. The questions that you need to ask will depend on what the child has presented with. Explain each step of any examination procedure and ensure that the patient and parent/carer understand and give consent.

The throat comprises the oral cavity, pharynx, and larynx. A fibre-optic nasendoscope is required to examine the larynx and pharynx. This is tolerated by only a minority of children, and often an examination under general anaesthetic is required.

However, it is possible to examine the oral cavity. Encourage the child to sit on his/her parent's/carer's knee for the examination, but if that is not possible, you can assist. The best position for the examination is if the child sits on the parent's knee facing the examiner. Advise the parent/carer to place one hand gently on the top of the child's head and the other arm across the child's chest. This position is comfortable for all concerned and reassuring for the child.

The most prevalent problem seen in paediatric ENT departments is a sore throat. Everyone has a sore throat at some time. It is important to elicit the symptoms of the sore throat to ascertain what the problem is. The questions to ask are:
• How long has the child had a sore throat?
• Where is the pain?
• How often does the child have this pain?
• Is it associated with pyrexia?
• Is the child able to tolerate diet and fluids when the pain is present?

Examination

Look in the child's mouth with a light. If necessary, use a tongue depressor to obtain a satisfactory view. If the child's sore throat is associated with general malaise and pyrexia, the indications are that it is infectious in origin. Most children with a sore throat can be managed in primary care, but refer to a specialist service if the following symptoms are present:
• peri-tonsillar abscess (quinsy)
• unilateral swelling of the tonsil
• the swelling of the tonsils is causing an upper airway obstruction
• the child has a history of sleep apnoea

Further reading

Drake-Lee, A. (1996). *Clinical otorhinolaryngology*. Churchill Livingstone, Edinburgh.
🖥 www.nice.org.uk

Jo Williams, Birmingham Children's Hospital NHS Trust

Examination of the nose

Before physical examination of the nose, listen to the patient, elicit symptoms, and take a careful history. The questions that you need to ask will depend on what the child has presented with. Explain each step of any procedure of examination and ensure that the patient and parent/carer understand and give consent.

History

A general health history will ascertain whether the child has any bleeding disorders or systemic disease that may be applicable.

Questions to ask

The following key questions should be asked when taking a nasal history

General

- How long have the symptoms been present?
- Is there any bleeding?
- From which side does the bleeding occur?
- How frequently does epistaxis occur?
- Is there any history of trauma?
- Is there any pain?
- Is there a history of foreign body insertion?

Blockage

- Is the nose blocked?
- Which side?
- Is the blockage present all the time or does it fluctuate?

Running

- Does the nose run?
- Is it bilateral or unilateral?
- What colour is the discharge?
- Does the discharge smell offensive?

Sneezing

- Does the child sneeze a lot?
- Does sneezing occur at a particular time of the day?

Examination

Encourage the child to sit on his/her parent's/carer's knee for the examination, but if that is not possible, you can assist. The best position for the examination is if the child sits on the parent's carer's knee facing the examiner. The parent/carer should then be advised to place a hand gently on the top of the child's head and the other arm across the child's chest. This position is comfortable for all concerned and reassuring for the child.

- Look at the face. Is there any asymmetry?
- Look at the nose. The position and development of the nasal bones are very variable. Is the nose straight or deviated? It is often useful to stand behind the patient and look down at his/her nose from above to ascertain whether it is straight.

Jo Williams, Birmingham Children's Hospital NHS Trust

The tip of the nose can be lifted gently and the vestibule can be inspected, showing the front of the nasal septum.

Airflow through the nose can be assessed by holding something metal, such as a tongue depressor or a spoon, just below the vestibule and watching the misting pattern. The patency of each side may be assessed separately by placing a thumb underneath each nostril in turn and judging the airflow through the other side of the nose.

A baby's nose can be assessed by holding a small piece of cotton wool under the nostril to see if it moves as the air is expelled through the nostril.

A nasal speculum can be used to examine the anterior nasal cavities, although in practice children are not keen! However, you can use an otoscope by placing it gently in each nostril; children will usually tolerate this method of examination.

Further reading

Ellis, P. (1996). *A companion to ENT for medical students and general practitioners*. Blueprint, Cambridge.

www.medicdirect.co.uk

Haematology and immunity problems

The blood

Blood makes up 7–8% of the body weight.

Functions

- Transports: O_2 and nutrients to cells
  CO_2 and waste from cells
- Communication: Hormones
  Cytokines
- Infection control: Leukocytes
  Igs
- Haemostasis: Platelets
  Clotting factors
- Helps maintain body temperature

Plasma

Straw-coloured clear fluid, 55% of total blood volume, carries blood cells and platelets. Plasma = 95% water + salts, sugars, lipids, vitamins minerals, hormones, blood clotting factors, enzymes, antibodies, and other proteins.

Red blood cells

- Also called erythrocytes: 4–6 million/mm^3; 40% of total blood volume. Large microscopic cells, no nucleus, biconcave disc, which change shape to squeeze through capillaries.
- Transport O_2 from lungs to all body tissues and transport some CO_2 away.
- Short life span of 120 days, but continuously produced by the bone marrow.
- 95% of the red blood cell is haemoglobin, an O_2-carrying iron-rich protein.

White blood cells

- Also called leucocytes: 5000–10 000/mm^3; only 1% of total blood volume. Life span 18–36 hours. There are two groups.
  - The *phagocytes* are made up of the granulocytes (neutrophils, eosinophils, and basophils) and the macrophages, and are produced by the bone marrow. Primary defence against bacterial infection.
  - The lymphocytes are made up of T lymphocytes and B lymphocytes. Their production is in two stages: initially produced in the bone marrow or the thymus, and then in the lymph nodes and spleen following exposure to an antigen. Produce antibodies.

Platelets

Thrombocytes: 150 000–350 000/mm^3; produced by the bone marrow. They are small and disc-shaped with no nucleus, and essential for haemostasis. They adhere to the walls of a damaged blood vessel, where they release coagulating chemicals, leading to the production of a clot. Life span of 9–10 days.

Gill McEwing, University of Plymouth

Immune protection in children

Babies are born with the ability to protect themselves against a variety of infections; this ability is described as 'immunity' (latin *immunitas*, freedom from). The immune system has three phases in the overall response to attack:

- phase 1: immediate response—innate immunity
- phase 2: the inflammatory response
- phase 3: the specific immune response.

The first phase, responsible for over 95% of defence, is predominantly preventive, stopping organisms which might cause harm to the human body from establishing themselves either in or on the body. This phase includes cell-mediated mechanisms (neutrophils and macrophages) humoral mechanisms (immune proteins in blood and tissue fluids), and barrier mechanisms. Barrier mechanisms are particularly responsible for protecting infants and young children.

If harmful micro-organisms have avoided the barrier mechanisms and become established in the body, they will start multiplying. Fortunately the immune system is prepared, and within minutes of any invasion by micro-organisms through the body's defence barriers, the inflammatory response is initiated. The classical signs of this phase are heat (localized and fever), swelling, redness, and pain. Many common conditions seen in childhood are manifestations of the inflammatory response, e.g. tonsillitis, otitis media, appendicitis, and eczema.

The specific immune response is targeted against specific antigens (substances capable of provoking an immune response). In addition, the specific immune system is involved in protection from diseases such as cancer, or if it malfunctions, it is the cause of diseases such as type 1 diabetes mellitus and arthritis. The immune system in infants has to 'learn' the specific antigens.

Specific immunity has a very long memory. It has two main arms: cell-mediated (T lymphocytes and B lymphocytes) and antibody-mediated immunity. Antibodies (immunoglobulins) produced from B lymphocytes are complex proteins found predominantly in mucus, blood, and lymph, and have a vital role in immune protection. Vaccination helps the child's specific immune system to learn about the antigens in the vaccine. Thereafter, the immune system will react vigorously to protect the child in future meetings with that antigen.

Maureen Harrison, University of Southampton

nnate immunity in young children

Barrier mechanism in innate immunity	Means of breaching	Measures to promote immune protection
Skin: commensal bacteria protect by inhibiting harmful bacteria from colonizing	Handling baby with incorrectly washed hands	Thorough hand hygiene. Promote skin-to-skin contact between mother and baby
Skin secretions that limit growth of commensal bacteria	Reduced production of sebum and sweat in young children	Regular washing of areas (e.g. nappy region) that are particularly prone to micro-organism colonization
Skin layers: outer stratum corneum of epidermis is very thin and under-developed in babies	Puncturing skin with Venflon or needle, cuts, and abrasions	Rigorous use of clean, non-touch, or aseptic technique during invasive procedures. Monitoring of skin around any device that breaches skin barrier for inflammation
Skin dermis richly supplied by blood capillaries and nervous tissue. Factors in blood protect the whole body from micro-organisms	Strictures that occlude flow of blood to skin, such as tight clothing, bandaging, or strapping	Ensure no structures are applied too tightly. Good circulation is indicated by a peripheral refill of 1–2 s
Eyes are protected by tears	Tear glands are prone to blockage in young children	Clean each eye separately, wiping eye lid from area near nose to other side. This action releases tears that clean the inner eye
Mucous membranes of respiratory and gastrointestinal tracts contain immuno-globulins that prevent attachment of micro-organisms	Reduced numbers of immunoglobulins in infancy. Produced as part of specific immune system that is still developing	Promote breast-feeding because breast-milk contains many immuno-globulins that protect mucous membranes
Saliva in mouth is limited until 4 months, after which time large amounts are produced. Saliva contains many protective properties	Babies who are bottle-fed are prone to mouth infections if equipment used is inadequately cleaned	Promote breast-feeding because milk from mother is sterile and contains many protective properties

Anaemia

Anaemia in childhood can be described as reduction of red blood cells or haemoglobin concentration in the blood caused by disease or injury. Therefore anaemia is not a disease itself but a manifestation of a pathological process.

Although there are many types of anaemia, there are three main classifications.

- Hypoproliferative anaemia resulting from defective red blood cell production, e.g. iron-deficiency anaemia and aplastic anaemia.
- Anaemia due to haemorrhage and therefore decreased number of red blood cells.
- Haemolytic anaemia resulting from excessive destruction of red blood cells (haemolysis), e.g. 📖 sickle cell anaemia (p. 570) and 📖 thalassaemia (p. 580).

Iron-deficiency anaemia

Iron-deficiency anaemia is the most common haematological disorder in childhood and is most frequent between the ages of 6 months and 2 years.

Clinical manifestations

Although any reduction in the amount of haemoglobin lessens the O_2-carrying capacity of the blood, the child may be asymptomatic while the anaemia is mild or may present with some symptoms on exertion.

The child with moderate or severe anaemia will be pale, lethargic, listless, and irritable, and may be breathless and tachycardic.

Reaching a diagnosis

A diagnosis is made from the history, clinical presentation, and the laboratory data. A full blood count examines bone-marrow function, red blood cells, white blood cells, and platelets. The haemoglobin content is included and a low haemoglobin confirms the diagnosis of anaemia (📖 Normal blood values).

Repeated investigations can detract from the normal lifestyle for these children and in some cases could lead to long-term psychological problems. It is important to PREPARE the child fully for blood sampling:

- **P**rofessional responsibility as child's advocate
- **R**eassurance of child and family
- **E**xplanations—age-appropriate
- **P**arental involvement
- **A**pply topical anaesthetic creams
- **R**anges of play/distraction techniques
- **E**ncourage, reward, and praise the child

Nursing management

The medical management is to treat the underlying cause and thus reverse the anaemia. Iron preparations will be used to correct the deficiency.

- Work in partnership with the child and family and with a multidisciplinary approach to care.

Jayne Price, Queen's University, Belfast

If the child has severe anaemia, he/she may require O_2 therapy, blood transfusion, IV fluids, and rest.

Educate the child and family regarding diet, introducing foods rich in iron, e.g. meat and vegetables. Enlist the expertise of a dietician.

Educate the family regarding medication to be administered and its safe storage.

Use distraction and play techniques during blood sampling and/or blood transfusion. Enlist the help of the play specialist.

Ensure follow-up appointment and that follow-up community care is available; inform the health visitor/GP on discharge.

Further reading

Hand, H. (2001). Blood and the classification of anaemia. *Nursing Standard*, **15**(39), 45–53.
MacDonald, A. (1999). Iron deficiency in infants and children. *Primary Health Care*, **9**(6), 17–24.
www.patient.co.uk/showdoc/40000529/

Sickle cell disease (SCD)

- Autosomal recessive inheritance.
- Normal haemoglobin has two α-chains and two β-chains.
- SCD has two β-globin genes in which there are single amino acid substitutions (glutamine for valine on codon 6 of the β-chains).
- HbS is less soluble than HbA.
- Inheritance of a single mutation results in the sickle trait in which 40% of the haemoglobin is HbS, which offers protection against malaria.
- Common in people of African-Caribbean descent but also people from the Mediterranean, Middle East, Far East, and parts of India.

Pathogenesis

- HbSS: the haemoglobin molecule becomes deformed (insoluble) in the deoxygenated state.
- Cells: characteristic sickle shape.
- Sickled cells life span ↓ and they become trapped in the microcirculation → thrombosis and ischaemia.
- Exacerbated by ↓ O_2 tension, hypoxia, dehydration, cold, and infection

Symptoms in children

Rarely displayed before 3–6 months; can occur at any age and range in severity.

- The hallmark clinical manifestation of SCD is the acute vaso-occlusive event or painful episode. This pain can start from as young as 6 months of age and recurs unpredictably over the lifetime, requiring treatment with opioids.

Acute complications

- Unpredictable pain in various body parts, including painful swelling of the hands and feet.
- Enlarged spleen and splenic sequestration.
- Fatigue and shortness of breath.
- Stroke occurs in approximately 10% of patients before the age of 20 years. Early detection and prevention is now possible.
- Haematuria.
- Priapism occurs from approximately 12 years of age.
- Bones and joints are often the site of vaso-occlusive episodes, and chronic infarcts may result and avascular necrosis may occur.
- Acute chest syndrome presents with chest pain, cough, fever, and tachypnoea, with clinical and radiological changes.
- Patients have chronic haemolytic anaemia, with a high reticulocyte count.
- Vulnerability to infection caused by encapsulated bacteria such as those that cause pneumonia and meningitis.

Janet Kelsey, University of Plymouth

Long-term complications

Infection is a major complication of SCD; the single most common cause of death is *S. pneumoniae*.

Acute chest syndrome presents with chest pain, cough, fever, and tachypnoea, with clinical and radiological changes.

Hyposthenuria may become evident in childhood as enuresis and dehydration.

Eye problems: occlusion of small retinal vessels, with neovascularization, is asymptomatic until haemorrhage occurs within the vitreous. Detachment of the retina may occur in late disease.

Between 10% and 20% of patients aged 10 years and upwards may develop leg ulcers.

Delayed growth.

Cardiac problems.

Renal problems.

Musculoskeletal changes.

Dysfunction of the liver and biliary tract. 40% of adolescents with SCD will have gallstones.

Transient red blood cell aplasia preceded or accompanied by a febrile illness.

Mortality and morbidity

85% of those affected survive to 20 years.

Main risk of death in the first 3 years is infection.

Life expectancy is 50 years.

Screening

Implementing antenatal screening for SCD should be commissioned by primary care trusts; in the UK by the end of 2004/2005 a more effective and appropriate screening programme for women and children should be available.

Further reading

www.nhlbi.nih.gov/health/prof/blood/sickle/index.htm

omni.ac.uk/browse/mesh/D000755.html

Management of sickle cell disease

Management of acute problems
- Hydration with IV fluids
- Oxygenation
- Warmth
- Early antibiotic therapy for suspected infection
- Analgesia, often with opiates

More severe crisis
- Blood transfusion for sudden marked fall in haemoglobin
- Exchange transfusion is an option for cerebral or pulmonary infarction

Long-term management
- Education of child and family is paramount.
- Of vital importance are avoiding the cold and dehydration, early recognition of febrile illness, respiratory distress, jaundice, and splenic enlargement, assessment and management of pain, and maintaining penicillin prophylaxis and immunizations.
- Steady-state anaemia, uncomplicated painful episodes, and minor surgery should not be treated with transfusions. Clear indications for therapy are acute chest syndrome, heart failure, multi-organ failure syndrome, stroke, splenic sequestration, and aplastic crisis. Chronic anaemia is not an indication for giving blood transfusion.
- Aim to keep HbS between 30% and 50%, depending on the individual child.
- Penicillin prophylaxis.
- Hib and MenC vaccine.
- Consider the possibility of iron overload.
- Hydroxyurea is a valuable adjunct in the treatment of severe SCD, but it must be used carefully with full consideration of its toxicity and long-term adverse effects.
- Folic acid for those with chronic haemolysis.
- Transfuse prior to major surgery.
- Genetic counselling.
- Psychological support.
- Haematopoietic cell transplantation is reserved for patients experiencing significant complications of SCD.

Adolescents with sickle cell disease present with unique needs, including delayed sexual development, avascular necrosis of the hip, gallstones, priapism, proteinuria, pulmonary hypertension, and the onset of retinopathy. Ongoing counselling is required for issues of sexuality, drug use, birth control, and educational performance.

Further reading
- www.nhlbi.nih.gov/health/prof/blood/sickle/index.htm
- omni.ac.uk/browse/mesh/D000755.html

Janet Kelsey, University of Plymouth

Haemophilia

Haemophilia is a genetic bleeding disorder caused by a defect in the blood-clotting mechanism. No family history of the condition is found in one in three children diagnosed with haemophilia.

Types of haemophilia

The two main factors that affect blood clotting are factor VIII and factor IX. Thus haemophilia can be classed as:
- haemophilia A—caused by deficiency of factor VIII, which accounts for 85% of cases
- haemophilia B—caused by deficiency of factor IX, also known as Christmas disease.

Haemophilia: the facts

- The abnormal gene responsible for this condition is carried on the X chromosome; therefore girls are carriers of the condition and boys suffer from the disorder.
- 1 in 10 000 boys have haemophilia A.
- 1 in 50 000 boys have haemophilia B.
- Haemophilia is classified by the level of severity: mild, moderate, and severe, depending on the level of clotting factors in the blood. The severity of the disorder is also inherited.

Symptoms

- The most common symptom of the disorder is excessive uncontrollable bleeding.
- It is a common myth to believe that children with haemophilia bleed faster; in reality they bleed for a longer time.
- The symptoms may appear more evident when an infant becomes mobile.
- Other symptoms include:
  - bruising
  - bleeding into a joint
  - bleeding into a muscle.

Treatment

- Haemophilia is a lifelong condition with no known cure, although it can be managed by treatment.
- Treatment involves IV replacement of the missing blood clotting factor.

Jayne Price, Queen's University Belfast
Fionnuala Diamond, Royal Belfast Hospital for Sick Children

Nursing care

Holistic care for the child with haemophilia must include:

Advice about dietary needs, dental care, and avoidance of anti-inflammatory drugs

Emergency care: educate the child and family about procedure if a bleed occurs

Maintenance of normal lifestyle within school

Offer genetic counselling

Play: to explain the illness and procedures to the child, and as a distraction

Home care education programme: the wider family

Identify emotional/support needs: promote a normal lifestyle

Liaise with multidisciplinary team: the haemophilia nurse specialist has a key role here

Information needs: e.g. the Haemophilia Society has a wide range of literature

Avoidance of overprotection and providing age-appropriate independence.

Further reading

Haemophilia Society 🖳 www.haemophilia.org.uk

Eisman-Shaw, A., Harrington, C. (1999). Haemophilia—the facts. *Nursing Standard* **14**(3), 39–46.

Butler, V. (2000). Factors for life. *Nursing Standard* **14**, 52–61.

Henoch–Schönlein purpura

Henoch–Schönlein purpura is an inflammatory disorder, with vasculit[?] affecting the capillaries of the skin, gastrointestinal tract, kidneys, joint[?] and, rarely, the lungs and CNS.

It is the most common form of vasculitis in children, although it is sti[?] quite rare. It is more common in boys than girls.

Henoch–Schönlein purpura is commonly preceded by a respiratory o[?] throat infection, although the exact causes are still unclear.

Common symptoms
- Rash. This presents initially as red macules and papules, becoming increasingly purple over time. Generally in clusters over lower extremities, buttocks, and lower abdomen.
- Abdominal pain.
- Nausea and vomiting.
- Joint pain and oedema, predominantly in the large joints.
- Inflammation of the kidneys, resulting in some degree of haematuria and/or proteinurea.
- Diarrhoea.

Serious complications
These complications are rare but should be considered:
- end-stage renal failure
- intussusception
- pancreatitis
- bowel perforation.

Treatment
Henoch–Schönlein purpura is generally a self-limiting and mild conditio[?] requiring little intervention. However, the symptoms can last a month o[?] more. Therefore treatment is symptom-based.
- Anti-inflammatory analgesics, e.g. ibuprofen, for joint pain. Should not be used if there is significant renal involvement.
- Steroids can be used for significant abdominal pain or kidney disease, to reduce the inflammation.

Nursing management
Regular urinalysis
Daily initially; then less frequently as indicated. Observe for signs o[?] protein or blood in urine; many children will have these present, but it [?] important to ensure that these are not increasing.

Blood pressure
Advised initially on diagnosis, then weekly to monthly if blood or prote[?] is present in urine.

Children will require re-assessment if:
- urine contains frank blood
- consistent high protein in urine
- mobility limited by joint swelling

Michelle Fuller, Southampton University Hospitals NHS Trust

increasingly severe abdominal pain
bile-stained vomiting
bloody stools
swollen testicles
consistently raised blood pressure.

urther reading

www.nlm.nih.gov/medlineplus/ency/article/000425.htm
www.emedicine.com/emerg/topic845.htm

Idiopathic thrombocytopenic purpura (ITP)

Definition

ITP is also known as immune thrombocytopenic purpura. It is:
- an autoimmune disease; platelets are destroyed in the spleen
- the most common causes of thrombocytopenia (a low platelet count) in children
- segregated into two categories, acute and chronic:
  - acute ITP usually resolves within 6 months
  - chronic ITP persists for longer than 6 months

Epidemiology

- Annual incidence of 3–8 cases per 100 000 children, including both acute and chronic cases.
- Peak incidence between the ages of 2 years and 5 years, usually resolving spontaneously within the first few months.
- Acute ITP affects both boys and girls equally.
- Chronic ITP affects more girls than boys and is more prevalent in adolescents. Remission often occurs within 5 years.

Causes

Unknown, has been linked to:
- viral infection present 3 weeks before manifestation of the acute disease
- live measles vaccination.

Some patients with chronic ITP have been found to have other underlying autoimmune disorders (e.g. inflammatory bowel disease or systemic lupus erythematosus).

Signs and symptoms

- A low platelet count will be evident by conducting a full blood count.
- Mucosal and/or cutaneous bleeding may be evident:
  - mucosal bleeding manifests as epistaxis, gingival bleeding, wet purpura, and menorrhagia
  - cutaneous bleeding manifests as petechiae and ecchymoses (bruising).
- Bleeding into the CNS is rare but predominantly fatal.

Investigations

- Full blood count and clotting.
- Examination of the peripheral blood smear.
- A full history to include any recent infections, immunizations, family history, any previous bleeding, and medication record.
- Physical examination to include examination of the skin, urine, and stool and examination for lymphadenopathy and hepato-splenomegaly.

Anna Oddy, Central Manchester and Manchester Children's Hospitals NHS Trust

If ITP persists for longer than 6 months, a bone marrow aspirate may be considered.

Virology investigations may also be considered.

Treatment

Treatment depends on the type of ITP and its severity. Platelet transfusion will not improve the condition because the patient's immune system will attack the platelets that have been transfused. Treatment for acute ITP is:
- IV Ig
- steroids
- anti-Rho (D) Ig.

None of these therapies will cure the disease, but they will help to resolve the platelet crisis as the body recovers.

Patients with chronic ITP who have significant episodes of bleeding may require splenectomy. This is only recommended in children over the age of 2 years, but over the age of 5 is preferable. Long-term follow-up after splenectomy can show a high rate of reappearance of ITP.

Prognosis

The prognosis of ITP depends on how quickly the disease is identified and treated, and the severity and type of ITP.

Further reading

www.itppeopple.com/aboutitp.htm

Thalassaemia

Introduction and definition

Thalassaemia is an inherited blood disorder in which there is a defect the structure of haemoglobin. It is most common among Middle Easter Indian, and Mediterranean populations and throughout Southeast As including southern China, Thailand, and Malaysia.

Haemoglobin is a protein that is contained in red blood cells. It responsible for the transportation of O_2 from the lungs to the tissues of th body where it is needed. A person who does not have enough haem globin is anaemic. Haemoglobin molecules contain four protein chai (two α-globin chains and two β-globin chains). Different genes a responsible for producing each chain. In thalassaemia there is an inherite defect in one of these genes, resulting in either α-thalassaemia β-thalassaemia, depending on the chain affected. The pattern of inher tance for thalassaemia is autosomal recessive.

There are a number of different types of thalassaemia within these tw groups.

Signs and symptoms

- Between birth and 3 months the thalassaemic child will seem normal and quite healthy.
- Gradually signs of anaemia begin to show: pale, not sleeping, reduced appetite, and vomiting.

Diagnosis

- Blood tests: to measure the size of red blood cells and amount of haemoglobin.
- Babies can be tested at 1 year old to give a clear diagnosis of carrier status.

Treatment

- Regular blood transfusions every 4–6 weeks.
- Treatment of iron overload caused by blood transfusions. Two drugs are used; Desferrarl® (desferrioxamine) and Ferriprox® (deferiprone) Some patients take both drugs.
- Bone-marrow transplant. This is the only cure for thalassaemia and is best done when the child is fairly young, before iron build-up. This procedure is painful and although success rates are improving, they ar unpredictable.

Without treatment a child may die between the ages of 1 year an 8 years.

Further reading

Beutler, E., Lichman, M.A., Coller, B.S., Kipps, T.J., Seligsohn, U. (2001). *Williams Hematolo* 6th edn. McGraw-Hill, New York.
Sidwell, R., Thomson, M. (2000). *Concise paediatrics*. Alden Press, Oxford.
▣ www.nhsdirect.nhs.uk

Sarah Jane Woolliscroft, Central Manchester and Manchester Children's Hospitals NHS Trust

Thrombocytopenia

Definition

Thrombocytopenia can be defined as a decreased circulating platelet count below the normal range of 150–400 $\times$ 10^9/litre.

Aetiology

Thrombocytopenia is a symptom associated with many disorders. The platelet count can be affected by three differing causes:

- decreased or impaired production of platelets in the bone marrow
- increased platelet consumption or destruction
- a problem with the distribution of platelets in the body.

Some of the disorders associated with thrombocytopenia

- ITP
- Drug-induced (commonly NSAIDS and antibiotics)
- Infection-related disorders
- Disseminated intravascular coagulation (DIC)
- Leukaemia
- Metastaic infiltration of bone marrow by malignant tumours
- After chemotherapy and radiotherapy causing bone-marrow suppression
- Aplastic anaemia
- Neonatal problems
- Hypothermia
- Hypersplenism
- Hereditary disorders (including Fanconi's anaemia)

Signs and symptoms

The most common symptom of a thrombocytopenic patient is bleeding. Bleeding without injury usually only occurs when the platelet count falls below 10–20 $\times$ 10^9/litre. Therefore those with counts higher than this may be asymptomatic so may only be diagnosed from a routine full blood count. Bleeding can include:

- epistaxis
- gingival bleeding
- purpura
- menorrhagia in adolescent girls
- petechiae
- prolonged bleeding from minor trauma
- intracranial haemorrhage.

Investigations

- Complete history and physical examination, including examination of skin and for hepato-splenomegaly and lymphadenopathy
- Full blood count
- Blood film to exclude malignant cells, disease, and other disorders that may indicate a need for bone-marrow aspiration
- Bone-marrow aspirate, if indicated from other tests
- Virology blood tests

Gemma Pritchard, Central Manchester and Manchester Children's Hospitals NHS Trust

Treatment

Treatment of thrombocytopaenia depends on the diagnosis.

Immunoglobulin infusions and steroids may be used to treat ITP.
Platelet transfusion is used for decreased bone-marrow production (threshold of <10–20 × 10⁹/litre), but this may be higher if the risk of bleeding is higher.
Bone-marrow transplant may be indicated to correct certain disorders, including severe aplastic anaemia and Fanconi's anaemia.
Treatment of malignancy to clear marrow and restore normal bone-marrow production.

Complications

Bleeding after surgery or invasive procedures.
Platelets consumed at a higher rate with fever.
Risk of intracranial bleed with platelet count <10 × 10⁹/litre commonly leading to fatality.
Premature infants or children with brain tumours who are thrombocytopenic, usually due to chemotherapy treatment, are at higher risk of intracranial bleeding, so may require a higher threshold to be set for platelet transfusion.
Advice should be given to avoid contact sports and NSAIDs.

Further reading

ggins, C. (2000). *Understanding laboratory investigations*. Blackwell Science, London.
ine, N., Tomlinson, D. (2005). *Paediatric oncology nursing*. Springer, Germany
www.cancerbacup.org.uk

HIV infection

The HIVs are retroviruses, the effects of which were first noted i 1981. They act principally by damaging the immune system, which ca lead to the development of AIDS. This leads to the infected perso suffering from recurrent opportunistic infection. The virus is blood- born and infection is transmitted through this route. HIV is diagnosed usin virological blood tests and identification of typical signs and infections.

Exposure to HIV can occur via five routes.
- Sexual transmission: unprotected sexual activity.
- Drug use: injecting drug users.
- Mother-to-infant transmission: can occur *in utero* or during or after delivery; improvements in care have resulted in this route being responsible for <2% of cases in the UK.
- Iatrogenic transmission: via infected blood products, organ transplantation, contaminated medical equipment, or infected health personnel.
- Occupational exposure.

Infection control
Achieved through the use of general universal precautions. Transmissio through normal social contact is impossible.

Natural history
Young children have a developing immune system so the course of th infection tends to be rapid, whereas young people with a competer immune system have an infection that may evolve over years.

HIV principally affects and eventually kills specific white bloo cells—CD4 T lymphocytes—which are a vital part of the immun response. As the HIV infection worsens, more of these cells are kille and the immune function progressively worsens. The patient suffers fron increasingly frequent infection, to the point of severity where AIDS ca be diagnosed.

Immunization
Children with HIV infection should be fully immunized. Because the immune system is damaged, they may not achieve full active immunit and may need passive immune protection after exposure to som childhood infections.

Breast-feeding
This brings many advantages for child health. However, because vertica transmission of HIV (from mother to baby) is possible through breas milk, breast-feeding is not recommended in the developed world wher there is a safe alternative.

Jim Richardson, University of Glamorgan

Social dimensions

HIV has carried something of a social stigma and this may be a dimension that affects children and their families. Every effort must be made to prevent this becoming a factor in the child's illness experience.

The young person with HIV infection should have information and guidance on the principles of safer sex.

Therapy

Management of HIV infection is through the following.
- Antimicrobial therapy against specific infections.
- Antiretroviral therapy, which is a prophylactic approach (i.e. the drugs must be taken regularly and consistently). These drugs inhibit the replication of the HIV virus. New drugs in this category are continually being developed.

Further reading

Pizzo, P.A., Wilfert, C.M. (1998). *Pediatric AIDS: the challenge of HIV infection in infants, children and adolescents.* Williams & Wilkins, Baltimore.

Pratt, R.J. (2003). *HIV and AIDS: a foundation for nursing and healthcare practice,* 5th edn. Arnold, London.

www.aidsmap.com

Primary deficiencies of the innate immune system in children

Definition
Unlike the acquired immune system, we are born with a functioning innate immune system. It consists of physical, mechanical, and chemical barriers, as well as certain white blood cells, such as neutrophils, monocytes, tissue macrophages, etc., but not lymphocytes.

Deficiencies in any part of the innate immune system can cause problems. We will consider just one deficiency.

Severe congenital neutropenia (Kostmann's syndrome)

Epidemiology
Affecting males and females, it appears within the first year of life, often immediately after birth.

Incidence
Rare, although neutropenia as a secondary immunodeficiency is more common.

Cause
Autosomal recessive disease, but the underlying mutation is unknown.

Clinical features
Consists of three characteristics:
- arrest to bone marrow granulocyte maturation
- severe chronic neutropenia (<200 neutrophils/µl)
- increased susceptibility to acute myeloid leukaemia.

Signs and symptoms
- Infection, including cellulitis, perirectal abscess, peritonitis, stomatitis, and meningitis
- Failure to thrive

Differential diagnosis
- Any immunodeficiency—primary or secondary
- Leukaemia

Investigations
- Neutrophil count
- Full white blood count
- Immune function tests

Management and treatment
- Prevent infection.
- Symptomatic treatment of infection.
- Infusion of recombinant granulocyte-colony stimulating factors (G-CSFs). G-CSF is produced naturally by our bodies to stimulate the production of granulocytes, a part of our immune defence, and so this treatment increases the production of granulocytes (including neutrophils).

Peter Vickers, University of Hertfordshire

Improve nutrition: this often improves with the absence of infection.
Very strict hygiene.
Counselling and support for the family.
Genetic counselling.

Prognosis

Was always fatal at an early age, but since children have been treated
with G-CSF, the number of infections, as well as the number of days
spent in hospital, has been reduced and the life expectancy of the
children has increased.[1]

Unfortunately there have been a few occasions when children treated
with G-CSF have developed acute myeloid leukaemia as a result of the
treatment.[1]

Further reading

Nairn, R., Helbert, M. (2002). *Immunology for medical students*. Mosby, Edinburgh.

Stiehm, E.R., Ochs, H.D., Winkelstein, J.A. (ed.) (2004). *Immunologic disorders in infants and children*, 5th edn. W.B. Saunders, Philadelphia.

Antibody deficiencies in children

An absence or deficiency of the production of antibodies (Igs) Antibodies are part of the acquired immune system and are produced b B lymphocytes in response to specific infectious micro-organisms. Ther are many different forms of antibody deficiency, and we will look at jus one: Bruton's X-linked agammaglobulinaemia (XLA).

XLA

This is a deficiency of IgG, which affects boys only and has an incidence c between 1 in 100 000 and 1 in 200 000[1]. The deficiency is diagnosed i infancy.

Cause

XLA is an autosomal recessive genetic disorder, and is caused by mutation of the *Btk* gene on the X chromosome. Boys inherit it from carrier mother with a 1:2 chance of being affected. (There is also a 1: chance of any daughters being carriers.)

Signs and symptoms

The Primary Immunodeficiency Association[1] has listed 10 warning signs c a primary immunodeficiency:

- eight or more episodes of otitis media within 1 year
- two or more episodes of severe sinusitis within 1 year
- ≥2 months on antibiotics, with little effect or no effect
- two or more occurrences of pneumonia within 1 year
- failure to thrive/grow normally in an infant
- recurrent deep skin or organ abscesses
- persistent oral or skin thrush after 1 year of age
- infection that will not clear without IV antibiotics
- two or more serious infections, such as meningitis or sepsis
- family history of a primary immune deficiency.

Differential diagnosis

- Any other primary immunodeficiency
- Secondary immunodeficiency
- Transient hypogammaglobulinaemia of infancy

Management and treatment

- Prophylactic antibiotics
- Aggressive antibiotic therapy when the child has an infection
- Ig replacement therapy: IV or subcutaneous
- Genetic counselling
- Counselling and support of child and family

Complications

- Serious infection, including meningitis
- Chronic lung damage due to infection
- Septic arthritis

Peter Vickers, University of Hertfordshire

ognosis

e prognosis of affected children is very good as long as they are gnosed early enough and have the correct treatment, including Ig erapy.

rther reading

rn, R., Helbert, M. (2002). *Immunology for medical students*. Mosby, Edinburgh.
ehm, E.R., Ochs, H.D., Winkelstein, J.A. (ed.) (2004). *Immunologic disorders in infants and children*, 5th edn. Elsevier Saunders, Philadelphia.

rimary Immunodeficiency Association. 🖳 www.pia.org.uk/

Severe combined immunodeficiencies (SCIDs) in children

SCIDs occur when there are problems with either T-cell or both T-cell and B-cell lymphocytes. There are several different types of SCID, but we will concentrate just on one, X-linked SCID, as an example.

X-linked SCID

Definition
X-linked SCID is an inherited immunodeficiency with an absence of mature T-cell lymphocytes, natural killer T-cell lymphocytes, and immunoglobulins.

Incidence
X-linked SCID has an estimated incidence of 1 in 150 000 to 1 in 200 000 live births, with only boys being affected and girls being carriers.

Clinical features/signs and symptoms
Boys usually present during the first months of life with:
- many severe, and often opportunistic, infections
- oral thrush
- persistent diarrhoea
- failure to thrive
- possibly interstitial pneumonia (*Pneumocystis jirovecii*)
- skin rash
- severe lymphopaenia
- agammaglobulinaemia.

Management and treatment
- Prevention of infection: reverse barrier isolation/prophylactic antibiotics and antifungal drugs.
- Very strict adherence to hygiene and skin care.
- Treat infection very aggressively with the correct antimicrobial drugs.
- Nutrition: total parenteral nutrition.
- Replacement immunoglobulin therapy.
- Replacement red blood cells and platelets where required (all blood products should be CMV-negative if the child is the same).
- No live immunizations.
- Support and counselling for the family.
- Genetic counselling regarding future children.
- Bone-marrow/stem-cell transplants (definitive cure).
- Now the possibility of gene-replacement therapy as a cure.
- Ongoing psychological, nursing, and medical support following successful treatment—there are many psychosocial problems following a cure.

Prevention
- Genetic counselling.
- Prenatal diagnosis, with the possibility of abortion of the fetus if found to be affected.

Peter Vickers, University of Hertfordshire

Prognosis

Without successful definitive treatment (bone-marrow/stem-cell transplant or gene-replacement therapy), this form of SCID is a fatal disease, with death occurring before the end of the first year of life. Palliative treatment—isolation antimicrobial therapy etc.—is only of marginal value in the long term and can only marginally prolong survival at best. However, the outlook for those children who do survive because of the curative treatment is very good.

Further reading

Nairn, R., Helbert, M. (2002). *Immunology for medical students.* Mosby, Edinburgh.

Primary Immunodeficiency Association. ⌨ www.pia.org.uk/

Stiehm, E.R., Ochs, H.D., Winkelstein, J.A. (ed.) (2004). *Immunologic disorders in infants and children,* 5th edn. W.B. Saunders, Philadelphia.

Care of the immunosuppressed child

Definition
There are two categories of immunosuppressed child: those whose immune system is damaged as a result of genetic/hereditary factor primary immunodeficiencies), and those whose immunosuppression is the result of an external factor (secondary immunodeficiency). Immuno suppression can refer to the absence or loss/diminution of function of any part of the immune system.

Epidemiology
There is no age limit as to when secondary immunodeficiencies may affect children, but most primary immunodeficiencies are present from birth or shortly afterwards. Most cases of immunodeficiency are secondary to an external cause, but the number of children identified as having primary immunodeficiencies is rising as a result of better diagnosis.

Causes of secondary immunodeficiencies
- Cancers/leukaemias
- Drugs
- Infections (including AIDS)
- Radiation
- Malnutrition

Clinical features
The major signs of immunosuppression/immunodeficiency, whether secondary or primary, are frequent, including severe infection, often by opportunistic micro-organisms (e.g. CMV), which e.g., and may produce atypical features.

Care and treatment
- Most important care is related to preventing the immuno-compromised child from becoming infected. Children who are severely immunocompromised will require isolation, and all immunosuppressed children should avoid people with infections.
- Prophylactic antibiotics and antifungal drugs may be given.
- Avoid crowded spaces.
- If the child does become infected, the infection is treated aggressively with antibiotics, antiviral drugs, and antifungal drugs, which may be administered via an IV route or central line.
- Contact with chickenpox requires zoster Ig ZIg.
- Nutrition maintained: may require total parenteral nutrition.
- Very strict adherence to hygiene.
- No live vaccines should be given to the child, and similarly the child should not come into contact with anyone who has recently had a live vaccine.
- If the child is CMV-negative, any transfused blood products must also be CMV-negative.
- If problems with antibodies, Ig infusions can be given.
- Support the child and family.

Peter Vickers, University of Hertfordshire

- Family/child counselling, particularly for severe immunodeficiency, e.g. HIV/AIDS.
- Genetic counselling for primary immunodeficiency.
- Educate the child/family/health professionals.
- Apart from the drugs above, the treatment depends upon the cause of the immunosuppression.
- If possible, remove any secondary cause, e.g. improve nutrition or successfully treat cancer.
- HAART therapy for HIV/AIDS.
- If possible, bone-marrow/stem-cell transplant for leukaemias and severe primary immunodeficiencies.
- Gene-replacement therapy for a very few severe primary immunodeficiencies, e.g. ADA SCID, X-linked SCID.

Complications

The major complication for the immunosuppressed child is death from infection.

Further reading

Stiehm, E.R., Ochs, H.D., Winkelstein, J.A. (2004). Immunodeficiency disorders: general considerations. In *Immunologic disorders in infants and children*, 5th edn (ed. E.R. Stiehm, H.D. Ochs, and J.A. Winkelstein), pp. 289–355. W.B. Saunders, Philadelphia.

Vickers, P.S., Brennan, V., Cochrane, S., et al. (1997). *Information for nurses, midwives and health visitors*. Primary Immunodeficiency Association, London. ☐ www.pia.org/publications.htm (accessed May 2005)

☐ www2.mc.duke.edu/depts/hospital/9200bmt/NeutropenicP.htm

Oncology

Related physiology

Oncology involves the investigation, diagnosis, and treatment of cancers (maligant tumours). Any abnormal growth of cells within the body is termed a tumour. Some are benign (i.e. self-limiting). Malignant tumours enlarge and/or spread to distant sites (metastasize) in an uncontrolled fashion: the cells repeatedly divide in an unlimited fashion due to mutation in the genetic material in the cell. Cells usually need to accumulate several mutations over several generations before they become cancerous.

Carcinogenesis (the development of cancerous cells from normal cells) is mediated by:
- oncogenes (which promote cancer if they are activated)
- tumour-suppressor genes (which allow cancer to develop if they are deactivated).

The characteristics of cancer cells
- Proliferate (increase in number through cell division) at an escalated rate.
- Differentiation (cell specialization) is generally decreased.
- Evade apoptosis (programmed cell death).
- Have unlimited growth potential—can divide repeatedly.
- Self-sufficient in growth factors and insensitive to anti-growth factors.
- Infiltrate neighbouring tissues because of loss of contact inhibition (the ability of the cell to recognize if other cells are the same as them or different).
- Able to promote angiogenesis (blood vessel growth).
- Able to metastasize (spread to distant sites via the lymphatic and blood vessels).
- The cancer acts like a parasite and, unless it is eradicated, usually causes death.

Mutations in the genetic material of cells [1]
- These take place during cell division and include:
  - deletions—material is left out
  - insertions—material is added
  - inversions—the material splits into three, the middle part turns through 180°, and the parts then rejoin
  - substitutions—incorrect material replaces the correct material
  - translocations—breaking and then inappropriate merging of two different chromosomes.
- Cells that divide most frequently (e.g. stem cells) have a higher risk of mutating than those that divide less frequently (e.g. neurons).
- The mutations may be triggered by environmental factors, such as cytotoxic chemicals, viruses, and radiation.
- If the mutated cell is not removed by the immune system, it will become a cancer.
- It is possible to look at mutations that have occurred in cancer cells and predict the probable behaviour of the disease.

Louise Holliday, Royal Aberdeen Children's Hospital

entences to illustrate different types of genetic mutations

'he cat sat on the mat'
'he dog had a bone'

eletion
laterial is left out:
'he cat the mat'

isertion
laterial is added:
'he cat sat a bone on the mat'

iversion
he material splits into three, the middle part turns through 180°, and
ie parts rejoin:
'he cat no tas the mat'

ubstitution
icorrect material replaces correct material:
'he dog sat on a bone'

ranslocation
ireaking and inappropriate merging of two different chromosomes:
'he cat sat'
'On the mat the dog had a bone'

urther reading

omlinson, D., Kline, N.E. (ed.) (2005). *Pediatric oncology nursing. Advanced Clinical handbook.* Springer, New York.

The child with cancer

As advances in treatments progress and survival rates increase, the need for expert professional care heightens. Although comparatively rare, every year in the UK approximately 1 in every 650 children develop cancer in the first 15 years of life.

- Childhood cancer ranks second in causes of death in childhood.
- There are approximately 1700 new cases of cancer in children (up to the age of 15 years) each year throughout the UK.
- Childhood cancer that affects different parts of the body responds differently to treatment.

Childhood cancer

Distribution of major cancers in children.

Childhood cancer

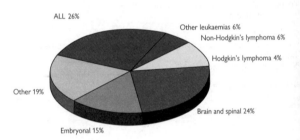

ALL 26%

Other leukaemias 6%
Non-Hodgkin's lymphoma 6%

Hodgkin's lymphoma 4%

Other 19%

Brain and spinal 24%

Embryonal 15%

Source: National Statistics 2004

The two most commonly occurring cancers in children are:

- leukaemia
- brain and spinal tumours.

Epidemiology

The cause of childhood cancer is unknown, although there are many theories about the causation. Collaborative research is currently studying a number of possible causes, including:

- environmental factors, e.g.
  - clustering of cases in small geographical locations
  - proximity to power lines, electromagnetic fields, and radiation
  - exposure to sunshine without adequate protection

Wendy M. McInally, Napier University Edinburgh

Individual factors and lifestyle, e.g.
- age and sex
- genetic predisposition (inherited abnormal gene or mutation)
- infection (Epstein–Barr virus, CMV, etc.)
- mobile phone usage
- dietary factors
- lack of exercise.

Survival rates

Since the 1960s there have been great advances in treatment. Currently the overall 5-year survival for childhood cancer is in the region of 65–70%, whereas in 1966 the average survival for childhood cancer was 30%.
- Survival rates are largely attributable to the introduction of intensive multi-agent chemotherapy, combined with radiotherapy and surgery as required.
- In 1977 the UK Children's Cancer Study Group (UKCCSG) was set up and centralization of specialist care evolved.
- At present there are 21 specialist centres around the UK, providing care for the child and family.

Future challenges

The prime focus for the medical and nursing profession is to provide optimal care to ensure quality survival for children with cancer. The main issues to be considered are:
- late effects (to minimize the late effects of treatment, especially for curable cancers)
- quality of life for the child with cancer
- to sustain the improvements in survival rates.

Further reading

Gibson, F., Evans, M. (1999). *Paediatric oncology acute nursing care*. Whurr, London.

Gibson, F., Soanes, L., Sepion, B. (2005). *Perspectives in paediatric oncology nursing*. Whurr, London.

Stiller, C., Quinn, M., and Rowan, S. (2004). *The health of children and young people childhood cancer*. The Office for National Statistics and the National Registry of Childhood Tumours, Oxford. ▪ www.statistics.gov.uk/children/

Paediatric brain tumours

Brain tumours are the most common solid tumour of childhood accounting for 20–30% of all paediatric tumours. In the UK about 30 children are diagnosed each year.

These tumours arise from the neuroglia (supportive tissue of nerve cells) or from nerve cells, which are immature (embryonal) in origin.

They occur anywhere within the brain or spine, but the most common site in childhood is the infratentorium (posterior fossa). Tumours are unlikely to spread elsewhere in the body, but the brain is often a site for secondary tumours.

The cause is unknown. Children with neurofibromatosis type 1 and tuberous sclerosis are at increased risk.

Signs and symptoms
- These are often delayed as a young child is unable to describe symptoms.
- Symptoms can be vague and mirror common childhood ailments.
- Signs and symptoms are predicted by the location of the tumours:
  - ataxia—posterior fossa
  - visual disturbances–optic nerve tract or posterior fossa
  - Seizures—temporal lobe
  - behavioural change—frontal lobe
  - hormone imbalance (precocious puberty)—pituitary gland.
- Raised ICP.

Investigations
- Medical history
- Full medical examination
- CT and/or MRI scan

Hazards
- If symptoms of raised ICP are not recognized or treated, death will occur.
- It is not possible to operate on tumours found in the brainstem, thalamus, motor area, and deep areas of the grey matter.

Treatment
- High-dose dexamethasone to reduce cerebral oedema.
- Surgery:
  - principal aim is to relieve hydrocephalus and reduce raised ICP by tumour resection
  - to obtain tissue samples for diagnosis
  - to remove as much tumour as possible without causing further damage to the child
  - complete resection has a better prognostic outcome.

Frances Northeast, Nottingham University Hospitals NHS Trust

MRI scan within 72 hours of surgery to define any residual disease.
Chemotherapy:
- tumour-type-specific protocols
- scan assessments.
Radiotherapy.

Nursing management
PICU immediate post-operative period
Support and explanations
Neurological assessment
Wound management
Rehabilitation
Nutrition
Multidisciplinary approach:
- discharge planning
- equipment needs
- package of care
- financial support
Parental education about the side effects of treatment
Child's schooling—may need Statement of Special Needs
Regular medical reviews
Endocrine support
Neuropsychological assessment

Further reading
www.cancerbacup.org.uk/Cancertype/Childrenscancers/Typesofchildrenscancers/Braintumours
www.nottingham.ac.uk/genetics/ChildrensBrainTumours/disease_info.html

Bone tumours

Definition

The two most common types of bone tumour in childhood ar osteosarcoma and Ewing's sarcoma.

Osteosarcoma

The most common type of bone cancer in childhood. It usually arises i the metaphysis of the long bones, with the most common sites being th distal femur, proximal tibia, and proximal humerus. Metastases occu most commonly in the lungs. The cause is unknown; however, there is genetic predisposition to osteosarcoma in children with hereditar retinoblastoma. Osteosarcoma can also develop as a secondary tumou following previous radiotherapy or chemotherapy.

Ewing's sarcoma

A small round-cell tumour that arises from bones or soft tissue. The commonly arise in the diaphysis of the long bones but can also occur i the pelvis and chest wall. If they start in soft tissue, they are called prim tive neuro-ectodermal tumours (PNETs).

Incidence

Osteosarcoma affects about 30 children a year in the UK, and the inc dence of Ewing's sarcoma is slightly less. Both tumours occur in th teenage years and can be associated with the adolescent growth spur There is also a higher incidence among boys than girls.

Presenting features

Both tumours present with similar symptoms: pain and swelling in th affected area. Occasionally the tumour weakens the area, which ca result in a fracture. As the symptoms occur at an age when growing pain are common, this can cause delays in diagnosis.

Diagnostic investigations

- X-ray of the site to identify a tumour.
- Biopsy of the tumour.
- Chest X-ray, bone scan, bone-marrow aspirate, and MRI and CT scans are used to assess the spread of the disease.

Staging

Bone tumours are graded in stages 1–3, where 1 is low grade or slo growing and 3 is high grade or rapidly growing. Both osteosarcoma an Ewing's sarcoma tend to be high-grade tumours.

- Stage 1A: low grade, within the hard coating of the bone.
- Stage 1B: low grade, extending into the soft tissue around the bone.
- Stage 2A: high grade, within the hard coating of the bone.
- Stage 2B: high grade, extending into the soft tissue around the bone.
- Stage 3: low or high grade, either within the bone or extending to the soft tissue. The tumour has spread to other parts of the body not directly associated with the affected bone.

Louise Viljoen, Southampton University Hospitals NHS Trust

Treatment

For both tumours:
- treatment depends on the size, position, and stage of the tumour
- initial treatment is chemotherapy to shrink the primary tumour followed by surgery to remove the tumour
- this can be complete amputation of the limb if the whole limb is affected or limb-sparing surgery if just part of the limb is affected
- limb-sparing surgery can replace the bone with either a prosthesis or a bone graft from another bone
- surgery is then completed, with final courses of chemotherapy to eliminate cells that have been missed by surgery.

For Ewing's sarcoma that has had a poor response to the initial chemotherapy, high-dose chemotherapy and a peripheral blood stem-cell transplant is used. Radiotherapy can also be used in the treatment of Ewing's sarcoma, and it is usually given before or after surgery, or if surgery is not possible, e.g. pelvic tumours.

Prognosis

In both cases, the 5-year survival rate is about 65% for children with localized disease. However, if the disease has spread, the survival rate is about 30%.

Further reading

Gibson, F. et al. (2000). *Paediatric oncology - acute nursing care*, pp. 363–74. Whurr Publishers Ltd, London.

St Jude Children's Research Hospital: Osteosarcoma or Ewing's sarcoma family tumours: 🖳 www.stjude.org/disease-summaries/0,2557,449_2167_2995,00.html

🖳 www.cancerbacup.org.uk/Cancertype/Childrenscancers/Typesofchildrenscancers/Ewingssarcoma

Neuroblastoma

Definition

Neuroblastoma is a cancer of the neural crest cells in the sympathetic nervous system. The tumour can, therefore, occur wherever these cells occur in the body. The primary site is most commonly in the abdomen, generally arising in the adrenal glands.

Incidence

Around 100 children are diagnosed with neuroblastoma in the UK every year. The majority of these children are aged < 5 years and most are around 2 years old.

Signs and symptoms

The initial symptoms depend on the site of the primary tumour, and because the most prevalent site is in the abdomen, an abdominal mass is the most common presenting sign. Children also present with weight loss, lethargy and malaise, bone or joint pain, anaemia, fever, constipation, difficulty in passing urine, neurological complications in their legs, and breathlessness if the tumour is in the chest.

Diagnostic investigations

- X-rays and ultrasound.
- Urine tests for levels of the urinary metabolites homovanillic acid (HVA) and vanillyl mandelic acid (VMA), which are increased in children with neuroblastoma.
- CT and MRI scans, which can be used for staging.
- Bone scan and meta-iodo-benzyl-guanidine (mIBG) scan (this is a radioactive substance that is taken up by neuroblastoma cells).
- Biopsy of tumour.

Staging

- Stage 1: localized disease with no spread, can be removed by surgery
- Stage 2A: localized disease with no spread, cannot be removed by surgery
- Stage 2b: localized disease with spread to nearby lymph nodes
- Stage 3: disease spread to surrounding organs or tissues, but not distant areas
- Stage 4: disease spread to distant areas, i.e. lymph nodes, bone, bone marrow, liver, skin, or other organs
- Stage 4S: localized disease, as with stages 1, 2A, and 2B, with spread to skin, liver, or bone marrow

Treatment

- The treatment of neuroblastoma depends on the stage and position of the tumour at diagnosis.
- Stage 4S tumours occur in infants under 1 year old, usually resolving without any intervention, but low-dose radiation or chemotherapy and surgery may be required.

Louise Viljoen, Southampton University Hospitals NHS Trust

For those children whose tumour is still localized with no spread, often surgery is the only treatment needed.

If the tumour has spread at diagnosis, which is common due to the aggressive nature of neuroblastoma growth, highly intensive chemotherapy is required. Surgery is then used if resection of the primary tumour is possible, and radiotherapy can be used if resection is incomplete. The treatment of stage 4 disease also uses high-dose chemotherapy with peripheral blood stem-cell transplant.

Prognosis

Depends on the age of the child and the stage of the disease.
Stages 1, 2A, and 2B have a good prognosis.
More often the disease has spread widely by the time it is found and the prognosis is not so positive.
Stage 4: the prognosis is 20% survival rate at 2 years.

Further reading

Pinkerton, C.R., Cushing, P., Sepion, B. (1994). *Childhood cancer management*, pp. 152–60. Arnold, London.

www.cancerbacup.org.uk/Cancertype/Childrenscancers/Typesofchildrenscancers/Neuroblastoma (accessed May 2005).

www.patient.co.uk/showdoc/40000525

Rhabdomyosarcoma (RMS)

Definition

- The most common of the soft-tissue sarcomas in childhood.
- Sarcomas are malignant tumours of the connective tissue cells. RMS arises from embryonal striated muscle precursor cells.
- Two main types of RMS: embryonal and alveolar.
- Embryonal-type RMS includes 'botryoid tumours', so called because of their grape-like appearance, usually occurring in the mucosal-lined hollow organs, e.g. bladder and vagina.
- Overall survival rate for children with RMS is 75%, but the survival rate is lower in patients with alveolar-type RMS at unresectable sites.

Epidemiology

- RMS is more common in boys than girls.
- Fewer than 60 children are diagnosed with this type of tumour each year in the UK.
- RMS can present in children and young people from 0–19 years of age.
- A high incidence occurs at 1–4 years, falling to a lower rate at 10–14 years, and remaining steady at 15–19 years.

Causes

- The cause of RMS is unclear; it many occur sporadically.
- There may be a link with familial syndromes, e.g. neurofibromatosis and Li–Fraumeni syndrome, which is associated with a germ-line mutation on the p53 tumour-suppressor gene.

Clinical features

- Embryonal RMS more commonly occurs in the younger age group.
- Alveolar RMS can occur at any age.
- RMS occurs anywhere in the body that striated muscle is laid down, but can also occur in other areas.

Common sites for RMS			
Parameningeal	16%	Genito-urinary	22%
Ear		Paratesticular	
Mastoid		Prostate	
Nasal cavity		Bladder	
Paranasal sinuses		Vagina	
Orbit	9%	Extremity	18%
Other head and neck	10%	Other	25%

Symptoms and signs

- Unexplained unresolved painless/painful swelling.
- Symptoms that are specific to the site of the tumour, e.g.
  - bladder—haematuria, and urine retention
  - ear—chronic otitis media, haemorrhagic discharge, and cranial nerve palsy.

Margaret Parr, Nottingham University Hospitals NHS Trust

Management

Referral to a paediatric oncology centre for investigations to determine a diagnosis:

- tumour biopsy
- Imaging—CT scan, MRI scan, ultrasound, and bone scan
- bloods
- bone-marrow aspiration and trephine, lumbar puncture (if tumour is parameningeal)
- pre-treatment investigations—echocardiogram, glomerular filtration rate.

• Children and young people diagnosed with RMS in the UK are recruited into clinical trials.

• Multi-modal treatment using chemotherapy, surgery, and radiotherapy.

Treatment (📖 p.622, Treatment regimens)

Further reading

McDowell, H.P. (2003). Update on childhood rhabdomyosarcoma. *Archives of Diseases in Children*, **88**, 354–7.

Pinkerton, C.R., Cushing, P., Sepion, B. (1994). *Childhood cancer management*. Arnold. London.

🔗 www.cancerbacup.org.uk/Cancertype/Childrenscancers/Typesofchildrenscancers/Rhabdomyosarcoma

Acute myeloid leukaemia (AML)

AML is an overproduction of the immature myeloid white blood cells. Leukaemia accounts for one-third of all childhood cancers, with approximately 400 new cases occurring each year in the UK. Less than one-quarter of these cases are AML. AML can affect children of any age and girls and boys are equally affected.

Causes

The exact cause of AML is unknown. Children with certain genetic disorders, such as Down syndrome, are known to have a higher risk of developing leukaemia. Brothers and sisters of children with AML also have a higher risk, although this is small. Other non-cancerous conditions such as aplastic anaemia, may also increase the risk of developing leukaemia.

AML is not infectious and cannot be passed on to other people.

Signs and symptoms

These are related to the lack of normal blood cells in the bone marrow:
- tiredness and lethargy
- bruising and bleeding
- recurrent infection.

In addition, the child may complain of any or all of the following:
- general feeling of being unwell
- aches and pains in limbs
- swollen lymph glands.

Treatment

Chemotherapy is the main treatment for AML. Usually a combination of drugs is given and the treatment has different phases.

Bone-marrow transplant is used for children who are at a high risk of occurrence or who have recurrent disease.

Side effects and nursing management

Many cancer treatments will cause side effects such as:
- hair loss
- anaemia
- bruising
- bleeding
- infection
- loss of appetite and weight
- nausea and vomiting.

Nursing management is related to side effects and the care required to enable the child and family to deal with the diagnosis of a possible life-limiting disease.
- Reduce anxiety:
  - give clear/concise information
  - build relationships

Helen Langton, Coventry University

Monitor effects of treatment:
- TPR and blood pressure
- fluid balance
- manage nausea and vomiting
- monitor weight
- drug-specific effects

Late effects:
- problems with puberty and fertility
- changes to the heart tissue
- small increase in the risk of developing a second cancer

Further reading

angton, H. (2000). *The child with cancer. Family centred care in practice.* Ballière Tindall, London.
www.cancernursing.org

Acute lymphoblastic leukaemia (ALL)

ALL affects the lymphocyte-producing cells in the bone marrow. Lymphocytes are white cells that produce antibodies and are vital part of the immune system. In ALL there is an accumulation in the bone marrow of immature lymphocyte precursor cells, called blast cells. Eventually the production of normal blood cells is compromised, resulting in the reduction in the number of red blood cells, normal white blood cells, and platelets in the blood.

ALL affects 1 in 25 000 children. Peak incidence is between 2 years and 4 years, with a higher male: female ratio. Event-free survival is 70–80%.

Characteristics of ALL
- Variable history.
- Anaemia → fatigue, limited capacity for exercise, and breathlessness.
- Thrombocytopenia → bruising, bleeding from mouth or nose, and blood in stools or urine.
- Low number of normal white blood cells, may have a high number of abnormal white blood cells with high metabolic rate → persistent infection, fever, painful joints, weight loss, and muscle wasting.
- Enlarged lymph nodes, spleen, and liver due to leukaemic infiltrates.
- Headaches, vomiting, cranial nerve palsies, and convulsions from CNS infiltration.

Hazards
- Infection risk due to lack of normal white blood cells. Avoid paracetamol because it masks raised temperatures, and PR drugs should also be omitted.
- Bleeding and associated problems with anaemia; check full blood count before major procedures.
- Avoid NSAIDs because they affect platelet function.

Diagnosis
Often suspected on full blood count but confirmed by bone-marrow examination, with cytogenetics and lumbar puncture.

Treatment
Should be undertaken in specialized centres using national protocols. Treatment is in the form of IV/oral/intrathecal chemotherapy, including steroids. This lasts approximately 2 years for girls and 3 years for boys and is broken into four sections:
- induction—to achieve remission
- consolidation—CNS prophylaxis
- intensification—to reduce the disease to a minimum and extend remission time
- maintenance—to maintain remission until the end of treatment.

Hazel Marriott, Nottingham University Hospitals NHS Trust

Nursing management

Reduce anxiety

Provide emotional support

Give consistent clear advice and information

Involve a social worker

Involve parents in decision-making and their child's care

Safety

Observe for anaemia and signs of bleeding → transfuse red blood cells and/or platelets.

Keep a strict fluid balance during induction on liberal fluids and administrate rasburicase or allopurinol to neutralize the effects of uric acid on the kidneys as the leukaemic cells break down.

Protect from sources of infection. Give prophylactic Septrin® and, if neutropenic, antifungals.

If pyrexial and neutropenic, treat with antibiotics according to hospital policy.

Be aware of the risks and side effects of chemotherapy to protect yourself, the child, and family.

Nutrition

Involve dietician

Monitor weight

Provide a highly nutritious diet

Pain relief

If the child is in pain, give codeine, not paracetamol.

Further reading

ssen, L.V., Enskar, K., Skolin, I. (2001). Important aspects of care and assistance for parents of children 0–18 years of age, on or off treatment for cancer. Parent and nurse perceptions. *European Journal of Oncology Nursing*, **5**(4), 254–64.

www.lrf.org.uk

Wilms tumour

- Also known as nephroblastoma.
- A type of kidney cancer in children.
- Arises from specialized cells known as nephroblasts, which are involved in the development of the kidneys in the embryo. These cells normally disappear at birth but can still be found in Wilms tumours.
- Can be unilateral (one kidney) or bilateral (both). Most cases are unilateral with 1 in 20 cases being bilateral.
- 70 new cases in the UK per year.
- Accounts for 1 in every 20 cancers in children under 15 years of age.
- Most children are under 5 years old at diagnosis.
- Overall survival rate is 90%.
- Relapse normally occurs within first 2 years.

Causes

- The cause is largely unknown. Links have been made to other congenital malformations.
- It is inherited in 1 out of 100 cases. Linked with a defect occurring on chromosome 11 and is autosomal dominant.
- Suggestions have also been made that the risk increases if the mother is exposed to radiation during pregnancy.

Signs and symptoms

- A firm, but not tender, swelling in the abdomen.
- Blood in the urine (haematuria).
- Occasionally patients may experience:
  - pain in the kidney area
  - hypertension
  - weight loss
  - lack of appetite
  - fever.

Diagnosis

- Urine and blood tests to check kidney function.
- Abdominal ultrasound.
- Abdominal CT scan.
- Scans of the liver and chest to check for spread. The most common site for metastasis is the lungs.
- Biopsy and histology of the tumour, i.e. a sample of the tissue is taken under general anaesthetic and sent to the laboratory for examination.

Histology tells us what type of cells the tumour consists of and therefore how advanced it is and how easy it may be to treat. Favourable histology indicates that there is a predominance of primitive cells, which normally give rise to mature kidney tissue. Unfavourable histology means that the predominant cells have features of other cells, e.g. muscle. This means a poorer prognosis.

- 90% of Wilms tumours have a favourable histology.

Jenny Freeman, Royal Devon & Exeter NHS Foundation Trust

Staging

In order for the right treatment to be planned and an estimation given on how successful treatment may be, tumours need to be staged. The lower the grading given to the tumour, the more successful treatment is likely to be.

  Stage 1: the tumour only affects the kidney and has not begun to spread; can be completely removed by surgery.

  Stage 2: the tumour has begun to spread beyond the kidney to nearby structures; still possible to remove the tumour completely by surgery.

  Stage 3: the tumour has spread within the abdomen and cannot be completely removed by surgery; may affect nearby lymph nodes.

  Stage 4: the tumour has spread to other parts of the body such as the lungs, liver, bone, or brain.

  Stage 5: there are tumours in both kidneys (bilateral).

Treatment

- Treatment depends on the stage of the tumour.
- Normally chemotherapy is given to shrink the tumour.
- Surgery is then performed, which involves removal of either the whole kidney (nephrectomy) or part of the kidney (partial nephrectomy).
- Because surgery cannot guarantee that all of the tumour has been effectively removed, and because some cancer cells may be found elsewhere, chemotherapy is then given to target any remaining disease.
- The most common drugs used are actinomycin, vincristine, doxorubicin, and etoposide.
- Treatment ranges from 6 months to 15 months.
- Radiotherapy is then offered to those with an unfavourable histology, or if the initial tumour was very large or there are signs of spread.

Nursing care

- Provide appropriate support and reassurance during diagnosis and treatment, which is an extremely stressful time for both the child and his/her family.
- Maintain nutrional, hygiene, and developmental needs for the child with cancer, as for any other patient.
- The care required will depend on the drugs used during treatment.

Further reading

www.cancerbacup.org.uk
www.ukccsg.org.uk
www.cancerindex.org

T-cell acute lymphoblastic leukaemia

Definition

ALL is a malignant disease arising from the haematopoietic tissues of the bone marrow and lymphatic system. T-cell ALL is a subtype of ALL that occurs during T-cell lymphocyte development; excessive numbers of immature T-cell lymphocytes (blasts) are produced. The high proliferation rate makes the disease acute in nature.

Incidence

T-cell ALL accounts for approximately 10% of the 300 cases of ALL diagnosed in the UK each year.

Symptoms and signs

Most symptoms are similar to those of ALL. However, there are additional symptoms specific to T-cell ALL.

Involvement of the thymus occurs in 60–70% of children with T-cell ALL. Infiltration by proliferating cells gives rise to an anterior mediastinal mass that is detected by X-ray; suspicion is raised by the following symptoms:

- cough
- shortness of breath
- pain
- dysphagia
- deviation of trachea
- respiratory distress.

Pressure caused by a mediastinal mass can cause superior vena cava obstruction. This is a serious, but rare, complication with the following symptoms:

- cough
- wheeze
- oedema of face, neck, and upper thorax
- dilation and prominence of vessels in the neck and upper thorax
- hypoxia
- reduced cardiac output.

Investigations

- Full blood count: pancytopenia or elevated white blood cell count may indicate leukaemia.
- Blood film: may identify blast cells.
- Bone-marrow aspirate: essential for diagnosis, >25% blast cells confirms a diagnosis of leukaemia.
- Lumbar puncture: detects blast cells in CSF to diagnose CNS involvement.
- Chest X-ray: for detection of a mediastinal mass.

Differential diagnosis

Immuno-phenotyping is used to distinguish the subtype of ALL. Haematopoietic cells express differing cell-surface antigens as they mature in the bone marrow. The antigen type can be used to differentiate between the subtypes of ALL, e.g. common ALL, null-cell ALL, B-cell ALL, or T-cell ALL.

Gemma Pritchard, Central Manchester and Manchester Children's Hospitals NHS Trust

Treatment

Children in the UK follow the Medical Research Council's ALL trial. Treatment is intensified according to risk-stratification criteria, such as age, initial response to treatment, cytogenetics, and highest pre-treatment white blood cell count. Treatment is not adjusted for the T-cell sub-type of ALL.

Complications: acute tumour lysis syndrome (ATLS)

T-cell ALL carries a higher risk of ATLS due to the large tumour burden. At the start of treatment, the rapid breakdown of large numbers of cells releases large quantities of metabolites into the circulation.

Characterized by:
• hyperkalaemia
• hyperphosphataemia
• hyperuricaemia
• hypocalcaemia.

Leading to:
• kidney obstruction
• numbness
• confusion
• weakness
• cardiac arrhythmias
• renal failure
• seizures
• possibly death.

To prevent ATLS, hyperhydration (to facilitate excretion of metabolites by the kidneys) and uric acid reduction with allopurinol or rasburicase (to prevent hyperuricaemia) are commenced before treatment of ALL. Rasburicase should be considered for those with a mediastinal mass.

Close monitoring of U+Es, uric acid, and phosphate is essential for early detection of ATLS—up to 6-hourly in the first days of treatment.

Relapse

Relapse occurs in 30–40% at patients with T-cell ALL, compared with 20% of those with common ALL. Further chemotherapy on a more intensive trial and possibly a bone-marrow transplant will be required.

Further reading

Fochtman, D., Foley, G.V., Patterson, Kelly, K., Rasco Baggott, C. (2002). *Nursing care of children and adolescents with cancer*, 3rd edn. W.B. Saunders.
Kline, N.E., Tomlinson, D. (2005). *Paediatric oncology nursing*. Springer, Berlin.
www.cancerbacup.org.uk

Lymphoma

Lymphomas are cancerous tumours arising in the lymphatic system

Incidence

The most common types of lymphoma seen in children in the UK are:
- non-Hodgkin's lymphoma, affecting approximately 80 children/year
- Hodgkin's lymphoma, affecting approximately 60 children/year.

Signs and symptoms

These depend on where the tumour is located and will include:
- painless lymphadenopathy—cervical masses are common in Hodgkin's lymphoma
- breathlessness and cough
- pyrexia
- lethargy
- weight loss and anorexia
- night sweats and pruritis—associated with Hodgkin's lymphoma
- bowel obstruction—associated with non-Hodgkin's lymphoma

Diagnosis

Children are referred to one of the 21 UKCCSG centres for diagnosis. Investigations to confirm diagnosis and determine the spread of disease will include:
- biopsy—to confirm the type of cancer cells
- chest X-ray—to locate chest disease
- body scan—to determine the spread of the disease
- blood tests, haematology, and blood chemistry
- bone-marrow biopsy—if bone-marrow infiltration is suspected
- lumbar puncture—children with non-Hodgkin's lymphoma may have cerebral disease.

Treatment

Dependent on type and spread of disease. Treatment is standardized throughout the UK. All children receive chemotherapy as their first line of treatment. Some have radiotherapy and/or high-dose chemotherapy which is followed by infusion of the child's pre-collected peripheral blood stem cells to 'rescue' the bone marrow.

Management

This alters during the treatment pathway, is always multidisciplinary, and should include the child and his/her parents whenever possible. Management plans will include:
- observing for complications associated with the disease—airway obstruction due to bulky chest disease, tumour lysis syndrome, or bowel obstruction
- managing side effects of the treatment—immunosuppression, nausea and vomiting, mucositis, and weight loss
- managing long-term side effects—poor growth, infertility, and heart disease.

Angie Tims, University Hospitals Coventry and Warwickshire NHS Trust

Further reading

Hoffbrand, A., Petit, J. (1997). *Essential haematology*, 3rd edn. Blackwell Science, London.
www.cancerbacup.org.uk/Cancertype/Childrenscancers/ (accessed July 2005).

Bone-marrow transplantation

What is bone-marrow?

The bone-marrow is the factory that makes blood, platelets, and white blood cells and is found in the centre of all large bones. Red blood cell carry O_2 around the body, platelets help to stop bleeding, and white blood cells fight against infection. Bone-marrow transplant is require when disorders of the blood occur.

Why is a bone-marrow transplant needed?

During bone-marrow transplant the patient's marrow is destroyed b chemotherapy, sometimes in conjunction with radiotherapy, and replace with healthy marrow from a donor.

Indications
- The most common indication for bone-marrow transplant is where the marrow is affected by a malignant disease, usually leukaemia.
- Sometimes it is performed when the bone marrow is failing to make normal blood; e.g. thalassaemia, where the marrow fails to make normal red blood cells.
- In certain metabolic disorders donor bone marrow is transplanted as a source of a deficient enzyme.

Types of transplant
- When the patient is transplanted with cells from a donor, this is called an *allogeneic transplant* and is the more common type of paediatric transplant.
- In *autologous transplant*, the patient receives his/her own pre-donated marrow or peripheral blood stem cells. It is usually performed in order to give high-dose chemotherapy to patients with solid tumors.

Allogeneic donors

The donor must be a tissue-type match of the recipient. The closer the match, the more successful the transplant. The most closely matche donor is usually a sibling, because children inherit their tissue type from both parents, but the chance of two siblings being matched is only one i four. If the parents are related, it may be possible to find a match within the extended family. Otherwise, an unrelated donor can be found on a donor panel or, alternatively, cord blood can be used from a from a cor bank.

The transplant

- Conditioning therapy is given to ablate the recipient immune system and bone marrow.
- The donated marrow is given intravenously via a central venous catheter.
- The patient will usually be nursed in protective isolation for approximately 2–3 weeks because of the risk of infection. Visitors will usually be limited and a 'clean diet' will need to be consumed.
- During this period the patient many suffer with severe mucositis and require high-strength analgesia and enteral or parental feeding.

Lynne Barnes, Central Manchester and Manchester Children's University Hospitals NHS Trust

Complications and risks of bone-marrow transplantation

There is risk in bone-marrow transplant and this risk must be offset against the underlying disease. The risks are principally due to:
• infection while the new immune system engrafts
• graft-versus-host disease, where the new marrow rejects the host
• organ damage from the high-dose chemotherapy or radiotherapy.

There are also some long-term effects on growth and fertility.

Further reading

Dannie, E. (1998). Care of bone marrow transplant patients. *Nursing Standard,* **13,**24–5.
Leukaemia Research Fund (2005). *Bone marrow and stem cell transplant.* LRF, London.

Care and preparation of children and young people undergoing investigation prior to and during treatment for cancer

Investigations form a key part of the diagnosis and treatment of children and young people with cancer. They are used to 'stage' the cancer, assess general health, study progress, and check for side effects of some treatments.

Type of investigations
- Biopsy
- Blood tests
- Bone-marrow aspirate
- Lumbar puncture
- Urinalysis
- X-rays
- Ultrasound tests
- Bone scan
- CT scan
- MRI scan

Preparation
- The key to preparation is to give information about the test—its relevance, what will happen during the test, and any special requirements prior to, during, or after the test.
- This information needs to be given in an age-related way.
- Play therapy prior to an investigation for younger children.
- Informed consent by child and family.
- May require preparation for a general/local anaesthetic or sedation, either because the investigation is painful/unpleasant or because it requires the child to be still.
- May require preparation for isolation if radio-isotopes are to be used.

During investigation
Many children and young people dislike investigations as much as, if not more than, treatment. Anticipatory nausea and vomiting can be common. The use of distraction therapy, guided imagery, sedation, and anti-emetics can alleviate anxiety and other symptoms. Assessment and relief of pain may also be essential.

Nursing management post-investigation
- If sedated, check and maintain ABC.
- Monitor vital signs.
- Pain assessment.
- Check wound site for bleeding/infection.
- Manage fluid balance as necessary.

Helen Langton, Coventry University

- Discuss the experience with the child and family to assess whether preparation was successful.

Key issues

- Many of these investigations are invasive.
- Investigations during treatment give indication as to whether the disease is under control or spreading.
- Preparation for and care during investigation is often linked to breaking bad news.
- Results can take several days to come back, which is very stressful for one child/family.
- Occasionally diagnosis is not straightforward.

Further reading

Langton, H. (2000). *The child with cancer. Family centred care in practice.* Ballière Tindall, London.

www.teenagecancertrust.org

Treatment regimens for children and young people with cancer

- Most children with cancer in the UK are cared for in specialized centres, which are members of the UKCCSG.
- Care is often shared with local hospitals and/or professionals working in the community.
- Many young people aged 15 years and above are cared for by adult services.
- Many patients enter clinical trials to establish the effectiveness of different treatment protocols. There is national and international collaboration in developing treatment protocols.
- Duration of treatment depends upon the disease and on the individual's response.
- Treatment regimens normally include two or more of the following.

Surgery

May be undertaken:
- for diagnostic biopsy of tissue
- to insert a central venous access device
- for the excision of a solid tumour and lymph nodes to which cells may have spread
- to insert a CSF shunt for some brain tumours.

Chemotherapy

May be undertaken:
- in an attempt to eradicate cancer cells
- to shrink tumours prior to surgery
- for the palliative control of disease.

Treatment aims to achieve an optimal balance between maximum kill of tumour cells and minimum damage to rapidly dividing healthy cells.

Radiotherapy

May be undertaken:
- to attack tumour cells in targeted sites
- for total-body irradiation prior to bone-marrow transplantation
- for the palliative control of disease.

All rapidly dividing cells are affected.

Haematopoietic stem-cell and bone-marrow transplants

- The child's own stem cells are harvested before high doses of chemotherapy or radiotherapy are given. After treatment they are transfused back into the child to allow the bone marrow to recover.
- If stem cells are diseased (e.g. leukaemia), stem cells or bone marrow may be given from a matched donor. This may prevent recurrence of the disease.

Louise Holliday, Royal Aberdeen Children's Hospital

Further reading

bson, F., Soanes, L., Sepien, B. (ed.) (2004). *Perspectives in paediatric oncology nursing*. Whurr, London.

omlinson, D., Kline, N.E. (ed.) (2005). *Pediatric oncology nursing. Advanced clinical handbook*. Springer, New York.

Health and safety of chemotherapy

There is a risk that cytotoxic drugs could be inhaled, ingested, absorbed through the skin or mucous membranes of a handler.

Reducing exposure to cytotoxic material

- Preparation should be performed by competent personnel in a special unit in the pharmacy, using protective clothing and laminar airflow cabinets.
- During transport the drug should be:
  - packaged to avoid leakage or tampering
  - labelled as cytotoxic, stating sender and recipient
  - kept at required temperature.
- On receipt, the drug should be stored as instructed on the label.

Administration of chemotherapy

- By competent staff, with knowledge of drugs and side effects.
- Follow guidelines for administering medicines.
- Use protective gloves and aprons.
- Cover cuts to reduce risk of infiltration if gloves are damaged unknowingly.
- Avoid carpeted rooms, if possible.
- Spillage kits with instructions, expert advice, and backup must be available.

If spillage occurs:
- use spillage kit and follow instructions
- remove contaminated clothing and wash separately in washing machine as soon as possible
- wash contaminated skin with soap and cool water
- irrigate mucous membranes or eyes with water or 0.9% saline.

Complete an incident form and inform occupational health and pharmacy departments of any spillage or any local or systemic symptoms after handling chemotherapy.

Disposal of cytotoxic material

- Contaminated excreta:
  - may be deposited into sewer
  - protect mattresses and pillows with plastic covers
  - for contaminated linen—in hospital follow linen policy, and at home wash separately in washing machine as soon as possible
  - for 1 week following last dose of cytotoxic medicine, staff or family should wear protective clothing for handling excreta (usually nitrile or latex disposable gloves and plastic disposable apron)
  - use disposable nappies, bedpans, urinals, sick bowls, and macerator in hospital
  - use scales for measurement of excreta (1 g = 1 ml) to reduce aerosol formation

Sue Danby and Louise Holliday, Royal Aberdeen Children's Hospital

Use 'cin bin', labelled as cytotoxic and lined to absorb splashes, for used medicine containers, spoons, syringes, infusion bags and giving sets, and protective apron and gloves used in administering cytotoxic medications

Send unused drugs to the pharmacy departments for incineration. Transportation back to the pharmacy should be as for transport from the pharmacy, except that the temperature does not need to be kept at any particular level

urther reading

oyal College of Nursing (2005). *Chemotherapy competencies: an integrated competency framework for training programmes in the safe administration of chemotherapy to children and young people.* RCN, London.

ancer-Chemotherapy-Completed Frameworks - Skills for Health. ☑ www.skillsforhealth.org.uk/viewcomp.php?id=2746

Assessing the needs of the child and young person with cancer, including family and siblings

Effective communication between hospital(s) and community, and between all professionals involved in the child's or young person's care, is essential in assessing the needs of the child or young person and avoiding fragmented care. It is useful to identify a named nurse who can establish a rapport with the child or young person and his/her family, including any siblings or grandparents, and oversee continuity of care.

The admission assessment should help the nurse build a picture of the child or young person and their family. An ongoing process of assessing, planning, implementing, and evaluating care should be used to identify their unique and changing needs and priorities and to guide nurses and others in attempting to meet the needs and priorities thus identified.

Some potential needs are listed below. They are divided here into separate categories, but in practice these needs are often interlinked.

Physical needs
- Prevention, or prompt detection and treatment, of infection.
- Control of symptoms such as pain, nausea, vomiting, diarrhoea, constipation, breathlessness, and convulsions.
- Nutrition and hydration, rest, mobility, and hygiene, including oral and skin care.

Emotional needs
- Support in coping with the emotional impact of the disease and treatment.
- Support in maintaining normal activities, returning to school, and making the transition from active treatment to the off-treatment phase.

Cognitive needs
- Provision of appropriate and consistent information at times when they are ready and able to receive and digest it.
- Use of an interpreter *other than a family member*, if the child or young person or members of their family are not fluent in English.

Social needs
- Accommodation for families in or near hospital.
- Opportunity to relax with peers/friends.
- Time for parents to be with all their children, not just the sick child.
- Advice about benefits, insurance claims, parental leave, and travel expenses.
- Domiciliary support.

Louise Holliday, Royal Aberdeen Children's Hospital

piritual needs

Support from the chaplaincy team and external ministers (if requested).
Access to a peaceful space for prayer/reflection.
Recognition of beliefs and values.

urther reading

ibson, F., Soanes, L., Sepien, B. (ed.) (2004). *Perspectives in paediatric oncology nursing*. Whurr, London.
www.clicsargent.org.uk

Information-giving to a child or young person and his/her family

Communication as the key to information-giving

Communication will be effective if it is clear, direct, and honest. Clear communication implies that what is said is understandable and what is heard is understood. When giving information, determine that the information given is complete and in words that the patients and families can understand. Because of the emotion involved in a cancer diagnosis, it is often necessary to repeat information.

Parental involvement in information giving

Parents are generally the experts on their children. The cancer diagnosis has a profound impact on the entire family. There is new information to be learned and treatment decisions to be made. There is also the difficulty for parents in deciding how much of this information they need or want to give to their child in order for them to feel comfortable and secure. For young people, there is also the added tension between parental rights and the rights of the young person to be told.

Tips for giving information

- Give accurate age-appropriate information about cancer. Do not be afraid to use the word 'cancer' and tell them where it is in the body, otherwise they may invent their own explanations, which can be more frightening than the facts.
- Explain the treatment plan and what this will mean to them.
- Prepare children for any physical changes they might encounter throughout treatment, e.g. hair loss.
- Answer children's questions as accurately as possible.

Strategies for information-giving

Age-appropriate, to include:
- use of resources, such as story books, 'dolls', and equipment
- creative input through drama, role play, drawing, and art work
- videos/DVDs/CDs
- internet information
- charity-funded information booklets.

Multidisciplinary involvement in information-giving

Children with cancer have access to many professionals. Team work is vital if information-giving is to be handled well. Specialists such as play, music, and art therapists can all contribute in different ways in this area.

Conclusions

- Do not give wrong information.
- Ensure that the team members are consistent in their information-giving and are aware of what information has been given, to whom, and when.

Helen Langton, Coventry University

urther reading

ngton, H. (2000). *The child with cancer. Family centred care in practice.* Ballière Tindall, London.
zo, P.A., and Poplack, D.E. (2002). *Principles of paediatric oncology,* 4th edn. Lippincott
  Williams & Wilkins Philadelphia.
  www.cancernursing.org

Endocrine and metabolic disorders

The endocrine system: related anatomy and physiology

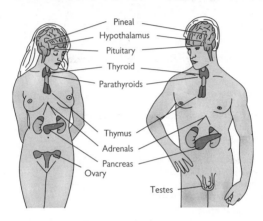

Hypothalamus

The hypothalamus is located in the brain at the base of the optic chiasma. It secretes hormones that stimulate or suppress the release of hormones in the pituitary gland.

Hormones are chemical 'messengers' and are either proteins, consisting of amino acid chains, or steroids, derived from cholesterol. Functions controlled by hormones include:
• activities of entire organs
• growth and development
• reproduction
• sexual characteristics
• usage and storage of energy
• levels of fluid, salt, and sugar in the blood.

The pineal body

The pineal body is located below the corpus callosum, a part of the brain. It produces the hormone melatonin.

Pituitary

The pituitary gland is located at the base of the brain. No larger than a pea, the gland controls many functions of the other endocrine glands.

Catherine Macfarlane, Royal Hospital for Sick Children, Edinburgh

Thyroid and parathyroids

The thyroid and parathyroid glands are located in front of the neck, below the larynx (voice box). The thyroid has an important role in the body's metabolism. Both thyroid and parathyroid glands have a role in the regulation of the body's calcium balance.

Thymus

The thymus is located in the upper part of the chest and produces T lymphocytes (white blood cells that fight infection and destroy abnormal cells).

Adrenal glands

The pair of adrenal glands are located on top of both kidneys. Adrenal glands work hand-in-hand with the hypothalamus and pituitary gland.

Pancreas

The pancreas is located across the back of the abdomen, behind the stomach. It plays a role in digestion, as well as hormone production.

Ovaries

A woman's ovaries are located on both sides of the uterus, below the opening of the Fallopian tubes (which extend from the uterus to the ovaries). In addition to containing the egg cells necessary for reproduction, the ovaries also produce oestrogen and progesterone.

Testes

A man's testes are located in a pouch that hangs outside the body. The testes produce testosterone and sperm.

Further reading

Griffin, J.E., Ojeda, S.R. (ed.) (2004). *Textbook of endocrine physiology.* Oxford University Press.
🖥 www.umm.edu/endocrin/anatomy.htm

Type 1 diabetes mellitus in childhood and adolescence

Definition
Diabetes mellitus is a metabolic disorder characterized by chronic hyperglycaemia due to defective insulin secretion, insulin action, or both.

Epidemiology
- Type 1 diabetes mellitus is the predominant form of diabetes mellitus in young people.
  - Incidence increases with age and is rising worldwide.
  - Age of onset: major peak at age 10–14 years.
- Type 2 diabetes mellitus used to be uncommon in children.
  - Incidence rising due to increasing rates of obesity worldwide.

Characteristic features of type 1 and type 2 diabetes mellitus are compared below.

Diagnosis of type 1 diabetes mellitus
- Should be made without difficulty and with urgency.
- The symptoms of thirst, excessive drinking, and urination (polydipsia and polyuria) should prompt *immediate* confirmatory tests.

Recommendation
Children and adolescents presenting with the above symptoms should be referred immediately to the local paediatric diabetes mellitus team for confirmation of diabetes mellitus by a venous blood sample.

Diagnostic criteria
Fasting plasma glucose: ≥7 mmol
2-hour (post-prandial) plasma glucose: ≥11 mmol

Recommendation
As children and adolescents diagnosed with type 1 diabetes mellitus are dependent on insulin for survival, insulin therapy must be started as soon as possible after diagnosis to prevent diabetic ketoacidosis.

Aims of management
- To provide sufficient insulin throughout each 24-hour period to cover basal requirements.
- To deliver higher boluses of insulin in an attempt to match the glycaemic effects of meals.
- To self-monitor blood glucose at frequent intervals in order to improve the quality and stability of glycaemic control.
- To encourage distribution of food energy and carbohydrate intake to balance insulin-action profiles and exercise.
- To encourage moderate-to-high-intensity exercise.
- To provide diabetes mellitus education by healthcare professionals with specialist training in diabetes mellitus, who have a clear understanding of the special and changing needs of young people and their families.

Kirsten Jones, Royal Devon and Exeter NHS Foundation Trust

- To fit management and education plans to suit each individual's age, stage of diabetes mellitus, cognitive ability, maturity, and lifestyle.
- Education in the management of diabetes mellitus should be a continuous process and should be repeated for it to be effective.

Main aims of treatment

Through agreed local and national guidelines and protocols:
- to maintain optimal health and prevent the risk of short-term (hyperglycaenia/hypoglycaemia) complications
- to ensure that all young people with diabetes mellitus will receive regular screening to prevent risk of long-term (microvascular/macrovascular) chronic complications of diabetes mellitus.

Further reading

ISPAD Guidelines (2000). *Consensus guidelines for the management of type 1 diabetes mellitus in children and adolescents* (ed. P.G.F. Swift), pp. 11–26. Medforum.

Department of Health (2002). *National Service Framework for Diabetes: Standards*, pp. 2–46. Department of Health, London.

www.ispad.org

Diabetic ketoacidosis (DKA)

A serious and potentially fatal metabolic complication, which occurs in young people with type 1 diabetes mellitus, caused by insulin deficiency. This leads to high blood glucose levels, ketosis, and, if untreated, ketoacidosis.

Morbidity and mortality rates are high for children and adolescents with DKA.

Incidence
- Significantly higher in children under 5 years old, and the greatest cause of deaths in people with type 1 diabetes mellitus who are aged under 30 years.
- There is a 5–10% mortality rate associated with DKA in Western countries.

Causes
- Previously undiagnosed diabetes mellitus
- Interruption of insulin treatment
- Stress of an intercurrent illness

Clinical features/characteristics
The patient may present with:
- thirst
- weight loss
- polyuria
- polydipsia
- tiredness
- weakness
- fatigue
- nausea
- vomiting
- abdominal pain
- difficulty breathing, as a result of metabolic acidosis (usually deep rapid breathing, known as Kussmaul respiration)
- symptoms of precipitating cause (e.g. intercurrent illness)
- ketotic breath
- drowsiness
- coma.

Hazards
- Under-insulination: the most common error is omission or reduction of insulin if the patient is vomiting or nauseated, and feels unable to eat.
- Hypotension: due to severe dehydration, which may lead to renal failure.
- Coma: insertion of a NG tube is required to prevent aspiration because gastric stasis is common.
- Hypothermia.
- Cerebral oedema: this is most common in children and may be related to hyperosmolarity.
- Lack of local DKA protocol/guidelines.

Julie Kitchen, Royal Devon and Exeter NHS Foundation Trust

Causes of death in children in DKA
- Aspiration of vomit.
- Electrolyte disturbance (hypokalaemia).
- Iatrogenic hypoglycaemia.
- Cerebral oedema, which is unpredictable and occurs more frequently in younger children and new diabetics.

Treatment
- Initial treatment:
  - adherence of medical staff to local DKA protocol or alternative algorithm for management of DKA.
- Subsequent treatment:
  - IV fluids and insulin are continued until the patient is able to drink and tolerate diet
  - subcutaneous insulin is given before the next meal and the IV fluids and insulin infusion are discontinued, usually 30 mins *after* the meal (depending on the type of insulin administered subcutaneously)
  - look for the cause
  - advise on how to avoid recurrence.

Prevention of DKA
- Earlier diagnosis
- Better patient communication
- Better access to specialist advice and protocols
- Better patient education on sick-day management

Prevention of deaths from DKA
This is possible when:
- symptoms are detected earlier and treated more promptly and effectively
- metabolic abnormalities are corrected slowly, minimizing the risk of cerebral oedema.

Further reading
Palmer, R. (2004). An overview of diabetic ketoacidosis. *Nursing Standard*, **19**(10), 42–5.
Williams, G., Pickup, J.C. (1999). *Handbook of diabetes*, 2nd edn. Blackwell Science, Oxford.
www.diabetes.org.uk

Management of DKA

DKA is a potentially life-threatening condition caused by insufficient insulin production, leading to high blood glucose levels. The body tries to remove the excess glucose by passing it out in the urine, causing dehydration and increased thirst. As water is removed from body cells to try and dilute the levels of glucose, electrolytes become affected. Despite the large amounts of glucose in the blood, the body cannot use the glucose for energy, because of the lack of insulin, and so it begins to break down fats to use as an alternative source of energy. As fats break down, acidic ketones are released into the bloodstream.

If left untreated, the high levels of acidic ketones, dehydration, and electrolyte imbalance can lead to coma and, eventually, death.

Clinical history and signs
- Polyuria
- Polydipsia
- Vomiting and dehydration
- Abdominal pain (can be severe)
- Confusion
- Kussmaul breathing (deep sighing respiration)
- Smell of ketones (sweet-smelling breath)
- Lethargy

Biochemical signs
- Elevated blood sugar >11 mmol
- Ketonuria
- Glucosuria
- Ketonaemia
- Acidosis
- Low bicarbonate

Treatment
- Slow dose of IV insulin (0.1 U/kg body weight/hour). Decreases glycaemia, suppresses lipolysis and ketogenesis, and corrects acidosis.
- Maintenance fluids to correct dehydration. Remember, as potassium is pulled back into the cells its blood level will decrease.
- Use 0.9% saline until blood sugar <15 mmol; then use 5% dextrose and 0.45% saline. If blood sugar falls below 6 mmol, use 10% dextrose.
- If potassium level is low, add 20 mmol potassium to each 500 ml bag of saline.

Never stop insulin infusion—the patient needs insulin or he/she will quickly become ketotic again.

Sarah Mitchell, Royal Aberdeen Children's Hospital

Monitoring

Hourly blood sugars.

Hourly pulse, respiration, blood pressure, and SaO_2.

Hourly neurological observation.

Cardiac monitoring, because low/high potassium can affect T wave.

Accurate hourly fluid balance (patient may need urine catheter if reduced level of consciousness).

Regular blood gases to check pH and bicarbonate levels.

Be aware of cerebral oedema as a complication of DKA. It requires urgent recognition and intervention. Mannitol should be given immediately if there is any neurological deterioration. Remember to exclude low blood sugar.

Further reading

British Society of Paediatric Endocrinology and Diabetes (2004). Recommended DKA Guidelines. www.diabetes.org.uk

Davies, J., Hassell, L. (2002). *Children in intensive care: a nurse's survival guide*. Churchill Livingstone.

Palmer, R. (2004). An overview of diabetic ketoacidosis. *Nursing Standard*, **19**(10), 42–4.

Type 2 diabetes mellitus

- Type 2 diabetes mellitus is linked to childhood obesity and lack of exercise.
- Presents at or around puberty.
- The body is unable to maintain normal blood glucose levels because of a failure of adequate insulin secretion over time.
- Caused by either pancreatic exhaustion or a genetic defect in insulin secretion unmasked by increasing insulin resistance.
- High blood insulin levels lead to insulin resistance.
- Problems include a varying degree of hyperglycaemia, hypertension, coronary heart disease, and other vascular complications.
- High prevalence in minority groups, namely African, Hispanic, and Asian populations.

Assessment and diagnosis

- Clinical findings similar to type 1 diabetes mellitus in childhood; can be milder and develop slowly, and unrecognized as type 2 diabete
- Type 2 diabetes mellitus distinguished by the presence of insulin resistance

Characteristics

- Hyperglycaemia leads to glysuria with osmotic diuresis and symptoms of polyuria and polydipsia.
- Increased appetite and weight loss.
- Recurrent infection.
- DKA can occur, with symptoms of nausea, vomiting, abdominal pain, tachypnoea, and lethargy.

The clinical presentation of type 1 and type 2 diabetes mellitus may b indistinguishable. However, as the number of children with type 2 diabete mellitus increases, it becomes increasingly important to classify the diabetes mellitus correctly so that appropriate therapy may be institutec

Diagnosis is confirmed if fasting blood glucose concentrations ar >7 mmol/litre on two separate days or if random glucose concentration are 11 mmol/litre on two separate occasions. Urinalysis may reveal keto uria and glycosuria.

Nursing care and management

There is a limited amount of evidence on which to base treatme strategies, because type 2 diabetes mellitus is a relatively new phenome non in children's nursing.

Diet

Some children can be managed effectively with a diet that is sufficient balanced to meet the needs for normal growth but moderately restricte in calories and low in fat.

Exercise

Increased physical activity helps the body use insulin more efficient Exercise → weight loss → decreases insulin resistance. In the long ter exercise is beneficial in helping reduce cardiovascular risk factors.

Phil Morrow, Queen's University Belfast

Drug therapy

If diet and exercise are not sufficient for glycaemic control, give oral hypoglycaemics.

These drugs have not been tested for safety and efficacy in children.

If glycaemic control is still not achieved, give insulin.

Care and management is similar to that for type 1 diabetes mellitus.

Early screening

Because of the long-term complications, carry out preventive measures/screening for at-risk children/families, i.e. those with:

a positive family history of type 2 diabetes mellitus

obese children

children of a particular race or ethnic group

those who present with signs of insulin resistance.

Fasting blood glucose should be assessed every 2 years, starting at the age of 10 years or the onset of puberty.

Health promotion

Prevention and management of obesity requires a range of coordinated policies.

Be aware of the risk associated with obesity, because early investigation and treatment may delay the onset of complications.

Further reading

Department of Health (2003). *National Service Framework for Diabetes: Standards.* 🖳 www.dh.gov.uk
Wiggins, C. (2002). Childhood obesity and diabetes. *Biomedical Scientist*, May, 474–6.
www.diabetes.org.uk
www.nice.org.uk

Maturity-onset diabetes mellitus of the young (MODY)

MODY is a rare form of diabetes mellitus in children, occurring a result of gene abnormalities. It has four main characteristics.

- Diabetes mellitus presents at a young age.
- Runs in families through several generations: a parent with MODY has a 50% chance of passing on MODY to their child. This is called autosomal dominant inheritance.
- Children with MODY do not always need insulin treatment and can often be treated with oral glycaemic therapy or meal planning alone.
- Children with MODY do not produce enough insulin. This is different from type 2 diabetes mellitus where the individual produces sufficient insulin but does not respond to it.

The clinical spectrum is broad, ranging from asymptomatic hyperglycaemia to a severe acute presentation. MODY has been reported in all races and ethnicities.

Diagnosis is based on molecular testing, which is currently not available to all. Until such testing becomes commonplace, children with MODY should be classified as having the type of diabetes mellitus that best fits their clinical picture, which requires appropriate care, management, education, and ongoing support and follow-up.

Further reading

Glasper, E.A., Richardson, J. (2005). *A Textbook of chidren's nursing*, Elsevier.
Department of Health (2003). *National Service Framework for Diabetes: Standards.* ⊡ www.dh.gov.(
⊡ www.diabetes.org.uk
⊡ www.nice.org.uk

Phil Morrow, Queen's University Belfast

Hypothyroidism

Definition
Abnormally low levels of thyroid hormones circulating in the blood stream.

Background
- TSH, which is secreted by the pituitary gland, stimulates the thyroid gland to make the thyroid hormones thyroxine (T_4) and triiodothyronine (T_3).
- Thyroid hormones control the metabolic rate by acting directly on cells all around the body.
- Plasma levels of thyroid hormones within the normal range are essential for normal brain development during infancy and skeletal growth during childhood.
- Untreated hypothyroidism in infants causes severe mental retardation.

Types of hypothyroidism
Primary
Failure of thyroid gland. This can be congenital or acquired.
- Congenital: during early fetal development the thyroid gland is formed from the pharynx, and by 12 weeks' gestation it descends to just below the Adam's apple at the front of the neck. This process is interrupted in 1 out of 3500 children and the thyroid gland is either completely absent or ectopic (incorrectly positioned). In both cases the gland does not function.
  - Guthrie test at 6–10 days after birth screens for increased levels of TSH—resulting from the pituitary gland trying to stimulate the non-functioning thyroid gland.
  - If positive, a venous blood sample is taken as soon as possible.
- Acquired: autoimmune disorder. Familial, and more common in girls than boys. Clinical features may include poor growth, dry skin, coarse hair, constipation, tiredness, slow pulse, and low blood pressure.

Secondary
Due to lack of thyrotrophin-stimulating hormone.
- Babies/children with a small or absent pituitary gland.
- Increasing numbers of children with hypothalamic/pituitary damage following surgery or radiotherapy for oncological conditions.

Diagnosis
Made by measurement of plasma TSH and thyroid hormones.

Treatment
- Hormone-replacement thyroxine—lifelong.
- In congenital hypothyroidism, treatment should be commenced within the first few weeks of life to prevent neurological impairment.
- Out-patient monitoring of growth, thyroid function tests, and developmental/educational progress through to adulthood.

Pauline Musson, Southampton University Hospitals NHS Trust

Nursing care
Explain the condition and importance of thyroxine replacement.
Teach how to administer thryoxine: tablets need to be crushed and
given directly from a spoon. A suspension is *not* recommended—it has
a shelf-life of only 3 weeks, needs refrigeration, and, if not shaken well
to ensure mixing, dosages are unreliable and blood levels fluctuate.
Explain the need for, and give support during, frequent venesection.

Further reading
ine, J.E., Donaldson, M.D.C., Gregory, J.W., Savage, M.O. (2001). Thyroid disorders. In *Practical
endocrinology and diabetes in children*. Blackwell Science.
www.bsped.org.uk
www.thyroidmanager.org

Short stature

Any child significantly below the average height for a child of the same age, sex, race, or family.

In the UK, the nine centile cross-sectional growth charts produced by the Child Growth Foundation are most frequently used to record height and weight.

Recommendations for referral for growth assessment are:
- children whose height is below the 0.4 centile
- children over 5 years of age whose growth curve crosses *two* centile lines
- children aged 2–5 years whose growth curve crosses *one* centile

Some causes of short stature

Non-endocrine
- Inherited and genetic factors.
- Malnourishment, rickets, and malabsorption disorders.
- Chronic diseases, such as congenital heart disease, kidney diseases, asthma, sickle cell anaemia, and thalassaemia.

Differential diagnoses

Differential diagnoses of short stature and slow growth:
- familial and constitutional short stature
- endocrine disorders, e.g. hypothyroidism and growth hormone deficiency
- intra-uterine growth retardation/prematurity/Russell–Silver syndrome
- chromosomal disorders, e.g. Turner syndrome
- metabolic disorders, e.g. glycogen storage disease
- chronic disease
- psychosocial deprivation
- malnutrition
- skeletal dysplasias
- iatrogenic, e.g. chemotherapy, radiotherapy, or steroids.

History and examination

Most children referred with short stature are normal.

Child's history

Pre-natal and post-natal
- Intra-uterine growth retardation (IUGR)
- Birth hypoxia (may cause hypothalamic hypopituitarism)
- Neonatal hypoglycaemia may imply growth hormone deficiency
- Fetal alcohol syndrome

Past medical history
Child's early health, medical conditions, and treatment (e.g. glucocorticoids); short stature for age identified.

Catherine Macfarlane, Royal Hospital for Sick Children Edinburgh

Family history

Parental heights; history of short stature or pubertal delay in parents or rest of family

Social deprivation, drug/alcohol abuse, and emotional or relationship difficulties.

Examination

Accurate measurement and plotting on growth chart

Pubertal staging and testicular volume

Fundoscopy to exclude hypothalamic tumour

Thorough physical examination to disclose features of recognized syndromes

Blood pressure

Investigations

Screen for:

full blood count, erythrocyte sedimentation rate, U&Es, liver function tests, and thyroid function tests

chronic diseases, such as congenital heart disease, kidney diseases, asthma, sickle cell anaemia, thalassaemia, juvenile rheumatoid arthritis, and diabetes mellitus

malabsorption disorders, such as coeliac disease and IBD

chromosome karyotype

X-ray: bone-age study (X-ray films of the left hand and wrist).

Specific investigations (when indicated):

endocrine: pituitary function tests and growth hormone test

MRI scan.

Treatment

Depends on the underlying aetiology of the short stature, but includes:

hormone replacement, e.g. growth hormone, thyroxine, cortisol, oestrogen, and testosterone

GnRH analogues (to suppress precocious puberty)

surgery: tumour removal and leg lengthening

dietary: gluten-free diet for coeliac disease.

Management

The importance of previous history, growth data, parents' heights, and pubertal history cannot be overemphasized in the management of children with short stature, in addition to accurate sequential growth measurements plotted on appropriate growth charts.

Further reading

Kelnar, C.J.H. (1999). *Growth disorders: pathophysiology and treatment*. Chapman & Hall.

Pandeva, H.S. and Bouloux, P.M.G. Evaluation of short stature. ⬛ www.studentbmj.com/back_issues/0500/education/143.html (accessed 13 June 2005).

www.childgrowthfoundation.org (accessed 13 June 2005).

Tall stature

Definition

In the UK, the nine centile cross-sectional growth charts produced by the Child Growth Foundation are most frequently used to record height and weight. Children whose height exceeds the 99.6 centile can be defined as being of tall stature.

Causes

Non-endocrine

- Tall parents: both parental heights have equal influence on their child's height
- Obesity
- Homocystinuria (inborn error of metabolism)

Endocrine

- Thyrotoxicosis
- Marfan's syndrome
- Soto's syndrome
- McCune–Albright syndrome
- Klinefelter's syndrome
- Fragile X syndrome
- Precocious puberty
- Congenital adrenal hyperpalsia
- Growth-hormone-secreting tumour
- Pituitary tumour

History and examination

- Early growth pattern of child
- Family history of tall stature

Examination

- Assess parental heights
- Assess child's standing and sitting height and arm span (in Marfan's syndrome leg length exceeds trunk length and arm span exceeds height)
- Measure child's head circumference (markedly increased in Soto's syndrome)

Investigations

- Growth hormone level (gigantism/growth-hormone-secreting tumour)
- TSH level
- Bone-age X-ray
- Amino acid screen (homocystinuria)
- Chromosome karyotype (Klinefelter syndrome or fragile X syndrome)
- 17-Hydroxyprogesterone (congenital adrenal hyperplasia)
- Glucose (Beckwith–Wiedemann syndrome)
- Androgen and oestrogen levels (precocious puberty)

Catherine Macfarlane, Royal Hospital for Sick Children, Edinburgh

Treatment

Depends on the underlying aetiology of the tall stature, but includes the following.
- Counselling: shortened life span and genetic risk to offspring.
- Patient with Marfan's syndrome should consider avoiding competitive sport (due to potential for fatal aortic dissection and rupture).
- Consider early introduction of prophylactic β-blockers (reduce mortality rate from aortic rupture) and aortic valve graft/replacement surgery in Marfan's syndrome.
- Surgery: removal of tumours.
- GnRH analogues: to suppress precocious puberty.

Management

The importance of previous history, growth data, parents' heights, and pubertal history cannot be overemphasized in the management of children with tall stature, in addition to accurate sequential growth measurements plotted on appropriate growth charts.

Further reading

pe, F.M. (2003). In *Oxford textbook of medicine*, 4th edn, (ed. D.A. Warrell *et al.*). Oxford University Press.
www.fpnotebook.com/END47.htm

Inborn errors of metabolism

An inborn error of metabolism is said to exist when an enzyme necessary for a stage of metabolism is missing. Most nutrients are broken down in number of steps. At each step, an enzyme or biological catalyst is necessary so that the process can proceed to the next step. Each metabolic process, e.g. the metabolism of protein to its constituent amino acids may involve many steps.

Inborn errors of metabolism are mainly autosomal recessive genetic conditions, and there may be a family history of early childhood difficulties or even death. There are many different inborn errors of metabolism and individually they tend to be rather rare conditions.

Inborn errors of metabolism cause difficulties because the product of metabolism at the stage at which the process is interrupted may be toxic and, as its level builds up in the blood, may result in damage that produces symptoms. If metabolism of a compound is interrupted, a deficiency of the end product of the nutrient concerned may also cause problems.

Presenting problems might include:
- faltering growth
- vomiting
- electrolyte imbalance
- jaundice
- neurological symptoms, including fits
- developmental delay

Inborn errors of metabolism can be treated in several ways:
- a special diet to restrict intake of a compound that the child cannot metabolize
- administration of another substance (e.g. a coenzyme) to partly replace the action of the missing enzyme.

Phenylketonuria (PKU) is an example of an inborn error of metabolism and illustrates the principal points. The enzyme necessary to break down phenylalanine, a constituent of many foods, is not produced, so the level of phenylalanine builds up until it reaches a toxic level, at which it starts to damage the CNS. This is particularly destructive in the infant and small child, because the CNS is immature but developing rapidly, and can result in learning disability. PKU is detected using the Guthrie test, which is only effective when the infant has been taking milk feeds for at least 5 days and will have ingested enough phenylalanine for the level to be detected.

Treatment of PKU includes a diet that contains a much lower level of phenylalanine. This diet must be used throughout childhood and probably throughout life. Frequent monitoring of the blood level of PKU is important.

Further reading

Lissauer, T., Clayden, G. (2001). *Illustrated textbook of paediatrics*, 2nd edn. Mosby.
Neill, S., Knowles, H. (2004). *The biology of child health.* Palgrave, Basingstoke. The Society for the Study of Inborn Errors of Metabolism. 🖳 www.ssiem.org

Jim Richardson, University of Glamorgan

Phenylketonuria (PKU)

PKU is the most common inherited metabolic disorder of prote
metabolism. It occurs in all racial groups, but is most common in Turke
and Ireland, and is rare in Asian populations. Inheritance is autosom
recessive.

Incidence

Approximately 1 in 10 000 in UK.

Causes

PKU is caused by mutations within the gene for phenylalanine hydrox:
lase, resulting in decreased enzyme activity within the liver. This results
failure to convert phenylalanine to tyrosine, leading to accumulation c
phenylalanine and relative tyrosine deficiency. Different mutations lead t
different levels of residual enzyme activity, resulting in varying degrees c
hyperphenylalaninaemia.

Clinical features

Infants with PKU are normal at birth. The accumulation of phenylalanin
prevents normal post-natal brain development. Signs of serious develo;
mental delay only become apparent from a few months of age. Unfortu
nately subsequent treatment cannot reverse brain damage that ha
already occurred. Untreated PKU leads to severe learning difficultie
hyperactivity/autistic features, lack of speech, and seizures.

Investigations

Newborn screening for PKU is undertaken in most developed countrie
(introduced in the UK in 1969) to enable diagnosis before the onset c
symptoms.

Management

Early diagnosis (by 20 days) and subsequent dietary management t
control blood phenylalanine levels within age-related limits enables ind
viduals with PKU to develop normally and obtain a final IQ within th
normal range. Current UK recommendations for the management c
PKU were published by the MRC in 1993.

Dietary treatment aims to:
• control blood phenylalanine levels to prevent toxic effects of high
  levels, while providing sufficient levels for normal growth and
  development (phenylalanine is an essential amino acid)
• ensure diet is nutritionally adequate, palatable, varied, and compatible
  with a normal lifestyle.

The principles of dietary management are as follows.
• Avoid high-protein foods, e.g. meat, fish, eggs, dairy products, pulses,
  nuts, soya, ordinary flour, and aspartame (artificial sweetener
  containing phenylalanine).
• Daily allowance of phenylalanine from foods containing smaller
  amounts of protein. Allowance varies depending upon phenylalanine
  tolerance.

Fiona White, Central Manchester and Manchester Children's University Hospitals NHS Trust

* Phenylalanine-free protein substitute, with added tyrosine, to ensure adequate total protein.
* Phenylalanine-free foods low in protein to provide normal energy requirements and variety in the diet, e.g. fruit, some vegetables, sugars, fats, and specially manufactured low-protein prescription products such as flour, bread, pasta, biscuits, and milk substitutes.

Outcome

Cognitive outcome is closely related to blood phenylalanine control, particularly in infancy and childhood. Current recommendations are to maintain a phenylalanine-restricted diet for life. This is particularly important for women because strict blood phenylalanine control is crucial pre-conception and throughout pregnancy to prevent adverse effects on the developing fetus, e.g. cardiac malformations, microcephaly, and growth retardation.

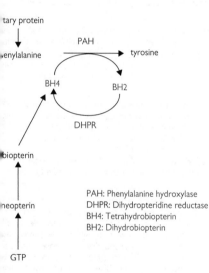

PAH: Phenylalanine hydroxylase
DHPR: Dihydropteridine reductase
BH4: Tetrahydrobiopterin
BH2: Dihydrobiopterin

Galactosaemia

Galactosaemia is an autosomal recessive inherited metabolic disorder carbohydrate metabolism, affecting metabolism of galactose (from the m sugar lactose). There are three inborn errors of galactose metabolism (s figure opposite). Classical galactosaemia due to deficiency of the enzym galactose-1-phosphate uridyl transferase (Gal-1-PUT) is commonest.

Incidence

Classical galactosaemia has an incidence of approximately 1 in 45 00 children UK.

Causes

Classical galactosaemia is caused by mutations within the gene fe Gal-1- PUT, resulting in an absence of, or markedly decreased, enzym activity in the liver and thus inability to breakdown galactose normall Consequently galactose-1-phosphate (gal-1-P) accumulates.

Clinical symptoms

Galactose (as lactose) is a constituent of breast milk and normal modifie infant formulas. Most infants present in the neonatal period. Commo features include lethargy, poor feeding, poor weight gain, vomiting, diarrhoe liver disease, encephalopathy, septicaemia (especially *E. coli*), and catarac Cessation of milk feeds and initiation of IV fluids improves symptoms.

Investigations

Depending upon symptoms, investigations include liver function tests, U&E clotting, and septic screen. Diagnostic investigations include the following.
- Measurement of the enzyme Gal-1-PUT in red blood cells (false negatives can occur within 3 months of a blood transfusion).
- Measurement of red blood cell gal-1-P levels.
- DNA analysis: approximately 60% of UK patients with classical galactosaemia are homozygous for the common mutation Q188R.

Management

If galactosaemia is suspected, dietary galactose must be excluded. Follow ing initial supportive therapy, the main treatment is exclusion of dietar galactose by a strict milk-free diet (see table opposite) for life. Despit recent reports of concerns over the effects of phyto-oestrogens, whic are present in soya beans, on later reproduction, soya-based infant for mulas remain the milk substitutes of choice because they are completel lactose free (British Inherited Metabolic Disease Group/Galactosaemi Support Group). Care must be taken to ensure the diet is nutritionall adequate. Calcium is a particular nutrient at risk. On a minimal galactos diet, symptoms resolve and gal-1-P levels fall, but not to normal levels probably because of endogenous galactose production.

Outcome

Despite early introduction and maintenance of dietary charges, long-term complications can include learning difficulties, speech abnormalities, an ovarian dysfunction in girls.

Fiona White, Central Manchester and Manchester Children's University Hospitals NHS Trust

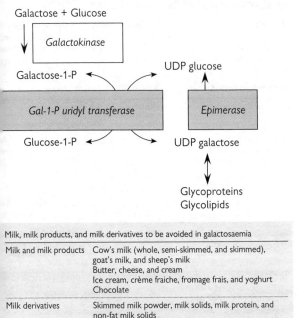

Galactose + Glucose

Galactokinase

Galactose-1-P ⟵ ⟶ UDP glucose

Gal-1-P uridyl transferase   *Epimerase*

Glucose-1-P ⟵ ⟶ UDP galactose

Glycoproteins
Glycolipids

Milk, milk products, and milk derivatives to be avoided in galactosaemia	
Milk and milk products	Cow's milk (whole, semi-skimmed, and skimmed), goat's milk, and sheep's milk Butter, cheese, and cream Ice cream, crème fraiche, fromage frais, and yoghurt Chocolate
Milk derivatives	Skimmed milk powder, milk solids, milk protein, and non-fat milk solids Casein, hydrolysed casein, caseinates, sodium caseinate, and calcium caseinate Whey, hydrolysed whey, whey syrup sweetener, hydrolysed whey sugar, vegetarian whey, and margarine containing whey Lactose, milk sugar, and hydrolysed milk sugar Buttermilk, milk fats, butter fat, animal fat (may be butter), artificial cream, cheese powder, and ghee
Lactose may be used as a filler in:	Flavourings, table-top or tablet artificial sweeteners, and tablet medication

Further reading

Walter, J.H. *et al.* (1999). Recommendations for the management of galactosaemia. *Archives of Disease in Childhood.*, **80**, 93–6.

Dixon, M. (2000). Disorders of carbohydrate metabolism. In *Clinical paediatric dietetics*, 2nd edn, (ed. V. Shaw and M. Lawson), pp. 303–8. Blackwell Science.

European Galactosaemia Society. 🖳 www.galactosaemia.com

The mucopolysaccharidoses (MPS)

The MPS are a group of disorders characterized by the storage of glycos aminoglycans (GAGs) within the cells of the body. This storage is caused by the lack of a lysosomal enzyme. Therefore a different enzyme is missing in each MPS disorder.

MPS type	Eponym	Stored GAG	Enzyme deficiency
I	Hurler, IH/S, Scheie	HS, DS	α-L-Iduronidase
II	Hunter	HS, DS	Iduronidate sulphatase
IIIA	San Filippo	HS	Heparan N-sulphatase
IIIB	San Filippo	HS	N-Acetyl-α-D-glucosaminidase
IIIC	San Filippo	HS	Acetyl CoA: α-glucosaminidase N-acetyltransferase
IIID	San Filippo	HS	N-Acetylglucosamine-6-sulphate sulphatase
IVA	Morquio	KS	Galactose 6-sulphatase
IVB	Morquio	KS	β-Galactosidase
VI	Maroteaux–Lamy	DS	Arylsulphatase B
VII	Sly	HS, DS	β-Glucuronidase
VIX	Natowicz	HYAL	Hyaluronidase

DS, dermatan sulphate; HS, heparan sulphate; KS, keratan sulphate; HYAL, hyaluronic acid.

Because the type of GAG stored and the enzyme deficiency differs in each MPS subtype, so does the area affected. GAG can be stored in the brain, eyes, skeleton, heart valves, liver, and spleen. The ear, nose, and throat are often affected in this condition, and the resulting facial feature and skeletal deformities mean that the patient has a shortened airway, in addition to stored product in the underlying tissue.

The patients have skeletal changes particular to the condition, known a dystosis multiplex, including lumbar gibbus, hip dysplasia, and genu valgum.

Treatment [1]

Treatments involve replacing the missing enzyme. This can be done by bone-marrow transplantation, where the new bone marrow make the enzyme (but this is only currently used in MPS I), or replacing the enzyme in a recombinant form. Currently the only enzyme replacement available for MPS is laronidase (Aldurazyme®) for MPS I. This treatment was licensed in June 2003 and aims to ameliorate the symptoms of the

Jean Mercer, Central Manchester and Manchester Children's University Hospitals NHS Trust sease. In a clinical trial, it has been shown to improve endurance and espiratory function. Galsulfase (Naglazyme®) was approved by the US ood and Drug Administration (FDA) in June 2005 for use in MPS VI, and linical trials of enzyme-replacement therapy in MPS II are at an advanced tage.

or other MPS disorders, palliative care services are of great importance. ll of the conditions can be diagnosed pre-natally.

Further reading

criver, C.R., Beaudet, A.L., Sly, W.S., Valle, D. (1995). *The metabolic and molecular bases of inherited disease*, Vol. 2, 7th edn McGraw Hill.
www.mpssociety.co.uk

Blood glucose monitoring

Self-monitoring of blood glucose (SMBG) is an essential tool in the management of childhood and adolescent diabetes mellitus, because it:
• helps to monitor immediate and daily levels of control
• detects hypoglycaemia
• assists in the safe management of hyperglycaemia
• has educational value in assessing blood glucose responses to insulin, food, and exercise.

A finger-prick blood test, using a blood glucose meter, measures the actual level of glucose in the blood at the time of the test.

Results are measured in mmol/l. The result will indicate if the blood glucose is too high (hyperglycaemia), too low (hypoglycaemia), or within the optimal target range (4.0–9.0 mmol/l) at that time.

Equipment
• Meters should meet individual needs in terms of:
  • visual acuity and manual dexterity of the child/adolescent
  • the amount of blood needed and the potential to test at alternate sites.
• Most blood glucose meters are quick and easy to use.
• Because there are many different blood glucose meters on the market, the individual meter instructions and blood test techniques will vary, depending on the type of device.
• In order to obtain accurate test results and prevent errors:
  • educate the patient in the use and maintenance of blood glucose meters.
  • provide written guidelines for blood testing techniques and correct use of individual meters, ensuring that they are understood and followed.

Timing of SMBG
Customize the number of tests taken and regularity of blood glucose monitoring for each patient, depending on:
• acceptance by the young person
• the type of insulin regimen
• availability of equipment.

Evidence shows that recording and acting on blood glucose results enables individuals to maintain better control of their diabetes mellitus.

Blood glucose is best measured:
• at different times of the day, to show the level of blood glucose in response to the action profiles of insulin, food intake, and exercise
• to confirm hypoglycaemia and monitor recovery
• during intercurrent illness, to prevent hyperglycaemic crises/DKA
• in association with vigorous sport or exercise.

Kirsten Jones, Royal Devon and Exeter NHS Foundation Trust

Trouble shooting

What if blood glucose results are outside normal values, with no obvious cause?

Some reasons for unexplained high or low results may include:
- not calibrating the meter
- not washing hands before testing
- not providing enough blood for a sample
- using out-of-date or wrong test strips
- incorrect storage of test strips or meters.

Action

- Repeat the test if an unexplained high or low result occurs.
- Contact a healthcare professional for advice if the problem persists.

Risk management

Records of serial numbers of meters provided to patients should be kept in case of recall or hazard warnings.

Further reading

Swift, P.G.F. (ed.) (2000). *Consensus guidelines for the management of type 1 diabetes mellitus in children and adolescents*, pp. 34–39. ISPAD Guidelines. Medforum.

Owens, D. et al. (2005). The continuing debate on self-monitoring of blood glucose in diabetes. *Diabetes and Primary Care*, **7**(1), 9–21.

www.accu-check.co.uk

Calculating insulin dosages and insulin types

Principles of insulin therapy

Children and young people with diabetes mellitus and their families need to be knowledgeable, skilled, and motivated to manage the condition. Insulin therapy cannot be considered in isolation from diet and exercise.

In people without diabetes mellitus, insulin is continually produced on demand by the pancreatic islet cells in response to increasing blood glucose levels. Insulin therapy aims to mimic this process, providing sufficient basal insulin to cover the 24-hour period, in combination with higher boluses of insulin to cover meal-time hyperglycaemia.

The choice of insulin regimen and daily insulin dose is dependent on many factors

- Age
- Weight (kg)
- Pubertal stage
- Duration and phase of diabetes mellitus
- Personal preference of the child/young person with diabetes mellitus and his/her family
- Nutritional intake and distribution
- Exercise and activity levels
- Daily routine
- Intercurrent illness

Aim of insulin therapy

Insulin therapy aims to achieve good metabolic glycaemia control (HbA$_{1c}$ < 7.5%). The insulin dose requires adjustment until target blood glucose levels are achieved: pre-prandial 4–8 mmol/l and post-prandial <10 mmol/l. Ongoing education and advice from the paediatric diabetes mellitus care team is essential to optimize diabetes mellitus management.

Guidelines for calculating insulin dose

Insulin dosages are individual, vary over time, and require regular review and assessment. Insulin treatment is started as soon as possible after diagnosis to prevent metabolic decompensation and DKA.

- After diagnosis: insulin requirements are based on 0.5 IU/kg body weight/day.
- Post-diagnosis: a partial remission phase is experienced (honeymoon period) when the daily insulin dose is often <0.5 IU/kg body weight/day.
- Pre-pubertal children: insulin requirements (outside the remission phase) are usually 0.7–1.0 IU/kg body weight/day.
- During puberty: insulin requirements may increase substantially to 1–2 IU/kg body weight/day.

Caution

Never stop insulin. If the child/young person is unwell, refer to local sick-day rules for insulin management.

Yvonne Davies, West Wales General Hospital, Carmarthen

Insulin concentration

The insulin concentration available within the UK is 100 IU/ml. Other concentrations are available. Occasionally the insulin concentration needs to be diluted for infants/young children, and special diluents can be obtained from the manufacturer for this purpose.

Insulin preparations

Insulin preparation	Onset of action	Duration of action
Rapid-acting	5–15 min	2–5 hours
Short-acting	30–60 min	Up to 8 hours
Intermediate-acting	1–2 hours	16–35 hours
Long-acting	1–2 hours	24 hours

Insulin regimens and preparations

One, two, or three injections/day: rapid-acting or short-acting insulin, pre-mixed or self-mixed with intermediate-acting insulin.
Basal bolus regimen (more than three injections daily): rapid-acting or short-acting insulin with long-acting or intermediate-acting insulin.
Insulin pump therapy: rapid-acting or short-acting insulin.

Dose distribution

Twice daily regimens are normally split: two-thirds dose in the morning and one-third dose in the evening. These ratios vary individually and change with the young person's age and maturity.
Basal bolus regimens incorporate 30–50% of the total daily dose as a long-acting (or intermediate-acting) insulin analogue with the remainder as a rapid-acting or short-acting insulin and are divided into three meal-time boluses. Often bolus doses are calculated according to the carbohydrate portion eaten at each meal.

Further reading

National Institute for Clinical Excellence (2004). *Type 1 diabetes: Diagnosis and management of type 1 diabetes in children and young people.* Guidelines 15. National Institute For Clinical Excellence Clinical.

International Society for Pediatric and Adolescent Diabetes (2000). *Consensus guidelines for the management of insulin-dependent diabetes in childhood and adolescence.* Freund Publishing House.

Neonatal problems

Neonatal assessment at birth

Birth is a traumatic event for all newborns, with periods of hypoxia during uterine contractions.

Although cyanosed at birth, a healthy baby will have good tone and will be pink after a few minutes; however, a less well baby will remain blue longer, have poor tone, and may have a heart rate of <100 bpm. A sick baby will be pale, floppy, and apnoeic bpm with a slow or very slow pulse (<60 bpm).

One method of assessing the neonate is by using an Apgar score. The neonate is assessed using five components:

• heart rate
• respiratory effort
• muscle tone
• response to stimuli
• colour.

These are graded by an assessor, with 2 points awarded for normal, 1 point for poor, and 0 for bad. A score of <7 indicates moderate neurological/cardiorespiratory depression and a score of <3 indicates severe depression.

On the basis of the Resuscitation Council (UK) Guidelines (2000)[1], the following series of events should occur, depending on the severity of the neonate's condition. The baby's colour, tone, breathing, and heart rate should be re-assessed every 30 s throughout.

• Drying, covering, and assessing: drying the baby will reduce the risks of hypothermia, while providing stimulation also provides an opportunity to observe and assess the newborn baby.
• Airway: if necessary place the baby on his/her back with head in a neutral position—the neck is neither flexed nor extended. If the baby is particularly floppy, chin lift and jaw thrust may be required.
• Breathing: if the baby is not breathing adequately by 90 s, give five inflation breaths. Chest movement should be seen, together with an increase in the apex. If the apex increases but the baby does not start breathing, continue with 30–40 breaths/min until baby breathes spontaneously. If no increase in the apex, either the chest has not been inflated—repeat inflation breaths—or the baby needs more help—chest compression.
• Chest compression: if the apex remains <60 breaths/min despite good chest movement, start chest compressions. In babies, the most efficient method of delivering chest compressions is to grip the chest in both hands in such a way that the thumbs can press on the sternum at a point just below an imaginary line joining the nipples, and with the fingers over the spine at the back. Compress the chest quickly and firmly in such a way as to reduce the antero-posterior diameter of the chest by about one-third. The ratio of compressions to inflations in newborn resuscitation is 3:1, which is different from any other time of life.
• Drugs: in a very few babies, inflation of the chest and effective chest compressions will not be sufficient to produce an effective circulation.

Debra Broom, Royal Gwent Hospital, Newport

In these babies drugs may be helpful. Drugs are only needed if there is no significant cardiac output despite effective lung inflation and effective chest compression.

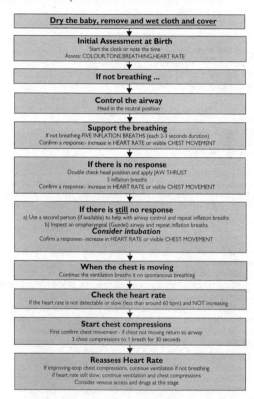

Dry the baby, remove and wet cloth and cover

↓

Initial Assessment at Birth
Start the clock or note the time
Assess: COLOUR, TONE, BREATHING, HEART RATE

↓

If not breathing ...

↓

Control the airway
Head in the neutral position

↓

Support the breathing
If not breathing-FIVE INFLATION BREATHS (each 2-3 seconds duration)
Confirm a response:- increase in HEART RATE or visible CHEST MOVEMENT

↓

If there is no response
Double check head position and apply JAW THRUST
5 inflation breaths
Confirm a response:- increase in HEART RATE or visible CHEST MOVEMENT

↓

If there is still no response
a) Use a second person (if available) to help with airway control and repeat inflation breaths
b) Inspect an oropharyngeal (Guedel) airway and repeat inflation breaths
Consider intubation
Cofirm a response:- increase in HEART RATE or visible CHEST MOVEMENT

↓

When the chest is moving
Continue the ventilation breaths it no spontaneous breathing

↓

Check the heart rate
If the heart rate is not detectable or slow (less than around 60 bpm) and NOT increasing

↓

Start chest compressions
First confirm chest movement - if chest not moving return to airway
3 chest compressions to 1 breath for 30 seconds

↓

Reassess Heart Rate
If improving-stop chest compressions, continue ventilation if not breathing
if heart rate still slow, continue ventilation and chest compressions
Consider venous access and drugs at this stage

AT ALL STAGES, ASK ..... DO YOU NEED HELP ?

In the presence of meconium, remember:
Screaming babies :- have an open airway
Floppy babies :- have a look

Produced by kind permission of the Resuscitation Council UK

Acknowledgement

Much of the detail contained on this topic and the algorithm has been produced by kind permission of the Resuscitation Council (UK). [1]

Further reading

Rennie, J.M., Roberton, N.R.C. (2002). *A manual of neonatal intensive care*, 4th edn. Arnold.

Resuscitation Council (UK) Newborn Life Support Guidelines (2000). ◻ www.resus.org.uk (accessed 27 October 2005).

The fetal circulation

In the fetus, the umbilical and placental circulations, ductus venosus, foramen ovale, and ductus arteriosus are temporary systems that are essential for growth and development. Changes take place at birth that transfer the function of gas exchange from the placenta to the lungs.

Oxygenated blood and blood rich in nutrients

- Transported from maternal placenta to the fetus by the umbilical vein.
- A high volume of blood flow is directed away from the liver by the ductus venosus towards the inferior vena cava and into the right atrium.
- From here, it is shunted across to the left atrium via the foramen ovale and flow is continued down into the left ventricle and into the ascending aorta.
- This flow of blood ensures that the most heavily oxygenated blood is directed to the heart and brain rather than the organs in the lower part of the body.

Less oxygenated blood

- Returns from head and neck through the superior vena cava, and blood that has passed into the liver returns through the inferior vena cava.
- Enters the right atrium, but it is directed through the tricuspid valve into the right ventricle and thus into the pulmonary artery.
- The collapsed fetal lungs and pulmonary capillary network present with very high resistance and blood is reflected back down the pulmonary arterial circulation, causing the pressure to rise beyond that in the descending aorta.
- This results in blood being shunted from the pulmonary artery through the ductus arteriosus into the descending aorta. Blood is distributed to abdominal and pelvic vicera and lower limbs.
- A greater portion of blood is returned to the placenta via the hypogastric arteries (branches of the internal iliac arteries). The hypogastric arteries are known as the umbilical arteries when they enter the umbilical cord. They return blood to the placenta for oxygenation and replenishment.

Phil Morrow, Queen's University Belfast

Circulation in the fetus before birth

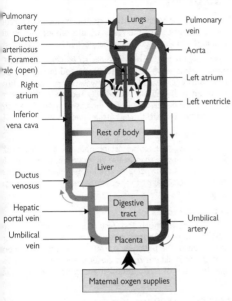

Foetal circulation (simplified)

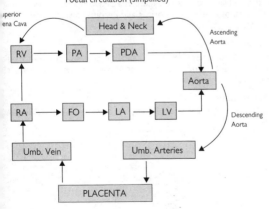

Further reading

Chamley, C.A., Carson, P., Randall, D., Sandwell, M. (2005). *Developmental anatomy and physiology of children*, Elsevier.

Changes at birth

The modifications that occur at childbirth to transform the fetal circulation to the neonatal circulation are the result of interruption of the placental circulation and the beginning of pulmonary activity.

At birth, the baby's first breaths cause the lungs to expand. Inspired O₂ dilates the pulmonary vessels, which results in a marked increase in pulmonary blood flow, thus decreasing pulmonary vascular resistance. Pressure in the right atrium and ventricle is markedly reduced. At the same time, occlusion of the umbilical circulation increases systemic arterial pressure, which is reflected back to the left atrium and ventricle.

Closure of the foramen ovale

As the circulation continues to become established, the pressure in the left atrium reaches values higher than in the right atrium, causing occlusion of the foramen ovale. The higher pressure in the left atrium presses the flap of the foramen ovale against the septum secundum and functionally closes it soon after birth.

Closure of ductus arteriosus

The increased O_2 content of the blood results in constriction of the ductus arteriosus. Closure of the ductus arterious occurs when pressure in the aorta exceeds that of the pulmonary artery. In addition, reduction in maternal prostaglandins facilitates ductus closure. The ductus is closed functionally within 24 hours of birth, although anatomical closure takes longer.

Constricture of ductus venosus

When the umbilical cord is cut, there is a reduced blood flow through the ductus venosus. In time, it shrinks and becomes a small band of connective tissue.

Umbilical vessels

The intra-abdominal aspects of the umbilical arteries form the medial umbilical ligaments. The intra-abdominal part of the umbilical vein becomes the ligamentum teres.

Further reading

Chamley, C.A., Carson, P., Randall, D., Sandwell, M. (2005). *Developmental anatomy and physiology of children*. Elsevier.

▣ www.uclan.ac.uk/facs/health/nursing/sonic/scenario

Phil Morrow, Queen's University Belfast

Post-natal circulation

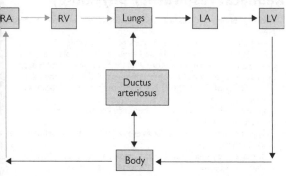

Circulation in the neonate after birth

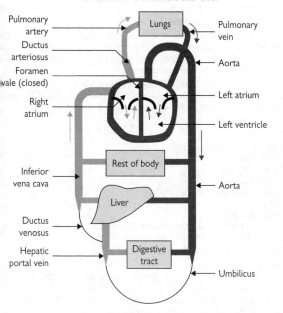

Neonatal respiratory physiology

Knowledge of neonatal respiratory physiology is essential for the neonat nurse.

- Pre-natally, exchange of gases occurs via the placenta.
- Following delivery of the baby and expulsion of the placenta, it is essential that normal respiratory effort is maintained at all times.
- Even at rest, newborn O_2 consumption is twice that of the adult.
- The majority of O_2 (85–90%) is transported around the body as oxyhaemoglobin, with a small amount dissolved in solution (approximately 10–15%). O_2 is used in cell respiration for the production of ATP.
- CO_2 is the waste product of cell respiration. It is transported in the blood in three ways:
    - it reacts very quickly with water, resulting in about 85% being carried as bicarbonate, which is formed as follows:
    $CO_2 + H_2O \rightarrow H_2CO_3 \rightarrow HCO_3^- + H^+$.
    - some is dissolved.
    - the rest is combined with proteins as carbamino compounds.
- O_2 and CO_2 pass across the alveolar–capillary membrane by the process of passive diffusion.

Neonatal respiratory disease

The most common respiratory problem in the newborn period is surfactant-deficient lung disease (SDLD), most commonly seen in the premature infant. SDLD is caused by a deficiency in the quantity and composition of surfactant (📖 p.672, Respiratory distress).

Surfactant is a lipoprotein that lines all mammalian alveoli, preventing collapse and maintaining functional residual capacity. Produced by type pneumocytes, it is not prominent until around 24 weeks' gestation.

Signs of SDLD

- Tachypnoea
- Sternal intercostal recession
- Nasal flaring
- Expiratory 'grunt'
- Cyanosis
- Reduced air entry on auscultation
- Hypotonia
- Hypotension
- Blood gas analysis will typically show respiratory acidosis due to retention of CO_2 associated with poor gas exchange

Treatment and nursing care

- Maintain thermal regulation.
- Respiratory support: give supplemental O_2 to maintain adequate SaO_2 levels or, if respiratory distress is severe, consider mechanical ventilation. Exogenous surfactant should be given to all premature infants requiring artificial respiratory support.
- Maintain fluid and electrolyte balance.

Jacqueline Baker, Maelor Hospital Wrexham

Maintain blood pressure.
Maintain haemoglobin.
Consider prophylactic antibiotics.
Maintain skin integrity.
Positive touch and diurnal cycles.
Keep parents fully informed; involve them in all aspects of care.

Respiratory distress

An infant may present with respiratory distress for a variety of reason symptoms of which include:
- tachypnoea
- grunting: an audible noise on expiration
- apnoea
- nasal flaring
- intercostal and subcostal retractions; if severe, the sternum appears to draw back against the spine
- cyanosis
- decreased activity; the work of breathing expends all available energy.

The pathophysiology of any respiratory disorder is directly related to th development of the fetus and will therefore influence management care.

Fetal development

17–27 weeks' gestation
Key respiratory development factors.
- Rich vascular supply and capillaries form closer to the epithelial cells c the airway.
- Production of surfactant by type II pneumocytes, which determines th surface tension in the lungs; detectable from 25 weeks' gestation, but insufficient for alveolar stability.
- Surfactant reduces surface tension, which means the alveoli do not collapse after expiration; opening pressure decreases, thereby increasing lung compliance and alveolar stability.
- Bronchioles are developing.

28–35 weeks' gestation
Key respiratory development factors.
- Surfactant production increases slowly initially and then more quickly from about 32 weeks' gestation.
- Alveoli multiply and capillaries move closer to the thinning surface of the epithelium of the air sacs.

General nursing features
- Minimize overhandling
- Monitor SaO_2, TPR and blood pressure, differential temperature, and arterial gases
- Oxygenation/ET tube management, nasal cannulae, and nasal prongs
- Temperature management, humidification
- Fluid and electrolyte management
- Nutritional management
- Maintain skin integrity
- Prevention of infection
- Support the family
- Provide developmentally supportive care
- Pain management

Janice Watson, University of Southampton

Conditions that interfere with surfactant production.

Decreases surfactant production	Increases surfactant production
Hypoxia	Catecholamines
Acidaemia	Glucocortisoides
Shock	Stress—IUGR baby
Overinflation of lungs	
Underinflation of the lungs	
Hypercapnia	
Pulmonary oedema	
Mechanical ventilation	
Hypothermia	
Insulin	

Common causes of respiratory distress

Respiratory distress syndrome (RDS)
Transient tachypnoea of the newborn (TTN)
Meconium aspiration syndrome (MAS)
Congenital pneumonia
Pneumothorax
Pulmonary hypertension

Consider systemic illness, such as:
  anaemia
  hyperviscosity

Consider malformations, such as:
  pulmonary hypoplasia
  diaphragmatic hernia
  choanal atresia
  Pierre Robin syndrome

Later onset, >4 hours:
  sepsis
  pneumonia
  pulmonary haemorrhage
  aspiration
  cardiac failure

Further reading

Maxwell, G. (2000). *Neonatal intensive care nursing*. Routledge.
Merenstein, G.B., Gardner, S.L. (2002). *Handbook of neonatal intensive care*, 5th edn. Mosby.
Stephenson, T., Marlow, N., Watkin, S. Grant, J. (2000). *Pocket neonatology*. Churchill Livingstone.
www.cps.ca/english/statements/FN/fn05-01.htm

Common respiratory disorders

Respiratory distress syndrome (RDS)

An acute illness, usually of pre-term infants, presenting within 4–6 hour of delivery, caused by surfactant deficiency and characterized by:

- respiratory rate ≥60 bpm
- dyspnoea or respiratory distress
  - intercostal/subcostal recession
  - sternal retraction
  - tracheal tug
  - nasal flaring
  - grunting
  - cyanosis without O_2

Chest X-ray after 4 hours: appearance of 'ground glass'.

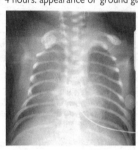

Chest X-ray showing RDS

Key management features

- Use of corticosteroids 1–7 days prior to delivery
- Surfactant-replacement therapy initiated at delivery
- Management of ventilation and perfusion:

Ventilation	Perfusion
O_2 delivery via headbox/nasal cannula	Management of ventilation: ventilate and sedate
CPAP via ventilator/infant flow driver	Blood pressure support: dopamine and dobutamine
Mechanical ventilation: IMV, SIMV, PTV	Correct metabolic abnormalities
High-frequency oscillatory ventilation	Vasodilate with drugs such as nitric oxide

Transient tachypnoea of the newborn

Delayed clearance of lung fluid caused by:

- lack of labour and consequently compression of the thorax during delivery, as in Caesarean section deliveries
- increased protein content because of aspiration of amniotic fluid durin asphyxia
- possible surfactant deficiency

Janice Watson, University of Southampton

key features

Term or near-term infants
Associated with:

- hypoproteinaemia
- birth asphyxia
- breech
- boys
- Caesarean section delivery

Tachypnoea up to 120 bpm, sometimes with tachycardia
Grunting and retraction minimal
Peripheral oedema
Crackles on auscultation
Hyperinflation
Intercostal bulging of pleura
Prominent peripheral vascular markings

key management features

Lasts 1–4 days
Prolonged if associated with mild asphyxia
Increased pulmonary vascular resistance has been described
Provide respiratory support
IV antibiotics
Withhold enteral feeds until tachypnoea subsides

Meconium aspiration

Meconium is passed *in utero*, inhaled, and damages the lung.
- Limited to mature infants; inhalation can occur pre-delivery or post-delivery.
- Causes airway obstruction, air trapping, overdistension of the lungs, air leak, and chemical pneumonitis.
- WCC is often raised.
- Hypoxia is a greater problem than hypercapnia.

Key management features

- Suck out mouth above and below the vocal cords at delivery.
- Ventilate if severe:
  - often need paralysing agent and sedation
  - longer expired time with low PEEP levels
  - high O_2 levels, which act as vasodilator
  - may be a candidate for extracorporeal membrane oxygenation
- Management of persistent pulmonary hypertension of the newborn which is characterized by cyanosis and shunting of deoxygenated blood through the ductus arteriosus and foramen ovale:
  - hyperventilate
  - nitric oxide

Further reading

Boxwell, G. (2000). *Neonatal intensive care nursing*. Routledge.
Merenstein, G.B., Gardner, S.L. (2002). *Handbook of neonatal intensive care*, 5th edn. Mosby.
www.rcpch.ac.uk/publications/clinical_docs/GGPrespiratory.pdf

Neonatal hyperbilirubinaemia

To understand the causes of hyperbilirubinaemia, it is necessary to understand bilirubin metabolism.

Bilirubin is derived from the breakdown of red blood cells, specifically the haem portion. The bilirubin combines with albumin (unconjugated) and transported to the liver. Unconjugated bilirubin is fat soluble and can pass through the blood–brain barrier. High levels are neurotoxic and can lead to kernicterus, which has a high rate of mortality or severe learning difficulties and disability in survivors.

Bilirubin is metabolized in the liver and then excreted via the kidneys or gastrointestinal tract as conjugated bilirubin (water soluble). The enzyme β-glucuronidase is found in the intestine of the newborn, which can convert conjugated bilirubin back to unconjugated bilirubin (entero hepatic circulation) and can add significantly to the bilirubin load.

Causes of hyperbilirubinaemia

High bilirubin production

- High haemoglobin levels in the newborn, short life span of red blood cells, and increased haemolysis
- ABO/rhesus incompatibility
- β-glucuronidase in the gut of the newborn (enterohepatic circulation)
- Bruising/cephalohaematoma
- Haemolytic anaemias

Poor bilirubin metabolism

- Low albumin levels
- Poor albumin binding
- Acidosis
- Free fatty acids (lipids)
- Drugs
- Possibly low levels of the carrier proteins and *UDP* glucuronyl transferase
- Infection affecting the liver: hepatitis and CMV
- Hypothyroidism
- Galactosaemia

Poor excretion of conjugated bilirubin

- Biliary atresia
- Cystic fibrosis
- Tumours

Breast milk jaundice

- Low fluid intake and calorific intake
- Slower gut transit time, allowing action of β-glucuronidase
- Possibly free fatty acids and pregnanediol in breast milk, but this is unproven

Diagnosis

- Clinical assessment—visible jaundice occurs once bilirubin levels reach 80–85 µmol/l

Janice Watson, University of Southampton

- <24 hours, usually pathological—investigate
- 1–7 days, usually physiological
- >7 days, usually pathological, e.g. sepsis—investigate

Serum bilirubin estimation via capillary blood sample

Family and obstetric history

Management of care

The aim of treatment is to prevent bilirubin levels rising to a level at which they can cause kernicterus.

- Ensure adequate fluid and calorific intake
- Phototherapy
- Exchange transfusion

Phototherapy is the most common mode of treatment and is the use of light (white-to-blue end of the light spectrum), which results in bilirubin being less lipotrophic and able to be excreted without the need for conjugation. The bilirubin serum level at which phototherapy is indicated varies according to length of gestation and age, and many units use the following graph to decide on treatment.

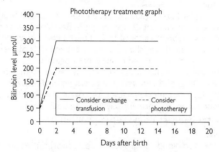

Key nursing considerations for the infant undergoing phototherapy

- Explain and fully support the family; this can be a distressing time.
- Eyes need to be covered—risk of retinal damage.
- Expose the baby fully and turn regularly.
- Skin integrity–infant has loose dark-green stools; observe for rashes (local histamine release) and do not use any creams, oils, or lotions.
- Monitor fluid balance and refer to unit protocol on the use of increased fluids.
- Monitor temperature—risk of unstable temperature.
- Take a minimum of daily bilirubin level estimations.
- Treatment stops when levels fall below reference levels—refer to unit protocol.

Further reading

Stephenson T., Marlow N., Watkin S., Grant J. (2000). *Pocket Neonatology*, Churchill Livingstone.
www.emedicine.com/ped/topic1061.htm

Neonatal physiology: haematology

- It is essential that there is lifelong production of all the haemopoietic cells. The liver is the principal organ of fetal haemopoeisis.
- Fetal haemoglobin is produced from about 4–5 weeks' gestation. An increasing amount of adult haemoglobin is produced throughout gestation. At term, about 70–80% is fetal haemoglobin and the remainder is adult haemoglobin. It follows, therefore, that the more pre-term the infant haemoglobin is, the more fetal haemoglobin he/she will have compared with adult haemoglobin.
- Due to its different structure, fetal haemoglobin has better O_2 carrying capacity and O_2 affinity than adult haemoglobin. Although this is perfectly appropriate in the hypoxic intra-uterine environment, it means that, following delivery, the high O_2 affinity of fetal haemoglobin adversely affects the rate at which O_2 can be unloaded to the tissues. Thus, over the first few months fetal haemoglobin is replaced with adult haemoglobin, which has a lower O_2 affinity and facilitates unloading at the tissues.
- Following birth, red blood cell production falls, probably due to the increase in the amount of circulating O_2. Red blood cells production begins several weeks after birth, and by 3 months of age full production of red blood cells should be apparent and all fetal haemoglobin should have been replaced by adult haemoglobin.
- The infant born at full term will normally have a haemoglobin level of between 15 and 21 g/dl. The infant born prematurely will have a slightly lower haemoglobin level. The circulating blood volume of a newborn infant is approximately 85 ml/kg body weight.

Neonatal haematology: some problems

Anaemia

- Reduced red blood cell production, particularly in the pre-term infant.
- Increased red blood cell destruction; the life span of a neonatal red blood cell is 70 days compared with 40 days in the preterm infant and 120 days in the adult. Haemolytic anaemia, enzymopathies, or haemoglobinopathies
- Blood loss; may be at delivery or due to a large amount of iatrogenic blood letting.

Polycythaemia

- Chronic intra-uterine hypoxia
- Delayed cord clamping
- Twin-to-twin transfusion
- Fetal–maternal transfusion
- Infants of diabetic mothers

Coagulation disorders

- The normal coagulation cascade is relatively inefficient in the newborn particularly in the premature infant
- Thrombocytopenia
- Vitamin K deficiency
- Disseminated intravascular coagulation, a serious complication of sepsis, shock, asphyxia, and viral infections

Jacqueline Baker, Maelor Hospital Wrexham

Treatment and nursing care
- Treatment will depend on the condition: treat the underlying problem.
- Maintain a thermoneutral environment.
- Maintain haemoglobin levels.
- All nursing care associated with blood transfusion.
- Keep parents fully informed and involve them in all aspects of care.

Neonatal hypoglycaemia

Neonatal hypoglycaemia is defined as a blood glucose <2.6 mmol/l; the majority of babies will be asymptomatic. Prolonged symptomatic hypoglycaemia can have serious effects on neurodevelopment; however, doubt still exists to the risk posed by asymptomatic hypoglycaemia.

Glucose homeostasis

In utero the fetus receives a continuous supply of glucose via the placenta and begins to lay down stores of glycogen from the first trimester. However, it is only in the third trimester that this process accelerates. At birth, the supply of glucose is severed and the infant has to switch to gluconeogenesis and glycogenolysis to maintain blood glucose levels particularly if feeding or fluids are delayed. Usually there is a fall in blood glucose in the first 4 hours before the regulatory hormones that trigger glucose production take effect.

Presenting symptoms are non-specific but can include:

- apnoea
- lethargy
- poor feeding
- hypothermia
- hypotonia
- seizures

Causes of hypoglycaemia

Depleted or exhausted stores	Prematurity
	Delayed feeding
	IUGR
	Hypothermia
	Asphyxia
	Sepsis
Impaired glucose metabolism	Inborn errors of metabolism
	Galactosaemia
	Glycogen storage disease
	Enzyme deficiencies
Hyperinsulinaemia	Infant of diabetic mother
	Beckwith–Wiedeman syndrome
	Erythroblastosis fetalis
Other causes	Exchange transfusion
	Congenital hypothyroidism
	Maternal drugs
	Interrupted feeding—IV extravasation
	Liver disease

Janice Watson, University of Southampton

Key nursing management

Prevention

- Avoid hypothermia
- Early feeding or, if contradicted and infant is at high risk, start IV 10% dextrose at 60 ml/kg body weight
- Monitor and measure blood glucose regularly (every 3–4 hours or refer to unit policy) until glucose levels stable and feeding established.

Blood glucose <2.6 mmol/l

If blood glucose <2.6 mmol/l on laboratory results, feed and consider NG or cup feed and if, on rechecking, blood glucose is still <2.6 mmol/l, commence IV infusion and investigate for cause.

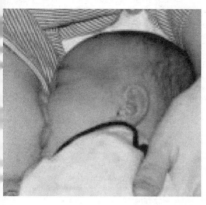

Note

Some babies may need an increased glucose concentration of 12%, 15%, or even 20%, which can cause serious tissue damage if extravasation should occur. Careful IV management is vital and preferably a central line should be used where possible.

Further reading

Boxwell, G. (2000). *Neonatal intensive care nursing*. Routledge.

Cowett, R.M., Loughead, J.L. (2002). Neonatal glucose metabolism: differential diagnoses, evaluation, and treatment of hypoglycaemia. *Neonatal Network*, **21**(4), 9–18.

www.cps.ca/english/statements/FN/fn04-01.htm

Temperature control in the neonate

Maintaining thermal control in the pre-term neonate is a vital nursing responsibility and requires the nurse to understand heat gain and ways to prevent heat loss. At 30 weeks' gestation the infant acts as if he/she is poikilothermic (his/her temperature alters with the environmental temperature). The aim is to maintain a thermoneutral environment, which is the temperature at which minimal rates of O_2 and energy are expended to maintain a normal body temperature. The normal range is considered to be 36.5–37.5°C; however, some units use different ranges, (36.2–37.2°C or 36.6–37.3°C).

Heat gain

- Non-shivering thermogenesis: the secretion of norepinephrine, release of thyroxine, and the metabolism of brown fat to product heat. Depends on a source of glucose, fatty acids, and O_2. This is the primary source of heat.
- Vasoconstriction.

Heat loss

Four main routes:

- Convection: the difference in air temperature between the infant and environment. The infant loses heat to the environment and this is exacerbated by the large body surface area to volume ratio of the newborn.
- Radiation: the difference in temperature between the baby and surrounding surfaces.
- Evaporation: insensible water loss from the surface of the skin. Transepidermal water loss increases greatly with increasing prematurity. At 2 weeks, a pre-term infant will have the transepidesmal water loss of a full term infant following rapid maturation of the skin.
- Conduction: the transfer of heat from one object to another when in contact, e.g. bedding and equipment surfaces.

Contributing factors:

- large body surface to area ratio
- poor deposits of insulating fat
- immature central control
- decreased physical activity
- poor stores of brown fat
- poor ability to shiver
- immature skin.

Preventing heat loss

- Ensure skin is dried thoroughly at delivery. Use warmed towels/ blankets.
- Nurse in an incubator, double-walled if possible, on air mode.
- Humidify air/gases for at least the first week initially, using highest level of humidity in the incubator that can be reached for the infant <30 weeks/kg body weight.
- Dress baby in a hat and wrap or dress as much as possible.

Janice Watson, University of Southampton

- Reduce drafts.
- Heat air/gases surrounding and entering baby.
- Unit temperature to be 24–25°C.
- Warm blankets/sheets prior to putting in contact with the baby.
- Warm X-ray plates.
- Allow fluids to reach at least unit temperature prior to administrating or feeding, or give warm feeds.

Consequences of hypothermia

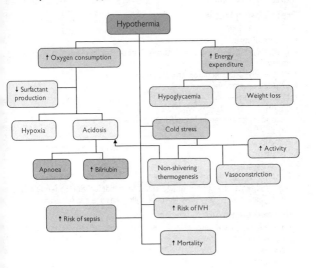

Further reading

Merenstein G.B., Gardner S.L. (2002). *Handbook of neonatal intensive care*, 5th edn, Mosby.
Stephenson, T., Marlow, N., Watkin, S., Grant, J. (2000). *Pocket neonatology*. Churchill Livingstone.

Hypocalcaemia

- Hypocalcaemia can be described as a serum calcium level below 1.7–1.75 mmol/l.
- Calcium is essential for bone mineralization, the control of muscle and neural activities, and blood clotting; it is the most profuse mineral in the body.
- Hypocalcaemia is commonly seen in the neonatal period, and can occur with or without symptoms.

Predisposing factors

- Pre-term infants
- Infants of diabetic mothers
- During first 24–48 hours in critically ill neonates: perinatal stress and asphyxia
- Potentially after exchange transfusion
- Hypoalbuminaemia
- Hypomagnesaemia
- Secondary to maternal hypercalcaemia
- Secondary to maternal hyperparathyroidism
- Alkalosis
- Bicarbonate therapy
- Malabsorption
- Hyperparathyroidism and hypoparathyroid syndromes (rare)
- Maternal vitamin D deficiency
- Rare: presents at 5–7 days of age in full-term babies, due to feeding with cows' milk; uncommon now formula milk feeds are readily available

Signs and symptoms

- Jitteriness and twitching
- Irritability
- Apnoea
- Convulsions
- Cardiac arrhythmias and tetany during exchange transfusion
- Laryngospasm
- High-pitched cry
- Heart failure: cardiac contractions become very weak and may fail altogether

Also:
- Lethargy
- Poor feeding
- Vomiting

Treatment

- Symptomatic hypocalcaemia: emergency correction, with 10% calcium gluconate by slow IV infusion, under ECG control; bradycardia and asystole may occur if correction is too rapid.
- Asymptomatic hypocalcaemia: correct with infusion of diluted 10% calcium gluconate over 24 hours.

Debra Broom, Royal Gwent Hospital Newport

- Monitor and observe IV site for signs of extravasation; may result in tissue necrosis and subcutaneous calcium deposits.
- Check magnesium level: correct hypomagnesaemia.
- Oral calcium supplementation may be necessary.
- Investigate underlying cause if not apparent.

Further reading

Rennie, J.M., Roberton, N.R.C. (2002). *A manual of neonatal intensive care*, 4th edn. Arnold.

Taeusch, H.W., Ballard, R.A., Gleason, C.A. (ed.) (2005). *Avery's diseases of the newborn*, 8th edn. W.B. Saunders.

Neonatal infection

Neonatal infection can usually be divided into two categories: early onset (48–72 hours) and late onset (after first week of life).

Early-onset infection
Presentation
- Pallor
- Temperature instability
- Lethargy
- Respiratory distress (including grunting, nasal flaring, rib recession, and insuction)
- Poor feeding
- Vomiting
- Irritability
- Apnoeic episodes
- Poor perfusion
- Tachycardia

Micro-organisms that can cause early-onset infection
- Group B streptococcus
- Other Gram-positive organisms
- E. coli
- Other Gram-negative organisms
- Listeria

Predisposing factors
- Maternal health and well-being during pregnancy
- Maternal condition at delivery (prolonged rupture of membranes, HVS positive to group B streptococcus, need for interpartum antibiotics, offensive liquor, chorionamnionitis, and maternal fever)
- Pre-term labour
- Prolonged labour
- Instrumental delivery
- Fetal distress

Treatment
IV penicillin combined with an aminoglycoside (e.g. gentamicin) as a first-line antibiotic regimen, following completion of surface swabs and blood cultures.

Late-onset infection
Presentation
As with early onset but also potentially:
- subtle changes in colour, tone, and activity
- deterioration in stability of vital signs (bradycardias, apnoeic episodes, and desaturations)
- feeding intolerance
- increased respiratory effort
- ?convulsions
- bulging fontanelle
- abnormal clinical markers
- abnormal white blood cell count
- unexplained metabolic acidosis
- hyperglycaemia
- >CRP

Nichola Maggs, Royal Gwent Hospital Newport

Organisms that can cause late-onset systemic infection

Gram-positive organisms:
- coagulase-negative staphylococci
- *S. aureus.*
- enterococci

Gram-negative organisms:
- *E. coli*
- *Klebsiella* spp.
- *Pseudomonas* spp.

Fungi:
- Mainly *Candida*

Predisposing factors

Prematurity
Intubation
Central/peripheral access
After surgery
Cross-infection/nosocomial infections
Meconium aspiration

Investigations

Full blood count
U&Es
Creative protein
Blood cultures

- Blood gas
- Chest X-ray
- Lumbar puncture
- Surface swabs

Treatment

Usually IV flucloxacillin and an aminoglycoside (e.g. gentamicin) would be used as a second-line antibiotic regimen following completion of the above investigations and stopped when blood cultures are confirmed as negative or altered to treat any confirmed positive blood culture—usually after 48 hours.

Nursing considerations for both early-and late-onset infection

Close observations of vital signs; report any deviations from normal to medical colleagues.
Safe administration of antibiotic therapy and care of IV site.
Maintain infant's comfort.
Ensure parents are aware of infant's condition and regularly updated of changes.
Maintain precise written documentation of nursing care.

Further reading

Rennie, J.M., Roberton, N.R.C. (ed.) (2005). *Textbook of neonatology*, 4th edn. Churchill Livingstone.
Taeusch, H.W., Ballard, R.A., Gleason, C.A. (ed.) (2005). *Avery's diseases of the newborn*, 8th edn. W.B. Saunders.

Necrotizing enterocolitis

- This is an acute intestinal necrosis syndrome of unknown aetiology, although bacterial infection and hypoxia appear important.
- Commonly occurs in the ileum but may affect any part of the gut from the stomach to the rectum.
- Although cases have been reported in term infants, necrotizing enterocolitis is almost exclusively a disease of the premature.
- Characterized by mucosal necrosis, with possible progression to intestinal infarction and perforation.

Incidence

Estimated at 0.3–2.4 cases per 1000 live births. Occurs in 2–5% of a neonatal admissions and in 5–10% of very low birth weight infants.

Risk factors

The small intestine is served by the superior mesenteric artery, which divides further to supply the submucosa and mucosa. This arterial network is vulnerable to underperfusion and therefore reduced oxygenation, which leads to ischaemia. During hypoxia, gut perfusion is reduced in order to maintain adequate blood flow to the vital organs. Therefore risk factors include:

- prematurity
- umbilical catheterization
- exchange transfusion
- polycythaemia
- patent ductus arteriosus
- perinatal asphyxia/hypoxia
- early enteral feeding
- maternal use of cocaine
- maternal pre-eclampsia.

Clinical signs

Symptoms generally present within the first 12 days of birth. However, if enteral feeding is delayed, symptoms can occur after feeding is commenced:

- distended/tense abdomen
- bile-stained vomit/aspirate
- blood in stools.

Non-specific symptoms

- Lethargy
- Temperature instability
- Bradycardia
- Apnoea
- Poor peripheral perfusion
- Hypotension
- Low platelet count

Diagnosis

Abdominal X-ray will show gas in the bowel wall, together with dilated thickened areas of bowel. The bowel may or may not be perforated.

Kathryn Martin, Maelor Hospital Wrexham

Management

Continual vital sign measurements
Abdominal girth measurements
Accurate fluid balance (BD)
Abdominal X-rays
Maintenance of systolic blood pressure
Blood count
U+Es
Blood cultures
Sedatives
Surgical opinion if perforation suspected

Treatment

NBM for 7–10 days, to rest the gut in order to minimize the risk of
perforation
Parenteral nutrition via a central line
NG tube on free drainage plus hourly aspirates
Antibiotics, usually for 7–10 days
Respiratory support, may need ventilation
Platelets (FFP)
Surgical intervention for perforated/necrosed bowel will involve
resection, with possible anastomosis

Further reading

Horton, K.K. (2005). Pathophysiology and current management of necrotising enterocolitis. *Neonatal Network*, **24**(1), 37–46.

McAlmon, K.R. (2004). Necrotising enterocolitis. In *Manual of neonatal care*, 5th edn (ed. J.P. Cloherty, E.C. Eichenweld, and A.R. Stark), pp. 634–50. Lippincott–Williams & Wilkins.

Breastfeeding

Breast milk is the perfect food for babies and helps protect them against infection. However, in order to breast feed successfully, mothers require practical advice and psychological support. In 1989 the United Nation Children's Fund established a global baby-friendly initiative to promote good practice. Children's nurses must give consistent and up-to-date advice. Health professionals who give mothers individual help and support can, and do, help breastfeeding succeed. Below are some actions to promote breastfeeding and the reasons for these. [1]

Action	Rationale
1. All staff must be made aware of locally written and agreed policy, based on current best evidence, and be trained in the skills to implement it	Effective care is consistently provided
2. Provide accurate advice about the benefits of breastfeeding and effective breastfeeding management	Mothers can make informed choices
3. If hospitalized, allocate infant a cubicle or a bed space that can be screened with curtains. Have 'Please do not disturb!' notices available	Respect privacy, enabling mother to relax
4. Offer appropriate advice about positioning and attachment	Promote infant and mother's well-being
5. Ask if mother wishes to use a foot stool or pillows to support her back/arms or to raise her infant	Promote comfort
6. Allow mother to sleep beside infant	Promote demand feeding
7. Provide mother with adequate fluids, encourage regular meals	Promote/maintain milk supply
8. Advise mother regarding hot showers, breast massage, and analgesia	To reduce discomfort of engorgement
9. If infant unable to feed on demand, support and encourage mother to express 6–8 times in 24 hours (every 3–4 hours during day and at least once overnight)	To establish/maintain lactation
10. Simultaneous bilateral expression may be required	For twins and to increase milk supply

Lynn Findlay, Rhona Stuart, Fiona MacDonald, and Louise Holliday, Royal Aberdeen Children's Hospital

Contd.

Action	Rationale
11. Advise mother to hand express first, even if using a pump	To stimulate milk-ejection reflex
12. Provide sterile equipment to collect, store, and administer breast milk	Uncontaminated milk
13. Label bottle of breast milk with infant's name, date of birth, unit number, date, and time expressed	
14. Follow local guidance about storage. Ideally store in body (not door) of designated refridgerator, with a temperature alarm, at 2–4°C for up to 24 hours	
15. Never use a microwave to thaw/warm breast milk	It heats unevenly, creating hot spots; immunoglobin A and lysozyme activity is reduced
16. If infant is unable to breastfeed, use NG/cup/spoon feeding	Using an artificial teat might interfere with the infant learning to breastfeed
17. Respect mother's informed wishes about using dummies	Using a dummy may interfere with demand feeding

Further reading

Royal College of Nursing (1998). Breastfeeding in paediatric units—guidance for good practice.
www.babyfriendly.org.uk

Bottle feeding

- **B**ottle
- **O**bservation
- **T**emperature
- **T**echnique
- **L**isten
- **E**ducation

- **F**eeding
- **E**quipment
- **E**vidence
- **D**emonstrate
- **I**ndividual
- **N**utrition
- **G**uidance

Generally, bottle feeding refers to the use of a bottle and teat when feeding an infant milk formula instead of using the breast. However, human milk may be expressed and fed with a bottle in some instances, e.g. for a premature baby. Although breastfeeding is superior for babies, infant milk formulas are intended to replace human milk if a mother has opted to bottle feed her baby. However, it is recommended that infant milk formulas are used only on the advice of an identified health professional, e.g. midwife.

Observation and equipment

- Important observations should be made regarding recommended milk formulas, e.g. measure water prior to adding milk powder to ensure accuracy (follow manufacturer's preparation instructions). Ensure safe water supply, handwashing, and storage of milk.
- Equipment needed before making up feeds includes either sterilizing liquid and cold water or a steam sterilizer.

Temperature and evidence

- Test temperature of feed before offering to infant; do not warm feeding bottle in the microwave because there is a risk of burns.
- Decisions in health care should be based on best evidence; reliable practice knowledge, up to-date literature, and common sense.

Demonstrate technique

- Demonstrate an angled bottle to decrease the need for burping; keep teat full of milk to avoid infant taking in air.
- Do not bottle feed infant lying flat, because infant could choke on vomit.

Listen to individual

- Bottle feeding seems to have become a negative experience for mothers and health professionals.
- The mother's choice must be respected; professional advice regarding bottle feeding should not be allowed to disappear.

Doris Corkin, Queen's University Belfast

ducation, nutrition, and guidance

Effective education of parents and ongoing support is essential.
Infants are immature and therefore totally dependent upon adults to
feed them safely; adequate nutrition is vital to promote growth and
development.
Mothers who choose to bottle feed need clear guidance in meeting
their infant's needs.

Average fluid requirements.

Age of infant	Total fluid in 24 hours
Newborn	30 ml/kg body weight
2 days	60 ml/kg body weight
3 days	90 ml/kg body weight
4 days	120 ml/kg body weight
5 days	150 ml/kg body weight
1 week to 8 months	150 ml/kg body weight

urther reading

is, M., Kanneh, A. (2000). Infant nutrition: part two. *Paediatric Nursing,* **12**(1), 38–43.
ehir, B. (2005). Stop hitting the bottle. *Nursing Standard,* **19**(52), 28–9.
www.healthpromotionagency.org.uk

Genetic and congenital problems

Mendelian inheritance

- Our genetic information is packaged as *chromosomes*.
- There are 23 pairs of chromosomes in every cell except egg/sperm cells, which have 23 single chromosomes.
- Chromosomes are numbered according to size: 1 being the biggest and 22 being the smallest. These are known as *autosomes*.
- The 23rd pair (sex chromosomes) determine the gender of the baby: XX female and XY male.
- We inherit one copy of each chromosome from each of our parents (see figure opposite).
- Chromosomes are made up of *genes*.
- Genes are coded instruction that govern development from fertilized egg to baby and how humans function following delivery.
- Each gene can be present in different forms known as *alleles*.
- Whether a person displays a trait or disease inherited from a parent depends on the two alleles (copies) of the gene present.
- The three most common modes of inheritance are *dominant*, *recessive*, and *X-linked*.

Dominant inheritance

- One of the two alleles is altered.
- This is sufficient for the individual to show the effects, e.g. neurofibromatosis, Huntington's disease, and tuberous sclerosis.
- The faulty copy *dominates* the other gene (see figure opposite).

Recessive inheritance

- Both alleles need to be altered in order for the individual to have the condition, e.g. cystic fibrosis (CF), sickle cell disease, and thalassaemia.
- Often the person carrying one altered allele will have no clinical manifestations of the condition (see figure opposite).

X-linked inheritance

- Eggs of the female will have 22 autosomes and an X chromosome.
- Sperm cells will have 22 autosomes and either an X or a Y chromosome.
- Eggs fertilized by a sperm with a Y chromosome will be male.
- A female carrying an altered gene on her X chromosome will have a second copy of the gene on the other chromosome and so is unlikely to have symptoms of the condition.
- A male has only one X chromosome and, not having a second copy to compensate, will have the condition, e.g. Duchenne muscular dystrophy (DMD) and haemophilia (see figure opposite).

Further reading

British Society of Human Genetics. 🖳 www.bshg.org.uk/

Kirk, M., Parker, E. (2005). Inherited conditions and the family. In *Textbook of children's nursing* (ed. A. Glasper and, J. Richardson), pp. 611–26. Elsevier.

Skirton, H., Patch, C. (2002). *Genetics for health care professionals a lifelstage approach*. BIOS.

Emer Parker, University of Glamorgan

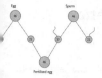

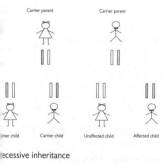

location of chromosomes to form zygote

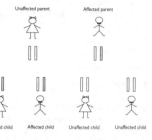

ominant inheritance

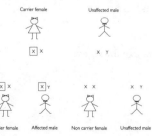

ecessive inheritance

-linked inheritance

Cystic fibrosis (CF): a genetic condition

The facts

- CF is the most common life-threatening genetic disease in the UK.
- 1 in 2500 babies born in the UK will have CF.
- 1 in 25 people in the UK carry a single faulty CF gene.
- CF occurs when both parents pass on a faulty gene.
- If both parents carry a faulty CF gene, in each pregnancy they have a 1 in 4 chance of producing a child with CF.

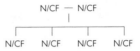

- There are many different ways in which the CF gene can be faulty.
- Over 1000 different mutations of the CF gene have been discovered.
- The most common mutation in the UK is called delta F508: 75% of people with CF in the UK carry two delta F508 genes; 94% of people with CF in the UK have this mutation as at least one of their faulty CF genes.

What does the gene do?

- The fault occurs on the gene called the CF transmembrane conductance regulator (CFTR).
- CFTR is responsible for transport of sodium and chloride (salt) across epithelial cell membranes that line the lungs and digestive system.
- In CF, transport of sodium and chloride across epithelial cell membranes is abnormal. Usually, it gives out too much chloride (salt) and not enough water. This leads to the secretions in the body becoming thick and sticky.
- The sweat of a person with CF is excessively salty. A test for CF is a sweat test to look at the amount of salt.

How does this affect the functioning of the body?

- Thick and sticky secretions in the lungs:
  - infection and inflammation
  - lung damage
  - respiratory failure.
- Thick and sticky secretions in the digestive system:
  - malabsorption
  - malnutrition
  - poor growth and weight gain.

Sarah Elworthy, Royal Devon and Exeter NHS Foundation Trust

Also:
- liver problems and liver failure
- diabetes mellitus
- constipation or bowel blockages.

These are a few of the complications associated with CF. All the body's secretions are affected. Therefore complications can occur anywhere in the body that secretions are found.

Further reading

Cystic Fibrosis Trust patient information leaflets. ▣ www.cftrust.org.uk
Hill, C.M. (1998). *Practical guidelines for cystic fibrosis care.* Churchill Livingstone.

Basic nursing care for a child with cystic fibrosis

Chest infection in CF

- Problem: increased shortness of breath and sputum production *or* identification of bacteria in the airway.
- Goal/objective: to establish cause and give appropriate treatment to encourage recovery.

Care planned	Rationale
Obtain sputum sample/cough swab for microscopy, sensitivity, and culture before starting antibiotic treatment	To enable the best choice of antibiotics for the treatment
Repeat sputum sample/cough swab culture weekly and at the end of the treatment or if condition deteriorates	To monitor for change in bacteria or sensitivity and asses whether bacteria have been eradicated
Record spirometry at the start of the treatment. Repeat at least weekly and at the end of treatment or if condition changes.	To assess condition and monitor for improvement or deterioration
To be assessed by a physiotherapist at the start of the treatment and daily. Support with chest physiotherapy regimen as prescribed	To encourage airway clearance
Give mucolitics, as prescribed, at the appropriate time in relation to chest physiotherapy	To thin viscosity of sputum and aid airway clearance
Ensure patient is in a good state of hydration	To avoid thick sputum
Monitor blood SaO_2 levels and give O_2 therapy as prescribed/required	To maintain satisfactory O_2 level
Give high-dose antibiotic therapy as prescribed	To reduce or eradicate bacteria from the lungs
Monitor sputum daily and record colour, amount, and consistency	To assess effectiveness of treatment
Monitor vital signs as required	To assess effectiveness of treatment
Give nebulized antibiotic as prescribed	To reduce or eradicate bacteria from the lungs
Give inhaled bronchodilator as prescribed	To dilate airway
Give inhaled steroids as prescribed	To reduce airway inflammation

Sarah Elworthy, Royal Devon and Exeter NHS Foundation Trust

Malabsorption in CF

Problem: potential/actual poor nutritional state due to malabsorption.
Goal/objective: improve and maintain nutritional status.

Care planned	Rationale
Ensure patient is taking prescribed enzyme supplement with all food and milky drinks	To optimize absorption of the nutrients consumed
Ensure patient is taking prescribed fat-soluble vitamins	To supplement poor absorption of these vitamins
Monitor and record bowel movements	To assess efficiency of digestive process
Refer to dietician	To advise and educate on maximizing nutritional intake
Discuss dietary habits and preferences with patient/family	To advise and educate on maximizing nutritional intake
Offer snacks and/or supplements and record amount taken	To maximize nutritional intake
Give gastrostomy/NG feed as/if pre-scribed	To maximize nutritional intake
Weigh twice weekly	To monitor weight gain/loss

Further reading

Hill, C.M. (1998). *Practical guidelines for cystic fibrosis care*. Churchill Livingstone.
Cystic Fibrosis Trust patient information leaflets: 🖥 www.cftrust.org.uk

Achondroplasia

Achondroplasia is one of the most common genetic causes of disproportionate short stature, occurring in approximately 1 in 25 000 births. Children with this condition have short limbs compared with their body length. It is mainly a physical condition, with affected individuals having normal IQ.

Characteristics

- Short stature.
- Normal trunk (body) length, shortened limb length, and other tissues unaffected, which can make the limbs appear bulky.
- Lumbar lordosis (curvature of lower spine).
- Prominent forehead (frontal bossing) with depressed nasal bridge.
- Broad short hands and feet, with a gap between the middle and third fingers (trident hand).
- Bowing of the lower legs.
- Possible overcrowded teeth and poor alignment of upper and lower jaw.
- Limited elbow extension.
- Normal IQ.
- Normal life expectancy.
- Expected adult height about 1.22 m (4 feet).

Affected babies develop motor skills and mobility more slowly than their contemporaries, because of the combination of a heavier head and shorter arms and legs, but ultimately achieve development within the normal range.

Complications

- Glue ear and hearing impairment
- Speech impairment
- Hydrocephalus
- Risk of sudden infant death
- Small pelvic dimensions; women will require delivery by Caesarean section
- Low back and leg pain and joint problems
- In late adolescence, spinal claudication can cause bladder spasticity and weakness after exercise.

Genetics

- Autosomal-dominant condition, with little or no variation in expression.
- Affects girls and boys equally.
- Caused by a point mutation in one copy of the fibroblast growth receptor gene on the short arm of chromosome 4, which causes the amino acid glycine to change to arginine.
- It occurs 'out of the blue' in 80–90% of cases, and so the recurrence risk is low (but not zero).
- The risk increases with increased paternal age.

Gilly Bromilow, Royal Devon and Exeter NHS Foundation Trust

If two affected people have children, there is a 25% chance that their child will receive two copies of the mutation (homozygous), which is lethal soon after birth.

Pre-natal testing is available where one or both parents are affected.

Treatment

Treatment of complications as they arise; usually involves surgical procedures to relieve pressure.

Further reading

American Academy of Pediatrics Committee on Genetics (1995). Health supervision for children with achondroplasia. *Pediatrics*, **95**, 443–51.

Gooding, H.C., Boehm, K., Thompson, R.E., Hadley, D., Francomano, C., Biesecker, B. (2002). Issues surrounding prenatal genetic testing for achondroplasia. *Prenatal Diagnosis*, **22**(10), 993–40.

Contact a Family. ⊞ www.cafamily.org.uk

Little People of America. ⊞ www.lpaonline.org

Duchenne muscular dystrophy (DMD)

- X-linked condition.
- Most common form of muscular dystrophy in males, affecting 1 in 3000–4000 live births; about one-third of these are new mutations.
- Generally diagnosed in boys between the ages of 1 year and 4 years by a muscle biopsy, showing the absence of dystrophin and very elevated serum creatinine kinase levels.
- Girls can also be affected, but very rarely.
- DMD is a progressive and degenerative disease, with most of the affected boys dying in their late teens or early twenties from heart failure and restricted breathing.

Characteristics

- Onset in early childhood
- Walking often delayed
- Calves initially large and firm
- Progressive proximal muscle weakness
- Large muscles are progressively replaced by fatty tissue
- Very high serum creatinine kinase level
- Abnormal muscle biopsy, showing absence of dystrophin protein
- Occasional mild learning and/or behavioural difficulties
- Often requiring a wheelchair by the age of 12 years

Management

Affected individuals will require:
- neurological and orthopaedic assessment and treatment
- physiotherapy and active exercise
- prevention of curvature of the spine
- treatment of chest infection and heart failure
- mobility aids
- home modifications
- appropriate schooling
- support for the family
- genetic counselling.

Genetics

- X-linked recessive condition caused by mutations in the dystrophin gene on the short arm of the X chromosome.
- These can be deletions, mis-sense mutations, or non-sense mutations, and are often individual to each family.
- If there is no family history, two-thirds of mothers of affected boys will be carriers, with a high risk of recurrence for themselves and other female relatives.
- Carriers can be detected by DNA analysis if the mutation can be identified in the affected child. If not, linkage analysis and creatinine kinase levels may be informative in the family.
- Carrier detection is important because female relatives are at potentially high risk (50%) of having affected sons.

Gilly Bromilow, Royal Devon and Exeter NHS Foundation Trust

DMD remains a challenge for accurate risk assessment in some families if the mutation cannot be identified.

Pre-natal testing using a chorionic villus sample for DNA analysis is available where the mutation is known. Otherwise, sex selection can be offered.

Aspects of nursing care

Provide support for the family and the child, particularly at the time of diagnosis when the mother may be feeling guilty and to blame for this devastating diagnosis. It is important to emphasize that it is no-one's fault; we all carry genetic faults of one sort or another.

Practical advice and help can be obtained through the regional muscular dystrophy family care workers. Make contact details available for both staff and families.

Further reading

Robinson, T., Tuckett, J., Harpin, P. (1998). Occupational therapy and Duchenne muscular dystrophy. In *Occupational therapy and children with special needs*. Whurr.

Muscular Dystrophy Association. 🖥 www.musculardystrophy.org/information_resources/factsheets/medical_conditions_factsheets/duchenne.html

Contact a Family. 🖥 www.cafamily.org.uk/Direct/d36.html

Down syndrome

Down syndrome is a chromosomal condition that affects roughly 1 700–900 births. It is the result of an extra chromosome 21. It is al important to understand that there are several types of Down syndrom

- Trisomy 21: each cell has 47 chromosomes (three chromosomes 21). Usually linked to increased maternal age (over 35 years). Non-disjunction at gamete production.
- Translocation 21: a segment of one chromosome 21 is attached to another chromosome (usually chromosome 14, 21, or 22). Usually inherited from one parent, but can be a spontaneous translocation. Not related to maternal age.
- Mosaic 21: fault occurs after fertilization, creating a mixture of norma and trisomy cells. The extent the child is affected depends on the percentage of trisomy cells.

Pre-natal diagnosis

Amniocentesis or chorionic villus sampling.

Characteristics

Children who are affected by this syndrome will have physical charact istics, medical problems, and developmental problems. Not all childr with Down syndrome will suffer with all the medical and physical chara teristics listed.

Medical characteristics

- Higher risk of hearing and sight problems
- Increased incidence of:
  - heart defects
  - infections
  - leukaemia
  - thyroid disorders

Physical characteristics

- Face and occiput flattened (brachycephaly)
- Eyes slant upwards and outwards
- Eyelids: an extra fold of skin (epicanthic fold)
- Hypotonic and hyperextensibility; usually improves with age
- Short stature
- Hands and fingers short; single palmar crease
- Small mouth cavity
- Slightly larger tongue; difficult to feed as infant
- Short broad neck with excess skin at back

Developmental problems

- Delayed motor skills (sitting, crawling, and walking)
- Delayed cognitive skills (speech and language acquisition and short-term memory abilities)

Sarah Wiggins, Royal Devon and Exeter NHS Foundation Trust

Diagnosis
Confirmed by chromosomal analysis.

Care/treatment
For independent and fulfilled lives of 50–60 years:
- education
- therapy
- social support
- effective health care.

Further reading
www.down-syndrome.info
www.dsa-uk.com/DSA_NewParents.aspx
www.psychnet-uk.com/ dsm_iv/downs syndrome.htm

Turner syndrome

- Named after the American endocrinologist Henry Turner.
- Chromosomal abnormality affecting only females.
- Caused by complete or partial deletion of an X chromosome.
- Incidence of 1 in 2000 live female births.

Normally cells in the body have 23 pairs of chromosomes that make up a to of 46 chromosomes. One pair of these chromosomes comprises the s chromosomes and will normally determine the sex of the individual. In t male there will be XY (46XY) and in the female there will be XX (46XX).

In Turner syndrome there is usually only one X chromosome (repr sented as XO). The missing X chromosome will have been lost duri sperm or egg production, and, following conception, will result in 46XC classic Turner syndrome.

Variations in the karyotype (chromosome analysis) for Turner syndrom can occur, e.g. the X chromosome will only be missing from some of th body cells (known as Turner mosaic), or a small part of a Y chromoson may have drifted across on to the X chromosome (known as mixe gonadal dysgenesis).

Although confirmation of a diagnosis of Turner syndrome is by kary type, initial diagnosis can be made by observing a series of characterist physical features:

- the neck has increased skin folds that give the appearance of webbing
- the chest can be very broad and the nipples widely spaced
- the hairline can be low
- lymphoedema of the hands and feet can be present.

Diagnosis can be made at birth if the child needs surgery for coarctatic of the aorta, another possible characteristic. Pre-natal diagnosis can als be made using chorionic villus sampling, amniocentesis, or ultrasound.

However, diagnosis usually takes place in early childhood when the chi fails to follow the normal growth centiles and later when there is a absence of puberty. These two characteristics are the main feature associated with Turner syndrome.

The term 'syndrome' is used to describe a collection of features that ma result from a single causative factor. It must be remembered that not a these features may be present in any one person. Listed below are som of the other features that can make up the syndrome:

- low-set ears
- droopy eyelids
- short fourth toe and short fingers
- high-arch palate (giving rise to feeding problems in neonates)
- high blood pressure
- small lower jaw
- myopia and problems with straightening the elbow (cubitus valgus).

Treatment

Endocrine intervention for both growth and puberty, and possibly IVF fo fertility.

John Bastin, University of Plymouth

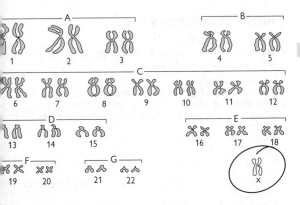

haracteristic karyotype

urther reading

www.tss.org.uk

Neurofibromatosis type 1

- Birth incidence: 1 in 3000
- Dominant-inherited condition: misprint on long arm of chromosome 1
- 50% are spontaneous mutations

Diagnostic criteria

Two or more of the following are required:
- six or more café au lait macules (>0.5 cm in children)
- two or more cutaneous/subcutaneous neurofibromas or one plexiform neurofibroma
- axillary or groin freckling
- optic pathway glioma
- two or more Lisch nodules (iris hamartomas seen on slit-lamp examination)
- bony dysplasia (sphenoid wing dysplasia and bowing of long-bone pseudoarthrosis)
- first-degree relative with neurofibromatosis type 1.

Initial diagnosis confirmed by:
- family history
- skin examination
- skeletal examination
- general physical and neurological examination
- ophthalmology assessment.

Cognitive deficits are present in 30–60% of people with neurofibromatosis type 1. These can be short-term memory problems, poor concentration, eye–hand coordination difficulties, difficulty in planning and executing task, poor visual tracking ability. Behavioural difficulties include sleep disturbance and poor interpretation of social clues.

Recommended annual clinical assessment

- Height/weight and head circumference
- Blood pressure
- Skin examination
- Skeletal examination (checking for signs of scoliosis or underlying plexiform neurofibroma)
- Neurological assessment if specific symptoms
- Pubertal development (precocious or delayed)
- Fundoscopy and visual acuity
- Educational progress (educational psychology and occupational therapy can help)

Rationale for these observations

- 30% have short stature
- 45% have macrocephaly (>97th centile)
- 44% will have cutaneous neurofibromas
- 82% will have Lisch nodules
- Scoliosis presents in 12–20% of cases
- Optic gliomas occur predominantly in children under 7 years of age

Rona Ross, Royal Aberdeen Children's Hospital

Renal artery stenosis in 1–2% of cases
Phaeochromocytomas are rare complication of neurofibromatosis
type 1

Encourage patient to report

Any of the following associated with a neurofibroma or plexiform neurofibroma:
• persistent pain for month
• new neurological deficit
• change in texture from soft to hard
• rapid increase in size
• changes in sensory or motor deficits, coordination, or sphincter
  disturbance.

Overall lifetime risk of malignant change in a plexiform neurofibroma is
~10%.

Headaches on waking, morning vomiting, and altered consciousness are
suggestive of raised ICP and need urgent assessment.

Further reading

Evans, D.G.R., Baser, M.E., McGaughran, J., Sharif, S., Howard, E., Moran, A. (2002). Malignant
    peripheral nerve sheath tumours in neurofibromatosis 1. *Journal of Medical Genetics*, **39**,
    311–14.
Ferner, R., Thomas, N., Partridge, L., Towers, R. (2003). *Clinical guidelines for the management of
    individuals with neurofibromatosis 1.* Neurofibromatosis Association UK.
North, K.N. (1998). Clinical aspects of neurofibromatosis 1. *Seminars in Pediatric Neurology*, **5**,
    231–42.

Osteogenesis imperfecta

Osteogenesis imperfecta, commonly known as 'brittle-bone disease', is a hereditary genetic disorder. Its primary manifestations include fractures, bone deformity, and bone pain. Children with osteogenesis imperfecta have reduced mobility, require increased parental/caregiver assistance, and may need significant adaptations to their home and social environment.

Characteristics

The Silence classification separates the disorder according to clinical presentation into types I–IV. Further types V and VI and rhizomelic osteogenis imperfecta have also been reported.

Type I
- Most common/mildest form
- Fractures occur occasionally
- Normal/near normal stature
- Bone deformity minimal or absent
- Brittle teeth
- Some hearing loss
- Collagen structure normal, but less than normal

Type II
- Most severe form
- Growth retardation during pregnancy
- Lethal at birth, or soon after, because of complex respiratory problems
- Numerous fractures, long bones crumpled and bowed, with ribs appearing beaded
- Collagen abnormal

Type III
- Bones fracture easily
- Fractures present at birth
- Several crush-fractured (squashed) vertebrae
- Short stature
- Brittle teeth and hearing loss
- Barrel-shaped rib cage
- Triangular face
- Bony deformity severe and spinal curvature present
- Collagen abnormal

Type IV
- Bones fracture easily (especially younger children)
- Shorter stature
- Crush-fractured vertebrae
- Some bowing of long bones
- Brittle teeth and hearing loss
- Collagen abnormal

Brian Silverwood, Healthcare Commission

Treatment

Aim: minimizing fractures and maximizing function and independence.
Medical management:
- bisphosphonate drugs—work by improving the thickness of bone (pamidronate given intravenously or risedronate given orally).

Surgical management:
- expanding intramedullary rod fixation (long bones)
- acute management of fractures.

Physiotherapy.
Occupational therapy (aids, adaptations, and special wheelchairs).

Nursing considerations

Babies and infants

Toys soft and easy to handle
Avoid lifting by ankles
Support head, trunk, and buttocks evenly
Make your movements slow, methodical, and gentle
Openings on clothes should be generous
Reposition child frequently to avoid flattening of the back of head
Give small frequent feeds (may be a poor feeder)
Ensure adequate hydration (prone to constipation)

Older children

Very independent; offer assistance
Appreciate normal adult conversation

Parents

Experts on their child's care
Listen to what they have to say

Further reading

Hill, C. et al. (2003). Recent advances in the management of osteogenesis imperfecta. *Current Paediatrics*, **13**, 151–7.
Iverwood, B. (2001). Osteogenesis imperfecta: care and management. *Paediatric Nursing*, **13**(3), 38–42.

Meningocele

Definition

Meningocele is a form of spina bifida cystica (spina bifida meaning 'split spine' and cystica meaning 'cyst-like'). There is a defect in the spinous process, together with herniation of the meninges through the defect which forms a cystic mass on the back.

The mass may be covered by a thick skin, with little risk of rupture or infection; alternatively, there may be a thin transparent membrane. There is no myelodysplasia or cord within the cystic mass in pure cases of meningocele and so the child is considered neurologically normal.

Because there is no cord displacement, hydrocephalus is not usually present.

Fetal development

The CNS and spine develop between the 14th and 28th day after conception. Spina bifida occurs when there is a failure of development of the bony canal that surrounds the brain and spinal cord.

The affected vertebrae of the spine have a posterior defect, which may occur in one or more of the vertebrae, most commonly lumbar vertebra 5 to sacral vertebra 2 (L5–S2).

Clinical manifestation

There is a notable bulging defect low down on the back. This contains tissues (meninges) which cover the spinal cord and CSF. There is usually no damage to the nerves; therefore there may be little or no disability.

Incidence

- Meningocele is the least common form of spina bifida.
- It accounts for 5% of all cases of spina bifida cystica.
- The number of cases has declined significantly in the past 30 years, now occurring in approximately 0.8 out of 1000 total births.

Cause

- Unknown.
- Perhaps due to a combination of genetic and environmental factors.

Prevention

Folic acid supplement 1 month before conception to the end of 12th week of pregnancy reduces the risk by up to 70%.

Risk

A person with an affected child or an affected person has a 1 in 25 chance of having an affected child.

Sue Swift, Royal Aberdeen Children's Hospital

Pre-natal screening

Alpha-fetoprotein in maternal serum is best detected at 16–18 weeks, but this may not detect closed defects such as meningocele.
Ultrasound: spina bifida is usually visible from 16 weeks to 20 weeks, but this may be missed in the L5–S2 region.

Treatment

Surgery is required to close the defect. There is little or no risk of neuro-logical damage but, as with all surgery, there are risks to the child.

Further reading

Goldberg, G. (2003). Nutrition in pregnancy, the facts and the fallacies. *Nursing Standard*, **17**(19), 39–42.
www.asbah.org
www.patient.co.uk/showdoc/40000439

Myelomeningocele

Definition
- Myelomeningocele is a form of spina bifida cystica. There is a defect in the spinous process and the spinal canal is incomplete, which allows the spinal cord, nerve roots, and meninges to protrude as a mass on the child's back.
- The spinal cord is damaged or not properly developed; this always results in some paralysis and loss of sensation below the damaged region.
- Most people have bowel and bladder problems because of the damage to the nerves that feed these areas.

For fetal development, cause, prevention, and screening, 📖 Meningocele (p. 714).

Incidence
Myelomeningocele accounts for approximately 75% of all cases of spina bifida.

Signs and symptoms
- The child has a visible mass low down on the back at birth.
- There will be partial or complete paralysis of the legs, with partial or complete lack of sensation.
- There is a strong possibility that the child will have problems with bowel and bladder control.
- Hydrocephalus is likely to be present (Arnold–Chiari malformation).
- The child may have dislocated hips at birth.

Complications
- Difficult delivery, with problems subsequent to traumatic birth (cerebral palsy and hypoxia)
- Permanent disability
- Loss of bowel/bladder control
- Frequent UTIs
- Meningitis
- Coexisting defects (hydrocephalus and congenital dislocated hips)

Treatment [1]
- Early surgical repair to close the defect is usually recommended to minimize the risk of rupture to the mass and infection. Occasionally surgery will be delayed to allow the baby to tolerate the surgery better.
- If surgery is delayed, the baby must be handled with extreme care to avoid damage to the exposed spinal cord, because any damage could increase paralysis. All aspects of care need to be considered, from positioning to feeding and all hygiene needs.
- Surgical intervention is often required for the treatment of hydrocephalus, which will require the insertion of a shunting device, such as a ventricular peritoneal shunt.

Sue Swift, Royal Aberdeen Children's Hospital

The baby will often require intervention from orthopaedic surgeons and physiotherapists: their involvement often increases as the baby develops into childhood and the extent of the musculoskeletal problems become more obvious.

Recent advances

In 2003 a world conference was informed that intra-uterine myelo-meningocele repair results in fewer UTIs, improved leg function, cognitive development and less need for CSF shunt. However, there is much debate about the suitability and safety of such surgical intervention.

Further reading

www.asbah.org
www.nlm.nih.gov
www.patient.co.uk/showdoc/40000439

Hydrocephalus

Hydrocephalus occurs when there is an abnormal accumulation of CSF within the ventricles of the brain.

Causes

- Non-communicating hydrocephalus occurs when there is a blockage within the CSF pathways, preventing the flow of CSF, e.g.
  - tumour
  - aqueduct stenosis
  - congenital abnormality: spina bifida, Arnold–Chiari malformation, and Dandy–Walker cyst.
- Communicating hydrocephalus occurs when there is inadequate reabsorption of CSF into the bloodstream, e.g.
  - meningitis
  - brain haemorrhage.

Signs and symptoms

Infant

- Increasing head circumference
- Tense bulging anterior fontanelle
- Dilated scalp veins
- Irritability
- High-pitched cry
- Vomiting
- Drowsiness
- Poor feeding
- Sunsetting eyes

Older child

- Headaches
- Vomiting
- Drowsiness/decreased conscious level
- Papilloedema
- Ataxia
- Bradycardia
- Unequal sluggish pupil response
- Photophobia
- Visual disturbance

Investigations

- Neurological examination
- Cranial ultrasound scan (babies)
- MRI scan
- CT scan

Treatment

The most common treatment is insertion of a shunt, a tube with a valve to control the rate of CSF drainage. The shunt diverts the CSF from the ventricles to a point distal to the blockage, where it can be absorbed into the bloodstream. The peritoneal cavity is the preferred drainage site

Carmel Geoghegan and Anne Squire, Central Manchester and Manchester Children's University Hospitals NHS Trust

ventricular peritoneal shunt), although the right atrium of the heart can also be used (ventricular atrial shunt). In most cases, a shunt is required for life.

An alternative treatment is third ventriculostomy. This involves opening the floor of the third ventricle, using an endoscope, to divert the flow of CSF. This treatment is not suitable for all types of hydrocephalus.

Nursing management

Once a diagnosis of hydrocephalus has been made, surgery will be performed.

Pre-operative care
* Close neurological observation and treatment of symptoms.

Post-operative care
Includes:
* neurological observation
* assess fullness/tenseness of fontanelle and measure head circumference daily in babies
* nurse the patient flat and gradually elevate
* observe abdominal girth when a ventricular peritoneal shunt is inserted

Complications
* If left untreated, the signs and symptoms of raised ICP will progress and become life threatening.
* Complications following insertion of a shunt include:
  * infection.
  * blockage of the shunt.
  * haemorrhage.
  * seizures.
* Third ventriculostomy is not always successful and in such cases the child requires insertion of a shunt.

Further reading
Hickey, J.V. (1997). *The clinical practice of neurological and neurosurgical nursing*, 4th edn. Lippincott.
Lindsay, K.W., Bone, I. (1997). *Neurology and neurosurgery illustrated*, 3rd edn. Churchill Livingstone.
 www.asbah.org

Cleft lip and palate

Cleft lip and palate is one of the most common congenital disorders with an incidence of approximately 1000 births in the UK each year. Therefore it is probable that most paediatric nurses will care for a child with this condition at some point in their career.

Classification

- Cleft lip only
- Cleft lip and alveolus
- Cleft lip and palate
- Cleft palate only

Cleft lip and/or palate may be unilateral or bilateral.

Cleft palate involves the soft palate and may extend into the hard palate.

The palatal cleft may be narrow or wide.

Isolated cleft palate is more likely to be associated with other congenital abnormalities or syndromes, such as DiGeorge syndrome and Stickler syndrome.

Pierre Robin sequence

This happens where the baby has micrognathia, as well as a wide U-shaped cleft palate. There may be feeding and respiratory difficulties because of a retro-displaced tongue. The baby will need to be monitored in hospital in the early weeks.

Treatment

Children are cared for at regional centres by a multidisciplinary team. This includes surgeons, nurse specialists, speech and language therapists, orthodontists, paediatric dentists, audiologists, psychologists, geneticists, and paediatricians.

- All children will follow a national protocol of care which is dependent on their type of cleft.
- Cleft lip and/or palate are generally repaired in the first year of life.
- For children born with cleft palate, the emphasis for the first 5 years is on audiological assessment and speech and language development prior to school entry.
- Children with an alveolar cleft will require further surgery (alveolar bone graft) between the ages of 8 years and 10 years to enable adult dental development. At this point in their treatment, children will be under the continuing care of an orthodontist, paediatric dentist, and maxillofacial surgeon.
- All young people up to the age of 20 years will remain under the care of the regional centre. They will be seen by members of the multidisciplinary team and offered further treatment as appropriate.
- Adults above the age of 20 years may continue to be seen as necessary.

Annie Cole and Jayne Tomlinson, Birmingham Children's Hospital NHS Trust

Nursing management

Newborn

- Diagnosis of cleft type.
- Assessment of baby, to determine nursing management.
- Method of feeding will be decided by the cleft type and parental preference. Guidance will be given by the nurse specialist.
- Offer emotional support to the parents, in order for them to come to terms with the diagnosis.

Subsequent care

The child will require the input of different nurses in a variety of settings as they progress through their treatment. These will include nurse specialists, ward-based nurses, paediatric community nurses, and health visitors. They will provide support regarding feeding and airway management, give pre-operative and post-operative advice around the time of surgery, and also monitor the child's general growth and development.

Further reading

Martin, V., Bannister, P. (ed.) (2004). *Cleft care: A practical guide for health professionals on cleft lip and/or palate.* APS Publishing.

Watson, A.C.H., Sell, D.A., Grunwell, P. (ed.) (2001). *Management of cleft lip and palate.* Whurr.

🖳 www.clapa.com

Omphalocele and gastroschisis

Definition

These are similar forms of abdominal wall defects. In omphalocele associated with other anomalies, there is a protrusion of abdominal contents but in gastroschisis (also referred to as antenatal rupture of omphalocele), these are not covered with a translucent sac of amnion and thus are exposed to amniotic fluid. This can cause damage to the bowel *in utero*.

Fetal development

The gastrointestinal system develops between the 7th and the 11th weeks of gestation.

Clinical manifestation

There is a visible protrusion of the abdominal contents, and the infant is generally premature and of low birth weight.

Incidence

- Combined incidence of these anomalies is 1 in 10 000 births, and this is increasing.
- Omphalocele is the most common form.
- Commonly occurs in first-born infants

Cause

May be a combination of genetic and environmental factors; disruption of blood supply in early pregnancy.

Prevention

No known prevention.

Pre-natal screening

Detected in pre-natal ultrasound scanning from about 14 weeks gestation.

Management

- Prevent fluid loss, electrolyte imbalance, and hypothermia.
- Primary repair or staged repair.
- Gastroschisis: abdominal contents are covered with saline packs or wrapped in surgical cling film to prevent infection.
- Small abdominal cavity: a pouch is created and suspended above the infant to allow gravity to place the contents inside the abdomen.
- NBM with NG tube *in situ*.
- IV feeding.
- Parental support to promote attachment and reduce anxiety.
- When the pouch is in place, abdominal wall is sutured.
- If there is insufficient skin to cover, a patch of silicone meshing or a Gortex patch is stitched to the skin. The skin grows over the patch.

Nettie Dearmun, Oxford Brookes University

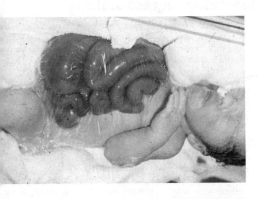

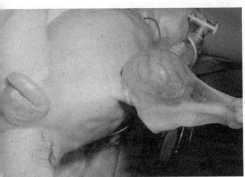

Photos reproduced with kind permission of Mr David Burge.

Complications

- Fluid/electrolyte imbalance
- Infection
- Hypothermia

Prognosis

- Omphalocele: mortality is approximately 40%
- Gastroschisis: mortality is approximately 10%. Infants have a better prognosis.

Further reading

Wong, D.L., Hockenbury, M.J. (2003). *Wong's Nursing care of infants and children*, 7th edn. Mosby.
☐ www.surgical-tutor.org.uk/system/hnep/gastroschisis.

Tracheo-oesophageal fistula

A tracheo-oesophageal fistula is a congenital malformation which consist of a link between the trachea and the oesophagus. There are five different types, the most common of which occur with oesophageal atresia (90%). There is no known cause.

Incidence
- Occurs in 1 in 3500 live births and equally in boys and girls.
- Usually a lower than average birth weight.
- Often with other anomalies, commonly VACTERL association.
- 10–20% mortality in premature babies or with other anomalies.

Diagnosis
- Antenatal polyhydramnios in 50% of cases.
- Noisy breathing and frothy saliva soon after birth.
- Choking, coughing, and cyanotic episodes, particularly on feeding.
- Abdominal distension owing to air in the stomach, confirmed by X-ray.
- Pulmonary problems if fed prior to diagnosis.

Management
- Maintain airway: frequent or continuous oral suction.
- Nursed with the child prone or on his/her side, and elevate the child's head to reduce gastric reflux.
- NBM with NG tube *in situ*.
- IV fluids.
- Surgical division and ligation of fistula. This may be staged.
- Provide parental support to promote attachment and reduce anxiety.
- Oral feeding, including breastfeeding, commenced once the child has fully recovered from surgery.
- Feed in an upright position when oral feeds are commenced.

Complications
- GOR is common and can be resolved by practical measures, such as an upright position during feeding, and prescribed medication.
- Tracheomalacia, leading to noisy breathing and respiratory difficulties.
- Strictures that can by made worse by reflux. These may need to be stretched under anaesthetic.
- Some children develop a characteristic cough, but this usually causes no problems. They can be prone to chest infections and asthma.
- Normal feeding programmes may take longer to achieve.

Prognosis
- This is related to the birth weight, associated anomalies, and time of diagnosis.
- Feeding difficulties and chest problems are common in the first 2 years but rare after 5 years.
- Normal life expectancy and abilities, notwithstanding other anomalies.

Ruth Davies, Royal Devon and Exeter NHS Foundation Trust

Further reading

Huband, S., Trigg, E. (ed.) (2000). *Practices in children's nursing guidelines for hospital and community.* Harcourt.
www.tofs.org.uk

Congenital heart defects

Defect	Anatomy and physiology	Signs and symptoms
Atrial septal defect	Opening between the left and right atria. This causes blood flow to shunt from left to right	Frequent chest infection Below average weight for age Acyanotic

Ventricular septal defect
Artery to left arm
Coarctation of the aorta
	Opening between the left and right ventricles. This causes blood flow to shunt from left to right	Murmur
		
		Breathlessness during feeds
		
		Sweating
		
		Frequent chest infection
		
		Large ventral septal defect:
		
		    failure to thrive
		
		    tachycardia
		
		    greyish complexion

Patent ductus arteriosus Patent ductus arteriosus Ventricular septal defect	The ductus sits between the aorta and pulmonary artery trunk and is necessary for the fetal circulation. Failure to close after birth equals a patent ductus arteriosus	Medium–large patent ductus arteriosus: Frequent chest infection Slow feeding Breathlessness on exercise Slow weight gain [1]

Sarah Baker, Royal Devon and Exeter Hospital NHS Foundation Trust

Contd.

Defect	Anatomy and physiology	Signs and symptoms
Coarctation of the aorta	Narrowing in the descending aorta causing restriction of blood flow to the lower regions of the body	Significant difference in upper and lower limb blood pressure Weak or absent femoral pulses Mottled lower body Increased respiratory rate
Tetrology of fallots		
Pulmonary stenosis	Narrowed pulmonary valve. Blood flow to the lungs is restricted	Severe pulmonary stenosis can cause: heart failure respiratory distress cyanosis
Aortic stenosis	Narrowing of the aortic valve. Systemic blood flow is decreased. Left ventricular workload is increased	Poor feeding Heart failure Respiratory distress Low SaO₂
Transposition of the great arteries	The aorta stems from the right ventricle and pulmonary artery from the left ventricle. This causes two completely separate circulations and results in no oxygenated blood reaching the body	Cyanosis Low SaO₂ Respiratory distress Acidosis

Contd.

Defect	Anatomy and physiology	Signs and symptoms
Tetralogy of Fallot	Four defects are present in tetralogy of Fallot: right ventricular outflow tract obstruction enlarged right ventricle overriding aorta ventricular septal defect	Cyanosis Respiratory distress Heart failure 'Spelling' 'Squatting'

Further reading

Farrelly, R. (2000). Systems and diseases: congenital heart disease–1. *Nursing Times*. **96** (24) 47–50.

Horrox, F. (2002). *Manual of neonatal and paediatric heart disease*. Whurr.

Congenital adrenal hyperplasia (adrenogenital syndrome)

Genetic disorder: autosomal recessive; affects boys and girls equally incidence of in 1 in 18 000.

A group of disorders relating to the lack of the enzyme 21-hydroxylase which is needed by the adrenal glands to make the hormones cortisol and aldosterone; leads to an overproduction of androgen. This is a male sex hormone that causes inappropriate appearance of male characteristics.

Symptoms

In girls
- Ambiguous genitalia, enlarged clitoris (internal reproductive organs normal)
- Early appearance of pubic and axillary hair
- Facial hair
- Deep voice
- Failure to menstruate

In boys
- Early development of masculine characteristics; puberty at 2–3 years old
- Well-developed musculature
- Enlarged penis
- Small testes
- Early appearance of pubic and axillary hair

Boys and girls will be tall as children because of accelerated bone growth but short as adults.

Diagnosis

- Decreased blood levels of aldosterone and cortisol
- Raised urinary 17-ketosteroids
- Decreased or normal blood levels of 17-hydroxycorticosteroids
- Raised blood levels of 17-hydroicy progesterone and serum dehydro-epiandrosterone sulphate
- X-ray shows advanced bone age
- Abnormal salt levels in blood and urine
- Genetic testing

Adrenal crisis

- Occurs in extreme forms in the newborn because of salt loss
- Symptoms develop soon after birth
- Vomiting
- Dehydration
- Electrolyte changes
- Cardiac arrhythmias
- Hyponatraemia
- Shock

Gill McEwing, University of Plymouth

reatment and nursing care

Gender of baby determined by karyotyping.
Psychological support for parents, with advice not to state gender of child until determined to avoid embarrassment.
Reconstructive surgery for girls performed at the age of 1–3 months.
Daily cortisol (dexamethasone, fludrocortisone, or hydrocortisone) to maintain normal hormone levels.
Instruction about the need to increase medication if the child is ill or stressed. Not to stop medication suddenly
(→ adrenal insufficiency).
Advice on the side effects of steroid therapy.
Genetic counselling.
Pre-natal diagnosis for some types: chorionic villus sampling.
Newborn screening: heelstick, not widely available.

upport groups

The National Adrenal Disease Foundation ⊡ www.medhelp.org/nadf/
Congenital Adrenal hyperplasia Research, Education, and Support Foundation. www.caresfoundation.com/

Complications

Tumours of testes in men
High blood pressure
Low blood sugar
Side effects of cortisol treatment

Prognosis

Short stature
Men will have normal fertility; women will have a small vaginal opening and reduced fertility
Medication must be continued for life

Further reading

Cull, M.L. (2005). A support group's perspective. *British Medical Journal*, **330**, 341.
www.nlm.nih.gov/medlineplus/ency/article/000411.htm

Mental health

Anorexia nervosa

- Incidence: 0.8–8 in 100 000 individuals per year.
- Peak age of onset: 15–19 years.
- Prevalence: 0.1–1% in adolescents, with a higher prevalence in girls; the ratio of girls to boys is 10 : 1.
- There is a higher prevalence in higher socio-economic classes, in specific groups, e.g. ballet dancers and models, and in the White population of the Western world.

Aetiology

Multifactorial:
- genetic factors
- socio-cultural factors
- familial factors
- physical illness
- sexual abuse
- personality
- neurotransmitters.

Diagnosis

- Body weight 15% below expected weight. BMI (weight (kg)/height^2 (m^2)) >17.5.
- Weight loss self-induced by avoidance of fattening foods and one or more of the following:
  - self-induced vomiting or purging
  - excessive exercise
  - use of appetite suppressants, diuretics, or laxatives.
- Body image disturbance and fear of fatness as an overvalued idea, leading to a self-imposed low weight threshold.
- Amenorrhoea in girls and loss of sexual interest in boys.
- Diagnostic criteria: ICD-10 and DSM-IV.

Physical signs and complications

- Emaciation, with hypotension and bradycardia
- Hypothermia, sensitivity to cold, peripheral cyanosis, and peripheral oedema
- Cardiac arrhythmias, heart failure, and cardiac arrest
- Dehydration, renal failure, and impaired liver and renal functions
- Lanugo hair, osteoporosis, and pathological fractures
- Reproductive system atrophy and infertility
- Constipation, ileus, acute gastric dilatation, delayed gastric emptying, and abdominal pain on eating
- Muscle wasting and proximal myopathy
- Reduced growth and delayed puberty

Chris Taylor, Southampton University Hospitals NHS Trust

Common blood abnormalities

- Hypokalaemia
- Hypoglycaemia
- Metabolic alkalosis
- Hypomagnesaemia
- Hypophosphataemia

- Raised serum amylase
- Low T_3
- Leucopenia
- Low gonadtrophins
- Low gonadal steroids

Management

In-patient management is no longer deemed essential. Out-patient care may yield greater compliance and a similar good outcome at 1 year. Admission should preferably be to a specialist eating disorders unit.

Indications for in-patient management:
- medical: BMI <13.5 kg/m^2, syncope, proximal myopathy, hypoglycaemia, severe electrolyte imbalance, and platelet suppression
- psychiatric: risk of suicide, comorbid impulsive behaviour, breakdown of family/social situation, and failure of out-patient treatment

Priority is to address medical complications:
- full physical examination and blood tests
- NG feeding may be required, but beware of re-feeding syndrome
- strict bed rest initially → programme of gradually increasing activity
- all meals/snacks supervised.

Longer-term aims include:
- restoration of a healthy eating pattern, and gaining insight into and alleviation of contributing psychological factors
- out-patient management involves monitoring weight, supportive nutritional psycho-education, CBT, group work, and family therapy
- the role of psycho-pharmacological treatment is small.

Prognosis

Anorexia nervosa is often a chronic severe disorder in which morbidity and mortality are high. Outcome figures vary between studies. Overall, 50% make a full recovery, 30% have persisting, but not severe, symptoms, and 20% remain ill. Mortality at 20 years is 20%. Cause of death is a direct complication of the eating disorder in 50% of patients; 27% commit suicide.

Further reading

Kaplan, H., Sadock, B. (ed.) (2002). Eating disorders. In *Synopsis of Psychiatry*, 8th edn, pp. 720–31. Waverly.

Lask, B., Bryant-Waugh, R. (ed.) (2000). *Anorexia nervosa and related eating disorders in childhood and adolescence*, 2nd edn. Psychology Press.

Eating disorders helpline (🖥 www.edauk.com).

Bulimia nervosa

Incidence

At some time in their lives, 3 out of every 100 women. Peak age of onset in women is 16–40 years of age. Commonly starts in early or mid twenties. Bulimia nervosa may develop from anorexia nervosa, which has a slightly earlier age of onset.

Aetiology

There is currently no definite known cause of bulimia nervosa.
- Genetic factors
- Familial factors
- Cultural factors
- Physical and sexual abuse
- Psycho-social factors

Diagnosis

Recurrent episodes of binge eating characterized by:
- Eating in a discrete period of time (any 2-hour period) an amount larger than most people would eat during a similar period of time in similar circumstances.
- A sense of lack of control over eating during episodes.
- Recurrent inappropriate compensatory behaviour in order to prevent weight gain, such as self-induced vomiting, use of laxatives, diuretics, or other medications, fasting, or excessive exercise.
- A minimum of two binge-eating episodes and inappropriate compensatory behaviour per week for at least 3 months.
- Self-evaluation is unduly influenced by body shape and weight

Diagnostic criteria: ICD-10 and DSM-1V.

Physical signs and complications
- Binge eating. This involves eating large quantities of fattening food in a very short space of time
- Normal weight (unless associated with anorexia nervosa, when weight is low)
- Irregular periods
- Vomiting and excessive use of laxatives
- Dental decay
- Irregular heart beat, palpitations, and chest pain
- Kidney damage
- Hoarseness and throat bleeding
- Diarrhoea, which leads to loss of minerals and bowel tone; chronic constipation, leading to further laxative dependence
- Acid reflux, chronic regurgitation, stomach pains, and stomach rupture

Management
- Usually out-patient management.
- Priority is to get the sufferer back to a regular pattern of eating. The aim is to maintain a steady weight on three meals a day at regular times, without either starving or vomiting.

Anne Fothergill, University of Glamorgan

Dietician/dietary advice about what constitutes a healthy/balanced diet.
Psychotherapy/counselling, e.g. cognitive–behavioural therapy.
Antidepressant medication: serotonin re-uptake inhibitors (SSRIs).
Self-help: keeping diaries of their disordered eating patterns and
developing self-control.

ooper, P.J. (1995). *Bulimia nervosa and binge eating: a guide to recovery. A self help guide using cognitive behavioural techniques.* Constable and Robinson.

chmidt, U., Treasure, J. (1997). *Getting better bit(e) by bit(e). Survival kit for sufferers of bulimia nervosa and binge eating disorders: clinician's guide.* Psychology Press.

Enuresis

Definition
Enuresis is involuntary voiding of urine at an age when it is reasonable t
expect dryness.

Aetiology
- Genetics
- Developmental delay
- Lack of bladder sensation or decreased bladder capacity
- Psychological factors

Types of enuresis
- Diurnal enuresis: wetting caused by delayed control
- 'Giggle' micturition: child experiences bladder emptying on laughing
- Functional urinary incontinence: result of bladder or sphincter
  dysfunction
- Urge incontinence: caused by detrusor instability
- Lazy bladder syndrome: result of long-standing interrupted and
  incomplete voiding
- Hinman's syndrome: caused by learnt pattern of ineffective voiding and
  considered to be a behavioural problem
- Stress incontinence: wetness after exercise or abdominal straining
- Nocturnal enuresis: primary, the child has never been dry, or
  secondary, child wets again after being dry for 6 months

Effects
- Disrupts families
- Frustration
- Guilt
- Low self-esteem
- Secrecy
- Social stigmatization

Nursing assessment
- Chart baseline volume and frequency of voiding
- Record fluid intake
- Estimate functional bladder capacity
- Note previous UTIs
- Exclude constipation

Medical investigation
- Medical check and urine test
- Assess perineal sensation
- Check lumbo-sacral reflexes
- Inspect external genitalia
- Check spine for subcutaneous lipoma, skin discoloration, or hair
  growth
- Pre-micturition/post-micturition ultrasound scan of renal tract to
  detect abnormalities

Gerri Clay, University of Plymouth

Management

Oxybutynin, an anticholinergic and antispasmodic, reduces daytime wetting for children with detrusor instability.

Prophylactic antibiotics benefit children with recurrent UTIs.

Desmopressin (antidiuretic hormone) is useful for children with nocturnal enuresis.

Alarms more cost effective than pharmacological interventions, with the lowest relapse rate and highest success rate (56% at 12 months) compared with 16% with imipramine and 10% with desmopressin.

Cognitive bladder training teaches children how to void and when to void by means of education, motivation, and biofeedback.

Further reading

Norgaard, J. (1998). Standardization and definitions in lower urinary tract dysfunction in children. British Journal of Urology, **81**(3), 1–6.

Rogers, J. (1998). Nocturnal enuresis should not be ignored. Nursing Standard, **13**(9), 35–8.

Encopresis

Definition
- Encopresis is the repeated passage of faeces into inappropriate places.
- The soiling is developmentally inappropriate, and the child should be at least 4 years old (or equivalent if they have developmental delay).

Subtypes
Retentive
- In the retentive subtype, the child has constipation, with overflow incontinence.
- Typically, this involves the involuntary passage of small amounts of soft faeces into underclothes.

Non-retentive type
- This involves the voluntary passage of normally formed faeces.
- The child is not constipated, and there is no overflow incontinence.
- Faeces are often deposited in prominent places, and rarely into clothing.
- There is a small subgroup of children with non-retentive soiling who have problems with sphincter control and do not recognize the need to defecate in time.

Management
- Children are increasingly being managed in nurse-led clinics.
- The first task is to exclude constipation by taking a careful history.
- A faecal mass may be palpable on abdominal examination, and a plain abdominal X-ray should be considered.
- Educate the child and parents about healthy bowel functioning, including advice on diet, fluid intake, and exercise.
- The family needs a basic toileting programme, which involves regular toileting throughout the day (e.g. after meals), with the child being rewarded for appropriate behaviour. It is vital that the family takes a non-blaming approach to toileting if this is going to be successful.
- Close liaison with the child's class teacher and school is important.
- Laxative medication may be needed if a child does not improve.
- If you suspect that a child has significant emotional and behavioural difficulties, it is worth consulting a child mental health professional (e.g. nurse specialist).
- Associated child mental health problems (e.g. oppositional defiant disorder or anxiety disorders) are more commonly associated with the non-retentive type of encopresis.
- Finally, if it is not possible to resolve the encopresis on an out-patient basis, the child may need short-term admission to a paediatric ward.

Stephen Earnshaw and Andrea O'Donnell, Royal Liverpool Children's Trust (Alder Hey)

urther reading

uchanan, A. (1992). *Children who soil: assessment and treatment.* Wiley, London.

layden, G. *et al.* (2002). Wetting and soiling in childhood. In *Child and adolescent psychiatry*, 4th edn, (ed. M. Rutter and E. Taylor). Blackwell.

oyal College of Psychiatrists, *Mental health and growing up*, 3rd edn. Children who soil or wet themselves. Fact sheet 8. ⌨ www.rcpsych.ac.uk/mentalhealthinformation/mentalhealth problems/physicalillness/childrenwhosoilandwetthemselves.aspx

Depression

Much debate has taken place over recent years as to whether children and young people can experience depression and, if so, whether it manifests itself in different ways to the symptoms experienced by adults. Evidence would suggest that depression is experienced by people in similar ways, regardless of their age.

Major depression refers to one or more periods of depressed mood or loss of interest or pleasure, lasting at least 2 weeks and accompanied by at least four symptoms, including:
- change of appetite or weight loss or gain
- disturbed sleep
- physical agitation or retardation
- fatigue or loss of energy
- feelings of worthlessness or inappropriate guilt
- difficulty concentrating or incisiveness
- recurrent thoughts of death or suicide.

Somatic complaints and social withdrawal are also common among young children, and depression in pre-adolescent children frequently occurs in conjunction with attention deficit–hyperactivity disorders and conduct, anxiety, or eating disorders.

Assessment

Interviewing the young person alone, as well as with a parent/carer, is recommended because parents may be unaware of how their child is feeling. Open questions about mood, participation, and enjoyment of usual activities, relationships with friends and family, and feelings of self-worth are generally asked first, and then additional questions about associated symptoms, such as change in sleeping, eating, and suicidal ideas or intent, and recent life events, stressors, and losses.

Treatment

A useful starting point is explaining to the parent/carer—with the consent of, and in the presence of, the young person—how the child is feeling. This can open up a discussion of the nature of depression, which can be backed up by a booklet or fact sheet. Tailor treatment to the young person and family, perhaps including social and psychological interventions and medication. Social interventions may address sources of distress, reduce opportunities for self-harm, or provide practical help with issues causing distress, such as school examinations. Antidepressants alone are not generally a good idea.

Suicidal behaviour

Suicidal behaviour is rare in children under 12 years of age, but girls are more than four times more likely to attempt suicide than boys. The number of boys who attempt suicide increases after the age of 14 years. Many young people who self-harm do so after arguments with family, friends, and partners. The decision to attempt suicide is often a hasty one, and those who fail in their attempts often regret what they did. However, all attempts should be taken seriously, because 10% of young

Andrea Fairclough, South Devon Youth Offending Team

people who attempt suicide make further attempts. Young people who make an attempt on their life should receive a prompt assessment by a specialist worker.

Further reading

Aggleton, P., Hurry, J., Warwick, I. (2000). *Young people and mental heath.* Wiley.
Schroeder, C., Gordon, B. (2002). *Assessment and treatment of childhood problems: a clinicians guide*, 2nd edn. Guilford Press.
 www.rcpsyth.ac.uk

Deliberate self-harm

Defined as 'self-injurious behaviour without a fatal outcome', commonly by an overdose of tablets or cutting. It can also present as burning, abusing drugs and alcohol, and attempted hanging or strangulation. Also described as 'a way of dealing with difficult feelings'.

Prevalence

It is estimated that 1 in 130, or 446 000 people engage in deliberate self harm each year in the UK; 3–4 times more girls than boys. Self-harm is found most commonly in teenagers and young adults, and is rare under the age of 12 years.

Identifying at-risk adolescents

Multifactorial:

- associated with depression, drug/alcohol abuse, behavioural problems, physical illness, bereavement, and loss
- family difficulties, parental discord, violence, abuse, role models of suicidal behaviour, and mental illness
- bullying, educational difficulties, and models of self-harm in peers/media
- deficits in problem-solving, hopelessness, impulsivity, anger, and hostility.

Motives/reasons

To die, escape from unbearable anguish, get relief, escape from a situation, show desperation to others, change the behaviour of others, to get back at others/make them feel guilty, and mobilize help.

Assessment and management

All children and adolescents who have taken an overdose or engaged in deliberate self-harm should be referred to hospital for medical evaluation, admission, and subsequent assessment by a mental health professional.

- Assessment and management of the current episode
- Identification and management of associated problems
- Identification and promotion of child's/family's resources
- Prevention of repetition

Urgent referral to secondary CAMHS should be considered when there is a high risk of further self-harm or completed suicide. Referral for psychological therapies should be considered.

Summary points (child and family)

- Deliberate self-harm should always be taken seriously, even if suicidal intent is low.
- Steps must be taken to prevent access to methods of self-harming again.
- The adolescent should not be made to feel guilty or rejected.
- The episode should be talked about so that the adolescent feels listened to, not devalued or ridiculed.
- Helplines are available 24 hours a day.

Chris Taylor, Southampton University Hospitals NHS Trust

Further reading

Hawton, K. (1996). Suicide and attempted suicide in young people. In *Adolescent medicine*, (ed. A. McFarlane). Royal College of Physicians, London.
Mental Health Foundation, Self-Harm Factsheet. 🖥 www.mentalhealth.org.uk

Challenging behaviour

Behaviour that, because of its nature or the environment it occurs in, proves difficult for the person caring for the child to manage.

It is usually linked with learning disabilities or mental health but can be witnessed in all fields of nursing.

Behaviours that can be described as challenging:
- abusive, physically or verbally
- destructive
- violent
- unpredictable
- self-harming
- sexual behaviour.

Caring for a child who displays such behaviour can be extremely difficult, no matter how small he/she is.

Some behaviours may be organic, attached to a specific syndrome or condition such as epilepsy or autism.

Communication plays an essential part in managing a child's behaviour. If a child cannot communicate his/her needs or anxieties, his/her frustrations may be vented by behaviour that is seen as unacceptable.

Short-term care
- Talk with parents/carers and agree a care plan for all carers to comply with.
- Try to interpret the child's needs; assess the level of his/her comprehension.
- A total communication approach may be helpful; use verbal communication alongside gestures and objects of reference.
- Explain what is going to happen before it happens; this may need to be done several times for the child to process the information.
- Plan what you are going to do and have everything ready to hand.
- Think ahead. Anticipate situations that may cause the child to react in an unacceptable way and use distraction techniques to prevent an outburst.
- Provide a safe environment for the child and yourself.

Long-term care
- Multidisciplinary team approach, including all those involved with the child's care.
- Comprehensive assessment of the behaviour—is it organic in nature, linked to a condition, specific syndrome, or epilepsy, or is the behaviour learnt?
- Ascertain a baseline from which to work. ABC charts are useful to monitor the occurrence of the behaviour: looking at antecedents to the behaviour and consequences to it and what happens before, during, and after which may reinforce the behaviour, encouraging it to happen again.

Wendy Sanders, Royal Devon and Exeter NHS Foundation Trust

- Agreed care plan, which all involved must work to. This may involve different approaches, such as behaviour modification, cognitive therapy, gentle teaching, or positive-behaviour support.
- Empowerment of the child to manage his/her own behaviour in a socially acceptable way.

Working with challenging behaviour can be very stressful. Nurses must work as a team, supporting each other and recognizing each other's anxieties.

Reflective practice, critical incident analysis, and clinical supervision should be available to all of the team.

Further reading

Harris, J., Hewett, D., Hogg, J. () *Positive approaches to challenging behaviour*. British Institute of Learning Disabilities, London.
www.nau.edu/%7Eihd/positive/ovrvw.html
www.childlink.com.au/behaviours.htm

Attention deficit–hyperactivity disorder (ADHD)

Incidence
- 3–5% of all school-age children suffer from ADHD.
- More common in boys than girls.

Cause
ADHD is a dysfunction of the brain, possibly caused by an imbalance of neurotransmitters, one of which is called dopamine. If the frontal lobe of the brain does not receive enough dopamine, it is unable to process information sent to the brain, which can cause the child to behave inappropriately.

Other possible causes:
- genetic
- smoking during pregnancy can raise incidence by one-third
- low birth weight
- family problems and emotional stress during pregnancy
- having a serious accident during the first month of life
- having surgery within the first month of life.

Symptoms
- Restlessness
- Inattention
- Lack of concentration
- Distraction
- Impulsivity
- Fidgety
- Behavioural problems
- Academic underachievement
- Withdrawn and anxious

The child with ADHD:
- is difficult to care for
- is often in trouble at school and fails to achieve
- lives in a world in constant turmoil, with conflicting sounds and images that he/she finds difficult to process
- presents as naughty and rebellious

Diagnosis
A paediatrician or psychologist will assess the child. For a diagnosis of ADHD the child must meet the following criteria:
- has been showing symptoms for at least 6 months
- symptoms are clearly evident before the age of 7 years
- must have six or more symptoms of inattentive behaviour and/or six or more symptoms of hyperactivity.

Wendy Sanders, Royal Devon and Exeter NHS Foundation Trust

Conners' rating scale is often used to help with a diagnosis. This is a series of questionnaires given to parents and teachers who rate the child's behaviour in different situations.

Treatment

Drug therapy: methylphenidate is commonly used. It is a stimulant drug which increases nerve activity in the brain, enabling the child to concentrate more; behaviour is improved in most cases. The side effects are lack of appetite and difficulties in sleeping. Medication is often used in combination with behavioural therapy.

Prognosis

It is estimated that one-third of all children with ADHD will grow out of it, 7 out of 10 children will still need treatment into their teenage years, and approximately 6 out of 10 of these children will continue to need treatment into adulthood.

Further reading

Holowenko, H. (1999). *Attention deficit/hyperactivity disorder: a multidisciplinary approach*. Jessica Kingsley.

www.besttreatments.co.uk/btuk/conditions/10236.html

http://premium.netdoktor.com/uk/adhd/childhood/behaviour/article.jsp?articleIdent=uk.adhd.childhood.behaviour.uk_adhd_xmlarticle_004621

Autism

Autism is often referred to as a 'spectrum disorder' because the characteristics can be present in a variety of combinations, from quite mild to very severe. Each child is an individual.

The three main areas of disability are:
• communication
• social interaction
• imagination.

Reality for a child with autism can be confusing—a jumble of sounds, images, and movement without sense.
• Their fear, frustration, anxiety, and lack of understanding of what is happening to them can be shown as an outburst of energy and noise.
• 'Naughty' or 'challenging' behaviour, may be the child's response to things and situations he/she does not understand or cannot cope with.

Common behaviours areas follows.
• Good sense of balance, climbing, and jumping.
• Poor sense of balance and wary of unfamiliar surfaces.
• Fussy eaters, self-induced restrictive diets, e.g. mash, ketchup, and junk foods.
• Love of *Thomas the Tank Engine*, in all forms.
• Poor imaginative play, lining up cars, posting out of the window, stacking objects, and twirling things in fingers.
• Ritualistic behaviours; likes routine, but not changes in it.
• Hypersensitive to sensory stimulus (loud noises).
• Will tolerate affection on their terms, so they may come to you for a hug.
• Ecolalia: repeating back what was said to them without necessarily understanding.
• Liking of quiet music.
• Fixations: repetitive play or watching a video and, showing distress when it is finished.
• Loves water play, not necessarily a bath.

How to help a child with autism cope with a hospital stay
• Be aware of the child's special needs; it is unlikely that he/she would cope in a bay, so try to arrange a single room.
• He/she will need constant supervision, and parents need to be offered a break.
• Use any communication aid he/she uses: Makaton sign language, PECs (picture exchange books), objects of reference, body language, and tone of voice. Use simple language to help him/her understand key words.
• Ask the kitchen for foods that he/she is known to enjoy, or ask parents to provide such foods in the short term.
• Find out what comforts him/her.

Alison Hayes, Royal Devon and Exeter NHS Foundation Trust

Further reading

Howe, A. (2000). *The Autism Handbook*. National Autistic Society.

National Autistic Society 🖳 www.nas.org.uk

Public Autism Awareness 🖳 www.paains.org.uk

Anxiety

Anxiety is as much a part of life as eating and sleeping, and can be benefic under the right circumstances. Faced with an unfamiliar challenge, a perso is often spurred by anxiety to prepare for future events. Likewise, anxie or fear and the urge to flee are a protection from danger; anxiety heighter alertness and readies the body for action. However, fears are not norm when they become overwhelming and interfere with daily living.

Anxiety may present in a variety of forms.

• Separation anxiety: excessive anxiety—beyond that expected for the child's age—regarding separation from a significant attachment figure; prevalence is about 4% of children and young people.
• Generalized anxiety: excessive and persistent worry, not focused on any specific object or situation; prevalence about 3%.
• Specific phobias: a persistent fear of particular objects or situations; prevalence about 2–4%.
• Social anxiety: a marked and persistent fear of social or performance situations in which embarrassment may occur; prevalence about 2%.
• Post-traumatic stress: closely linked to anxiety states, although some differences.
• Obsessive–compulsive behaviour: closely linked to anxiety, although some differences; prevalence about 1%.
• School refusal: it is imperative to distinguish school refusal from truancy—peaks at ages 5–6 years, 11 years, and 13–14 years.

Assessment

Common symptoms include:
• unrealistic/excessive worry
• exaggerated startle reactions
• sleep disturbances
• muscle aches
• cold/clammy hands
• fatigue
• dry mouth
• lump in throat
• unrealistic fears
• flashbacks
• ritualistic behaviours
• trembling
• sweating
• dizziness
• tension
• racing heart
• tingling of hands, feet, or other body part
• diarrhoea
• high pulse
• increased breathing rate

Andrea Fairclough, South Devon Youth Offending Team

Questions to ask

To what degree is the anxiety interfering with the child's everyday functioning or causing distress?
Is it realistic that another child of a similar age would be anxious in the same circumstances?
Is the child exhibiting other symptoms?
How are family members responding to the anxiety? Are they unwittingly re-inforcing it?

Treatments

When anxiety symptoms are age and situation appropriate, reassuring parents/carers may be all that is necessary. Parents/carers should be warned that the child's anxiety may worsen when it is confronted, but as the child becomes better able to tolerate the object of fear, the anxiety will lessen. Generally, the child is exposed to the fear situation gradually, with pictures, role play, or at a safe distance, with the parent and child negotiating each stage. Other means of treatment may include:

* psycho-education
* training in monitoring symptomology
* exposure to feared stimuli
* relaxation skills
* cognitive restructuring
* reward systems
* family involvement
* school involvement
* individual work.

Further reading

Aggleton, P., Hurry, J., Warwick, I. (2000). *Young people and mental health*. Wiley,.
Schroeder, C., Gordon, B. (2002). *Assessment and treatment of childhood problems: a clinician's guide*, 2nd edn. Guilford Press.
www.rcpsych.ac.uk.

Conduct/antisocial disorder

All children are defiant at times, and refusing the requests from adults is a normal part of growing up. Conduct disorder is characterized by the persistent failure to control behaviour and the consistent breaking of age appropriate socially defined rules. Behavioural problems often start in early childhood, although for some this is longer lasting and of more concern. Prevalence of conduct disorder is between two and three times higher in boys than girls, with rates estimated between 0.8% and 16%. Substance misuse is often present, and mood, anxiety, and somatization disorders are also common.

Assessment

Complaints about children's behavioural problems are among the most frequent to specialist child and adolescent mental health services. The first consideration is whether such behaviour is 'age appropriate', e.g. is this 'normal naughtiness', or is it causing distress and/or impairment. More behaviours, earlier age of onset, and greater persistence indicate a more serious problem, often associated with ADHD and low school achievement.

Common symptoms include:
- cruelty to animals or people
- frequently bullies or intimidates others, including starting physical fights
- engages in illegal activities
- frequently tells lies
- frequently stays out late/overnight or plays truant before the age of 13 years
- serious violation of rules
- deceitfulness.

Treatment

Once a distinction is made between normal naughtiness and behaviour that cause distress or impairment, professional intervention can be helpful. However, treatment is likely to be most effective before a child is 8 years old, because antisocial habits will be less ingrained, and he/she is unlikely to be part of a deviant peer group. Whatever the underlying cause, multi-agency cooperation is especially important in dealing with conduct problems, because health, education, and social work can make valuable contributions to helping these children and their families. Unfortunately, in practice there are sometimes significant gaps, overlaps, and lack of clarity in service provision. Emphasizing some of the less blaming factors in the development of conduct problems will encourage parents/carers to engage in problem solving with professionals and the young person. Finding out what parents/carers have done that works, can also be affirming and lead to more problem-solving strategies and less blaming.

Oppositional defiance disorder

This is a recurrent pattern of negativistic, defiant, disobedient, and hostile behaviour towards authority figures, which is expressed by persistent stubbornness, resistance to directions, and unwillingness to compromise.

Andrea Fairclough, South Devon Youth Offending Team

ve in, or negotiate with adults or peers. It is sometimes seen as a pre-
ursor of conduct disorder; the age of onset is usually before 8 years and
efore puberty, but about equal afterwards, with prevalence rates of
–16% reported in different studies.

Further reading

ggleton, P., Hurry, J., Warwick, (2000). *People and mental health*. Wiley.
chroeder, C., Gordon, B. (2002). *Assessment and treatment of childhood problems: a clinician's
    guide*, 2nd edn. Guilford Press.
www.rcpsych.ac.uk

Substance misuse

Many young people drink alcohol, smoke cigarettes, and experiment with drugs and solvents for fun, curiosity, or as part of a peer group. Although substance misuse in young people should be considered in the context of 'normal' adolescent risk-taking and experimentation, it can also be symptom of an underlying psychological or social problem that requires treatment, and it can occasionally be fatal, so should be taken seriously.

Assessment

When identifying children's substance-related needs, it is important to establish their level of knowledge and understanding of substances, the level of their usage, and the impact substances have on the young person's life. Information should be gathered holistically through positive engagement, and consideration needs to be given to issues of confidentiality and consent. Awareness of the young person's understanding, in addition to the unpredictability of what may arise and the influence of substances during assessment, need to be taken into account.

Children presenting with substance misuse often do so through the instigation of others and may present with a range of signs and symptoms from each of the following categories.
- Social: family conflict, divorce/separation, deteriorating educational performance, and participation in criminal activity.
- Psychological: mood changes, depression, irritability, psychosis, confusion, and deliberate self-harm.
- Physical: respiratory symptoms (smoking), oral and nasal lesions (inhalation/snorting), physical injury (intoxication), and, in more severe or long-term cases, agitation (prolonged or multi-drug use), needle tracks, thrombosis or abscesses caused by use, and withdrawal symptoms.

Substance misuse can be a symptom of an underlying psychological problem that needs more specialized assessment, including:
- deliberate self-harm (intoxication or overdose, which may not be accidental)
- mood, anxiety, eating, or psychotic disorders
- ADHD
- acute/chronic confusional state.

Treatment

- Encourage children to discuss their substance use with their parents/carers.
- Following identification of substance misuse, provide:
  - targeted education on safe usage and minimization of harm
  - advice and encouragement for reduction and cessation
  - access to services specifically aimed at young people that meet their individual needs.

Debbie Chant, South Devon Youth Offending Team

Refer to an appropriate agency for specialist treatment or assessment if the young person has:
- comorbid severe mental illness
- unstable social circumstances or child protection issues
- abuse of multiple substances
- frequent relapses of substance misuse
- severe physical illness.

Further reading

Britton, J., Noor, S. (2003). *First steps in identifying young people's substance related needs*. Home Office London.

Crome, I., Ghodse, H., Gilvarry, E., McArdle, P. (ed.) (2004). *Young people and substance misuse*. Gaskell.

www.drugscope.org.uk

Children and young people with chronic illness/disability

Key principles in caring for a child with complex needs

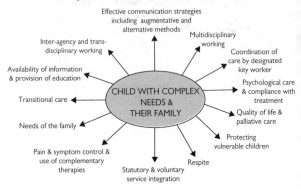

Caring for a child with complex needs.

Further reading

Townsley, R., Abbott, D., Watson, D. (2004). *Making a difference? Exploring the impact of multi-agency working on disabled children with complex health care needs, their families and the professionals who support them.* Hobson.

While, A., Forbes, A., Ullman, R., Lewis, S., Mathes, L., Griffiths, P. (2004). Good practices that address continuity during transition from child to adult care: synthesis of the evidence. *Child Care, Health and Development,* **30**(5), 439–52.

▣ www.jrf.org.uk

Debbie McGirr, Napier University, Edinburgh

Psychological effects of long-term illness: child, parents, and siblings

The diagnosis of a long-term illness has a profound effect upon the child, parents, and siblings. There can be feelings of loss, isolation, and being different; being treated as special, while craving normality. The child, parents, and siblings will have common and individual needs and concerns that must be addressed positively and realistically in an attempt to maintain family integrity and hope for the future.

Child

- Loss of identity; may be labelled, e.g. diabetic
- Socialization affected because the child is unable to participate in usual activities
- Absence from school leads to anxiety regarding academic work and isolation from friends
- Fears and concerns regarding future
- Fears
  - being different, e.g. having to leave class to administer medicine
  - disability
  - death
- Need to learn about condition and take responsibility for compliance with treatment regimes when appropriate

Parents

- Can feel frustrated in their role as protector/advocate for their child
- Need to keep responsibility for overall care of child, not only health care
- Can be concerned regarding discipline issues; important for child's security but should reflect child's health status
- Want professionals to treat the child as special, but also crave normality
- Family and social relationships can suffer because of awkwardness of all parties in not knowing what to say
- Holidays, outings, social activities, etc. can be affected, reducing time that the family can spend together

Siblings

- Can feel very protective of affected sibling
- Can be isolated if parents have the mistaken belief that absence, actual or psychological, can be made up later; excessive time spent with their ill child can cause deep-seated resentment
- Anxiety and loneliness can be profound, which is increased if exposed to rumour, gossip, and bullying
- Being excluded from situations, to protect them, can exacerbate problems
- Schooling may suffer because of anxiety and lack of parental support resulting from the demands of the affected child's condition

Irene McTaggart, University of Dundee

▶ There is no right thing to say! All family members should be encouraged to talk to one another, while professionals should enquire about the concerns and well-being of the whole family, not only the affected child.

Further reading

Cooper, C. (1999). *Continuing care of sick children; examining the impact of chronic illness.* Quay Books.

Goodley, D., Lawthorn, R. (ed.) (2005). *Disability and psychology: a reader.* Palgrave Macmillan.

Chronic pain in children

Acute pain associated with injury or following surgery usually disappears once healing has taken place, whereas chronic pain persists beyond this time span and may last several months or years. The pain can be persistent or recurrent, with fluctuations in severity, quality, regularity, and predictability. Children with chronic pain may suffer from poor quality of life, isolation from peers, sleep disturbance, and anxiety.

Common chronic pain conditions in children include:
- reflex sympathetic dystrophy
- headache
- abdominal pain
- neuropathic pain
- hip and knee pain
- pain associated with disease progression.

Aim of treatment

Early intervention is necessary. For some children, there is no medication or treatment to cure their pain. The aim of chronic pain management is to empower the child and family to manage their pain through psychological interventions, such as coping strategies; complete pain relief is not always the primary goal. A multidisciplinary team approach, involving psychology and physiotherapy, is necessary.

Assessment

- Comprehensive history and examination of child (exclude underlying disease).
- Pain assessment (note quality, quantity, intensity, location, and duration of pain).
- What makes the pain worse? What relieves the pain?
- Effect of pain on child's sleep, mood, appetite, and school performance.
- Past experiences of pain.

Range of treatments

Treatments are conventional and complementary; the physical pain cannot be treated in isolation. It is important to use a holistic, individual, and multimodal approach, taking into account the child's pain and family dynamics.
- Simple analgesics, such as paracetamol, and NSAIDs
- Opioids
- Tricyclic antidepressants and anticonvulsant agents
- Antispasmodic agents
- Sympathetic and peripheral nerve blocks
- Cognitive behavioural techniques, relaxation, and guided imagery
- Topical creams and heat therapy
- TENS and acupuncture
- Massage and reflexology
- Physiotherapy, graduated exercises, and hydrotherapy
- Parental and child education

Denise Jonas, University of Salford

Management
- Comprehensive plan of care, with long-term and short-term goals.
- Use the least invasive methods possible.
- Regular re-assessment of child's pain.
- Liaise with school services.
- Regular evaluation of effectiveness of treatment.
- Clear support plan for parents, with strategies for crisis events.

Munafo, M., Trim, J. (2000). *Chronic pain. A handbook for nurses.* Butterworth-Heinemann.
www.bath.ac.uk/pain-management/adolescent_service.htm

Transition from paediatric to adult services

Transitional care: 'the purposeful and planned movement of adolescents and young adults from child-centred to adult-orientated healthcare systems'. Transition involves the patient and his/her family and caregivers. Problems relating to transfer can occur for any of these groups.

- Problems for the young adult patient:
  - will be leaving a team they know well
  - may have to accept a new hospital, as well as new staff
  - will be expected to meet the professionals without their parents being present
  - may find an adult ward a very different environment, with more rigid rules (such as visiting) and older patients.
- Problems for the parents:
  - may feel excluded by the adult team
  - lose friendships and support from the paediatric team they have known over many years
  - fear how the child will manage without them.
- Problems for the paediatric team:
  - may feel a sense of loss for the patient that they have cared for and nurtured for many years.
- Problems for the adult team:
  - may feel adversely judged on any differences in approach to treatment
  - may be blamed by parents if there is deterioration in health.

What is needed for a successful transition

- A formal transition programme that includes planning care for all involved: patient, family, and paediatric and adult teams.
- An appropriate place to be transferred to.
- Flexible age of transfer: usually somewhere between 16 and 18 years of age. Disease stage and progress should be considered when deciding on the right time.
- The paediatric and adult teams need to work together and maintain good communication before, during, and after transition.
- There should be the opportunity to attend joint clinics between the paediatric team and the adult team.
- The young person should have the opportunity to visit the adult service facilities.
- In-patients require both appropriate environment and staff to meet their special needs.
- Young people need facilities that instill independence and allay boredom.

Further reading

Pownceby, J. (1996). *The Coming of Age Project: A study of the transition from paediatric to adult care and treatment adherence amongst young people with cystic fibrosis*. Cystic Fibrosis Trust.
RCN (2004). *Adolescent transition care: guidance for nursing staff*. RCNPublications.
🖳 www.rcn.org.uk/publications/pdf/adolescenttransitioncare.pdf

Sarah Elworthy, Royal Devon and Exeter NHS Foundation Trust

Respite care

Respite, or carers' breaks, can be defined as giving a carer a short break from the child or young person they care for, and the cared-for person break from them, which can be equally as important. There should be positive benefits for both.

When a family has a child with disability, caring for him/her at home can be a totally consuming role.

- Simple tasks, such as shopping or ironing, which are considered easy, can become almost impossible.
- It is extremely difficult to sustain the level of care required over a long period of time without the main carer becoming run down and exhausted.
- Parents often cope alone from day to day; this can be very isolating and not good for the child, especially because many children have single parents.
- Regular carers' breaks enable the family to continue caring for their child at home.
- To enable the family to give quality time to siblings. Within the family, the needs of the child with disability take precedence over the other children's needs, although parents are usually aware of this and try hard for this not to happen.

Parents of a child with disability are assessed by social services to determine their needs and those of the child; together they decide how best their needs can be met.

- The break can be provided in their own home or in a residential setting, depending on the needs of the child and family.
- This can be provided through the NHS, social services, or a private organization.
- Breaks can vary from a few hours each month to couple of weeks each year so that the family can go on holiday.
- Whatever is decided, ideally it should be a gradual process of introduction to this provision for the child, to reduce any anxieties he/she may have and for the new carers to get to know him/her.

Asking for help is difficult for parents, because they see it as a sign of failure; every effort should be made to support them. Once parents have experienced a break, they will realize the benefits to themselves and their child and continue to use this service.

Further reading
www.elsc.org.uk/briefings/briefing05
www.mencap.org.uk/

Wendy Sanders, Royal Devon and Exeter NHS Foundation Trust

Compliance/non-compliance with treatment

Definition

Compliance is seen as obeying, fulfilling, meeting terms, acting in accordance with, conforming to, abiding by, or submitting to the desires c professionals involved in care delivery. It implies an uneven relationship where the power base rests with the professionals involved, and children and their families defer to the decisions made by them regarding care o delivery of services. Non-compliance is recognized as a strategy for resistance by children and parents.

Motivation for compliance

- Belief that professionals know best
- Wish to secure services or custody arrangements
- Belief that there is no alternative
- Feelings of dependency upon the healthcare team

Reasons for non-compliance

- Resistance to diagnosis and/or treatment
- Child and/or parents wish to be partners in care
- Desire for their expertise, concerns, and opinions to be taken seriously
- Child dislikes treatment method, e.g. taste of medication, inability to swallow tablets, and discomfort related to physiotherapy
- Parents feel guilty if child is upset or suffering discomfort
- Parents feel ill-prepared to perform aspects of care required of them

Compliance is not always positive; children and parents have the right to make choices and decisions regarding treatment and care, while healthcare professionals are not infallible.

Recommendations

Children and parents are more likely to comply if they trust the professionals they are in contact with, rather than following a route of non-compliance that may be unknown to the professional and be detrimental to the child.

- Include the child and parents in decision-making processes, while providing them with support.
- Educate the child and parents, to enable them to be confident in participating in any technical care required of them.
- Give the child and parents an opportunity to ask questions, which should be answered honestly.
- Do not be afraid to admit you do not know answers, but make sure that you find out for them.
- Information is power—do not be afraid to share it with the child and parents, because they are more likely to comply if they know the reasons for your advice.

Irene McTaggart, University of Dundee

The child and his/her family may still take a non-compliant stance, but should trust you enough to make you aware of their actions and discuss their reasons for it.

Further reading

Alderson, P. (2000). *Young children's rights: exploring beliefs, principles and practice*. Jessica Kingsley.
Pendleton, D. et al. (2000). The compliance conundrum in cystic fibrosis. *Journal of Royal Society of Medicine*, **93** (suppl. 38), 9–13.

Working with the multidisciplinary team

In an age and culture where good health is taken for granted, it expected that children will remain well and survive their parents, bu there are many diseases that compromise the life expectancy of children with some 10–15% of children under 16 years of age being affected b chronic long-term conditions. These children face a lifetime of hospita appointments, diagnostic tests, and sometimes painful procedures. It also important to remember that a child's illness will affect every member of the family, who have a vital role in the integrated care of the child

Disease management

• Comprehensive
• Integrated approach to care
• Reimbursement based on the natural course of a disease

It requires a management approach that brings together:
• research evidence
• best practice
• inter-professional and inter-agency working
• continuity of care for individual patients
• structured coordination of care over time and across primary, secondary, and tertiary settings

Multidisciplinary teams are ideally suited to develop, lead, and implement evidence-based disease management programmes, because they have an essential role in the preventive, diagnostic, and therapeutic decisions for patients throughout the course of their disease.

ACT have developed a strategy in their integrated pathway for palliative care that encompasses the needs of all children with a chronic disorder In this, as their third standard, they state that 'every child should receive a multi-agency assessment of their needs as soon as possible after diagnosis or recognition, and should have their needs reviewed at appropriate intervals'. Their strategies emphasize the importance of a key worker to coordinate this multi-agency care plan.

Satisfaction for families and professionals can be achieved when members from all the involved agencies attend the multidisciplinary meetings. Everyone in the team knows the progress of all other teams, and the key worker is able to coordinate care very easily.

Further reading

ACT (2004). Integrated multi-agency care pathways for children with life-threatening and life-limiting conditions. www.act.org.uk

Jackie Imrie, Central Manchester and Manchester Children's Hospitals NHS Trust

'Contact a Family'

- Information for families and professionals across the UK who care for children with any disability or medical condition.
- A useful resource providing information to professionals, to enable them to advise and support families of children with disabilities.

What information do families need?

Medical information

The condition and its effect on their child and the information needed to care for their child, e.g. advice on physical lifting, managing difficult behaviour, and therapies to maximize their child's potential.

Welfare information

Access to financial benefits, educational support, short breaks, equipment, child care, leisure activities, etc.

Psychosocial support

To help them manage and adjust emotionally:
- Meet others through local groups where they share information, find solutions to common problems, and provide each other with practical and emotional support → empowerment and reducing isolation.
- The national condition support groups provide more specific information relating to the child's condition.
- The groups' newsletters have articles on how to overcome problems posed by the child's specific condition.
- Through these articles, parents hear how other families cope, and this can serve as a role model, giving them confidence that they too can cope.

Contact a Family provides

Medical information

Contact a Family directory of specific conditions and rare disorders, as well as signposting families to appropriate national condition support groups.

Welfare information

Free-phone helpline, written fact sheets, and national, regional, and London-based offices, and its network of parent volunteer representatives. Contact a Family can also help families find out where to access local support.

Psychosocial support

By putting families in touch with other families, through either local multi-disability parent groups, national condition support groups, or, in the case of a rare condition, linking families direct. Contact a Family can also support local groups and, in some areas, provide newsletters and workshops.

Helping families of disabled children to access information and support

Contact a Family can provide posters and samples of their fact sheets to display in clinics and other settings where families of disabled children go.

Sheila Davies, Contact a Family London

amilies are more likely to access support when suggested by a profes-
ional.

To order Contact a Family material: telephone 020 7608 8700 or email
nfo@cafamily.org.uk

Useful addresses

ree-phone helpline: 0808 808 3555; open Monday to Friday 10 a.m.–4 p.m.
or parents or professionals, language line available: text phone 0808 808
8556

Contact a Family website. 🖥 www.cafamily.org.uk

Email: help@cafamily.org.uk

All information is provided to families free of charge.

Palliative care

Breaking bad news

Breaking bad news is a task that most professionals have little experience with and find incredibly difficult. How this news is given will affect the adjustment and future coping mechanisms of the recipients.

Bad news = any information that adversely and seriously affects an individual's view of their future.

- Its impact depends on the gap between the patient's expectations and the reality of the situation.
- Religion, ethnicity, culture, and previous experiences of both patient and staff will affect how the information is given and received.
- Usually the doctor gives the information; this should be someone who will have ongoing involvement in the patient's care.
- The primary nurse should attend the interview: this enables you to support the family after the event and feed back to colleagues, because you will have knowledge of what information was given and the terminology used.
- Rarely will the recipient remember all the information given, so things may have to be repeated.
- Parents should be told together so they receive the same information and can support each other.

Although there are guidelines on how to break bad news, the approach used will need to be adapted on an individual basis.

Several steps are suggested for professionals to progress through when breaking bad news:

- Adequate preparation.
  - Time in a place that offers privacy and no interruptions.
  - Conduct interviews sitting down and face to face, without any physical barriers. This indicates that there is time to talk and eye contact can be maintained.
  - Introduce yourself to the family, if not already known, and ask family members how they wish to be addressed.
- Establish what the patient/parent already knows by asking questions.
  - It is important to know what information the family knows and what their needs are.
- Give a warning shot, e.g. 'The test results are back and they are not as good as we hoped'.
  - This may reduce the shock and allows the recipients to prepare for what they are about to be told.
- Breaking the news.
  - Avoid medical jargon.
  - Take cues on how to continue by observing the recipients' reactions.
  - Most families respond better to honesty; this strengthens the relationship between professional and patient.
  - Reassurance should be given that everything is being done, but false optimism should not be given.
  - Non-verbal cues will be picked up, in addition to what is said.

Jenny Freeman, Royal Devon and Exeter NHS Foundation Trust

Time for questions and to vent feelings.
- Patients may display a variety of reactions.
- It is important that time is given for feelings to be expressed and questions to be asked.

Further support.
- Before concluding the interview, the patient/parent must be aware of the plan for the future.
- Written advice should be given to support verbal information.

Further reading

Dias, L., Bruce, A., Lynch, T., Penson, R. (2003). Breaking bad news: a patient's perspectives. *Oncologist*, **8**(6), 587–96.

Kay, P. (1996). *Breaking bad news; a ten step approach*. EPL Publications.

Children, young people, and bereavement

Misconceptions
- Infants and toddlers are too young to grieve.
- Children should not attend funerals.
- If children do not cry, or say they are sad, they are not affected by the death.
- Not talking about the deceased to the children will diminish their sense of grief.

Children's responses to bereavement
A child's response depends on a number of factors, including:
- the nature of the relationship with the deceased person
- their age and understanding of death
- previous experience of serious illness and death
- the circumstances of the death
- their culture, religion, and personality
- the overall impact on the family unit, and their response and attitude.

Children's understanding of death at different ages
0–2 years
- Experience is of separation.
- No understanding of death.

2–5 years
- Death is seen as temporary, reversible, and like sleep. Dead people still have feelings and bodily functions.
- Death may be avoidable.

5–9 years
- Complete understanding of death being finite and permanent by age of 7 years.
- Keen to have factual details.
- Concern for others and themselves.

10 years to adolescence
- Long-term understanding of death and its consequences in terms of loss and adjustment. Able to reflect on life and death.
- Role within family/confused identity.

Signs of grief in children
- Sleep difficulties
- Disruptive behaviour
- Regressive behaviour (e.g. bedwetting)
- Anxiety
- Guilt—sense of responsibility for the death
- Sadness, longing, and anger
- Acting out death scene
- Psychosomatic disorders

Alison Tait, University College London Hospitals NHS Trust

Children need

Age-appropriate factual clear information.

Adults who are not afraid to use words such as death, dying, or died, and to explain what they mean.

Opportunities to ask questions (using open questions).

Avenues to express their thoughts and feelings: talking, drawing, and playing.

Advice on how to deal with reactions from their friends and family.

A break from grief-stricken relatives.

Their thoughts, questions, and feeling to be taken seriously.

To be involved and included.

A routine to cope with the adjustments and secondary losses.

Reassurance that the death is not their fault and that they are still loved.

Be aware

- Children often think that they have caused the illness or death.
- Without the appropriate information, they tend to imagine it to be far worse that it is.
- They may take what is said very literally, e.g. if talking about the body, they may worry what has happened to the head.
- Children try to protect their parents, just as their parents try to protect them.
- Expressions such as 'sleeping forever' can be hugely misinterpreted and damaging to the child in the long term.

Further reading

Dickenson, D., Johnson, M. (ed.) (1993). *Death, dying and bereavement*. Open University Press.
www.winstonswish.org.uk

What happens when a child or young person is dying

Physiological aspects

- Thready or thumping pulse; peripheral shutdown
- Large fluid loss, usually *per rectum*
- Adrenaline surge (unusual, but could involve suddenly sitting up when previously comatosed)
- Slow laboured breathing (2–6 breaths/min)/Cheyne–Stokes breathing
- Confusion/hallucinations

Practical aspects

- Individualized care is paramount.
- Ensure resuscitation status is discussed and documented.
- Prepare the family for all possible situations as death approaches (e.g. ?fitting/?lose consciousness/?bleeding).
- Encourage honesty within the family and with the dying child/young person.
- Support the family in telling other family and friends; they may need help and guidance in what to say (especially to siblings).
- Ensure privacy if possible: cubicle and time alone.
- Discuss supportive care (e.g. observations and blood products) within the medical/nursing team and with the family.
- Consider the family's religion. Is it appropriate for members of the hospital chaplaincy team to visit and support the family?
- Include and support the whole team on the ward. It may be the first paediatric death for at least one of the team (this may well be the doctor). Include the cleaning/domestic staff on the ward as part of the team.
- Inform the GP and health visitor of the child's death.

Emotional aspects

- Increased emotional stress in those dealing with palliative situations, giving rise to feelings of acute helplessness, inadequacy, and powerlessness.
- Awakens issues within us, and forces us to look at losses in our own lives.
- Forces us to examine our beliefs and views around own death.
- Loss of professional independence, with blurred boundaries.
- It is important to acknowledge that dealing with a dying child is incredibly draining for all those involved. It takes courage to be in the medical/nursing team supporting the child/family.
- Do not underestimate the impact that a child or young person's death may have on you; seek professional support.

Further reading

📖 www.cancer.org/docroot/NWS/content/NWS_2_1x_Discussing_Death_with_a_Dying_Child.as
📖 www.lpch.org/DiseaseHealthInfo/HealthLibrary/terminallyill/needs.html
📖 www.beachpsych.com/pages/cc87.html

Alison Tait, University College London Hospitals NHS Trust

Palliative care

Palliative care for children with life-limiting conditions is an active and total approach to care, embracing physical, emotional, social, and spiritual elements.

Palliative care for children and their families diagnosed with any life-limiting disorder starts at diagnosis, as the family come to terms with the news. Often the child has few symptoms and support is primarily emotional and social. Throughout subsequent years, whether a few or several decades, it is important to ensure that the child and family receive optimum care as and when needed.

Whatever the condition—cancer, neurodegenerative disease, HIV, etc.—palliative care needs are often the same.

Pain

Cognitive, behavioural, and emotional factors modify children's pain perception, so optimal pain control for children in palliative care requires drug and non-drug therapies.

Seizures

Although not all children develop seizures, they can be a major problem. Cataplexy (common in some neurodegenerative diseases) can usually be controlled; the drug of choice is imipramine.

Complex seizures can be very difficult to control, with the child often prescribed more than one anticonvulsant medication.

Swallowing problems

Swallowing difficulties invariably occur. Initially, drooling can be a problem because secretions are not swallowed and can be inhaled. This runs alongside difficulty with eating and choking episodes. NG or gastrostomy feeding is invariably needed. Excess secretions can be a problem. Hyoscine patches can be helpful in drying these up once the child is not eating. Alternatively glycopyrulate can be given via the gastrostomy.

Dementia

A major symptom that families find hard to cope with is dementia in the young person. The child gradually loses cognitive skills and so will not respond to behavioural therapies that may work in children with learning difficulties. The child may also have mood swings and behavioural disturbances that can be difficult to cope with. It is often at this stage that the family may gain support from a children's hospice.

Adolescents

It is important to recognize that these young people have their own issues, and palliative care needs to address the psychological issues that they face.

Jackie Imrie, Central Manchester and Manchester Children's University Hospitals NHS Trust

Further reading

McGrath, P.J., Finley, G.A. (1996). Attitudes and beliefs about medication and pain management in children. *Journal of Palliative Care*, **12**(3), 46–50.

Thornes, R. (2001). Palliative care for young people aged 13–24. ACT: 🖳 www.act.org.uk/act/start.asp

🖳 www.oxfordchips.org.uk/Palliative_Care.asp

High-dependency care

Assessing airway safety

Assessment of the airway

Initially, assess the child's responsiveness by asking 'Are you alright?' or applying a gentle painful stimulus. Although a meaningful reply may not be immediately forthcoming, the child who is crying or talking has some degree of airway patency and ventilation.

Assess airway patency by a look, listen, and feel approach. Place your ear over the child's nose, with your cheek over the mouth and look down towards the child's chest.

• *Look* for movement and symmetry of the chest/abdomen
• *Listen* for breath sounds/stridor
• *Feel* for expired breaths

Airway obstruction may be partial or complete and occurs at any level from the nose and mouth down to the trachea. Causes include:

• displaced tongue—unconsciousness, cardiopulmonary arrest, or trauma
• fluid—vomit, secretions, and blood
• foreign body
• laryngeal oedema—anaphylaxis or infection
• bronchospasm—asthma, foreign body, or anaphylaxis
• trauma
• pulmonary oedema—cardiac failure, anaphylaxis, or near-drowning

Whatever the cause of airway obstruction, prompt recognition and effective management are essential. Simple measures are usually all that are needed to open the airway, such as suction to remove secretions, head tilt/chin lift/jaw thrust manoeuvres, or insertion of a pharyngeal airway.

If the child is not breathing, his/her tongue may have fallen back, obstructing the pharynx. The airway can be opened using the head tilt/chin lift manoeuvre:

• Placing one hand on the child's forehead, gently tilt the head back.
• Place the fingers of your other hand under the child's chin and lift upwards.
• Care must be taken not to compress the soft tissues under the chin.
• A 'neutral' position in an infant and 'sniffing' position in a child are recommended (see figure).

The head tilt/chin lift manoeuvre is contraindicated in trauma because of suspected cervical spine injury, and in this instance the jaw thrust manoeuvre is recommended.

• Place two or three fingers of each hand under each side of the child's jaw and lift upwards (see figure).

Re-assess the success of the airway opening manoeuvre with a look, listen, and feel approach, as described above. The airway may need to be secured with a pharyngeal airway.

  Summon senior experienced help immediately because intubation may be necessary.

Ruth Trengove, South Devon Healthcare NHS Trust

patent airway does not ensure adequate ventilation. Deliver high-flow O_2 at 10–15 l/min via a face mask and non-rebreathe reservoir bag, which allows high concentrations of O_2 (up to 100%) to be delivered. If the child has a slow rate and weak respiratory effort, O_2 should be delivered and respiration supported via a bag–valve–mask device.

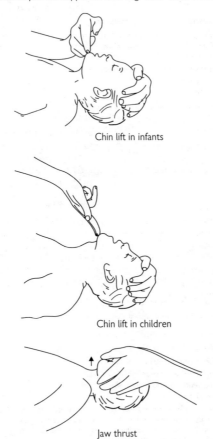

Chin lift in infants

Chin lift in children

Jaw thrust

Further reading

Advanced Life Support Group (2005). *Advanced paediatric life support: the practical approach*, 4th edn. Blackwell Publishing, London.

Jevon, P. (2004). *Paediatric advanced life support: a practical guide*. Butterworth Heinemann, London.

Assisting with tracheal tube intubation

Action	Rationale
1. Prepare for tracheal tube intubation	Whatever the indication, tracheal tube intubation should be carried out in a systematic controlled fashion
All necessary staff aware of impending intubation	
Appropriate tracheal tube intubation-sized equipment checked and ready	
Laryngoscope, blade, and handle: check that bulb is bright	
Infants: *straight blade*	The size of the blade depends on the size of the child
Children: *curved*	
Tracheal tube + one smaller	Tracheal tube tube size is critical for being able to ventilate optimally
Soft suction catheters (2 × tracheal tube width)	Term infants require 3.0 mm or 3.5 mm tracheal tube
Rigid suction catheter	1-year-old requires 4.0 mm tracheal tube
Oral and nasal airways	Above 2 years age use tracheal tube formula: 4 + age/4
Magill forceps	Uncuffed tracheal tube used in <8-year-olds because the narrowest portion of a young child's larynx is the cricoid, compared with the glottis in adults
Pre-cut tape to secure tube	
NG/orogastric tube	
Patent IV access	
Stethoscope	
Induction drugs to be used	
Paralysing/anaesthetic/analgesic	
Bag–valve–mask device with O_2	
Suction apparatus	
Monitoring equipment: ECG monitor, pulse oximeter, and CO_2 monitor	
Checked ventilator and circuit with humidification	
2. Once all equipment and drugs checked and intubating practitioner ready, position the infant/child supine, with the head positioned to open airway	Appropriate placement of the head allows for easier visualization of the epiglottis and vocal cords
Infant: *neutral*	
Child: *'sniffing'* (a folded towel under the head may facilitate positioning)	

Marion Aylott and Sarah Reed, University of Southampton

Contd.

Action	Rationale
If a cervical-spine injury is suspected, the neck should be stabilized in a neutral position	
3. Ideally an infant/child should be NBM for 4–6 hours prior to intubation. An NG/orogastric tube tube should be placed and stomach contents aspirated and discarded prior to intubation	NBM status or aspiration of gastric contents ↓risk of emesis and aspiration. A NG/orogastric tube is also useful to prevent insufflation of the stomach with air during bag–valve–mask procedure
4. Throughout procedure, monitor the child; inform intubating practitioner of bradycardia/desaturation	Instigate timely pre-oxygenation with bag–valve–mask to prevent hypoxia
5. Once the intubating practitioner has positioned the tracheal tube, note its length at the lips	Provides record for future tracheal tube intubation and detection of dislodgement
6. Assist the intubating practitioner with auscultation of breath sounds bilaterally over chest and stomach, while intubating provides ventilation via tracheal tube. Attach CO_2 monitor if available	Confirm TT placement until definitive tracheal tube chest X-ray obtained
7. Once tracheal tube confirmed, assist the intubating practitioner by securing tracheal tube in place using pre-cut tapes according to local protocol	↓ Risk of accidental extubation
8. Obtain chest X-ray	Formal and accurate confirmation of tracheal tube placement

Further reading

Advanced Life Support Group (2004). *Advanced paediatric life support: the practical approach*, 4th edn. Blackwell.

evon, P. (2004). *Paediatric advanced life support: a practical guide*. Butterworth Heinemann.

Insertion of a nasopharyngeal airway

Action	Rationale
1. Assess child's need to have the procedure undertaken	Need to establish artificial passage by separating the posterior pharyngeal wall from the tongue for airflow
2. Do *not* use if basal skull fracture suspected or evidence of coagulopathy	In basal skull fracture NP airway may penetrate cranial fossa. If coagulopathy exists, trauma to nasopharynx is likely to → haemorrhage
3. Position the infant/child supine, with a small blanket or towel roll under shoulders if necessary	Enable ease of insertion and correct placement
4. Select the correct size naso-pharyngeal airway; ~half the width nostril or diameter of child's little finger (sometimes a shortened ET tube is used)	Must be of a width that does not cause of sustained blanching of the alae nasae
5. Estimate correct length by measuring from the tip of nose to tragus of ear	Too short: ineffective Too long: intubation of oesophagus → distension and hypoventilation
6. Prior to insertion, ▶ secure a safety pin in to flange. If using a shortened ET tube, reattach blue connector	Prevent inadvertent inhalation of the airway
7. ◆ Lightly lubricate airway with K-Y jelly	Aid insertion; reduce risk of trauma
8. Insert airway gently through nostril in a posterior direction, perpendicular to the plane of the infant/child's face	Prevent accidental trauma and position appropriately
9. Continue to maintain correct alignment of airway and chin lift as necessary	Malposition of the infant/child's head will still obstruct the airway
10. Reassess airway and check for patency by assessment of adequate ventilation	To maintain adequate ventilation
11. Document event, including size of airway, length inserted, nostril used, and condition of alae nasae	Maintain documentation

Further reading

Advanced Life Support Group (2000). *Advanced paediatric life support: the practical approach.* BM
Jevon, P. (2004). *Paediatric advanced life support: a practical guide.* Butterworth Heineman, Londo
Resuscitation Council (UK) (2006). *Paediatric basic life support guidelines.* Resuscitation Coun
(UK), London: 🖳 www.resus.org.uk

Marion Aylott, University of Southampton

Assessing respiratory effectiveness

Action	Rationale
1. Determine respiratory effectiveness	
The hallmark of nursing care is assessment, monitoring, and evaluation	Once these three steps are completed, you must act on your findings. Monitor the trends of parameters because one particular measurement is more meaningful when compared with previous measurements
2. Wash hands	↓ Risk of cross infection
3. Gather supplies:	Avoid unnecessary interruption
Stethoscope	
Saturation monitor	
4. Without the child knowing, observe and count the respiratory rate over 60 s. Normal range: 12–40 breaths min depending upon age	▶▶ Awareness that breathing is being counted is likely to affect rate
	Assessment over 60 s is important in infants <6 months of age because ot periodic breathing
	Rate >60 is indicative of hypoxia
	Breathing rate alone does not provide sufficient information. Consider quality of breathing
5. Prior to hands-on respiratory assessment, explain procedure as appropriate for child's age and understanding, and parents if present	To enable self-regulatory behaviours
6. Observe respiratory depth. Stand at the child's head or feet and look down their midline. Note symmetry/asymmetry	Assess presence and equality of chest rise and fall incorporating the abdomen in children <8 years
It may be necessary to palpate respiratory movements if breathing is shallow. Place the palmar surface of each hand flat against the child's chest or back with thumbs in midline along the lower costal margin	Hands will move with the chest wall excursion
7. Auscultate lung field to determine whether breath sounds are: normal, abnormal, diminished, absent, or adventitious	Diminished or absent breath sounds are *always* abnormal. Report immediately. Monitoring the presence/absence of adventitious sounds guides therapeutic intervention

Marion Aylott, University of Southampton

Contd.

Action	Rationale
8. Assess work of breathing (WOB): Recession: intercostals, subcostal, substernal, clavicular, and suprasternal Accessory muscle use: nasal flaring, tripod positioning, and head bobbing	Work of breathing is an important clinical indicator of severity of respiratory compromise
9. If concerned, measure SaO_2. Report if <92% in air or <95% in O_2	◆ Mucous membrane and skin colour are unreliable SaO_2 <92% indicates hypoxia
10. Consider each of these findings in the light of the child's behaviour, conscious level, and haemodynamic variables	Any measure does not provide sufficient information in isolation
11. Document observations and repeat as indicated by intervention and child's condition	Maintain accurate records and provide a point of reference in the event of any queries

Further reading

Evans, D., Hodgkinson, B., and Berry, J. (1999). *Vital signs: a systematic review No. 4.* Joanna Briggs Institute: 🖥 www.joannabriggs.edu.au

Rajesh, V.T., Singh, S., and Kataria, S. (2000). Tachypnoea is a good indicator of hypoxia in acutely ill infants under 2 months. *Archives of Disease in Childhood*, **82**, 46–9.

Simoes, E.A., Roark, R., Berman, S., Esler, L.L., Murphy, J. (1991). Respiratory rate: measurement of variability over time and accuracy of different counting periods. *Archives of Disease in Childhood*, **66**(10), 1199–20.

Assessing perfusion

Action	Rationale
1. Assess need: monitoring tissue perfusion is important for early recognition of circulatory failure and in assessing response to therapy	Tissue survival depends on both oxygenation and the blood flow (perfusion) through the capillary bed
2. Wash hands	↓Risk of cross-infection
3. Explain procedure as appropriate for child's age and understanding, and parents if present	Enables self-regulatory behaviours and promotes partnership with family
4. Prior to assessment, consider the recent and current thermal environment of the child and ambient lighting. Capillary refill time (CRT) is better estimated on the skin of the forehead or chest than on the skin of the peripheral digits, i.e. fingers and toes	Skin blood flow is used as a marker of overall perfusion, but it is also affected by the thermal environment. Measurement reliability is also affected by room lighting
5. Apply pressure to skin with forefinger (sufficient to blanch the skin) for a period of 5 s	CRT is the rate at which blood returns to the capillary bed after it has been compressed digitally. Always use this reference standard
6. Release the pressure and count in seconds how long it takes for the skin to return to normal colour	Normal values have been published, and, in general, the skin reperfuses in <2 s (3 s in neonates)
☙7. If the CRT is >2 s (3 s in neonates) this reflects ↓skin blood flow. Consider reporting to medical practitioner immediately (see point 10)	☙Prolonged CRT is caused by vasoconstriction and is considered to be an early indicator of shock
8. Assess core–peripheral temperature differential. This is usually measured with a temperature probe in the axilla and a probe taped to the sole of the foot or abdomen	It has been shown that skin temperature correlates with peripheral perfusion and cardiac output.
☙9. If the core–peripheral gap is 2°C this reflects ↓ skin blood flow. Consider reporting to medical practitioner immediately (see point 10)	☙The greater the difference in core–peripheral temperature, the greater the reduction in peripheral perfusion and cardiac output. As the child responds to treatment, the temperature differential should return to normal
10. Consider core–peripheral temperature gradient and CRT findings in the light of other haemodynamic variables	Evidence suggests that these two measures do not provide sufficient information in isolation
11. Document observations and repeat as indicated by intervention and child's condition	Maintain accurate records and provide a point of reference in the event of any queries

Marion Aylott, University of Southampton

urther reading

ruse, L. (2004). Physiological measures in intensive care. *Paediatric Nursing*, **16**(9), 14–17.
bby, S.M., Hatherill, M., Murdoch, I.A. (1999). Capillary refill and core–peripheral temperature gap as indicators of haemodynamic status in paediatric intensive care patients. *Archives of Disease in Childhood*, **80**, 63–166.

Haemodynamic monitoring

This is the clinical assessment of the cardiovascular system, particularl heart rate, CVP, and arterial blood pressure.

Heart rate

- Usually continuously monitored by a screen at the patient's bedside, with either 3-lead or 12-lead ECG.
- Essential for cardiovascular assessment in the critically ill patient.
- Used to detect abnormalities in heart rhythm and also to detect evidence of myocardial ischaemia, electrolyte imbalance, drug toxicity, and other metabolic disturbances.

CVP

- Reflects the pressure of blood returning to or filling the right atrium.
- To assess blood volume.
- Guides fluid management of the critically ill by showing dehydration or overhydration.

Sites

Inserted into central veins, either superior or inferior vena cava, interna jugular, subclavian vein, or femoral vein.

Equipment

- Pressure infuser bag and fluid bag, with specific tubing attached to CVP line.
- Transducer, which is set to a level equal to patient's mid axilla (right atrium of heart).
- Transducer transfers data on to a monitor by the patient's bed.

Measurements

- Normal CVP is 5–10 mmHg if level at mid-axilla.
- A low reading indicates dehydration, and a high reading indicates overhydration.

Complications

- Injury during insertion
- Air embolus
- Infection
- Dislodgement
- Fluid overload
- Central venous thrombosis

Arterial blood pressure

- Continuous blood pressure monitoring
- Early recognition of haemodynamic changes in the critically ill
- Enables frequent blood sampling to analyse arterial blood gas

Sites

Most commonly used is radial artery, but brachial, femoral, or dorsali pedis arteries can be used.

Fiona Smith, Royal Aberdeen Children's Hospital

Equipment

- Pressure infuser bag and fluid bag, with specific manometer tubing and three-way tap to enable blood sampling.
- Transducer, as per CVP: same transducer used with a double-giving set.

Measurements

Continuous blood pressure measurement of mean arterial pressure.

Complications

- Haemorrhage
- Thrombosis
- Infection

Nursing care

CVP

- Close observation and monitoring of patient for early detection of complications.
- Ensure that the transducer is maintained at the mid-axilla level to maintain accurate readings.
- The system should be zeroed at each shift change to ensure that accurate readings are maintained.

Arterial blood pressure

- Cannula should be clearly marked as arterial.
- The cannula and limb, where the cannula is inserted, should always be visible to allow blood flow to the limb to be seen.
- Never inject any drugs into an arterial line.
- The patient should be nursed in a high-dependency unit or intensive care.
- Zero system, as per CVP.
- Ensure that the level is maintained at the mid-axilla.

Further reading

Garreston, S. (2005). Haemodynamic monitoring: arterial catheters. *Nursing Standard* [online], **19**(31). 🖳 http://gateway.uk.ovid.com/gw1/ovidweb.cgi (accessed 31 May 2005).

Woodrow, P. (2002). Central venous catheters and central venous pressure. *Nursing Standard* [online], **16**(26). 🖳 http://gateway.uk.ovid.com/gw1/ovidweb.cgi (accessed 31 May 2005).

Methods of non-invasive respiratory support

Definition

To increase alveolar ventilation without the need for ET intubation.

Advantages

- Avoids mechanical damage to airway
- Reduces occurrence of nosocomal infections
- Maintains natural humidification, filtration, and heating of air
- Increases patient morale

Indications

- Both chronic and acute conditions
- Respiratory insufficiency and infection
- Weaning off ventilator
- Neuromuscular degenerative diseases
- Sleep-related respiratory disorders
- Skeletal deformity

Prerequisites

- Patient should not be exhausted, should have adequate ventilation, and should be able to maintain their own airway.
- He/she must be able to breathe spontaneously and have swallow and cough reflexes.

Method of delivery	Advantages	Disadvantages	Mechanism of delivery
Face mask	Humidification and warming of O_2 *may* be required	Tight seal required	Ventilator
		Pressure areas over bridge of nose and forehead	
	Improved mobility	Discomfort	
	Improved speech ability	Cosmetic appearance	
		Claustrophobia	
	Improved dietary intake	Reduced communication	
		Drying of airway	
		Reduced ability to eat and drink	
		Reduced mobility if ventilator not portable or has large battery life	
Nasal mask	Humidification and warming of O_2 may be required	Tight seal required	Ventilator
		Pressure areas over bridge of nose and forehead	

Donald Todd, Royal Aberdeen Children's Hospital

Contd.

	Improved mobility	Discomfort	
		Cosmetic appearance	
	Improved speech ability	Claustrophobia	
		Drying of airway	
	Improved dietary intake	Ventilation reduced when mouth opened	
		Reduced mobility if ventilator not portable or has large battery life	
Nasal prongs	Improved mobility	Pressure areas around nostrils	Ventilator
	Improved speech ability	Drying of airway	
	Improved dietary intake	Inability to humidify or warm O_2	
		Discomfort	
		Ventilation reduced when mouth opened because there is no tight seal	
Iron lung/ tank	Improved speech ability	Immobile	Continuous negative extrathoracic pressure
	Improved dietary intake	Claustrophobia	
		Full body seal difficult	
		Inability to check skin integrity	
		Pressure areas around seal because of immobility	
Cuirass	Chest wall only covered	Sizing of cuirass to fit chest wall	Biphasic cuirass ventilation
	Full mobility	Pressure areas around seal	
	Improved speech ability	Discomfort	
	Improved dietary intake	Cosmetic appearance	
	Intermittent use		
	Physiotherapy mode		

Further reading

Shelly, M.P., Nightingale, P. (1999). ABC of intensive care: Respiratory support. *British Medical Journal*, **318**, 1674–7.
www.mediventintl.com

Invasive methods of respiratory support

Positive pressure mechanical ventilation
- Efficient uptake and delivery of O_2
- Elimination of CO_2
- Maintenance of acid–base balance
- Gas is pushed into respiratory tract using positive pressure
- Two main types: pressure control and volume control ventilation

Indications
- Respiratory failure
- Airway obstruction, fitting, facial/neck oedema, and thermal injuries
- Cardiac failure
- Severe head injury
- Cervical cord injury above C4
- Drug overdose
- Acute exacerbation of chronic lung disease
- Respiratory centre depression
- Chest wall trauma
- Asthma

Complications
- Airway: damage to nasal/oral mucosa, teeth, hard and soft palate, vocal cords, and subglottic region
- Pulmonary: barotrauma/volutrauma causing pneumothorax, fibrosis, etc
- Cardiovascular: impaired cardiac output, hypotension, reduced cerebral perfusion pressure, arrhythmias
- Gastrointestinal: stomach distension splinting of the diaphragm and reduced gut motility, gastrointestinal haemorrhage from stress ulceration, malnutrition, and metabolic disorders
- Renal: altered antidiuretic hormone secretion—fluid retention, pulmonary oedema, pleural effusions, ascites, and renal failure
- Others: sepsis endocrine dysfunction, multi-organ failure, pressure sores, psychological problems

High-frequency oscillation ventilation
- Delta P (small tidal volumes) delivered at a high rate
- Lungs kept open at constant airway pressure
- Oxygenation and CO_2 clearance adjusted separately

Indications
- Respiratory failure with conventional ventilation
- Barotrauma/volutrauma
- Ventilation–perfusion mismatch
- Acute RDS
- Reduced lung compliance, RDS, increased resistance

Andrea Macarthur, Central Manchester or Manchester Children's University Hospitals NHS Trust

Complications

As for conventional ventilation, plus:
hyperinflation/atelectasis
tracheal inflammation if gases not humidified.

Nitric oxide therapy

Principles

Inhaled gas, which causes pulmonary vasodilatation

Indications

Pulmonary hypertension
Acute RDS
Acute hypoxic respiratory failure

Complications

- Pulmonary oedema
- Hypoxia
- Methaemoaglobinaemia
- Bleeding disorders

- Unknown long-term effects on staff
- Difficult to scavenge waste gases
- Unknown effects on fetus
- Need to monitor environmental levels

Extracorporeal membrane oxygenation

Provides cardiorespiratory support while the patient is recovering from reversible cardiac or respiratory failure.

Indications

- Failure to respond to conventional ventilation, surfactant therapy, high-frequency oscillation ventilation, and nitric oxide therapy
- O_2 index (OI) > 40 (OI = (MAP × FiO_2 × 100)/PaO_2)

Complications

- Bleeding
- Hypoxia and haemodynamic instability
- Infection

- Technical problems
- Neurological problems
- Renal insufficiency

Liquid ventilation

- Total liquid ventilation: lungs filled with perfluorocarbon, 30 ml/kg, then ventilated with 'liquid ventilator'.
- Partial liquid ventilation: 30 ml/kg perfluorocarbon instilled, then ventilated with conventional ventilator.

Indications

- Acute RDS
- Ventilation–perfusion mismatch

- Meconium aspiration
- Pneumonia

Complications

- Pneumothorax

Further reading

Anaesthesia UK ⬚ www.frca.co.uk
⬚ www.med.umich.edu/liquid/what is lv.html

Care of the ventilated child

- Assess child at beginning of and throughout shift. Report and document changes in condition.
- Check bed space, equipment, ventilator settings, emergency equipment, and alarm settings each shift. Damp dust and remove unnecessary equipment. Document when checks are complete.
- Adhere to hospital policies, guidelines, and procedures.

Airway	Record ET/tracheostomy tube size and length. Check tapes are secure. Head in mid-line position. Suction as required and at least every 6 hours
Breathing	Regularly assess and record air entry, work of breathing, and compliance with ventilator. Analyse blood gases following changes in condition or ventilation settings. Liaise with physiotherapists. Obtain tracheal/nasopharyngeal aspirate for analysis as required
	Elevated position; prone when possible. Change position regularly
Circulation	Regularly assess and record heart rate and rhythm, pulse, arterial/cuff blood pressure, CVP, capillary refill time, core and peripheral temperatures. Report signs of shock. Monitor effects of inotropes. Change lines following unit guidelines
Neurology	Regularly assess neurological condition. Report signs of raised ICP, fitting, altered neurological state immediately. Head-injured child: follow hospital guidelines to minimize risk of secondary brain injury. Immobilize cervical spine. Log roll
Drugs	Check drug and IV fluid prescriptions and dose rates of all infusion pumps. Give drugs as prescribed. Evaluate effectiveness. Report and document side effects/allergic reactions. Check compatibility of drugs and infusions. Liaise with pharmacist. Label IV lines
Electrolytes	Analyse glucose, electrolytes, full blood count, clotting studies, organ function, etc. as required. Record results
Fluids	Calculate fluid requirements. Check infusion sites. Record IV pump pressures. Change lines regularly. Report dehydration, fluid overload, and capillary leak syndrome. Infuse colloid as prescribed and evaluate effect
Infection control	Adhere to trust guidelines. Hand washing: all staff and visitors. Strict aseptic technique. Septic screening as required
Renal	Calculate fluid balance regularly. Report reduced/excessive urine output. Administer diuretics as prescribed. Keep urine catheters clean and unblocked. Urinalysis as required. Renal replacement therapy: follow unit guidelines
Gastro-intestinal tract	Observe for abdominal distension. Listen for bowel sounds. Feed enterally as soon as possible. Liaise with dietician. Regular mouth care. Administer total parenteral nutrition, as prescribed, using aseptic technique. Weigh child regularly. Record stools. Report constipation/diarrhoea

Andrea Macarthur, Central Manchester and Manchester Children's University Hospitals NHS Trust

Contd.

Psychological	Involve parents/ carers as much as possible. Prepare child before interventions. Calm manner. Stroke, cuddle, and comfort child; may reduce need for sedation. Facilitate play as condition allows. Child-friendly environment
Parental support	Ensure parents are with child as much as they wish. Explain procedures, care, etc. in understandable terms. Reinforce information given. Facilitate parental involvement in child's care. Provide accommodation and necessary support, e.g. expressing breast milk. Liaise with multiprofessional support teams
Skin	Observe for rashes, marking, redness, bruising, and pressure sores. Use pressure-relieving mattress. Attend to hygiene needs. Liaise with tissue viability team

Further reading

Williams, C., Asquith, J. (2000). *Paediatric intensive care nursing*. Churchill Livingstone.

Complications of intubation and ventilation

Airways
- Damage to nasal and oral mucosa
- Damage to teeth
- Damage to hard and soft palates
- Damage to vocal cords and subglottic region
- Damage to upper airway with prolonged ventilation
- Repeated intubations may cause subglottic oedema/stenosis

Pulmonary
- Barotrauma/volutrauma, leading to pneumothorax, pneumomediastinum, or pneumopericardium
- Lung disease, such as fibrosis

Cardiovascular
- Impaired cardiac output with high PEEP
- Hypotension
- Reduced cerebral perfusion pressure
- Arrhythmias from high CO_2, low PaO_2, and vagal stimulation

Gastrointestinal
- Stomach distension
- Splinting of the diaphragm
- Reduced gut motility
- Gastrointestinal haemorrhage from stress ulceration

Nutritional
- Malnutrition
- Metabolic disorders

Renal
- Alterations in level of antidiuretic hormone secretion, causing fluid retention and leading to pulmonary oedema, pleural effusions, and ascites
- Fluid retention
- Renal failure

Others
- Sepsis
- Multi-organ failure
- Psychological problems
- Endocrine dysfunction
- Pressure sores

Andrea Macarthur, Central Manchester and Manchester Children's University Hospitals NHS Trust

Transfer and retrieval

The key to successful transport and transfer is preparation.

Transfer of an unstable ill child is potentially hazardous because of the risk of:

- deterioration from primary illness
- complications of therapy
- secondary insults of the transfer process itself.

Minimize these factors; ensure maximum stability is achieved.

For transfer or retrieval of a child requiring intensive care (level 3 care), a dedicated consultant-led retrieval service based within a tertiary (lead) centre should be utilized. Within the UK, an effective network of specialized teams are available.

Contact tertiary centre for advice; ensure the child is appropriately prepared for the journey. Use the centre's pro forma checklist, from centre or internet, for information required for referral and advice.

Mode of transport depends on:

- nature and severity of child's illness
- distance and geographical location of referring hospital
- proximity of referring and receiving hospitals to a helipad or airport
- weather and flying conditions
- number of personnel for transfer team.

Road ambulances are as effective as air transport for transferring critical or unstable patients up to 50 km and stable patients up to 150 km.

Helicopters are effective up to 150 km; over these distances fixed-wing aircraft should be considered. When using air transport, there is potential for significant physiological effects to the child as a result of variation in:

- altitude (changes in pressure)
- acceleration and deceleration forces
- temperature
- humidity
- noise/vibration.

Preparation and management will anticipate these effects.

Transfer within hospital

The transfer and transport within hospital must be planned and executed with the same preparation and expertise as with an external transfer.

Documentation

Contemporaneous concise documentation will inform all concerned. The following should be present:

- summary of all procedures
- transfer letter
- copies of the child's notes, X-rays, and charts should travel with the child
- any cross-matched blood available should also travel with the child; suitable containers can be obtained from the blood bank
- result of RSV status if appropriate

Neil Bloxham, Plymouth Hospitals NHS Trust

- results of investigations that become available later should be communicated to the receiving unit.

Do not forget the parents; keep them informed and up to date. Retrieval teams may not be able to permit parents to travel with the sick child but may ensure safe transport of the parents to the destination.

Equipment checklists

Wards and units are likely to have checklists regarding transport equipment and requirements on the basis of individual unit needs. Policies will also include the frequency of checking these preparations.

It is vital that all the transferring team are familiar with all aspects of the equipment to be used and the layout of the vehicle.

Checklist before moving patient

- Is the airway protected and ventilation satisfactory (substantiated by blood gases, pH, and pulse oximetry)?
- Is re-intubation equipment available?
- Is the neck immobilized?
- Is there sufficient O_2 available for the journey?
- Is there sufficient vascular access? Are all lines patent, secure, and labelled?
- Is there sufficient infusion fluid?
- If catheterized, is catheter secure and attached to urine measuring device?
- Will all pumps work by battery/sufficient battery life/spare battery packs?
- Are emergency drugs and saline flushes drawn up and labelled?
- Are drugs required en route drawn up and labelled?
- Are fractured limbs appropriately splinted and immobilized?
- Are appropriate monitors in use with spare batteries?
- Will the infant/child/young person be warm enough for the journey—use incubator/transport pod?
- Documentation available?
- Care discussed with receiving team—telephone prior to departure and provide an estimated time of arrival.
- Parents up to date?

Calculation of amount of O_2 required

[Pressure (lb/in^2) × 0.3]/flow (l/min) = minutes of O_2 available

Example

Size E cylinder reads 2000 psi and O_2 flow is set at 4 l/min:

$(2000 × 0.3)/4 = 150$ min of O_2 available.

Aim to have twice the required amount of O_2 available for the journey.

During transfer

- Secure infant/child/young person with available straps.
- Ensure all pumps and monitoring devices are secure and that you can easily see these devices.
- Ensure you use your seatbelt.
- Observe and record relevant parameters at a frequency appropriate to child's condition. Many units have specific transfer charts for recording observations and aspects of care.
- Maintain communication with receiving unit; if you need to stop/child's condition deteriorates, ensure they are kept up to date.

Do not forget yourself

- Be comfortable
- If motion nausea is a problem, consider appropriate medication and do not forget to take it!

- If transferring to another hospital, consider the return journey. You may need a travel warrant/fare if the ambulance is not returning that day

- Have emergency cash
- Transfer/retrieval is likely to involve considerable time so cater for the team's own refreshment needs
- Ensure that you have your hospital identity badge

Further reading

Mackway-Jones, K., Molyneaux, E., Phillips, B., Wieteska, S. (ed.) (2005). *Advanced Paediatric Life Support: The Practical Approach*, 4th edn. BMJ Books–Blackwell.
Neill, C., Hughes, U. (2004). Improving inter-hospital transfer. *Paediatric Nursing*, **16**(7), 24–7.
PICS (1996). *Standards for paediatric intensive care*. Paediatric Intensive Care Society.

Arterial line management and arterial blood gas sampling

Indications for arterial line insertion:
- Blood gas analysis
  - to evaluate the adequacy of ventilation
  - to assess the O_2-carrying capacity of the blood
  - to evaluate the child's response to ventilation changes
  - to monitor acid–base balance
- Arterial blood pressure monitoring
  - to evaluate the child's response to treatment/interventions

Line/site management

- Transduce set as per hospital guidelines/policy/procedure.
- Check arterial blood pressure alarm limits at beginning of each shift.
- Calibrate arterial line transducer each shift.
- Ensure sutures (if present) are intact and secure.
- Secure cannula with non-occlusive dressing.
- Ensure site is visible at all times.
- Check limb distal to arterial site regularly for signs of poor perfusion.
- Check site regularly for signs of bleeding/haematoma/infection.
- Ensure site and line are clearly labelled as arterial.
- Avoid injectable caps/ports.
- Immobilize joint if applicable.
- Minimize risk of infection by adhering to hospital guidelines/policy/procedure for accessing/sampling from arterial line.
- Change administration set regularly according to hospital guidelines/policy/procedure.

Complications

- Haemorrhage (from site or line disconnection)
- Arterial occlusion
- Lack of perfusion distal to arterial line
- Arterial spasm
- Air embolism
- Blood clot embolism
- Haematoma
- Infection
- Trauma to arterial wall

Procedure for sampling from arterial line

- Should only be performed by staff trained and assessed as competent.
- Universal precautions: follow hospital policy.
- Prepare equipment: follow hospital guidelines/policy/procedure.
- Prepare child and family by explaining procedure.
- Silence alarms on monitor if safe to do so.
- Remove 'waste': 3–5 times the volume from the sampling port to the distal end of the arterial cannula.
  - Reason: to avoid contaminated (dilute) sample, causing erroneous results—high sodium, low potassium, and haemoglobin.

Andrea Macarthur, Central Manchester and Manchester Children's University Hospitals NHS Trust

- Obtain sample: 0.5 ml blood in heparinized syringe.
- Expel air bubbles from sample and replace cap. Air bubbles cause erroneous results: high PaO_2, and low PCO_2.
- Anticoagulate sample: gently rotate syringe 20–30 times to prevent clot formation and damage to blood gas analyser.
- Flush arterial line following hospital guidelines/policy/procedure, observing site for retrograde flow and blanching.

Venous blood sampling

Venous blood can be obtained peripherally via direct venepuncture or centrally via a central venous access device. The goal is to obtain a representative sample without causing unnecessary discomfort and distress to the child and family.

Knowledge of the following is necessary to ensure that a quality sample is obtained:

- specific patient requirements, e.g. fasting or at rest.
- appropriate collection tubes required and recommended order for filling: for blood cultures, plain tubes with no additives; coagulation, use tubes with no additives.
- sample requirements, e.g. on ice, warmed, or stored in the dark.
- measures to avoid haemolysis, such as avoiding excessive pressure on syringe, gently transferring blood into the tubes, and inverting rather than shaking collection tubes.

General criteria

- Patient identity: check the patient's name, date of birth, and hospital number against his/her name band and the patient's notes. Samples labelled immediately and by the person obtaining the sample.
- Equipment: pressure in a vacuum system can cause small veins to collapse; therefore, the syringe method is preferable. All equipment should be intact and in date.
- Infection control: handwashing and wearing gloves and an apron are universal precautions to prevent the spread of infection.
- High-risk samples: treat all blood and bodily fluids as high risk; there is more danger from the ones not known about, because less care is taken. Clearly label high-risk samples to ensure relevant personnel are aware.
- Needle safety: handle sharps safely and dispose at point of source in an appropriate container. Consider the use of safety devices to reduce risk of accidental needlestick injury.
- Documentation: samples obtained, volume of blood taken, and any complications.
- Storage and transportation: immediately transfer blood samples to the laboratory or store in a refrigerator to avoid deterioration of the sample. Transport in an accepted biohazard container.

Specific criteria

Peripheral blood sampling

- The fear of needles is common in children and young people. Consider the use of strategies such as topical local anaesthetic products, preparation, explanation, empowerment, and diversional therapy. Positive reinforcement by means of a reward will enhance the child's perception of the procedure.
- Ensure patient is comfortable, preferably sitting or lying down, because fainting or a vasovagal response can occur.
- Avoid areas where a pulse is felt to prevent accidental arterial puncture. If arterial puncture is suspected (bright red blood), release

Jo Rothwell and Alison Hegarty, Central Manchester and Manchester Children's University Hospitals NHS Trust

pressure around the limb, remove needle, and apply direct pressure to the site for 5 min.

● Awareness of previous use, condition of the veins, and patient preference is beneficial. Hands, arms, feet, and scalp veins can all be used in paediatrics.

● A syringe with a butterfly is often easier and less threatening for paediatrics, as opposed to a standard straight needle. Manual syringe suction is more easily controlled than a vacuum system and allows small amounts of blood to be divided between collection tubes.

● Potential risks to the patient when using broken needles outweighs their benefits. Safer alternatives are available.

● Smallest gauge needle to minimize damage to the vein.

● If an infusion is in progress, stop the infusion 5–10 min prior to blood sampling and recommence immediately after. The puncture site should be distal to the location of the cannula.

● Clean venepuncture site with a 70% alcohol swab for 30 s and allow to air dry.

● To dilate the veins, apply circumferential pressure on the limb with hands or a tourniquet, whichever is the least threatening for the child/young person. Release pressure as soon as possible to prevent haemoconcentration through venous stasis.

● If unable to obtain blood after two attempts, refer to a more experienced practitioner.

● Remove needle if bruising/formation of haematoma occurs.

● Following removal of the needle, apply direct pressure, with a gauze swab, to the puncture site for at least 60 s. Do not bend arm during this period. Apply plaster in case of re-bleed.

Blood sampling via peripheral and central access devices

● Blood sampling via a peripheral cannula may provide a poor-quality specimen.

● Blood sampling for coagulation and drug levels should not be taken from an IV device. Medications can stick to the internal lumen of the catheter, with subsequent erroneous results.

● Blood loss through sampling in paediatrics should be no greater than 5 ml/kg in 24 hours. To minimize loss, consider utilizing the mixing or reinfusion technique rather than discarding.

● Following blood withdrawal, flush the device with 0.9% saline, utilizing a pulsatile positive pressure technique to clear the line of debris and prevent occlusion/infection.

Further reading

▶ Dougherty, L., Lamb, J. (ed.) (1999). *Intravenous therapy in nursing practice*. Churchill Livingstone.
RCN standards for infusion therapy, October 2003.

Total parenteral nutrition (PN)

Total PN is the provision of nutrients via the IV route. It is used when enteral feeding is either not feasible or is unable to meet the full nutritional requirements of the child.

The goal of total PN is to maintain the nutritional status and achieve balanced somatic growth until, in most cases, the enteral route is available.

Indications for use

- Prematurity
- Intestinal failure caused by conditions such as congenital defects, abdominal surgery, obstructions, and short bowel syndrome
- Trauma
- Burns
- Malignant disease
- Multiple organ failure
- Severe IBD

Routes of administration

Whenever possible, administration via a peripheral IV line should be avoided because there is increased risk of phlebitis, infection, thrombosed veins, and severe extravasation injury because of the hypertonic constitution of the solution.

Ideally, total PN should be administered via a central venous catheter, preferably a triple lumen, with the total PN having its own lumen to reduce the risk of interaction with other drugs and fluids.

Composition

- Protein: as amino acids, such as Vamin®
- Carbohydrate: as glucose (lower percentage used if peripheral administration)
- Fat: such as Intralipid®
- Water
- Electrolytes
- Trace elements

Ingredients are prescribed and titrated to each patient, taking account of the patient's condition, needs, fluid requirements, renal and liver functions, and serum electrolyte levels.

Monitoring

Check local policy for frequency of parameters to be monitored, but the following should be used as a guide.

- Prior to commencement of total PN, laboratory evaluation of blood glucose, urea, creatinine, calcium, phosphorus, magnesium, bilirubin, albumin, liver enzymes, and triglyceride.
- Weekly monitoring of the above thereafter.

Fiona Smith, Royal Aberdeen Children's Hospital

- Monthly monitoring of zinc, copper, selenium, and vitamins A and E.
- Initially, regular monitoring of blood glucose on ward, especially with infants and small children.
- Daily urinalysis for glucose.
- Careful observation of venous line site.
- Careful monitoring of fluid balance.
- Weigh patient weekly.
- Ensure strict aseptic technique by all when handling bag and line.

Complications

- Catheter-related complications, including thrombosis, embolism, pneumothorax, pleural effusions (extraverted solutions), cardiac arrhythmias, and haemorrhage
- Infection
- Electrolyte disturbances
- Metabolic disturbances
- Systemic complications such as *homeostasis* and cirrhosis (with long-term use).

Wherever possible, minimal enteral feeding, of 1–10 ml/hour (dependent on age), is recommended to maintain intestinal mucosa integrity, reduce bacterial translocation, and prevent biliary homeostasis.

Further reading

Horn, V. (2003). Paediatric parenteral nutrition. *Hospital Pharmacist*, **10**, 53–62.
Williams, C., Asquith, J. (2000). *Paediatric intensive care nursing*. Churchill Livingstone.

Inotropic support

Definition

An inotrope is a drug that increases the force of contraction of the heart. A combination of these drugs may be needed to achieve the desired effect, and they will not work adequately if the heart is not sufficiently volume-loaded.

Indications for use

- Low cardiac output following cardiac surgery.
- Pre-operative support of cardiac function.
- To ensure adequate cerebral perfusion following a severe head injury.
- Restoration of central circulating volume in septic shock.

Action

Inotropes act on three main receptors.

- Alpha receptors: vasoconstriction of most peripheral blood vessels; some increased myocardial contractility.
- Beta 1 receptors: increased heart rate, and rate of atrioventricular contraction, and myocardial contractility.
- Beta 2 receptors: peripheral vasodilation of vascular beds, such as some skeletal muscle, and bronchodilation.

Effects of stimulation

- Heart: increases rate and force of contraction (*alpha* receptors = constricts *coronaries* and *beta* receptors = dilates coronaries)
- Lungs and bronchi: dilates but, slightly constricts blood vessels
- Kidneys: decreases urine and renin secretion
- Basal metabolism: increases
- Abdominal systemic arterioles: constricts skin arterioles: constricts muscle arterioles; alpha receptors constrict, beta receptors dilate.

Common inotropes in use

- Dopamine
- Epinephrine
- Norepinephrine
- Digoxin
- Dobutamine
- Enoximone

Common side effects

- Nausea/vomiting
- Headache
- Hypertension
- Reduced renal perfusion
- Peripheral vasoconstriction
- Arrhythmias
- Sweating

Angela Ledsham, University of Southampton

Nursing considerations

- Must be given via a central IV line: IV site should be checked at least every hour because extravasation causes severe tissue damage.
- The drugs have short half-lives, so are usually administered via a syringe driver pump as a continuous infusion and weaned over a period of time as the child's condition allows.
- Usual monitoring required for a child receiving inotropes: ECG, blood pressure (usually via an arterial line for constant accurate measurement), CVP, urine output, and peripheral perfusion (skin temperature).
- Critically ill children receiving inotropes may be at risk of cardiovascular instability during routine changing of infusion. Latest evidence from the literature suggests the best way of managing this is by the quick-change method.
- Because more than one inotrope may be given via the same lumen of the central line, drug compatibilities should be checked with a pharmacist, and either a one-way valve system or three-way tap may be used.

Further reading

Arino, M., Barrington, J.P., Morrison, A.L., Gilles, D. (2004). Management of the changeover of inotrope infusions in children. *Intensive and Critical Care Nursing*, **20**(5), 275–80.

Horrox, F. (2002). *Manual of neonatal and paediatric heart disease*. Whurr.

Withholding and withdrawing life-sustaining care

Consideration might be given to withholding and withdrawing life-sustaining care in certain complex, difficult, and tragic situations.

- Withholding care: not introducing a therapy that could be used in the situation.
- Withdrawing care: stopping a treatment that has been used up to that point.

It is vital to remember the following.

- Withholding or withdrawing life-sustaining care does not mean ceasing care but is the start of palliative care.
- Any decision in this area is based on consideration of the best interests of the infant, child, or young person, while taking into account the family's needs and wishes.
- Every effort should be made to achieve as nearly as possible a consensus of opinion between child, family, and professionals.
- Such consensus can only be achieved through open supportive communication between child, family, and professionals.
- The child's wishes and views must, as far as possible, be ascertained and taken into account in any decision-making.

The Royal College of Paediatrics and Child Health define five situations where it might be appropriate to withhold or withdraw care that may be sustaining life but is not improving health or well-being or reducing suffering:

- brainstem death: as defined by existing criteria for the diagnosis of brainstem death
- the permanent vegetative state
- the 'no chance' situation—treatment that simply delays death
- the 'no purpose' situation—possible survival but with devastating impairment
- the 'unbearable' situation.

Ethical basis

Frameworks, such as that of Beauchamp and Childress, can be used in the analysis of the situation. The latter requires that four principles are the basis of consideration:

- respect for autonomy
- beneficence—doing good
- non-maleficence—avoiding harm
- justice.

Legal basis

Particularly difficult situations sometimes require the judgement of a court for their resolution. Decisions in this case are likely to be based on:

- Children Act 1989 (1995 for Scotland)
- Human Rights Act 1998

Jim Richardson, University of Glamorgan

- individual case decisions, such as the Charlotte Wyatt case in the Court of Appeal.

The UN Convention on the Rights of the Child might also exert an influence.

Further reading

Beauchamp, T.L., Childress, J.F. (2001). *Principles of biomedical ethics*, 5th edn. Oxford University Press.

Royal College of Paediatrics and Child Health (2004). *Withholding or withdrawing life-sustaining treatment in children: A framework for practice*, 2nd edn. RCPCH.

Commentary: the end of intolerability the Charlotte Wyatt case in the Court of Appeal
🖥 www.ethics-network.org.uk/comment/FosterWyatt.htm

Drugs in children's nursing

Pharmacology

Medical pharmacology is the science of drugs and how they interact with the human body. These chemical interactions can be divided into two areas for consideration:
- pharmacokinetics: how the body handles a drug
- pharmacodynamics: how a drug works (📖 Pharmacodynamics, p.826)

Pharmacokinetics

If a drug is to have an effect on the cells of the body, it must be in the right place, for the right amount of time, and at the right concentration. The concentration is very important if the drug is to be therapeutic:
- too high, it may well become toxic
- too low, it will be non-therapeutic.

Drugs are administered by a variety of routes, using a variety of formulations, in order to have a desired response. The desired response will only happen if a therapeutic level is maintained and this, in turn, relies on *bioavailability*. The bioavailability of a drug is defined as 'the proportion of the administered dose that reaches the circulation', e.g. IV drug administration would equal 100% bioavailability (see figure). Factors that will affect bioavailability should be considered in any situation where drugs are being used.

Drugs are usually metabolized within the liver by specific enzyme pathways. The time taken for the plasma level of the drug to be reduced by one-half is known as the half-life, $t_{1/2}$.

Pharmacokinetic data for a drug will tell us what dose to give, how often to give it, and what other factors to take into consideration.

Pharmacokinetic processes can be divided into four stages (see figure):
- Absorption: depends on many factors, e.g. whether the drug is water or fat soluble, how it is formulated, and what else is in the gut at the same time.
- Distribution: depends on quality of blood flow and binding of the drug to protein carriers, which is a real issue with polypharmacy because of carrier competition. Of particular importance in children:
  - the blood–brain barrier may be compromised in neonates
  - fat levels are low in the newborn
  - protein binding is also lower in the first few months of life.
- Metabolism in the liver will produce new products called metabolites; these are usually waste products, but for some formulations, they will be the active component of the drug. Factors such as blood flow through the liver and the size of the liver will be important, particularly in neonates.
- Elimination of the drug, usually via the kidney. ↓ Blood flow and poor kidney function will lead to a serious accumulation of drug or drug metabolites in the body. Administered drugs are also eliminated by the gut, sweat glands, and, sometimes forgotten with young babies, mother's breast milk, which may contraindicate the child's medication.

John Bastin, University of Plymouth

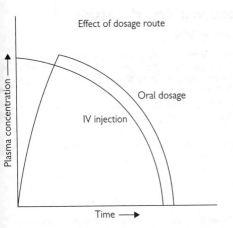

Effect of dosage route

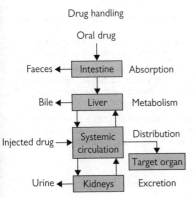

Drug handling

Further reading

Trounce, J. (1999). *Clinical pharmacology for nurses*, 16th edn. Churchill Livingstone.
www.druginfozone.nhs.uk

Pharmacodynamics: the study of how drugs work

Most drugs produce their effect by acting on proteins called receptors. These receptors are genetic in origin and allow cells to communicate with the outside or internally. Receptors usually respond to synaptic transmitters or hormones.

The interaction of the drug and the receptor depends on the fit of the drug molecule to the receptor. The better the fit, the more specific the drug.

Sometimes a drug molecule will affect more than one receptor and may produce unwanted side effects.

Action of drugs

Drugs act as follows.
- Replacing chemicals that are deficient—hormones, minerals, and vitamins.
- Interfering with cell functions and metabolic pathways by stimulating or inhibiting normal levels of activity—clotting disorders, inflammation, and hormone disorders.
- Acting against invading or abnormal cells—antibiotics and anticancer drugs.
- Interfering with the function of receptor sites themselves, enhancing responses (agonists) or preventing normal responses (antagonists).

Agonist drugs bind to the receptor site and improve the response to normal stimulation, thus producing a reaction that will result in improved cell function. e.g. metformin hydrochloride increases the receptor sensitivity to insulin in patients with diabetes mellitus.

Antagonist drugs bind to the receptor site and block normal function and cell activity, e.g. tamoxifen prevents the oestrogen molecule from docking with a receptor, thus preventing cell growth stimulation in breast tumours.

Prescribing for children

It is useful to use the following terminology:
- neonate: birth to 1 month
- infant: 1 month to 2 years
- child: 2–12 years
- adolescent: 12–18 years

Children are not 'mini-adults'. Paediatric doses should be calculated from paediatric baseline data and not just a modified adult dose.

Further reading

Neal, M.J. *Medical pharmacology at a glance*, 3rd edn. Blackwell Science.
Trounce, J. (1999). *Clinical pharmacology for nurses*, 16th edn. Churchill Livingstone.
🖳 www.druginfozone.nhs.uk

John Bastin, University of Plymouth

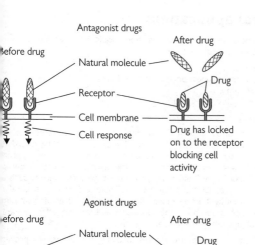

Topical applications

Skin thickness, sensitivity, and condition should be taken into accoun
when applying topical treatments.

Skin thickness:
- face: 0.12 mm, thinnest on lips and round eyes
- body: 0.6 mm
- palms and soles: 1.2–4.7 mm.

Emollients

Hydrate and soften the skin. Can be applied to all skin surfaces. Act as
barrier to water and external irritants for all dry or scaling disorders
Their effects are short lived so frequent applications needed. Applying
immediately after washing maximizes the hydration effect. Allow to
soak in for 20–30 min before applying other topical treatments, such as
steroids. The greasier the emollient (e.g. liquid and white soft paraffin
emulsifying ointments), the more effective it is. Some emulsifying ointments can also be used as soap substitutes and are very effective when
used in conjunction with a bath emollient.

Apply liberally in downward strokes following hair growth to prevent
folliculitis. Rubbing in should be avoided as this creates heat and irritation, and can cause damage to delicate skin cells.

Vehicle types	Description	Uses
Creams	Light emulsions with high water content (60%). Contain preservatives	'Wet' skin; easy to apply and well absorbed
Barrier creams	Water repellent, often contain silicone	Protection of intact skin, e.g. round stomas, pressure sores, and nappy area
	Easy to apply, not sticky	*Not* to be used over acute skin lesions
Ointments	Water-in-oil emulsions, greasy, and often in soft paraffin base	Chronic dry conditions (eczema); encourage hydration because they stay on skin longer so can be more effective; antipruitic
Gels	Consistency between creams and ointments; have high water content but can burn skin	Particularly suitable for face and scalp; antipruitic
Lotions (shake)	Alcohol base may cause stinging. Contain insoluble powders that leave deposit on skin	Cooling effect often preferred on hairy skin, e.g. calomine lotion; antipruitic
Pastes	Stiff preparations with high proportion of finely powdered solids. Impregnated bandages	Circumscribed, chronic licheni-fied lesions. Bandages may be left on for several days
Antiseptics and cleansing lotions	Care must be taken that correct dilution is used to avoid risk of burning and irritiation	Cleansing infected and weeping lesions

Di Keeton, Southampton University Hospitals NHS Trust

Topical steroids

- Treatment of inflammatory conditions, e.g. eczema.
- Apply no more than twice daily.
- Ointments provide better absorption and often less irritation; apply thinly following finger-tip units (FTUs).
- One FTU (500 mg) is sufficient to cover an area twice that of a flat adult palm.

Age	Number of adult FTUs				
	Face + neck	Arm + hand	Leg + foot	Trunk (front)	Trunk (back)+ buttocks
3–6 months	1	1	1.5	1	1.5
1–2 years	1.5	1.5	2	2	3
3–5 years	1.5	2	3	3	3.5
6–10 years	2	2.5	4.5	3.5	5

Potency classification	Example
Mild	Hydrocortisone 0.5%, 1%, and 2.5%
Moderate	Eumovate
Potent	Elocon, Betnovate (RD), Cutivate
Very potent	Dermovate (rarely used for children)

- 1% hydrocortisone is safe for infants under 1 year and on face for all ages.
- Occlusion increases potency up to 10-fold.
- Use the least potent preparation that is effective for severity of condition.
- Avoid prolonged use, especially on the face and around the eyes.

Side effects

- Mild to moderate potency is associated with few side effects. Absorption through skin rarely causes adrenal suppression.
- Locally, excessive and long-term use of potent strengths can result in:
  - Skin thinning
  - Striae
  - Talengectasis
  - Fine hair growth
  - Easy bruising
  - Peri-oral dermatitis
- Pigment changes are caused by eczema *not* by topical steroids.

Further reading

British Association of Dermatology. 🖳 www.bad.org.uk

Administration of ear medication

One method of treating an infection in the ear is to introduce ribbon gauze or sponge wick soaked with specified eardrops or ear ointment. This should be performed by an experienced practitioner.

On the other hand, simple eardrops can be administered by the child's carer, but it is important to explain to the child and carer how to administer eardrops for the medication to be effective.

The correct procedure for the administration of ear drops is as follows.
• Wash hands with soap and water; dry hands.
• Keep the eardrops clean. Avoid touching the dropper on the ear.
• If the drops are in a suspension, shake well before using.
• It is useful for the child to lie on his/her side, with the affected ear uppermost. The pinna should be gently pulled up and back, and the drops placed into the ear canal.
• Massage the tragus just in front of the ear. This will help propel the drops down the ear canal.
• The child should be advised to stay in that position for about 5 min to allow the drops to seep down to the eardrum. A good video/DVD for the child to watch while he/she is waiting is an idea!
• Wash hands with soap and water; dry hands.

Further reading

BMA and RPS (2005). British National Formulary. British Medical Association and Royal Pharmaceutical Society of Great Britain.
Daya, H., Crittenden, G. (1998). Inside ENT. Pale Green Press,
www.earcarecentre.com

Jo Williams, Birmingham Children's Hospital NHS Trust

Administration of eye medication

Action	Rationale
1. Assess need for medication, and check medication has been correctly prescribed	Eye medication is equally as important as other forms of medication
	If wrong medication or dose is given, it can be harmful to the patient
2. Gather supplies and wash hands	Prevent cross-infection and avoid unnecessary interruption of procedure
Tissues (clean) or gauze (not cotton wool)	
Eye medication	
3. Explain procedure as appropriate for child's age and understanding and to parents/carers if present	Promotes partnership with child and family
4. Select correct eye for instillation of eye medication, as per prescription	To ensure medication administered as prescribed
5. Position appropriately	To prevent injury and promote comfort
Swaddle infant	
Ensure head is flat and child is still	
If instilling eye drops	
6. Take off bottle top (check prescription)	
With the child's eyes closed, drop medication as prescribed into inner corner of the eye (next to the nose)	To prevent discomfort
Wait for drop to disappear. If it remains visible, gently pull down lower lid and watch drop roll in	
Wipe away excess medication	To prevent irritation
Drops can also be instilled as above if eyes are open	
7. Distract child if necessary to ensure they allow drop to be instilled	Can be an emotionally difficult procedure
If instilling eye ointment	
8. If using ointment, gently pull down lower lid and squeeze in 2 cm along the lower lid	For ease of administration
9. With the eyes closed, gently wipe with a clean tissue, if necessary	To aid comfort
10. Praise/congratulate the child	Can be emotionally difficult

Julie Kitchen, Royal Devon and Exeter NHS Foundation Trust

Contd.

Action	Rationale
1. Put the top firmly back on the bottle/tube	To prevent spillage or cross-infection
2. Wash your hands again	To prevent cross-infection
3. If several different eye medications are due, administer 5 min apart	To enable drops to be absorbed
4. Do not share bottles/drops with other patients	To prevent cross-infection
5. Store as directed, and discard according to instructions	To ensure safe practice is maintained
6. Report and document any reaction according to local protocol	To ensure safe care and prevent harm
7. Document on prescription chart	To prevent drug error

Further reading

Marsden, J., Shaw, M. (2003). Correct administration of topical eye treatment. *Nursing Standard*, **17**(30), 42–4.

Nursing and Midwifery Council (2002). Guidelines for the administration of medicines. NMC.

Administration of nose medication

It is important to explain to the child or carer how to instil nasal medication. Because of the shape of the nose, it is important that nasal drops are applied in such a way that they are able to reach the sinuses.

• Ask the child, or help the child, to blow his/her nose.
• Wash your hands with soap and water; dry your hands.
• Keep the nose drops clean. Avoid touching the dropper on the nose or anything else.
• Ask the child to lie, or place the child, on a bed with his/her head extended over the end of the bed. Drops can be placed in one nostril with the head slightly turned to that side. The head should be maintained in that position for 30 s and then the drops can be instilled into the other nostril.
• For an older child, it may be easier for him/her to stand with his/her head downwards and forwards. The drops can then be applied to each nostril.
• Both the above-mentioned positions ensure that drops do not simply trickle down the back of the nose into the throat.
• Wash your hands with soap and water; dry your hands.

Further reading

BMA and RPS (2005). *British National Formulary*. British Medical Association and Royal Pharmaceutical Society of Great Britain.
Daya, H., Crittenden, G. (1998). *Inside ENT*. Pale Green Press,
🖳 www.members.aol.com/pocketpeds/pages/drugs/pp72.htmm

Jo Williams, Birmingham Children's Hospital NHS Trust

Administration of nebulizers

Action	Rationale
1. Assess child's need for nebulizer	Nebulizer therapy enables the delivery of bronchodilators, steroids, antibiotics, mucolytics, epinephrine, and normal saline
2. Gather equipment	
Select appropriate nebulizer system for drug:	
Mouthpiece or mask	Mouthpiece increases aerosol delivery
	Masks need to be tight-fitting to avoid drug getting into eyes
	Drug delivery is reduced if mask held away from face
Appropriate compressor or gas source	In acute asthma, croup, and anaphylaxis, O_2 must be used because hypoxia can occur
	If there is a risk of CO_2 retention, e.g. cystic fibrosis, air should be used
Select appropriate flow rate	Most nebulizers work on 6–10 l/min; driving gas should be set at 6–8 l/min
Place compressor on firm surface	To avoid cold dusty air being drawn into compressor
3. Select required drug	
Dispense correctly—dilute, if necessary, with normal saline	2–2.5 ml fill is satisfactory for most nebulizers; however, delivery is maximized by a 4 ml fill, and this is recommended for steroids and antibiotics
	Diluting with water could provoke bronchospasm
4. Explain procedure to child and carer in age-appropriate language	Understanding will enhance compliance and reduce anxieties
If possible, child should sit up to keep the nebulizer upright	Level of drug delivery is reduced because of abnormal breathing pattern if child is crying
Discourage the child from talking or having a dummy in mouth during nebulization	To maximize delivery of drug
Encourage normal tidal breathing through the mouth	Duration of nebulization is important for compliance; should take no longer than 10 min
The end point is when spluttering occurs; tap pot and continue nebulizing for 1 min	Drug output remains high at this point

Celia Charlton, Royal Devon and Exeter NHS Foundation Trust

Contd.

Action	Rationale
5. At end of nebulization	
Turn off airflow and reassess condition of child	To detect any change in child's condition
Advisable to wash face if mask used, especially if steroids used	Promote comfort
	To avoid skin irritation from drug particles
6. Decontamination of nebulizer equipment after use	
Wash nebulizer and dry thoroughly	To prevent bacterial contamination
	To remove remnant drug crystals, which could block nebulizer nozzles

Further reading

Kendrick, H. *et al.* (1997). Selecting and using nebuliser equipment. *Thorax*, **52** (suppl. 2), S92–S101.

Silverman, M., O'Callaghan, L. (ed.) (2001). *Practical paediatric respiratory medicine.* Arnold, London.

Administration of oral drugs

Action	Rationale
1. Check prescriber has dated and signed prescription	Legislation
2. Check what is prescribed and when due	Give right medicine at right time
3. Check dose is appropriate for condition being treated and child's age, weight, and surface area A second independent check of calculations is recommended	Dosage accuracy
4. Check that child's name, date of birth, and identification number on identity band match those on prescription chart	Give medicine to right child
5. Confirm steps 2–4 with parent/older child if possible	Effective partnership
6. Offer choice of formulations (liquid/tablet/capsule) if available	Acceptance
7. Ensure storage of medication has been correct	Potency
8. Calculate volume of liquid/number of tablets/capsules If possible, avoid dividing tablets or dissolving/dispersing tablets in a specified volume of water and taking an aliquot	Dosage accuracy
9. Child may prefer a crushed tablet or contents of a capsule with a spoonful of yoghurt or ice cream. ▶ Modified-release preparations will lose their modified-release properties	Acceptance
10. Avoid adding drug to large quantities of drink/food	Accuracy and potency
11. Check container, label, expiry date. ▶ Liquids that have been reconstituted will have an expiry date based on date of reconstitution, in addition to an expiry date for the dry powder preparation	
12. Shake liquids before opening	Mix contents
13. If dose <5 ml, always draw up using a syringe	Dosage accuracy

Sue Danby and Louise Holliday, Royal Aberdeen Children's Hospital

Contd.

14. Do not draw up more than one medicine into the same syringe	
15. Explain treatment to child/parent	Concordance
16. Offer choice of delivery method (spoon, oral syringe, or medicine cup), if possible	Acceptance
17. Offer medicines to an infant before a feed, unless contraindicated	
18. Seek cooperation through play and patience	Compliance
19. If cooperation from young child unobtainable, sit child on adult's lap, with one arm tucked under the adult's arm and the other arm secured by adult's same arm and hand	Reduced risk of inhalation of medicine through struggling
20. Never threaten child with an injection as an alternative	Coercion
21. A drink may usually be given after medicine	To wash it down

Further reading

Royal College of Paediatrics and Child Health and Neonatal and Paediatric Pharmacists Group (2003). *Medicines for children*. RCPCH.
Royal Pharmaceutical Society. 🖳 www.rpsgb.org.uk

Procedure for administration of rectal medication to children

Aims
- To administer medication if rectal administration is the preferred/recommended route.
- To clear the lower bowel in cases of severe constipation.
- As medication to treat a pyrexia, pain, nausea, and vomiting.

Practice points
- This procedure should only be carried out by a competent and trained practitioner.
- The administration of rectal medication is an invasive procedure and may be contraindicated if:
  - there is any rectal bleeding
  - there is diarrhoea
  - the child has any anatomical anomaly of the anus or rectum
  - the child is extremely uncooperative.
- Two adults must normally be present when the procedure is performed (one as chaperone).

Objectives
- To minimize distress by preparing the child physically and psychologically and by preparing the family.
- To ensure safety by the use of an appropriate technique for administration of rectal medication.
- To ensure correct administration.
- To ensure appropriate disposal of equipment afterwards.

Equipment
- Prescribed medication
- Lubricating jelly
- Disposable gloves
- Tissues
- Disposable incontinence pad or equivalent

Michelle Fuller, Southampton University Hospitals NHS Trust

Procedure	Rationale
Preparatory phase	
Explain and discuss the procedure with the child using age-appropriate language	To ensure the child understands the procedure and gives his/her valid consent
Ensure privacy	To avoid unnecessary embarrassment and maintain privacy and dignity
Encourage, where appropriate and possible, the child to empty his/her bladder prior to the procedure	A full bladder may cause increased discomfort during the procedure
Wash hands or clean with gel rub and assemble equipment	To minimize the risk of cross-infection. To ensure all equipment is to hand
Position the child as follows: lying on left side, with knees well flexed and the upper leg higher than the lower leg	To ease the passage of the medication/suppository/tube into the rectum
Place disposable incontinence pad or equivalent under child's hips and buttocks to catch spillage	To reduce potential infection caused by soiling. To avoid embarrassing the child if medication ejected

Further reading

Rotherham Primary Care Trust. 🖳 www.rotherhampct.nhs.uk/policiesprocedures/nursing/default.asp

Administration of an intramuscular (IM) injection

Action	Rationale
1. Explain procedure to child and family	Increases understanding and decreases fear
2. Consider use of local anaesthetic cream	Decreases pain
3. Assess validity of prescription. Check that the dose and route are correct	Safe drug administration
	Limited drugs may be given intramuscularly
4. Gather equipment and wash hands	
Clean receptacle for syringe	Reduces risk of cross-contamination
Appropriate syringe. <2 ml advised for intramuscular injection	Decreases pain and facilitates absorption
21 g needle to draw up (23 g from glass ampoule)	Prevents shards of glass being drawn up
23 g or 25 g needle to inject	
Drug and appropriate diluent	
Sharps bin	Safer sharps disposal
5. Prepare and draw up drug. Change needle	Ensures needle is not blunted
Check with second nurse, as governed by local policy. Check child's nameband	Reduces risk of drug errors
6. Reassure child	Injection is more painful in tensed muscle
7. Choose site for injection	
8. Help child into a comfortable position, and uncover site	
9. Ensure area to be injected is socially clean	Prevents introduction of dirt
	Routine use of alcohol wipes is not recommended
10. Pull skin at injection site to one side (Z track technique)	Decreases leakage of drug into subcutaneous tissue
11. Rapidly plunge the needle into the muscle at 90°	To ensure muscle mass is penetrated
12. Aspirate for blood	Ensures injection not given into vein
If blood present, discard and start again	
13. Slowly inject fluid, approximately 1 ml per 10 s	Allows fluid to dissipate and reduces pain

Michelle Fuller, Southampton University Hospitals NHS Trust

Contd.

Action	Rationale
14. After a few seconds, withdraw needle	
Apply pressure	Prevents bleeding
Discard needle	
Ensure child settled	
Document procedure	

Sites for injection

Ventrogluteal	Consistent presence of muscle—can be used in emaciated/ young patients with little risk of injury
Vastus lateralis	Easily accessible, and little risk of injury
Deltoid	Little muscle mass—small volumes only
Dorso-gluteal	Risk of nerve/artery damage. Sizeable muscle—larger volumes
Rectus femorus	Painful but suitable for self-injection

Further reading

Hemsworth, S. (2000). Intramuscular (IM) injection technique. *Paediatric Nursing*, **12**(9), 17–20.

Pratt, R. *et al.* (2005). The need for skin preparation prior to injection: point-counterpoint. *British Journal of Infection Control*, **6**(4), 18–20.

Rodger, M., King, L. (2000). Drawing up and administering intramuscular injections: a review of the literature. *Journal of Advanced Nursing*, **31**(3), 574–82.

Administration of a subcutaneous injection

Action	Rationale
1. Explain procedure to child/family	Increases understanding and decreases fear
2. Consider use of local anaesthetic cream	Decreases pain
3. Assess validity of prescription. Check that dose and route are correct	Safer drug administration
4. Gather equipment and wash hands	
Clean receptacle to carry syringe	Reduces risk of cross-contamination
Syringe: <1 ml advised subcutaneously	
21 g needle to draw up (23 g from glass ampoule); 25 g needle to inject	Prevents shards of glass being drawn up with drug
Drug and appropriate diluent	
Sharps bin	Safe sharps disposal
5. Prepare and draw up drug. Change needle	Ensures needle is not blunted
Check with second nurse, as governed by local policy. Check child's nameband	Reduces risk of drug errors
6. Reassure child	Lessens distress of injection
7. Choose site, ensuring regular rotation	Decreases risk of skin irritation
Lateral aspects of upper arms	
Lateral aspects of thighs	
Abdomen	
Buttocks	
8. Help child into comfortable position and uncover site	
9. Ensure area to be injected is socially clean	Prevents introduction of dirt
	Routine use of alcohol wipes is not recommended
10. Pinch up chosen area	Ensures needle enters subcutaneous tissue
11. Rapidly plunge the needle in at 45°. Release skin pinch	Increased pain if injected into compressed tissue

Michelle Fuller, Southampton University Hospitals NHS Trust

Contd.

Action	Rationale
12. Slowly inject fluid	Allows fluid to dissipate, and reduces pain
13. After a few seconds withdraw needle	
Apply pressure	Prevents bleeding
Discard needle	Prevents sharps injury
Ensure child settled	
Document procedure	

Further reading

Pratt, R. et al. (2005). The need for skin preparation prior to injection: point-counterpoint. *British Journal of Infection Control*, **6**(4), 18–20.

Workman, B. (1999). Safe injection techniques. *Nursing Standard*, **13**(39), 47–53.

Administration of an IV bolus

Action	Rationale
1. Explain procedure to child and family	Increases understanding and decreases fear
2. Assess validity of prescription. Check the dose is correct and is suitable for IV use, and rate of IV bolus	Safe drug administration Only selected drugs may be given by IV bolus
3. Gather equipment and clean hands	
Consider wearing gloves/safety clothing	Prevent contact with toxic drugs
A clean receptacle in which to carry equipment	Reduces risk of cross-contamination
Two syringes, 5 ml or over, of appropriate size for drug and flush	Applies less pressure than smaller syringes
21 g needle to draw up (23 g from glass ampoule)	Prevents shards of glass being drawn up
Drug and appropriate diluent, and saline flush	
Sharps bin	Reduces risk of sharps injury
Alcohol wipe	
4. Prepare and draw up drug	
Draw up saline flush	Flush required to ensure line is patent and prevent adverse mixing of drugs
Discard needles in sharps bin	
Check with second nurse, as governed by local policy. Check child's name band	Reduces risk of drug errors
5. Reassure child	Lessens distress of IVs
6. Expose cannula site. Observe for signs of pain, redness, and swelling	To assess for signs of tissue irritation
7. Wipe port of cannula with alcohol wipe (30 s). Allow to dry for 30 s	Ensures port is clean
8. Introduce syringe of saline into port; unclamp line; apply gentle consistent pressure, observing for redness/swelling; give required volume of flush; clamp line; remove syringe	Lessens risk of tissue damage
9. Repeat above step with drug, delivering at recommended rate	Decreases risk of adverse drug reaction
10. Flush with saline	Clear line of drug

Michelle Fuller, Southampton University Hospitals NHS Trust

Contd.

Action	Rationale
11. Discard all material, as per local policy; re-dress cannula site	
12. Document that the drug has been given	To prevent drug error

Further reading

Dougherty, L. (2002). Delivery of intravenous therapy. *Nursing Standard*, **16**(16), 45–52.
Workman, B. (1999). Peripheral intravenous therapy management. *Nursing Standard*, **14**(4), 53–60.

Entonox® administration

Entonox® (nitrous oxide) is a homogeneous gas, containing 50% nitrous oxide and 50% O_2 compressed into a cylinder. It is a potent analgesic, with properties comparable to strong opioids.

Entonox provides effective analgesia for use in labour and can be used for short-term pain relief in children having a variety of painful procedures, such as joint injections, change of dressings, and venous cannulation. It is very soluble in the blood and so it is delivered very quickly to the brain to produce an analgesic effect.

Nitrous oxide is an anaesthetic gas and should always be administered following local set criteria and guidelines. It diffuses more rapidly than nitrogen and can expand in enclosed air-containing spaces within the body; therefore care should be taken with its use.

Entonox can be used as a form of self-administered analgesia, but the child must be able to cooperate by using the mouthpiece to release the demand valve and inhale the gas. If he/she is unable to do so, an alternative method of analgesia must be used.

Contraindications for use

- Age
- Airway abnormality
- Breathing problems
- Head injury with impaired consciousness
- Raised ICP
- Signs of basal skull fracture
- Intestinal obstruction
- Vitamin B_{12} deficiency
- Middle-ear obstruction
- Uncorrected congenital heart disease
- History of GOR

Nursing management

- If patient-controlled Entonox is being used, assess each child on an individual basis to determine appropriateness for use.
- Any member of staff involved in Entonox administration should be competently trained in its use and be aware of the safety issues surrounding its use, e.g. use in a well-ventilated room to avoid accumulation, risks for use during early pregnancy, monitoring requirements, concurrent sedatives in use, etc.
- Follow local guidelines regarding fasting recommendations for children before using Entonox.
- Complete a medical checklist before Entonox administration, and monitor appropriately throughout the procedure.

Further reading

Hee, H.I., Goy, R., Suah-Bwee, A. (2003). Effective reduction of anxiety and pain during venous cannulation in children: a comparison of analgesic efficacy conferred by nitrous oxide, EMLA, and combination. *Paediatric Anaesthesia*, **13**(3), 210–16.

Kanagasundaram, S.A., Lane, L.J., Cavalletto, B.P., *et al.* (2001). Efficacy and safety of nitrous oxide in alleviating pain and anxiety during painful procedures. *Archives of Disease in Childhood*, **84**(6), 492–5.

Catherine Trower, Royal Hospital for Sick Children, Glasgow

Patient-controlled analgesia (PCA)

PCA is the administration of analgesia, usually an opioid, by infusion from a hand-held button attached to a pre-programmed computerized pump. The pump is programmed with a suitable dose of analgesia, which is calculated on the child's age and body weight. This allows the child to have control over his/her own analgesia, which has considerable psychological benefits. It also allows the child the chance to anticipate painful procedures and self-administer appropriate analgesia. A maximum dose per hour and lockout time period are programmed into the pump to ensure that the child cannot overdose, thus ensuring safety. Previous studies have found that delivery of a continuous infusion alongside PCA for the first night following surgery can help to give the child a better sleep pattern. The handset is still available for use for breakthrough pain.

Considerations for patient selection

- Cognitive development: the child must be old enough to understand the concept of PCA.
- Understanding: must be able to understand how to use the PCA correctly, including the principles of the lockout time, allowing the analgesia time to take effect, and safety issues.
- Physical ability: those with physical disabilities or reduced conscious levels may not be suitable for PCA.

Safety issues

- Pump programming should be carried out by an appropriately trained person.
- Inappropriate use by parents or other family members. Clear explanation and information about PCA is essential.
- Accidental siphonage: a non-return anti-free-flow valve should be used to prevent free flow of opioid into the patient and reflux of drug up concurrent infusion lines.

Nursing management

- Close monitoring and observation by competently trained staff. Follow local policies for monitoring and recording.
- Monitoring may include:
  - pain scoring (at rest and on movement) to assess efficacy of analgesia and determine appropriate use
  - sedation, nausea, SaO_2, and respiratory rate recordings to ensure early detection and treatment of opioid-induced side effects
  - device check to ensure correct delivery of opioids and detect any potential problems that may occur.

Further reading

Walder, B.M. *et al.* (2001). Efficacy and safety of patient-controlled opioid analgesia for acute postoperative pain. A quantitative systematic review. *Anaesthesiologica Scandinavica*, **45**(7), 795–804.

Catherine Trower, Royal Hospital for Sick Children Glasgow

Epidural analgesia

Epidural analgesia is the administration of analgesics, normally local anaesthetic drugs with or without opioids, into the epidural space. This technique enables analgesics to be given close to the spinal cord and nerves and is a widely used method of managing acute pain in children. A catheter is introduced into the epidural space when the child is asleep, at such a level to ensure that the appropriate spinal nerves are blocked. The administration of epidural analgesia can be done by bolus dosing or continuous infusion. A steady analgesic effect may be difficult to maintain with bolus dosing, but it can be useful in some situations. Continuous delivery of drug agents, administered through an infusion pump, can provide a more consistent level of pain control, which is titrated to meet patients' individual needs.

Any staff involved in the care of a child receiving epidural analgesia must be appropriately trained.

Level of administration

- Thoracic: used in the treatment of pain after major abdominal and thoracic surgery.
- Lumbar: used to provide analgesia after orthopaedic and other limb surgery, and urological and pelvic surgery.
- Caudal: useful approach for younger children having various surgical procedures, e.g. circumcision, inguinal herniotomy, and lower abdominal surgery.

Suggested nursing care

- Regular monitoring is important for early detection of drug-related side effects and signs of epidural procedure complications, and to detect intensity of pain.
- Follow local guidelines for assessment and monitoring requirements of a child receiving epidural analgesia.
- Monitoring may include:
  - pain scoring (at rest and on movement), to assess efficacy of analgesia
  - sedation levels, heart rate, and respiratory rate
  - motor block
  - pulse oximetry, SaO_2 blood pressure
  - urinary pattern
  - device check.

Potential complications

- Motor blockade: can increase the risk of pressure sores in lower limb surgery
- Hypotension
- Dural puncture: can occur when the dura matter is accidentally punctured during the placement of the epidural catheter
- Catheter migration
- Urinary retention

Catherine Trower, Royal Hospital for Sick Children Glasgow

- Haematoma: from trauma to an epidural blood vessel during catheter insertion
- Epidural infection

Other complications if opioids are used:
- respiratory depression
- sedation
- nausea and vomiting
- pruritis.

Further reading

Pasero, C. (2003). Epidural analgesia for postoperative pain: excellent analgesia and improved patient outcomes after major surgery. *American Journal of Nursing* **103**(10), 62–4.
Royal Marsden NHS Trust (2004). Pain management—epidural analgesia. In *Manual of Clinical Nursing Procedures*, 6th edn (ed. L. Dougherty, S. Lisher), pp. 1–22. Blackwell.

Controlled drug administration

Definition

The control of drugs is defined by law within the UK through the Misuse of Drugs Act 1971 and regulations in 1985 and 2001. Five schedules of drugs are identified.

Drugs subject to control by nurses lie within Schedules 2 and 3. These drugs have stringent regulations regarding prescription, requisition, storage, administration, disposal and recording.[1]

Controlled drugs must be administered by a registered nurse and witnessed by another person, who also signs the ward drug record and the child's drug treatment chart, checking the stock balance is correct. The qualification of the second checker depends upon local policy. Within UK hospitals, local policies usually require storage within a securely locked cupboard inside another, with an identified key holder.

Controlled drugs: some uses in nursing children

These drugs are used to manage pain, enable procedures, or facilitate sedation. Some anticonvulsants are also included. Examples include using oral morphine solution for pain management in cancer care, an IV patient-controlled infusion pump for an older child following orthopaedic surgery, or the use of phenobarbital in the control of convulsions.

Issues in administering controlled drugs to children

Dose calculation

Doses are calculated using the child's weight to achieve an optimum dose and then the volume required is calculated. In areas where children may be prescribed single doses post-operatively or to manage pain in emergency departments, the drug dose will be drawn from a stock supply. Frequently, this is in small volumes from ampoules and magnitude errors (10 times the dose prescribed) are possible.

Complications of treatment

As with any medication, nurses must be aware of the nature of the drug given and the potential outcomes that may occur. Childrens' nurses are advised to use the paediatric formulary recommended by the Royal College of Paediatrics and Child Health[2] to ensure they are conversant with these.

Opioids

A number of drugs within the Misuse of Drugs Act Schedules 2 and 3 are opioids, which have specific considerations. Opioids can induce depression of the child's respiratory centre, making respiratory arrest a complication. This can be identified through monitoring and resolved using an opioid antagonist such as naloxone. The use of opioids can also induce nausea and vomiting as a side effect.

Carol Hall and Christopher Jones, University of Nottingham

Communication

Use of controlled drugs requires effective communication with children and their families. Parents may express worries that their child may become addicted to the drugs prescribed, and they need to be prepared for the effects of the drugs they may observe in their child.

Further reading

🔲 www.urban75.org/legaldrugs.html

1 Royal Pharmaceutical Society of Great Britain. Fitness to Practice and Legal Affairs Directorat. *Fact Sheet Two: Controlled Drugs and Hospital Pharmacy*. RPS, (2004).
2 Royal College of Paediatrics and Child Health (2003) *Medicines for children*, 2nd edn. RCPCH.

Commonly used medicines

Medicinal treatment is common in the care of children, in both hospital and community settings. Within the community, it is estimated that 200 million medicines were issued for children and young people during 2002.

Although medicinal treatment is common, associated practice is complex. Historical reluctance to include children during product development means that many medicines remain unlicensed. Medicines are given outside of existing product guidance or modified to make treatment palatable (off label). Research into efficacy and safety remains limited, and there are concerns about information, education, and concordance. It is essential to refer to paediatric formularies for information relating to medicines for children, even if they are commonly used.

Children's formularies

- BNFc (2005): a newly published annual formulary resulting from recommendations made within Standard 10 of the National Standards Framework for Children.
- Royal College of Paediatrics and Child Health (2003): this formulary precedes the BNFc but may be found in practice.

Common purposes of medicinal treatment for children

Therapeutic—to treat identified disease or reduce existing symptoms

- Treatments apply to a range of medicines administered to children, e.g.
  - a bronchodilator, e.g. salbutamol, to treat asthma
  - an antibiotic, such as amoxicillin, for a bacterial throat infection.
- Symptom relief, e.g. analgesics, such as paracetamol, ibuprofen, or morphine, for pain management

Diagnostic—to assist in determining the presence of disease

- Use of laxatives, e.g. sodium picosulphate, to clear the bowel for investigation
- Radio-opaque dyes, to provide contrast in radiography

Preventive—to prevent the onset or development of disease or symptoms

- The childhood vaccination programme
- Rifampicin to reduce secondary cases of meningococcal septicaemia
- Local anaesthetics, such as amethocaine, to prevent pain at venepuncture

Further reading

Costello, I., Wong, I.C.K., Nunn, A.J. (2004). A literature review to identify interventions to improve the use of medicines in children. *Child: Care, Health and Development*, **30**(6), 647–65.

Royal College of Paediatrics and Child Health (2003). *Medicines for Children*, 2nd edn. RCPCH, London.

▣ www.bnfc.org/

▣ www.rcpch.ac.uk/publications/recent_publications/Safer_Better_Medicines.pdf

Carol Hall and Christopher Jones, University of Nottingham

Calculating medicines

Calculating medicines

Prescription of medication to obtain therapeutic doses in children based upon a dose–weight relationship and will vary significantly through the developmental years as the child's weight increases. To accommodate this, pharmaceutical companies prepare many medications in liquid form so that different doses of medication can be drawn from one stock solution.

Although medical practitioners are legally responsible for the correct prescription of the medication, nurses are accountable for ensuring that the correct calculated dose is administered.

The metric system is used to describe the units of medication. If stock solutions are prepared in grams (g) and the prescription is in milligrams (mg), before a calculation can be made a conversion is necessary so that the prescribed and stock doses are in the same units. Some medications which exert a therapeutic effect at very low doses, may be prescribed in micrograms (µg) but supplied in mg in stock solutions. If conversion to similar units is not achieved, then a magnitude error in the calculation will occur, leading to overdose. Another conversion is now necessary to convert the quantity of medication (mg or µg) into a volume (mL) of the solution to be administered.

An equation can be set up to deal with both conversions at the same time:

$$\frac{\text{what is required (prescribed dose)}}{\text{what is available (stock dose)}} \times \text{available dilution (stock volume)}$$

A child is prescribed 125 mg of antibiotic from stock solution of 250 mg/5 mL:

$$\frac{125 \text{ mg}}{250 \text{ mg}} \times 5 \text{ mL}.$$

Divide the top and bottom of the equation by 125.

$$\frac{1}{2} \times 5 \text{ mL} = 2.5 \text{ mL}.$$

Units (mg) on the top and bottom of the equation are the same, and so they cancel each other.

A child is prescribed 800 µg of metoclopramide from a stock solution of 5 mg/5 mL. Because the units of the doses are different, one must be converted so that they are the same. There are 1000 µg in 1 mg. Therefore

800 µg 0.8 mg (by dividing 800 by 1000).

Christopher Jones and Carol Hall, University of Nottingham

There the equation becomes

$$\frac{0.8 \text{ mg}}{5 \text{ mg}} \times 5 \text{ mL}.$$

Divide the top and the bottom of the equation by 5:

$$\frac{0.8}{1} \times 1 \text{ mL} = 0.8 \text{ mL}.$$

Further reading

Hutton, M., Gardner, H. (2005). Calculation skills. *Paediatric Nursing*, **17**(suppl.).
Royal College of Paediatrics and Child Health (2003). *Medicines for children*. Royal College of Paediatrics and Child Health.
Nursing and Midwifery Council (2004). *Guidelines for the administration of medicines* www.nmc-uk.org

Medication calculations

This is a typical prescription chart used in children's wards. Calculate the amount of solution to be given from stock solutions.

REGULAR PRESCRIPTION			Administration Record			
Date			07/10	08/10	09/10	10/10
Drug Metronidazole		06	*(signed)*			
		08				
Dose **80 mg**	Route **i.v.**	Start date **07/10**	12	*(signed)*			
		14				
Additional instr.	Pharm *A.L.B*	18	*(signed)*			
		22				
Signature ⎯⎯*Jones*⎯⎯		24				

- *Question 1.* You have a stock vial of 5 mg in 1 mL.
- Answer…

- *Question 2.* You have a stock bottle of 50 mg in 1 mL, what volume would give for a dose of 280 mg?
- Answer…

- *Question 3.* You have a stock bottle of folic acid 2.5 mg in 5 mL, what volume would give for a dose of 3.5 mg?
- Answer…

- *Question 4.* You have a stock bottle of 4 mg in 5 mL, what volume would give for a dose of 6 mg?
- Answer…

- *Question 5.* You have a stock bottle of 5 mg in 5 mL, what volume would give for a dose of 800 µg?
- Answer…

- *Question 6.* You have a stock bottle of 50 µg in 1 mL, what volume would give for a dose of 80 µg?
- Answer…

Answers: (1) 16 mL; (2) 5.6 mL; (3) 7 mL; (4) 7.5 mL; (5) 0.8 mL; (6) 1.6 mL.

Christopher Jones and Carol Hall, University of Nottingham

Safe storage of medicines

Action	Rationale
All medicines should be stored and handled in a safe and secure manner	To ensure safety of the patient and to comply with the Medicines Act 1968
Storage methods include:	
Lockable cupboards, which are used to store tablets, capsules, and mixtures injections	
Refrigerators reserved solely for the storage of medicines marked with 'store in a refrigerator'. Refrigerators must be fitted with approved temperature monitoring	
Lockable medicine trolleys, for storing all the oral drugs in current use in the ward or department, except for drugs controlled by the Misuse of Drugs Act. Trolleys must be immobilized when not in use	
Lockable controlled drugs cupboard, which contains only those medicines controlled by the Misuse of Drugs Act and marked 'controlled drugs'. *No other drugs/items should be kept in this cupboard*	To ensure continuing safety of the patient and to meet the requirements of the Medicines Act 1968, Misuse of Drugs Act 1971, Use and Control of Medicines 1989, and the Control of Substances Hazardous to Health Regulations 2000
Lockable immobilized bedside medicine storage cupboards, for storage of the patient's own drugs and those supplied for that patient if appropriate	
Lockable security-sealed containers, for transportation or moving medicines	
Sterile fluids should be stored in a clean area designated only for this use	
Emergency boxes, for resuscitation purposes, should be stored in their sealed container with their tamper-proof seals intact, ideally in a closed drawer on the resuscitation trolley	
All cleaning materials must be stored in a separate locked cupboard	

Debbie Martin, Hertfordshire Partnership NHS Trust

Contd.

Action	Rationale
Entrances to pharmacies and other controlled areas should have solid doors, fitted with security locks and alarms	To ensure continuing safety of the patient and to meet the requirements of the Medicines Act 1968, Misuse of Drugs Act 1971, Use and Control of Medicines 1989 and the Control of Substances Hazardous to Health Regulations 2000
Stationery, such as order books and blank prescription forms, should be locked in a cupboard	
The senior nurse/midwife in charge has overall responsibility for the safe keeping of medicines in the ward/department. However, all staff handling medicines must be security conscious	
The medicine cupboard and trolley keys must be kept separate from all other keys and, if not in immediate use, should be held by the nurse in charge	
Keys for the controlled drug cupboard should be kept on a separate ring from keys to other medicine cupboards	

Further reading

Use and Control of Medicines (1989). Guidelines for the safe handling, administration, storage and custody of medicinal products in the Health and Personal Social services. DHSS, London.
Control of Substances Hazardous to Health Regulations (2000). 🖳 www.hse.gov.uk/coshh/

Professional issues

NMC competencies

NMC competencies for nursing practice fall into four key domains and apply to all branches of nursing. They are mandatory for registration as a nurse and encompass one of eight standards that govern nursing practice:
- professional and ethical practice
- personal and professional development
- care management
- care delivery

There are also two standards for post-registration education and practice (PREP), updated in August 2004:
- the PREP (practice) standard
- the PREP (continuing professional development) standard.

Competencies for nursing children and young people build on the core NMC standards to emphasize the wide-ranging principles of family-centred care and negotiation and empowerment for children, young people, and their families. The Royal College of Nursing (RCN) has outlined guidance for children's nurses in a framework for both core and specialist practices, using a broad evidence base.

The framework identifies 19 core role descriptors, which are related to both direct and indirect care. Each descriptor is classified against competency criteria for novice, advanced beginner, competent, proficient, and expert practices. Specialist competencies are also classified, such as paediatric diabetes mellitus nursing.

RCN role descriptors for direct care	RCN role descriptors for indirect care
Professional, ethical, and legal practice	Development of self and others
Care management	Leadership
Communication	Teaching and education
Teaching children, young people, parents and families	Research and evidence-based practice
Promotion of health	Health, safety, and security
Child and adolescent mental health	Equality, diversity, and rights
Protection of children and young people	Cultural competence
Support children, young people, parents, and families through change and difficult circumstances	Quality
Knowledge and information management	Service and practice development
Working with other professionals/agencies	

Geraldine Lyte, University of Manchester

Such work is vital to illustrate the scope of children's nursing practice and, crucially, to stress why children and young people need specially educated nurses. This factor has been highlighted in research to classify children's nursing competencies.

Further reading

Gibson, F., Fletcher, M., Casey, A. (2003). Classifying general and specialist children's nursing competencies. *Journal of Advanced Nursing*, **44**(6), 591–602.
NMC (2004). *Standards of proficiency for pre-registration nursing education*. NMC.
NMC (2004). *The PREP handbook*. NMC.
RCN (2004). *Services for children and young people: preparing nurses for future roles*. RCN.

Developing policies and guidelines

Within the hospital environment, a policy cannot be waived and provides the definitive course of action to be taken.

In the definition of a guideline, the Oxford English dictionary states that a guideline is a general rule, principle, or piece of advice. Any guidelines produced provide guidance, but if there is sufficient reason, they can be varied.

The system used for creating policies is the same as that used for creating guidelines, and therefore the following information can be applied to the production of both.

Identifying the need for a new policy/guideline

The need for new policies or guidelines can arise in a number of ways.

- Incidents highlight the need to address methods of practice.
- Complaints reflect concern regarding how practice is carried out.
- Staff need to be aware of how to use new equipment and carry out new procedures.
- Clinical uncertainty or controversy.
- Resource shortages, resulting in new methods of practice.
- Audit demonstrating need for change in practice.
- Quality of care issues perceived by patients/clinicians/managers.
- Professional/government directives requiring changes in practice.

Writing a policy/guideline

The role of the policies and guidelines facilitator is to draw together the information required for each new document and to ensure that each document reaches the highest possible standard before it is disseminated and implemented.

Once the need for a policy/guideline has been noted, the author(s) gathers the information required to create a new document. If there is an existing document, this can be used to form a framework for the new document. Research must be undertaken to ensure that the document is evidence based and conforms to the latest government and professional directives. Any departments or individuals, such as specialist nurses, ward managers, and medical experts, who have an interest in the document should be sent a draft copy for comment and feedback. This is to ensure that the document meets the standards set in all departments where the document will be used. Other departments with a specialist interest, such as infection control and risk management, should be involved where relevant. Staff representatives from the areas that are expected to implement the document should also review the draft document. In some trusts, this group might take the form of a practice development group.

Standardizing the new documents

Validation

It is essential to ensure that all documents meet the standards set. There are two considerations in forming a validation group.

- The validation group should be empowered to ratify the documents, with a suitably senior person as the chairperson of the group.

Karen Swanson, Southampton University Hospitals NHS Trust

- A minimum number of members for this group should be stipulated to ensure that a broad view of all documents is taken before validation.

A medical consultant will often chair the group, and other members may include a registrar, specialist nurses, a pharmacist, and the policies and guidelines facilitator.

It is important to keep a record of those who have seen and approved the document. The author(s) can be asked to sign and date a form to record this information. The policies and guidelines facilitator is responsible for ensuring that this document is held in case of any future queries. To ensure that the document is based on current evidence, the author may be asked to document the level of evidence that has been reached. One way to do this is to use a recognized method. Additionally, in order for a document to be approved, all members should be asked to review the documents prior to the meetings. This is to ensure that every opportunity is given to the members to provide feedback or clarify information. A monthly meeting can be held to discuss documents.

Once signed by the chairman of this group, the document can be disseminated to the relevant areas for implementation.

Dissemination

To provide readily accessible information to all staff, a folder containing all validated documents can be created. This can be maintained by the policies and guidelines facilitator, with the help of a link person from each unit.

Implementation

Implementation of any change in practice should be carefully planned and monitored and should involve representatives from all areas affected by the new document.

Reviewing the documents

To ensure that documents are regularly reviewed, every document validated should be issued with a review date, which is normally 1–3 years after it has been issued. The policies and guidelines facilitator can maintain a database to ensure that documents are reviewed by the original author(s) where possible before this date is reached. The validation committee can then approve any amendments arising from a review before they are incorporated within the document.

Further reading

Grimshaw, J.M., Russell, I.T. (1993). Effect of clinical guidelines on medical practice: a systematic review of rigorous evaluations. *Lancet*, **342**(8883),1317–22.

Woolf, S., Grol, R., Hutchinson, A., Eccles, M., Grimshaw, J. (1999). Clinical practice guidelines: the potential benefits, limitations and harms of recommending how to care for patients. *British Medical Journal*, **318**, 527–30.

The NSF for Children, Young People, and Maternity Services in England

The English NSF for Children, Young People, and Maternity Services sets new standards for children and young people across health and social care boundaries in England. This will be achieved through the introduction of 11 auditable standards, which are predicated upon best evidence-based practice in the care of pregnant women, children, and young people. The NSF is presented in three parts.

- Setting standards for well children and young people aimed at keeping them safe and healthy through the provision of optimum life chances.
- Setting standards for sick children and young people in the community and hospital, and for those with mental health problems, disabilities, and complex health needs.
- Setting standards for maternity services.

In his introduction to the NSF, Dr John Reid, the Secretary of State for Health, reinforces the reality that inequalities in healthcare and social care still impact on children and young people. His emphasis on child poverty and the effect this has on children and young people forms the backdrop to the whole NSF, commencing perhaps with standard 11 of the report 'maternity services', because it is known that much ill health and disease in adulthood has its origins before, during, and after pregnancy. The standards of the NSF cover many of the parameters of childhood, such as tackling the growing burden on health of obesity through recommendations to improve school meals and encouraging children to take 60 min of exercise daily.

The Right Start: The NSF for Children, Young People, and Maternity Services (🖳 www.doh.gov/childrenstaskforce), the first part of the NSF to be published, sets rigorous standards for children in hospital, which are grouped around three main themes:

- child-centred hospital services
- quality and safety of care provided
- quality of setting and environment.

Although the government envisages that full implementation of the NSF will take up to 10 years, it has also stressed that the NHS and local authorities charged with its implementation will be frequently assessed by the Healthcare Commission, the Commission for Social Care Inspection, and Ofsted, to ensure that they are compliant and making progress. The Association of Chief Children's Nurses will regularly post exemplars of good practice related to the NSF on its website (🖳 accnuk.org).

Further reading

Department of Health (2004). The National Service Framework for Children, Young People and Maternity Services. 🖳 www.doh.gov.uk

Alan Glasper, University of Southampton

The NSF for Children, Young People, and Maternity Services in Wales

The NSF for Children, Young People, and Maternity Services in Wales was published in September 2005, with the stated purpose that it should provide the template for the development of health services in Wales to ensure that 'children and future generations enjoy better prospects in life and are not landed with a legacy of problems bequeathed by us'. It sets out the quality of services that children, young people, and their families have a right to expect.

The NSF forms one part of a range of Welsh Assembly Government strategies aimed at improving the health and well-being of children and young people in the principality. All of these are guided by the United Nations Convention on the Rights of the Child and can be expressed in seven core aims.

To ensure that *all* children and young people:
• have a flying start in life
• have a comprehensive range of education and learning opportunities
• enjoy the best possible health and freedom from abuse, victimization, and exploitation
• have access to play, leisure, sporting, and cultural activities
• are listened to, treated with respect, and have their race and cultural identity recognized
• have a safe home and a community, which supports physical and emotional well-being
• are not disadvantaged by poverty.

The NSF has six sections.
• Key actions universal to all children
• Maternity services
• Children and young people with mental health problems and disorders
• Disabled children and young people (includes transitions)
• Children and young people in special circumstances
• Children and young people with acute and chronic illness or injury

These comprise 203 key actions, which are all explicit objectives that are all framed in the present tense—no 'should' or 'will'—as the strongest way of wording objectives. Of the key actions, 82 are 'flagged', which means that they have to be achieved by the last day of March 2006 'Unflagged' key actions must be achieved by 2014.

Each key action identifies who is responsible for ensuring that it is achieved, e.g. NHS trust, local health board, local authority, etc.

Achievement of the key actions will be audited by the children's and young people's framework partnerships in each local health board/local authority area. They will use an on-line self-assessment audit tool for this A 'balanced-score card' report can be produced annually to record progress across Wales.

Jim Richardson, University of Glamorgan

Further reading

Welsh Assembly Government (2005). *The National Service Framework for Children, Young People and Maternity Services in Wales*. Welsh Assembly Government, Cardiff.

The National Service Framework for Children, Young People and Maternity Services in Wales (document in English). 🖳 www.wales.nhs.uk/sites/documents/441/ACFD1F6.pdf

Fframwaith Gwasanaeth Cenedlaethol ar gyfer Plant, Pobl Ifanc a Gwasanaethau Mamolaeth yng Nghymru (document in Welsh).

🖳 www.wales.nhs.uk/sites/documents/441/NSFforChildren,YoungPeople&MaternityServices (welsh).pdfJim Richardson

A national framework for service change in the NHS in Scotland

Building a health service fit for the future

Key messages

In planning the future of the NHS in Scotland, a number of recommendations are made that are underpinned by the following key messages.

- Ensure sustainable and safe local services: redesign where possible to meet local needs and expectations—specialize where required, having regard to clinical benefit and to access.
- View the NHS as a service delivered predominantly in local communities rather than in hospitals; 90% of health care is delivered in primary care.
- Preventive, anticipatory care rather than reactive management: the NHS should work with other public services and with patients and carers to ensure that healthcare crises are prevented from happening.
- Galvanize the whole system: integrate the NHS more fully to meet the challenges.
- Become a modern NHS: use technology to improve the standard and the speed of care, connect clinicians, and support the research vital to future well-being.
- Develop new skills to support local services: generalists, as well as specialists, nurses and allied health professionals, and doctors—all with the right skills for patients.
- Develop options for change *with* people, not *for* them.

A health service fit for children

Key recommendations

- NHS Scotland adopts the guiding principle that the age of admitting children and young people to acute care in paediatric facilities is up to the 16th birthday, dependent upon their clinical need and patient choice. For young people between the ages of 16 years and 18 years there should be discussion with their clinician(s) regarding where their care is best delivered, recognizing their right of choice, unless there are clear clinical reasons that determine whether admission is to paediatric or adult services.
- Each NHS board area should review its services for young people and develop proposals for age-appropriate care and arrangements for transition from child to adolescent care and adolescent to adult care.

Specialized services

- The definition of specialized services underpins the future planning of children's health care, and the NHS adopts the Department of Health (DOH) specialist services definitions as they apply to children and as appropriate for Scotland.
- There is a framework for specialized critical care. This includes:
  - accident and emergency departments and in-patient services for babies and children should be supported by the capability to provide, at least short-term, critical care support for children.

Angela Horsley, NHS Grampian

- NHS Education Scotland (NES), with other stakeholders, should adapt the existing arrangements for training accreditation so that training can be provided through rotational posting across a number of sites within one service and develop accredited training for nurses to advanced practitioners.
- People: this information should be shared with NHS 24, primary care teams, out-of-hours' services, and the Scottish ambulance service.

Scottish policies: bridging the gaps

Since the formation of the Scottish Parliament in 1999, the Scottish Executive has introduced several pieces of legislation that have focused on the health and well-being of young people (Scotland Act 1999). These have reflected the key policy document issued by the United Nations (The United Nations Convention of the Child 1989) and the European Parliament (European Convention on Human Rights 1998).

The Children's (Scotland) Act 1995

This legislation incorporates the principles of the United Nations Convention of the Rights of the Child (1989) and gives children and young people the rights to express their views on a wide range of decisions.

Beattie Report (1999)

The Beattie Report (1999)—*Implementing Inclusiveness, Realising Potential*—aimed to increase both the participation and attainment of young people in post-school education and training.

Social Justice ... A Justice Where Everyone Matters (1999)

Set out the strategy aimed at improving opportunity for young people to make the transition between school and work life. The essence of the strategy is to ensure young people have the opportunity to participate to the maximum of his or her potential.

The Child Strategy Statement 1999

The focus of this statement was to encourage all departments within the Scottish Executive to review how individual policies impacted on the health and well-being of children and young people. It recommended that the views of children and young people should be sought, as well as adults. This has led to wider consultation being undertaken.

Our National Health: A Plan for Action, a Plan for Change (2000)

As well as setting out the priorities for the health of children and young people, this document strongly recommends that they should be included in any consultations that take place with the public.

The Policy Framework for Tackling Social Exclusion in Scotland (2000)

One in three children in Scotland live in relative poverty. This document outlines the Scottish Executive strategy for tackling social exclusion.

Equality Strategy: Working Together for Equality (2000)

The focus of this document relates to disadvantaged and discriminated young people. It aims to tackle discrimination, prejudice, and poverty in Scotland.

Kate Jackson, Napier University Edinburgh

Scottish Youth Parliament

The Scottish Youth Parliament was set up after devolution in 1999. It is an elective body of 200 14–25-year-olds, representing the young people of Scotland. It launched its first manifesto in 2003, *Getting the Message Right*, in which it sets out its hopes and expectations for the future citizens of the country.

The Commissioner for Children and Young People's Act 2003

Kathleen Marshall was appointed the first Commissioner in 2003. Her main responsibility is to promote and safeguard the rights of children and young people in Scotland.

Useful websites

- www.healthscotland.com/
- www.scottishyouthparliament.org.uk/
- www.childpolicy.org.uk/enghome/index.cfm

Other relevant policies

Represented here is a glimpse into government policy already in existence that will be of relevance to you as a registered children's nurse.

- Remember: each health organization/trust has its own approach to implementing and disseminating policy.
- Familiarize yourself with the systems and processes in place where you are currently employed. These may well be linked to a local Clinical Governance Framework.
- New or revised policies are appearing all the time, at both local and national levels. Therefore you have a responsibility for keeping up to date and ensuring that your nursing practice adheres to current policy and guidelines.
- Your employer also has a responsibility to inform you of changes in practice as a result of changing policy.

The United Nations Convention on the Rights of the Child (1989)

International legislation that is well respected, well used, and accepted across the world. Signed up to by the UK (1991). Stands alongside the Human Rights Act 1998 (DoH 2000) (📖 Children's rights, p. 884)

Historical landmark policies for children's health services

- *Platt Report* (HMSO 1959)
- *Court Report* (HMSO 1976)
- *Children's Act* (HMSO 1989)
- *Welfare of Children and Young People in Hospital* (HMSO 1991)
- *Allitt Inquiry/Clothier Report* (DOH 1994)

More recently:

- *Kennedy Report* (DOH 2001) into Bristol children's heart surgery
- *Redfern Report* (DOH 2001) into Liverpool Children's Hospital
- *Seeking consent: Working with children* (DOH 2001)
- *Laming Report* (DOH 2003) into the death of Victoria Climbie
- *Children's Bill* (DOH 2004)

However, government policy relating to healthcare more often relates to the NHS as an organization, in its entirety, and seeks to address issues, concerns, and/or introduce long-term and short-term changes to service provision that affect the entire population.

It then becomes important as a registered children's nurse to seek to use these policies to address issues, resolve disparities in healthcare, and highlight the specific and very different needs of children and, particularly, young people. Examples of these are:

- *NHS modern and dependable* (DOH 1997)
- *Health of the nation* (DOH 1998)
- *Essence of care* (DOH 2001)

Furthermore, it is important to understand that there are implications in adhering to and following policy associated with working in any one of

Krystyna Sutkowski, North East Wales NHS Trust Wrexham

the four countries that make up the UK (England, Scotland, Northern Ireland, and Wales), e.g. NSF for children and young people.

Government policy emanating from the Department of Health will either be adopted for use within Wales, Scotland, or Northern Ireland or each country may choose to instigate its own policy, e.g. 📖 child protection.

The way forward

For further information and to remain up to date.

- Ask your managers to outline the local policy system and to show you how to access copies. Check out your local intranet sites and clinical governance team for information relating to policy.
- Visit your local nursing/NHS library to scan relevant journals for notification of pending publications out for consultation or published.
- Log on to the following sites:
  - England and Scotland:
    - 🖥 www.doh.gov.uk
    - 🖥 www.scotland.gov.uk
    - 🖥 www.dfes.gov.uk
    - 🖥 www.scottish.parliament.uk
    - 🖥 www.parliament.uk/commons
    - 🖥 www.doh.gsi.gov.uk
  - Wales and Northern Ireland:
    - 🖥 www.wales.gov.uk
    - 🖥 www.dhsspsni.gov.uk
    - 🖥 http://childcomwales.org.uk
    - 🖥 http://investingforhealthni.gov.uk
  - Also:
    - 🖥 www.childpolicy.org.uk/news
    - Nursing and Midwifery Council. 🖥 www.nmc-uk.org
    - Royal College of Nursing. 🖥 www.rcn.org.uk
    - Association of British Paediatric Nurses. 🖥 http://abpn.org.uk
    - National Electronic Library for Health. 🖥 www.nelh.nhs.uk
    - National Institute for Clinical Excellence. 🖥 http://nice.org.uk
    - Royal College of Paediatrics and Child Health.
    - 🖥 http://rcpch.org.uk

Further reading

Muir, J., Sidey, A. (2000). *Textbook of community children's nursing*. Ballière Tindall/RCN publication.

Clinical judgements and decision-making: nursing diagnosis

The RCN has defined nursing as 'the use of clinical judgement in the provision of care to enable people to improve, maintain, or recover health, to cope with health problems, and to achieve the best possible quality of life, whatever their disease or disability, until death'.

Nursing diagnosis is a clinical judgement that describes how an individual or group of people respond to health problems or other health-related experiences. It forms part of any assessment process and provides the basis for nursing, collaborative, and/or client-led decisions for care. A medical diagnosis, by comparison, usually describes what the health problem is. Nursing diagnosis is recognized internationally as an essential element of both first-level and advanced practice roles.

There are North American and European classifications of commonly used nursing diagnoses, although with children and young people specific diagnoses have been less common until recently.

Below is an example of one child and young person nursing diagnosis, one of 28 that were developed with several practising children's nurses in a London NHS Hospital. You will see that it is the defining characteristics, related factors, and outcomes for care that validate the diagnosis for use with children and young people.

Child and young person nursing diagnosis (Lyte and Jones (2001) reproduced with the permission of the *Journal of Clinical Nursing*, Blackwell Publishing)

Diagnostic label
Fear of needles.

Definition
A feeling of dread related to the use of needles.

Geraldine Lyte, University of Manchester

Defining characteristics	Related factors	Outcomes for care
Infant/child/adolescent does not cope with needles	History of traumatic needle event	The infant's/child's/adolescent's fear will be reduced with family/carer and multidisciplinary team support
Family/carers do not cope well with child requiring a needle	Fear that treatment is punishment	The infant's/child's/adolescent's fear will be alleviated with family/carer and multidisciplinary team support
Child/adolescent verbalizes inability to cope with needles	Inability to understand use of needles	Selected interventions will be effective in aiding the child/adolescent and family/carers to cope with the use of needles
Family/carers verbalize own inability to cope with needles	Fear of pain from needle insertion	An alternative form of therapy will be provided whenever feasible
Family/carers verbalize infant's/child's/adolescent's inability to cope with needles	Relay fear from family/other	
Child/adolescent refuses needle		
Family/carers refuse needle on behalf of infant's/child's/adolescent		
Increased pulse rate		
Increased respiration rate		
Crying		
Sweating		
Anxiety		
Panic behaviour		

Further reading

Royal College of Nursing (2003). *Defining nursing*. RCN.

North American Nursing Diagnosis Association (2005). *Nursing diagnoses: definitions and classification 2005–2006*. NANDA.

Lyte, G., Jones, K. (2001). Developing a unified language for children's nurses, children and their families in the United Kingdom. *Journal of Clinical Nursing*, **10**. 79–85.

Record keeping

Importance of record keeping
- Provides objective written evidence of actions taken, advice given, observations, and plans made.
- Facilitates continuity and consistency of care.
- Provides an aide-memoire in the preparation of reports/statements.
- Contributes to audit of clinical care.

Professional accountability
- Documentation of the action is as important as the action itself.
- Failure of record keeping could be construed as failure of care (negligence).
- Any entry by a pre-registration student or nursing auxiliary/healthcare assistant must be countersigned by a registered nurse, who is professionally accountable for any consequence of this entry.

Involvement of child/family
- Records should ideally be written with the involvement of the child/family.
- Any decision to keep a supplementary record to which access by the child/family is limited or withheld must be justifiable. All the health-care team must be informed of its existence and be able to access it without compromising patient/client confidentiality.

Content and style
- Records must be legible, accurate, relevant, comprehensive, and factual.
- Any opinions or feelings must be clearly identified as such.
- Records should be contemporaneous (completed as near to the event as possible) and written in chronological order.
- If information is quoted from a third party, the source must be attributed.
- A clear care plan must be included, reviewed, updated, and evaluated.
- Abbreviations, jargon, meaningless/offensive phrases, and irrelevant speculation should be avoided.
- All entries must be signed, timed, and dated by the person recording the information.
- The person recording the information must print their name against their signature if writing in this record for first time.

Mistakes
- Information entered in the record must not be obliterated (e.g. with correction fluid).
- Errors should be crossed out with a single line (so they are still legible), dated, timed, and signed.
- The correct entry should then follow or an explanation about the error should be included (e.g. if the nurse wrote in the wrong records).

Louise Holliday, Royal Aberdeen Children's Hospital

Access to records
- Nurses have a duty to protect the confidentiality of the patient/client.
- Patients/clients usually have the right of access to their records.
- Records should be retained at least until the date of a child's 21st birthday.

Further reading
Nursing and Midwifery Council (2004). *Guidelines for records and record keeping.* NMC.

Children's rights

The value and need for children to be consulted, and have their views heard and respected, are clearly stated in many influential documents.

Respect

Show respect in your partnership with the child/young person and family. Every effort should be made to respect the child's need for privacy, explain what is happening, and ask permission.

Legal and ethical position

Through effective assessment and developing a rapport with the child and family, you should be aware of any potential conflicts between the interests of the child/young person and those of the parents. Although young people at the age of 16 years can give valid consent to treatment without regard to their parent's wishes, they do not have complete autonomy. Treatment refusal can be overruled by the court in respect of life-threatening situations. Discuss any concerns over the legal position with the multidisciplinary team involved in the child/young person's care and your organization's legal department.

Sharing information

Children/young people need access to accurate information that is understandable and ethically and culturally appropriate. A range of communication methods can be used, e.g. videotapes and storybooks.

Children/young people's opinions and views

Structures should be in place to allow children/young people to voice their opinions and views about their care and treatment. Public participation and involvement groups allow healthcare users the opportunity to do this. This is recognized as a standard for best practice.

Patient advisory and liaison services are available in every NHS trust. They provide help, advice, and information. Most NHS trusts have a representative for children/young people.

Environment

- Where admission is planned, children should be prepared through a pre-admission visit where information and orientation to the health-care setting is provided.
- Children/young people have a basic need for play and recreation. There is evidence that this reduces anxiety.
- Play should be used for therapeutic purposes to assimilate new information, adjust to and gain control over a potentially frightening environment, and prepare to cope with procedures and interventions.
- A child/young person-friendly environment, with age-appropriate facilities, is paramount for this.

Jan Orr, Royal Cornwall Hospital Trust

Planning care and discharge

It is well evidenced that children/young people recover more quickly at home. Discharge planning is a priority and should start as soon as the child/young person is admitted. Discharge planning and information should always involve the child/young person and be conducive to their understanding.

Further reading

Department of Health (2003). The *National Service Framework for Children, Young People and Maternity Services*. Stationery Office.

United Nations General Assembly (1989). *Convention on the Rights of the Child*. United Nations, New York. (Ratified by the UK Government in 1991.)

The role of the nurse advocate

Advocacy is a complex concept used to describe a range of actions that benefit others. There is a difference between acting in someone's best interests, which stems from beneficence, and advocacy, which stems from autonomy, the right to self-determination. Children's nurses frequently advocate for parents, carers, teenagers, and older children, all of whom are able to voice their hopes, values, and wishes in a way that is understandable to all. Advocating for babies and very young children is not possible. However, acting in their best interests is appropriate and essential, and a legal requirement under the Children Act 1989, but it is different from advocacy.

The essence of advocacy is to hear the voice of those not powerful enough to be heard and speak for them. In children's nursing, this means developing sensitive, age-appropriate, and culturally appropriate communication, to break the silence of those with little language or ability to communicate. Advocacy involves actively canvassing the opinion of such children in order to present and articulate their views. This involves allowing them the right to be free from interference and participate in difficult decisions about their own healthcare, safety, and protection, accepting or rejecting a proposed course of action. The advocate does not have to agree, and the child's voice will usually be one of several in the decision-making process, but the child's view needs to be heard, noted, and acknowledged.

In addition to health and child protection, children's views should also be sought in relation to the provision of health services. Too often, the user's view is that of the parents. They cannot represent the child themselves, and ways need to be found to ensure that the voices of children, even very young ones, are heard.

Further reading

Charles-Edwards, I. (2001). Children's nursing and advocacy: are we in a muddle? *Paediatric Nursing*, **13**(2), 12–16.

Helen Russell-Johnson, University of Hertfordshire

Consent

Consent is a patient's agreement for a health professional to provide care. To be valid, the patient must be competent to take the particular decision, have received sufficient information, and not be acting under duress. Consent for operative procedures and specific investigative treatments require a consent form to be completed. Healthcare providers should have local policies for this.

Consent is relevant to major decisions and smaller choices. The law requires that consent is gained on every occasion for routine intervention, such as blood taking, urine testing, and X–rays. This should be documented.

When a child who is not deemed old enough or competent to give consent is admitted to a healthcare setting, a discussion should take place with the parents/carers. If the parent/carer is with the child, consent should be sought prior to any procedure or intervention. If the parent/carer is not going to be present, then information about intended and probable interventions and consent must be gained in advance. This should be clearly documented. If the parent/carer specifies that he/she wishes to be asked before particular procedures are initiated, this must be done, unless the delay involved in contacting them is detrimental to the child's safety.

Can children consent for themselves?

Young people over 16 years are presumed to have the competence to consent for themselves. Younger children who understand what is involved in the proposed procedure can give consent. Ideally their parents/carer should be involved. If a competent child consents to treatment, a parent cannot override the decision. Legally a parent/carer with parental responsibility can consent if a competent child refuses.

If the child is too young or not deemed competent, an adult who has parental responsibility, or the court, can give consent and sign relevant documentation. When necessary, the courts can overrule a refusal by a person with parental responsibility. Advice should be sought from the healthcare provider's legal team if there are any concerns.

Contraception

Contraception, and the required advice, can be given to the child/young person under 16 years without their parent/carer's consent. The healthcare professional must be sure that the child/young person cannot be persuaded to inform his/her parents and is likely to go ahead and have intercourse with or without contraception. The child/young person must understand the advice that he/she is given.

Further reading

Gillick v West Norfolk and Wisbech Area Health Authority (1985). 3 All ER 402–3.

Jan Orr, Royal Cornwall Hospital Trust

Legal frameworks

The following standards give guidance and required action plans to promote standards of safe and good practice for the child/young person.

Every Child Matters: Change for Children (2004)

The Children Act (1989) changed the law relating to child protection. The framework required updating to strengthen services to children, young people, and their families. As a result, the Children Act (2004) is now in effect.

This new law requires that every organization caring for children has a designated lead member and director of children's services.

The Act gives guidance on common core skills and knowledge required for everyone working with children, young people, and families. These include:

• effective communication and engagement
• child and young person development
• safeguarding and promoting the welfare of the child
• supporting transitional care
• multi-agency working
• sharing information.

Published alongside this is a 'common assessment framework for children and young people', which is designed to help practitioners in all agencies to work more effectively and to provide early intervention when difficulties arise.

Human Rights Act (1998)

This law allows individual citizens who feel their rights, as outlined in the Act, have been abused or infringed to seek redress in the British courts. The Act is divided into articles, all of which are relevant to the healthcare professional.

Issues, such as a right to respect of private and family lives, freedom of thought, conscience, and religion, freedom of expression, freedom of assembly and association, and prohibition of discrimination, are paramount issues in caring for the child/young person and their family.

Parental responsibility

Changes in the law relating to parental responsibility came into effect in 2004.

The changes result from amendments to the Children Act (1989). The law states there will be two sets of parental responsibility arrangements for unmarried fathers. Those who do not register the birth of the child jointly with the mother will be in the same position as existing unmarried fathers. Fathers who register jointly will have automatic parental responsibility.

Care should always be taken when undertaking patient history and assessment to clarify who has parental responsibility. Any concerns should be discussed with your organization's legal team.

Jan Orr, Royal Cornwall Hospital Trust

The Victoria Climbié Inquiry (2003)

This report identified recommendations to reshape the way child protection cases are managed. The report, undertaken by Lord Laming, identified that systems in place were ineffective, lacked resources, and lacked documentation and communication between agencies. The RCN produced an action plan to increase the profile of child protection and make people take account of their own roles and responsibilities in relation to child protection. The main message is that every healthcare professional has a duty of care.

Convention for the Rights of the Child (1989)

This international convention highlighted that children and young people have rights that are not always understood and respected, and that they should be involved in decisions about their care. This influential document sets out standards of good practice with regard to valuing the child/young person.

Further reading

Chudleigh, J. (2005). Safeguarding children. *Paediatric Nursing*, **17**, 37–42.
Department of Health (1989). *Children Act*. HMSO.
Department of Health (2003). *The Victoria Climbie Inquiry*. Stationery Office.
Department of Health (2005). *Every child matters: change for children*. Stationery Office.
United Nations (1989). *Convention for the rights of the child*. UN, New York. (Ratified by the UK Government in 1991.)
Power, K. (2002). Implications of the Human Rights Act 1998. *Paediatric Nursing*, **16**, 28–9.

User involvement in planning and evaluating services

Children and young people who need to spend time in hospital may find it stressful. Both the NHS Plan and the Partnership for Care (government reports on making the NHS meet patients' needs better) say that involving patients and the public in developing the NHS is important. Doing so makes sure that the service is 'patient-centred'. It also gives patients and the public, including children and young people, a say in managing their local services. They can be more confident that the NHS will provide the health care they need.

The Kennedy Report (the public inquiry into children's heart surgery at Bristol Royal Infirmary) also recommends involving people. It says that the NHS should make sure it involves not only patients, but the public too. The NHS should do this in a way that it can to be open and honest.

The Health and Social Care Act 2001 makes sure that health organizations listen and respond to the views of patients and the public. It requires them to involve and consult patients and the public when they plan new services and change existing ones.

The Association of Chief Children's Nurses supports the idea of patient and family forums, which will give trusts the chance to involve and consult patients and the public fully when they:
- plan services that they are responsible for
- draw up and think about plans to change the way those services are provided
- make decisions that will affect how services work.

Setting up a patient forum
Forum members must include:
- children, young people, and their families who use, or have used, your service
- young people who have now moved on to adult services
- people from support groups for specific health conditions
- a non-executive director of the trust board or a senior member of the management team.

Working with members
- Give members of the forum a trust honorary contract and identification badge, which must be visible at all times.
- Provide forum members with an orientation programme.
- Make the most of forum members' skills and time.
- Give members any other training that they need, so they can help with the forum's work as much as possible.

Further reading
Department of Health (2000). *The NHS Plan.* Department of Health London.

Rory Farrelly, Derby Hospitals NHS Foundation Trust

Clinical governance in children's services

Clinical governance is about a culture shift to a child, young person, and their family-centred, accountable, and high-quality service in an open and questioning environment. It challenges traditional structures and ways of doing things, leading to creating a consistent and quality approach to health care. Clinical governance assists safe and high-quality care, and it is crucial that it is not used in isolation.

Key principles of clinical governance

- It has been a statutory duty since 1997 for all health organizations
- Staffing and staff management
- Research
- Information management
- Clinical audit
- User satisfaction
- Education and continuing professional development for all staff
- Risk management
- These principles have led to the creation of a widely used clinical governance model

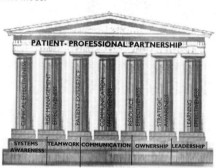

Dewar model of clinical governance

Key principles of quality improvement

- Needs of children, young people, and their families are central
- Quality needs to be measured
- Quality improvement needs to be continuous and ongoing
- Quality is best achieved through effective leadership and management
- Effective organizational communication
- Establish training and development programmes to meet needs
- Promote the development of clinical and non-clinical standards and clinical audit
- Effective organizational quality strategy
- All staff are responsible for quality

Rory Farrelly, Derby Hospitals NHS Foundation Trust

- Good incident reporting systems, taking the 'fair blame' approach and learning from mistakes
- Clear lines of responsibility and accountability for quality of clinical care

Questions to consider, helping you reflect on your day-to-day practice

- What does clinical governance mean to you in the area in which you work?
- What do you need to do differently?
- What does quality mean to you?
- What does quality mean to you when at work?
- What does the NMC mean by quality?

Conclusion

The expectation for providing high-quality health care has never been greater. The clinical governance process is a dynamic one, which will evolve further with better evaluation, sharing, and benchmarking of best-practice guidelines, quality indicators, and regular reviews of standards linked with outcomes of patient care. The major issue, having successfully met the basic requirements for clinical governance, is to maintain the momentum. As well as assuming responsibility and ownership, commitment to delivery will be essential. Quality is everyone's business and should been seen as a significant aspect in the evolution of health care in the 21st century.

Further reading

Royal College of Nursing (1999). *Realising clinical effectiveness and clinical governance through clinical supervision*. Radcliffe Medical Press.
Dewar, S. (1999). Clinical governance under construction. King's Fund.

Adverse-event reporting

Definitions

- An adverse event: any event that has led to unintended or unexpected harm to a patient.
- A near miss: an event that could have led to harm to a patient, but either the error was rectified before harm occurred or no harm occurred by chance.

Why is there an adverse-event reporting system?

- Government response to the Clothier (1990) and Kennedy (2001) reports, where inadequate reporting was identified as a factor in causing harm.
- Repeated serious incidents, e.g. administration of IV vincristine intrathecally in error.

Why report adverse events?

- To identify what is going wrong
- Chance to investigate root cause, rather than individual blame
- Opportunity to learn from mistakes

Why report a 'near miss'?

A near miss can be regarded as a 'free lesson'. An opportunity to learn from a mistake that has not harmed a patient but might do so if repeated.

How to report

- Each trust will have its own system of reporting. Sometimes clinical incidents are reported separately from non-clinical (e.g. health and safety and security). Find out how to report incidents in your department, who needs to see the report, and what happens to it afterwards.
- Serious incidents have an accelerated reporting pathway. Find out about your employer's serious incident policy and when to use it.
- When completing documentation, give date, time, description, people involved, and outcome. Give precise information, e.g. equipment machine number, batch number of disposables, drug name, and dose. Remember a judgement has to be made about the level of risk this event represents.
- Risk managers do not always have time to get back to you about individual reports. If you want to know what has happened, ask.

What happens next?

- The primary aim of the process is to prevent harm occurring, rather than blaming an individual.
- If you are involved in the incident, your employer should provide some support for you. Ask your mentor or manager about this.
- Reflect on the event yourself. It is known that human error cannot be eliminated, but is there a change that could help, e.g. avoiding giving drugs around shift handover, when communication errors may occur?

Pearl Mathews, Southampton University Hospital NHS Trust

- Your trust will pass on statistical details of the reported events to the National Patient Safety Agency and outcomes of any serious incidents investigations.

Further reading

Department of Health (2000). An organisation with a memory: *report of an expert group on learning from adverse events in the NHS chaired by the Chief Medical Officer*. Department of Health London.
Department of Health (2001). *Building a safer NHS for patients: implementing an organisation with a memory*. Department of Health London.

Dealing with complaints in the NHS

Complaints, verbal or written, need to be dealt with appropriately and sensitively. To ensure complaints are resolved as quickly and fully as possible, the Government has produced a framework and targets for responding to complaints.

The complaints procedure has three stages.
- Local resolution: the service provider attempts to resolve the complaint as directly and quickly as possible. Includes both informal responses from front-line staff and formal investigation and written responses.
- Independent review: from January 2005, the Healthcare Commission has taken on the role of dealing with these reviews. Information is requested about the original complaint and a decicision taken as to whether a review is appropriate.
- Ombudsman review: where an independent review is refused or the complainant is dissatisfied with the outcome, the ombudsman may be asked to consider the complaint.

Your role in dealing with complaints

Before a complaint occurs:
- familiarize yourself with your local complaints policy and how your department prefers to deal with complaints
- know how to contact key people and what they do, e.g. department complaint lead, PALS, and to whom written complaint should be addressed

When a complaint occurs
- Treat all complaints seriously. Do not become defensive or dismissive. It is the family's experience that must be addressed.
- Listen carefully so you can respond to the actual concerns. Ask what they want to achieve.
- Ensure you record the concern/complaint and any information given or action taken according to local policy.
- If you cannot resolve the complaint, pass it on to someone more senior.
- Inform your department manager or complaint lead of any unresolved complaint.
- If an specific incident has occurred or the family is very angry, complete an adverse-incident form according to local policy.

Be aware
- Confidentiality: this remains the same as when dealing with any clinical information.
- Accuracy: it is very important to be absolutely accurate and honest. If you give an incorrect answer and a subsequent investigation shows this to be wrong, the family may well become suspicious.

Further reading

Department of Health (2003). *NHS complaints reform: making things right.* Department of Health London.

Department of Health. Handling complaints in the NHS—*good practice toolkit for local resolution.* www.doh.gov.uk Gateway ref.2944

Pearl Mathews, Southampton University Hospital NHS Trust

Safeguarding children

Identifying and assessing harm, abuse, and neglect

Significant harm

The Children Act (1989) requires that local authorities make enquiries and assess what is happening to children if there are concerns that they may be suffering significant harm. Children are suffering significant harm if, in the best interests of the child, compulsory intervention in family life is deemed necessary to prevent abuse and neglect.

Abuse and neglect

Children may be abused in a family, institutional, or community setting, most commonly by someone known to them, in a number of ways.

- *Physical abuse* such as hitting, shaking, throwing, burning, suffocating, or by deliberately causing or fabricating symptoms of illness in the child.
- *Emotional abuse* or persistent ill-treatment that impairs children's emotional development by making them feel worthless, unloved, inadequate, frightened, or exploited.
- *Sexual abuse* involving forcing or coercing children to participate in sexual activities, such as rape or buggery, or non-penetrative acts, such as making children look at pornographic materials.
- *Neglect* or persistent failure to meet children's physical and/or psychological needs by depriving them of food, shelter, and clothing or being unresponsive to their basic emotional needs.

Assessing needs

The *Framework for the Assessment of Children in Need and Their Families*[1] advises that a triangular assessment framework can be used to safeguard and promote the welfare of children.

- Child's developmental needs: health, education, emotional and behavioural development, identity, family and social relationships, social presentation, and self-care skills.
- Parenting capacity: basic care, ensuring safety, emotional warmth, stimulation, guidance and boundaries, and stability.
- Family and environmental factors: family history and functioning, wider family, housing, employment, income, family's social integration, and community resources.

Responsibility for assessing needs

What to do if you're worried a child is being abused[2] identifies that anyone whose work brings them into contact with children and families is responsible for assessing needs, but highlights the particular responsibility of those working in social care, healthcare, education, and the criminal justice services. The document focuses on what practitioners should do when they have concerns that children are at risk of significant harm,

Gerri Clay, University of Plymouth

what happens once concerns have been reported, what further contributions practitioners may make to assessing, planning, working with, and reviewing children's progress, and, finally, the legislative framework in which children's welfare is safeguarded and promoted.

Further reading

Department of Health, Department of Education and Science (2004). *National Service Framework for children, young people and maternity services: core standards.* Department of Health London.
📖 www.doh.gov.uk/safeguardingchildren/index.htm

1 Department of Health, Department for Education and Employment (2000). *Framework for the assessment of children in need and their families.* Stationery Office.
2 Department of Health (2003). *What to do if you're worried a child is being abused.* Department of Health, London

What to do if you suspect a child is being abused or neglected

Practitioner has concerns

- The practitioner discusses the case with a senior colleague, supervisor, or manager.
- If concerns remain after the discussion, the practitioner refers the case to social services and documents concerns within 48 hours.
- Social services acknowledge the referral and decide on action within a working day.
- If action is deemed necessary, social services conduct an *initial assessment* (see below). If no action is necessary, they feed back to the referring practitioner and may make referrals.
- If there are concerns about the child's immediate safety, *emergency action* (see below) is taken.

Initial assessment

- The initial assessment is completed within 7 working days and may result in identification of a child in need. If no social services intervention is needed, the referring practitioner will be informed and other referrals may be made.
- Where *no actual or likely significant harm* is identified, the social worker discusses the next steps with the child, family, and colleagues. Discussion may identify a need for other services, in which case the social worker leads a core assessment, coordinates provision of services, records decisions, and reviews outcomes.
- Where *actual or likely significant harm* is identified, social services meet agencies such as police and healthcare professionals to discuss strategy and may initiate an *s47 enquiry* (see below).

Emergency action

- Immediate strategy discussion between social services and other relevant agencies.
- Following legal advice, decisions are made regarding immediate safeguarding of the child and information-giving to the family.
- If no emergency action is needed, a plan for the child's future safety and welfare is agreed with the family and other professionals, and the outcome is recorded.
- If emergency action is needed, an *s47 enquiry* is initiated.

s47 enquiry (Children Act 1989)

- Where concerns are substantiated and the child is at continuing risk of significant harm, the social work manager convenes a child protection conference within 15 working days.
- If risk of harm continues, the child's name is placed on the child protection register, a child protection plan is prepared, and a core group is formed.

Gerri Clay, University of Plymouth

Following the child-protection conference

- The core group meets within 10 days, specialist assessments are commissioned, and the core assessment is completed within 35 days.
- The key worker and core group members develop and implement the child protection plan and commission the necessary interventions for the child and his/her family.
- The first child protection review is held within 3 months. If there are no concerns about harm, the child's name is removed from the register and the reasons recorded.
- If concerns remain after the first review at 3 months, the child's name remains on the register and the child protection plan is revised, implemented, and reviewed within 6 months until the concerns are resolved.

Further reading

Department of Health, Department of Education and Science (2004). *National Service Framework for children, young people and maternity services: core standards*. Department of Health.
⊞ www.doh.gov.uk/safeguardingchildren/index.htm

Safeguarding children: policy for England

Policy for safeguarding children has developed dynamically over the past decade. Legislation and policies are now in place that enable and empower healthcare professionals to safeguard and promote the welfare of children. Recent legislation and policy have been formulated following the tragic case of Victoria Climbié. This case highlighted the disastrous consequences of professionals failing to act in their duty to safeguard a child in need of protection.

When attempting to safeguard children, healthcare professionals must be aware of, and have a duty to follow, relevant legislation and policy.

Legislative framework

The Children Act (1989) provides a comprehensive legal framework for the care and protection of children. Together with the Children Act (2004), it aims to ensure that children are a priority. This means that a health care professional *has a duty to safeguard and promote the welfare of the child* and prioritize the child's safety over and above the healthcare professional's relationship with other members of the family.

Children's services authorities for England are to be established following the Children Act (2004), with the intention of making arrangements for ensuring that each person and body has regard to the need to safeguard and promote the welfare of children. Local Safeguarding Children Boards will be formed to develop policies for safeguarding and promoting the welfare of children in the area of the authority. The Children Act (2004) also requires healthcare professionals to have regard to any guidance given on safeguarding children by the Secretary of State. *This means that if a healthcare professional decides to depart from the guidance, he/she must have clear reasons for doing so.*

Safeguarding and promoting the welfare of children is defined by the Act as:
- protecting children from maltreatment
- preventing impairment of children's health or development
- ensuring that children are growing up in circumstances consistent with the provision of safe and effective care
- creating opportunities to enable children to have optimum life chances and to enter adulthood successfully

Policy framework

Guidance has been given nationally in the publication *What to do if you're worried a child is being abused.* In addition, every healthcare professional has a duty to be familiar with, and follow, local policy for safeguarding children. Principles of policy include:
- believe the child
- discuss concerns with your manager and other appropriate agencies
- refer to social services or police
- record all aspects contemporaneously
- continue until your concerns are addressed

Rachel Carter, University of Plymouth

Further reading

Department of Health (2003). *What to do if you're worried a child is being abused*. Department of Health, London.

⊞ www.everychildmatters.gov.uk
⊞ www.doh.gov.uk/safeguardingchildren/index.htm

Child protection: policy for Wales

The statutory provision under the Children Act (1989) applies equally to children and young people in Wales; however, the way in which child protection policy has developed is unique, as a result of the following:
- devolved government to the National Assembly for Wales
- the unique involvement of the Children's Commissioner for Wales (the first one in the UK)
- a commitment to revitalizing the Welsh language and creating a bilingual Wales

The All Wales Child Protection Procedures[1] were developed in 2002 as a way of unifying child-protection throughout the principality.

The Welsh Assembly Government and local health boards take a strategic lead, on behalf of health services, for children's services and child protection, with particular emphasis on inter-agency working. The Care Standards Inspectorate Wales encompasses a wide range of services, including regulating social care.

One of the fundamental ways to improve outcomes, in terms of welfare and safety for children in Wales, is for statutory and voluntary agencies to work together to keep safe all the children who are most vulnerable.

Recent developments include the publication of *Safeguarding children: working together for positive outcomes* (Welsh Assembly Government 2004) as a companion document to *Working together* (Welsh Assembly Government 2000).

All agencies and professionals should:
- be alert to potential indicators of abuse or neglect
- be alert to the risks that individual abusers, or potential abusers, may pose to children
- share and help to analyse information so that an informed assessment can be made of the child's needs and circumstances
- awareness of routes of referral and activation of procedures
- contribute to whatever actions are needed to safeguard the child and promote his/her welfare
- regularly review the outcomes for the child against specific shared objectives
- work cooperatively with parents, unless this is inconsistent with the need to ensure the child's safety.

The Children Act 2004[2] will mean that a major revision of the All Wales Child Protection Procedures will be necessary.

---

1 All Wales Area Child Protection Committees (2004). *All Wales child protection procedures* 🖳 http://allwalesunit.gov.uk/index.cfm?articleid=298 (accessed 3 October 2005).
2 Children Act 2004: 🖳 www.dfes.gov.uk/publications/childrenactreport/ (accessed 3 October 2005).

Mary Smith, University of Glamorgan

Child protection policies and procedures in Scotland

Policies and procedures in Scotland are similar to those in the rest of the UK, but there are significant differences in the legislative process. This topic outlines:
* inter-agency child protection procedures
* national child protection policy developments
* the role of the Children's Hearing System
* relevant legislation.

Inter-agency child protection procedures

Within every local authority area, a child protection committee, with representation from all agencies involved, is responsible for ensuring that there are procedures that will be followed when a child is believed to be at risk of harm. These are detailed in each area's *inter-agency child protection guidelines* and include arrangements for referrals, child protection case conferences, registration, and child protection care plans. If the level of parental cooperation does not permit the necessary interventions, then emergency orders granted, in the first instance by a Sheriff, or longer-term legal measures (see the Children's Hearing System, below) may be necessary to secure the child's safety.

National policy developments

In 2002, the Scottish Executive undertook a national audit of child protection practice; the findings prompting the establishment of a child protection reform team. Policy developments to date include *the Charter* for the protection of children and young people and *the framework for standards*, which identifies how all professionals are expected to function and will be the benchmark for national inspection. The function and accountability of child protection committees has been addressed by the team's most recent policy, which will ensure that all child protection procedures are standardized and determine lines of accountability and reporting mechanisms.

The Children's Hearing System

Unique to Scotland since 1971, and reflecting awareness that a court-room setting was not the best place to meet a child's needs, this system utilizes highly trained lay people who sit on a children's panel. Panels work alongside a reporter, who has the responsibility of determining which cases referred should be heard within this legislative system and which may respond to voluntary processes. The panel can use its powers to, for example, legally oblige a parent to comply with social work supervision, and can determine conditions such as with whom a child may reside. Originally established under the Social Work (Scotland) Act (1968), the legislative powers of the system are now enshrined in the Children (Scotland) Act (1995).

Ruth Mitchell and Marjorie Keys, Napier University Edinburgh

Relevant legislation

The Children (Scotland) Act (1995), which states that legal orders should only be made if there is no other way to secure the child's welfare, provides specific orders for the emergency protection of children. Other legislation that is relevant to child protection policy includes the Age of Legal Capacity (Scotland) Act (1991), Data Protection Act (1998), and Protection of Children (Scotland) Act (2003).

Further reading

Daniel, B. (2004). An overview of the Scottish multidisciplinary child-protection review. *Child and Family Social Work*, **9**(3), 247–57.

Scottish Executive website also provides links to the Children's Hearing website. www.scotland.gov.uk

Child protection policies and procedures in Northern Ireland

In 2005, the four Area Child Protection Committees for Northern Ireland produced Regional Child Protection policies and procedures for the first time. This guidance is based on *Cooperating to safeguard children*.[1]

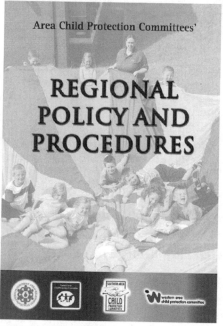

Reproduced with permission of Brenda Creaney, Directorate Manager/Principal Nurse, Royal Belfast Hospital for Sick Children.

Child protection procedures apply if you
- Work directly with children.[1]
- Work with adults who are parents or carers.
- Supervise, or are a colleague of, those who have contact with children or their parents/carers.
- Are a concerned member of the public.

Brenda Creaney, Royal Hospitals Northern Ireland

Principles
- The child's welfare must always be *paramount* and overrides all other considerations.
- Listening to and engaging children and their families is crucial to ensure their full *participation* when decisions are being made that affect them.
- Children and their families should receive responses and services that engage them as *partners* in problem-solving.
- Children and their families have a right to services that are designed to best meet their assessed need, regardless of their gender, racial group, age, religious belief, political opinion, or sexual orientation.

Definitions
- Child protection policies and procedures apply to all children and young people under 18 years of age, including arrangements for children upon their birth.
- Child abuse occurs when a child is harmed or not provided with proper care.

Types of abuse
- Physical abuse: deliberate physical injury to a child or wilful or neglectful failure to prevent physical injury or suffering.
- Neglect: the persistent failure to meet a child's physical, emotional, and/or psychological needs, which is likely to result in significant harm.
- Emotional abuse: the persistent emotional ill-treatment of a child such as to cause severe and persistent adverse effects on the child's emotional development.
- Sexual abuse: forcing or enticing a child to take part in sexual activities. The activities may involve physical contact, including penetrative or non-penetrative acts.

A child may be at risk of suffering from one or more types of abuse and abuse may take place on a single occasion or may occur repeatedly over time.

If in doubt, every professional and every agency has the responsibility to consult or to refer the child.

Child protection process
Four stages:
- cause for concern
- formal referral and investigation
- initial case conference and plan
- core group meeting and review of ongoing management of the case.

Further reading
Department of Health, Social Services and Public Safety (2005). *Area child protection committees Regional Policies and Procedures*. DHSSPSNI Belfast.
🖳 www.childrensservicesni.co.uk

1 Department of Health, Social Services and Public Safety (2003). *Cooperating to safeguard children*. DHSSPSNI Belfast.

Chapter 16

Religion, culture, and spirituality

Religious aspects of food

For some people, food has a spiritual significance. Certain foods may be prohibited and, as such, form a vital part of people's everyday life.

Religious restrictions may affect the diets of Hindus, Sikhs, Muslims, Jews, and Rastafarians.

Some religions may not only have dietary customs, but also strict rules about how foods should be prepared.
- Halal meat—meat that has been slaughtered and prepared in accordance with the Muslim faith.
- Kosher meat—meat that has been slaughtered and prepared in accordance with the Jewish faith.

Both faiths believe that eating meat that has not been slaughtered in their religious way is wrong.

Vegetarians do not eat meat, and vegans do not eat any meat or dairy products at all.

Food	Muslim	Jew	Sikh	Hindu	Rastafarian
Lamb	Halal	Kosher	Yes	Some	Some
Pork	No	No	Rarely	Rarely	No
Beef	Halal	Kosher	No	No	Some
Chicken	Halal	Kosher	Some	Some	Some
Cheese	Some	Not with meat	Some	Some	Yes
Milk/ yoghurt	Some	Not with meat	Yes	Some	Yes
Eggs	Yes	No blood spots	Yes	Some	Yes
Fish	Halal	With fins, scales, and backbone	Some	With fins and scales	Yes
Cocoa, tea, and coffee	Yes	Yes	Yes	Yes	Yes
Fast periods	Ramadan	Yom Kippur	No	No	No
Alcohol	No	Yes	No	No	No

Martin Firth, University of Nottingham

Culture

Any definition of culture must contain three basic ideas:
• there are typical patterns of emotional, social, and intellectual behaviours
• they derive from a shared set of beliefs and values, including religious ones
• these patterns are adaptive to the environment.

Some of these cultural differences will include skin care, bathing and toileting, diet, discipline, and the life stage rituals of birth, marriage, and death.

Culture can thus be extremely important for many of the different people living in the UK and in the world.

In the UK, various laws have been passed that will give everyone, irrespective of their cultural background, the same opportunities in society. This will give children an equal chance achieve, learn, socialize, and practice cultural activities chosen by their families. These laws are:
• Race Relations Act (Amendment; 2000)
• Sex Discrimination Act (1995)
• Equal Pay Act (1970)
• United Nations Convention on the Rights of the Child (1998)
• Human Rights Act (1998)
• Children Acts (1989 and 2004).

Every employer must ensure that their employment policies abide by governmental legislation regarding employment, religious, and cultural rights for every employee as an individual in their own right, and in hospital such policies must be available to read and be taught and understood by all staff working there.

Further reading

Watts, S. et al. (2004). Culture, ethnicity, race: what's the difference. *Paediatric Nursing*, **16**(8), 37–42.
Beaver, M. et al. (2001). *Babies and young children*. Nelson Thornes.
⌨ www.sdhl.nhs.uk

Communication and modesty

Obtaining consent from patients and families should feature in the initial stages of every communication exchange.

We all have different perceptions of modesty. We should always establish what is acceptable to children, young people, and families.

Tips

- Initiate contact; introduce yourself by name, title, and your relationship to them.
- Establish what name and form of address the child/young person wants to be called (cultural expectations).
- Avoid language that may offend; do not make flippant remarks.
- Decide on the best form of communication appropriate to the circumstances. Use different interpersonal skills, e.g. body language and empathy, to put the child/young person at ease. Identify what personal space is acceptable to all parties.
- Establish a rapport with the person using a common ground of communication.
- Through feedback, establish what the child/young person and their families have understood.

Caress, A.L. (2003). Giving information to patients. *Nursing Standard*, **17** (43), 47–54.

Hermione Montgomery, Birmingham Children's Hospital NHS Trust
Janet Hetherington, Birmingham Children's Hospital NHS Trust

Challenge	Solutions
Ensuring consistency through multi-professional working	Everyone uses the same words for body parts
	Information is documented
	Liaise with different agencies, e.g. youth worker
	Access appropriate training
Involving children/young people and their families in decision-making	Consult and listen to their views about their care, how they want to be cared for, and change practice accordingly
Recognize where verbal communication is not possible	Engage with children/young people using their preferred method of communication, e.g. Makaton or drawing
Ensuring family involvement, where appropriate, but also recognize child's/young person's independence	Offering child/young person a choice regarding whether their family is present
	Be sensitive to the family's contrbution
Recognizing what the child/young person considers embarrassing	Remove stigma through honest and frank dialogue
	Use jargon sparingly and explain meaning
	Use humour where appropriate
Developing mutual trust where information is freely exchanged	Establish boundaries regarding confidentiality. Create suitable environments, which create privacy
Identifying and establishing cultural expectations	Access knowledge and resources (internet, community) regarding cultural issues
	Ask the child/young person and their family about their cultural needs
Relating treatment and care to lifestyle choices	Listen and establish the child's/young person's lifestyle and support them by accessing appropriate resources
	Keep informed about national initiatives, e.g. sexual awareness and obesity
Establishing understanding	Ask pertinent questions
	Obtain the child's/young person's and family's perceptions of what is happening

Cultural issues with the dying child

Judaism

The medical professional is held in high regard. There is very little mystique about medicine within the Jewish community. Questions from relatives tend to be direct and practical.

• Cremation is forbidden (Orthodox Jews).
• The family may wish to recite psalms and prayers (the Kaddish).
• The body should be handled as little as possible and buried within 24 hours of death, delayed only by the Sabbath.
• The Sabbath begins on sunset Friday and ends Saturday evening.
• It may be difficult to contact the family and other members of the Jewish community during the Sabbath because they do not answer the phone or travel (specifically Orthodox Jews).
• Close the eyes after death and wrap the child in a clean sheet or shroud.
• The family will contact a Jewish undertaker and synagogue.

Muslim

A Muslim believes that whatever takes place is the consent of Allah.

• The family may wish to face the dying child to Mecca (south-east in the UK).
• Relatives will whisper prayers in the dying child's ear.
• Family will recite prayers around the bed.
• Organ donation is acceptable on religious grounds, but not popular.
• Post-mortems are only acceptable if demanded by the coroner (the body belongs to Allah and should not be cut).
• The child should not be touched by non-Muslims.
• The Muslim funeral takes place within 24 hours of the death.
• Muslim procedure requires that the body is straightened immediately. Turn the head to the right shoulder (which allows the body to be buried with the face towards Mecca).
• Wrap the child's body in a clean white sheet.
• Do *not* wash the body, or cut the hair or nails.

African-Caribbean

The main religion is some form of Christianity (Pentecostal/Methodist). The family may wish to say prayers and sing hymns. Families are often more demonstrative than the average white family and can feel inhibited and restricted in UK hospitals.

• Post-mortems only agreed to on request of the coroner.
• There may be many visitors.
• Wrap the child in a clean white sheet.
• A burial is more common.
• The body may be bought home for viewing prior to the funeral.

Christianity

Church of England

• No specific requirements.
• Cremation and burial are equally acceptable.
• Post-mortems and organ donation are acceptable.

Alison Tait, University College London Hospitals NHS Trust

Roman Catholics

- Practising Catholics may wish for a priest to perform the sacrament of the sick.
- Relatives may keep a vigil by the bedside and say the Rosary.
- If a young baby has not been baptised, the family may request this to be done.

Sikhs

- Post-mortems are only acceptable if legally unavoidable. No objections to organ transplantation.
- Close the eyes and mouth and straighten limbs.
- The body is washed and white clothes put on before cremation. Cover the body in a white sheet or shroud.
- Do *not* cut the hair or remove any religious objects from the body.

Hindus

- The family may wish to lay the child on the floor; a link with Mother Earth.
- Post-mortems and organ transplants are acceptable on religious grounds.
- Funerals are arranged within 24 hours of death. All adults are cremated and generally children under 5 are buried.
- Close the child's eyes and straighten limbs.
- Do *not* wash the body (relatives will do this).
- Do *not* remove any religious objects from the body, including sacred threads.

Further reading

Dickenson, D., Johnson, M. (ed.) (1993). Cultural issues of the dying child. In *Death, dying and bereavement*. Open University Press.

Trans-cultural nursing

The basics

Coping with a period of ill health can be a time of uncertainty. This can be helped by the nurse encompassing trans-cultural principles into care delivery by:
- showing respect by always being approachable
- getting to know and understand what is required
  - being comfortable with asking children, young people, and/or their families about their needs
  - accepting that you cannot know every diversity, but knowing where to find out.

Definition

A culturally competent field of practice that is centred on the patient and has a focus on research.

Considerations

- A holistic approach to care delivery requires you to take into account lifestyle dimensions while considering:
  - availability of interpreters
  - gender-sensitive issues
  - provision of culturally appropriate information and education
  - multicultural play
  - naming systems
  - nutrition practices
  - parenting styles
  - perceptions and reactions
  - privacy/socializing
  - religious preferences
- You are also required to take into account your own culture.
- The quality of the assessment interview will influence the effectiveness of care.
- A cultural assessment tool can assist you in developing awareness of the cultural needs of the child and family.

Within nursing, there is a need to strive to provide care that is fair for all, and to balance this with individualistic holistic care. When respecting the uniqueness of children and young people in our care, we often focus on trying not to make them feel different. Being comfortable with difference is at the heart of trans-cultural care, and staff who value diversity by respecting differences help ensure care is culturally appropriate for each child, young person, and their family.

There are complexities with interpersonal communication, and while an interpreter will help prevent isolation, the possibility of misunderstanding is always greater when we communicate across a cultural boundary.

Further reading

Giger, J.N., Davidhizar, R.E. (2004). *Transcultural nursing assessment and intervention*, 4th edn. Mosby.

Royal College of Nursing (2004). Transcultural health care practice: An educational resource for nurses and health care practitioners [Online] ▣ www.rcn.org.uk/resources/transcultural (accessed 1 June 2005).

Watt, S., Norton, D. (2004). Culture, ethnicity, race: what's the difference? *Paediatric Nursing*, **16**(8), 37–42.

Lucelia Mackay and Leanna Will, Robert Gordon University Aberdeen

Research with children

What is research?

These are exciting times for nurses, in that all the clinical decisions made should be based on sound evidence and new knowledge. This is expected to be drawn from *research*. Research, quite simply, is systematic enquiry to answer questions or solve problems. In this way, in terms of nursing practice, new care can be planned. This will affect all areas of nursing, such as education, informatics, practice, administration, and management.

Essentially, there are two broad approaches to research design: quantitative and qualitative.

Quantitative research

Seeks causes and facts, establishing the strengths of relationship between variables, thereby producing data in numbers. Consequently, quantitative analysis deals with statistics, systematic collection of data, and its interpretation. It is usually prospective (predicting something to happen) or retrospective (calculating something that has happened), but in both cases, it is very useful if you have an existing question. Key terms that are used are presented in the table opposite.

Qualitative research

On the other hand, qualitative nursing research is a mode of systematic enquiry concerned with understanding human beings and the nature of their transactions with other humans and their surroundings, thereby seeking to understand the interpretations and motivations of people, rather than to explain why. It produces in-depth information from a narrow and relatively small sample and is flexible because you can reflect and respond as findings emerge. Qualitative research is especially useful if little is known about the area of the study, because the research can reveal processes that go beyond surface appearances. Qualitative methods have been criticized for not investigating causal relationships or making predictions because there is no controlled or systematic design, but it involves areas where there is little theoretical or factual knowledge. Key terms that are used are presented in the table opposite.

Mixed designs

The types described above are often viewed as a continuum, with one type at each polar end, but there are also mixed designs—a combination of both qualitative and quantitative approaches. Decisions about which type to use depend on what you want to find out.

Further reading

Polit, D., Beck, C.T. (2004). *Nursing research: principles and methods*, 7th edn. Lippincott–Williams & Williams.

Polit, D.F., Beck, C.T., Hungler, B.P. (2001). *Nursing research. Methods, appraisal and utilization*, 6th edn. Lippincott.

Coad, J., Lewis, V. (2004). Eliciting children and young people's views in research. 🖳 www.necf.org

Jane Coad, University of West of England

Key terms used in qualitative and quantitative research

Key questions	Quantitative word	Qualitative word
Who undertakes the study?	Researcher	Researcher
	Principal investigator	Principal investigator
Who gives the information to the study?	Subject	Participant
	Respondent	Informant
What is being studied?	Variables	Attributes
	Constructs	Phenomena
	Concepts	Concepts
How is the study organized?	Positivist approach	Naturalistic approach
	Controlled	Descriptive
	Experimental	Exploratory
	Scientific	Interpretative
	Predictive	In-depth
	Systematic	Rich accounts
	Causal relationships	
How is the research question set up?	Hypothesis	Aims and objectives
How does the sampling occur?	Randomization	Purposeful
	Control	
What types of data collection are common?	Questionnaires	Interviews
How is the data analysis organized?	Results	Findings
	Using statistical analysis	Emerging themes
	(numerical values)	Narrative descriptions
How is the quality determined?	Empirical evidence	Dependability
	Reliability of tests	Credibility
	Validity	Confirmability
	Generalizability	Transferability
	Objectivity	
	Representation	

Involving children and young people in research

Participation of children and young people in service design, delivery, and evaluation is central to the Government's agenda. One way in which children and young people can have their say is through the use of methods that successfully elicit their views about services. While there are important philosophical issues that must guide the involvement of children and young people in research, this section will briefly outline a range of the commonly used techniques.

Overview of possible methods

Interviews: individual and focus groups

- This is by far the most favoured, effective, and economical technique and includes one-to-one, family, and group interviews.
- Interview schedules should be well planned and tried out (pilot) beforehand to ensure that open-ended questions are used as much as possible.
- In group interviews, the researcher should consider carefully the setting up of the room, group support, peer/adult influence, and sustaining the interview. Number and composition of the group is important; a group of between three and six children and young people appears optimal.

Questionnaires

- Questionnaires are commonly used, but the children and young people need to be able to read, write, and understand their meaning.
- Questions should be carefully thought out and layout appealing, e.g. including pictures and illustrations.
- Careful piloting, with a group of children and young people, will help test the tool.

Visual art based

- Many art-based methods are commonly used in research, which can provide a child-centred forum using a familiar medium (i.e. art materials) to enable children to express their feelings.
- Examples include draw and write, graffiti boards, clay work, paint, scrapbooks, video, and photographs.
- They can be used alone or with other techniques.

Observation

- Observational techniques have been used widely in child psychology and also by some nurse researchers, both on their own or with other methods.
- In the present context overt participant unstructured observation is the most frequent approach taken.

Role play, drama, and storytelling

- Children and young people may find it easier to communicate through drama and oral techniques such as role play, storytelling, drama, puppets, and music-making.

Jane Coad, University of West of England

- However, some children may find this type of research challenging if they do not want to perform or do not have the required cognitive listening abilities. Thus, the facilitator must have well-developed skills in order for quality evidence to be collected.

Further reading

Christensen, P., James, A. (ed.). (2000). *Research with children: perspectives and practices*. Falmer.

Kirby, P. (1999). *Involving young researchers: how to enable young people to design and conduct research*. JRF/Youth Work Press.

Coad, J., Lewis, V. (2004). Eliciting children and young people's views in research. www.necf/org.

Ethics of research involving children

Fundamental issues to consider.

- In terms of children and young people, their effective and active involvement can only be achieved in an environment that encourages their ongoing involvement, safeguarding, equity, valued feedback, and empowerment. This should be embedded in all child-centred research.
- In the NHS, currently all research on staff, patients, and their families must be agreed by a local research ethics committee (LREC approval) before it commences (if the research is to be at more than one centre, it is known as multi-research ethics committee or MREC approval).
- There are also many well-thought-out protocols and guides designed to protect children and young people from unwarranted intrusion by potential researchers. Informed consent 📖 is fundamental to research with children and young people. Three other important issues are highlighted here.

Protection: access/gatekeepers

In research involving a young child, someone usually acts as a gatekeeper, providing or withholding access to the child participant. In most cases, this will be the parent or carer, but somebody else, such as a nominated member of staff, may act as a gatekeeper. This will have been agreed by the ethics committee before the study commences.

Confidentiality and anonymity

Formal guidance on research methods usually stresses the importance of *confidentiality* (this means you must not disclose information about the participant or site where the research takes place). A researcher must guarantee *anonymity* in any written documentation (i.e. comments or views are not attributed in a way that could be traced back to a specific individual).

Recognition and feedback

Recognition of the child's/young person's involvement is crucial. Small token gifts, such as stickers, certificates, and/or small gifts, can provide a modest 'thank you'. In more substantial projects, researchers may give vouchers or token payment in exchange for their involvement (with parental agreement).

It is now widely recognized that participants should have the opportunity to receive feedback from researchers about the outcome of the study. With young children, feedback may be done through adults known to them, but older children and young people should be given their own feedback.

Further reading

Fraser, S., Lewis, V., Ding, S. *et al.* (2003). *Doing research with children and young people.* Sage, London. 🖳 www.necf/org

Jane Coad, University of West of England

Consent issues

The UN Convention on the Rights of the Child calls for state parties to 'assure to the child who is capable of forming his or her own views the right to express those views freely in all matters affecting the child, the views of the child being given due weight in accordance with the age and maturity of the child' (Article 12).

- *Consent* is when a person gives full and informed consent either for a procedure or to be involved in a research project. Consent may be given by the young person (in law this is usually 16 years of age) or by another on the child's behalf, such as a parent or guardian. The person giving consent will be asked to sign an approved document pre-set and agreed usually by the ethics committee.
- However, emphasis is placed on whether a person is *competent* to give consent. This is when a child or young person, who has the capacity to understand fully a decision affecting his/her life, automatically has the capacity to make that decision, unless statute law states otherwise. This is known as the *Gillick competence* test after the Gillick case (1985) concerning under-16-year-olds' right to contraception without the permission of their parents. The court found in favour of the GP. This set a precedent because it allowed under-16-year-olds to consent to medical treatment provided they could show 'sufficient understanding' and 'competence to make wise choices'.
- Assessing competence in children and young people can be difficult, so researchers often also use *assent*, which is taken to mean the child's agreement to participation in the process when another, e.g. a parent, has given consent.
- Consent is not in itself sufficient; *informed consent/assent* is needed. In order to give informed consent, the person needs:
  - information about the chance to participate
  - to know about a right to withdraw from the activity
  - to know what their role will be
  - to know what the outcomes are intended to be.
- To be able to respond to all the above four aspects of informed consent, the participant (or someone on their behalf) has to receive the information, understand, and respond. This means that obtaining informed consent may be a considerable undertaking and daunting to achieve.
- Many researchers ensure that the child or young person continually understands during the life of a project. Thus explicit continuation of assent enables a corresponding and genuine right to withdraw at any point.

Further reading

Alderson, P. (2000). *Save the children: young children's rights*. Jessica Kingsley. 🔲 www.necf/org

Jane Coad, University of West of England

Paediatric emergencies

Recognizing a seriously ill child

Early recognition of the seriously ill child is vital. Intervention given in the initial stages of illness improves outcomes and stops the progression to cardiorespiratory arrest. Rapid assessment using A = airway (cervical spine immobilization in trauma), B = breathing, C = circulation, and D = disability can save lives.

Action	Rationale
A = airway	
Check patency/maintain airway	Partially/fully obstructed airway may be the problem; opening the airway may start breathing
	Proceed to breathing if airway is assessed as open and effective
B = breathing	
Assess rate	Tachypnoea is the first sign of respiratory distress
	Trends in rate over time are more significant than single recordings
	Bradypnoea highly significant = pre-terminal sign of exhaustion/CNS depression
Assess air entry/breath sounds	Chest movement /airflow should be equal
	Listen for breath sounds → stridor = inspiratory noise upper airway → wheeze = expiratory noise lower airway → grunting = serious disease exhalation against partly closed glottis causing positive end expiratory pressure → slient/reduced noise = obstruction/exhaustion—it is a pre-terminal sign
Assess work of breathing	Intercostals/subcostal/sternal recession/retraction = ↑ work of breathing
	Accessory muscle use → head bobbing/see-saw breathing = inefficient respiration → nasal flaring seen in infants
Assess colour/record saturations	Hypoxia = vasoconstriction/skin pallor
	Central cyanosis is a pre-terminal sign seen on mucosae of the mouth/nail beds

Melanie Kelly, Royal Cornwall Hospital Trust

Contd.

Action	Rationale
C = circulation	
Assess heart rate	Tachycardia occurs to maintain tissue oxygenation, if this fails → hypoxia/acidosis → bradycardia = pre-terminal sign → cardiorespiratory arrest imminent
	Trends in rate over time are more significant than single recordings
Assess blood pressure	Caution: hypotension is a late sign of illness = pre-terminal → cardiorespiratory arrest imminent
Assess peripheral and central pulses	Peripheral pulse before ↓ central pulse → diminished central pulse = preceding cardiorespiratory arrest
Assess skin perfusion	Capillary refill time >2 s = early indicator of shock
	Progressive line of coldness/mottling: starts at digits, proceeds towards trunk = peripheral vasoconstriction
Monitor urine output	<1 mL/kg body weight/hours = inadequate renal perfusion
D = disability	
Assess mental state	Drowsy, agitated, lethargic = ↓ cerebral perfusion → ↓ consciousness level
	Do not ever forget glucose—check blood sugar levels

Further reading

Advanced Life Support Group (2002). *Advanced paediatric life support: the practical approach*, 3rd edn. BMJ.
European Paediatric Life Support (2003). *European Paediatric Life Support Course: Provider manual for use in the UK*, 1st edn. Resuscitation Council (UK).
🖵 www.erc.edu/index.php/doclibrary/en/viewdoc/83/3

Haemorrhage

Definition

The leakage of blood from blood-carrying vessels, because of traum
surgery, or clotting abnormalities. The volume of blood loss depends o
the size and origin of the vessel, i.e. arterial or venous.

Early haemorrhage indicators

- Tachycardia
- Normal systolic blood pressure
- Normal/reduced pulse volume
- Normal/increased CRT
- Skin pallor; reduced perfusion
- Tachypnoea
- Mild agitation

Late indicators

- Tachycardia/bradycardia
- Hypotension (pre-terminal sign)
- Reduced pulse volume
- Increased CRT
- Pale and cold skin
- Reduced respirations
- Minimal response to stimuli

Assessments of CRT and pulse volume (comparisons between centra
and peripheral pulse volumes) should be used in conjunction with othe
indicators above, because the former are not sensitive indicators in ch
dren. Assessments must account for variations in vital signs that occu
with children of different ages.

Early recognition and response to changes in vital signs prevents rap
progression to late indicators of reduced tissue perfusion. Early indicato
are comparable with hypoxia signs that are circulatory in origin, due t
trauma, surgery, or coagulopathy. Haemorrhage can compromise cardia
output for two reasons: tachycardia allows insufficient time for ventricle
to fill, and intravascular volume is reduced.

Later haemorrhage indicators are observed with progressive circulator
failure, hypoxia, acidosis, and poor organ perfusion, affecting the bra
(altered neurology), kidneys (anuria), and heart (cardiac contractili
reduced). The reduced circulating volume causes hypovolaemic shoc
requiring treatment and restoration.

Potential causes

Trauma

- Accidental injuries involving organs, e.g. ruptured liver or spleen
- Chest injuries (haemothorax) or bone fractures
- Head trauma or infant cerebral haemorrhages require specific
  management

Sarah Reed, University of Southampton

urgery

Post-operative bleeding, e.g. after tonsillectomy or prolonged spinal surgery

Bleeding from inadequate surgical repair (requiring return to theatre)

Acceptable blood losses are <5 mL/kg body weight/hour

lotting abnormalities

Bleeding secondary to liver failure

Haemophilia

Cardiopulmonary bypass (heparinization and dilution of clotting factors) for congenital heart surgery

Drug-induced, e.g. aspirin

Thrombocytopenia (platelet depletion)

Disseminated intravascular coagulation

Treatment

Assess airway and breathing; administer 100% O_2.

Secure venous (or intra-osseous) access.

Restore circulating volume:

- 20 mL/kg body weight bolus crystalloid/colloid assess response
- if no response, further 20 mL/kg body weight crystalloid/colloid bolus, reassess
- if no response, administer blood/packed cells (20 mL/kg body weight), with immediate surgical review. Cross-match patient's blood (time-dependent); administer blood type O-negative in real emergency.

- Check clotting and treat coagulopathy.
- Stem flow by applying direct pressure.

▶ Consider: the reduced O_2-carrying capacity following haemorrhage.

Nursing management

- Communicate effectively with multidisciplinary team; coordinate and document care.
- Evaluate response to resuscitation fluids; reassess frequently and report changes or stability.
- Assess and monitor blood loss from chest drains (mL/kg body weight/hour).
- Observe cannulae puncture sites and wound sites for blood oozing.
- Weigh blood-stained dressings if profuse loss.
- Reassure both the child and family throughout the episode, providing analgesia as required.

Further reading

Advanced Life Support Group (2001). *Advanced paediatric life support. The practical approach*, 3rd edn. BMJ Books.

Horrox, F. (2002). *Manual of neonatal and paediatric heart disease*. Whurr.

Sudden infant death syndrome (SIDS)

SIDS or 'cot death' is defined as the 'sudden and unexplained death of a infant under 1 year of age'; it most commonly occurs in children und 6 months. This term was invented in 1969 to acknowledge that, whi unexplained, most of these deaths are natural, with no blame placed o parents, who are already burdened by this bereavement. Over 300 babie still die each year as a result of cot deaths in the UK. It is particular traumatic because the infant is usually depicted as being previously well.

Today, UK statistics show that SIDS is the single largest cause of death i this age group.

Known risk factors include:
- prematurity, particularly birth weight <2500 g
- low birth weight for gestational age
- male babies
- low Apgar score
- CNS disturbances
- respiratory disorders.

More recently, other risk factors, namely overheating, prone sleeping maternal smoking, and co-sleeping have been recognized as risk factors A study commissioned by the Foundation for Study into Infant Death found that bed-sharing greatly increases the risk of infant death if the parent is a smoker, has drunk alcohol, or has taken drugs.

Bacterial infection is also thought to be a risk factor; this and the 'prone sleeping position' not only increased bacteria in nasal secretions, but also resulted in a temperature rise in the nasal tissues to 37°C or greater in previously healthy infants.

It is not possible to prevent these tragedies occurring, but 'reducing the risks' campaigns have been found to be effective, and the number o babies dying of cot death has fallen by approximately 75%.

Strategies include the following.
- Ensure the baby is put to sleep on his/her back, with light bedding and wearing nothing other than a Baby Gro and nappy.
- Avoid the baby's head accidentally getting covered, by sleeping the baby 'feet to foot', with the feet at the bottom of the cot, and with the clothes tightly tucked in. Using a sleeping bag avoids the risks associated with using a duvet and may reduce the risk of overheating.
- Smoking cessation—a mother smoking during pregnancy, or either parent smoking in the vicinity of the child once he/she is born, will also substantially increase the risk of cot death.
- Advise parents to seek prompt advice when the baby is unwell.
- A significant change is the recommendation that babies should sleep in the same room as the parents for the first 6 months of life.

Mair Sinfield, University of Glamorgan

Care after SIDS

Support the family during the acute grieving period.

Counsel the parents and reassure them that they are not responsible for their child's death.

Gently make them aware that the police may want to interview them.

Employ therapeutic listening skills to assist parents in the grieving process.

Allow privacy for the parents to be with their child.

Refer parents to appropriate resources, such as a funeral director, or support services.

Involve parents in the 'care of the next infant' scheme.

Further reading

eming, P.J., Blair, P.S., Sidebotham, P.D., Hayler, T. (2004). Investigating sudden unexpected deaths in infancy and childhood and caring for bereaved families; an integrated multi-agency approach. *British Medical Journal*, **328**, 331–4.
www.sids.org.uk

Near-drowning in children and adolescents

- Drowning: death by asphyxia caused by submersion in a liquid medium
- Near-drowning: the immediate survival after asphyxia caused by submersion.

Drowning has a worldwide incidence of over 100 000 per year; 40% of cases involve children under 5 years of age.

Risk of drowning/near-drowning is highest in the under-5 age group and male adolescents aged 15–19 years. In adolescents, predisposing factors include alcohol, drugs, suicide, trauma, and epilepsy.

Definitions

- Dry drowning (15%): laryngospasm will prevent water entering the lungs.
- Wet drowning (85%): reflex gasping will lead to aspiration of water into the lungs causing alveolar damage and pulmonary oedema. There is no significant difference in the effects of salt water and fresh water.
- In both dry and wet drowning, the resultant hypoxia can lead to bradycardia and cardiac arrest.

Main problems

Hypoxia, hypothermia, and cardiac arrest may have occurred.

Nursing interventions

- Assess ABC and start CPR if necessary; may need to continue for a long period of time if the child is cold.
- Protect the cervical spine if trauma is involved.
- Ventilate with 100% O_2.
- Pass a NG tube to relieve gastric dilatation: large amounts of water are usually ingested, which the child may vomit and aspirate.
- Monitor core temperature and re-warm as appropriate; monitor cardiovascular status closely; anticipate a drop in blood pressure as re-warming occurs.
- Record U&Es, blood gases, and haemoglobin.
- No evidence to support use of prophylactic antibiotics and/or steroids.
- If well, the child will still need observation for a minimum of 6 hours for signs of developing respiratory distress.

Support for family

The outcome of near-drowning events can range from a full recovery to severe neurological damage. Submersion time is the most important factor in predicting outcome. The effects can be devastating for the family.

Primary prevention

The majority of near-drownings in the under-5 age group occur in the child's home, in garden ponds, baths, swimming pools, or hot tubs.

Caroline Williams, West Wales General Hospital Carmarthen

osen, L.M., Koch, T. (2002). Submersion and asphyxial injury. *Critical Care Medicine*, **30**(11), S402–8.

uominen, P., Baillie, C., Korpela, R., Rautanen, S., Ranta S., Olkkola, K.T. (2002). Impact of age, submersion time and water temperature on outcome in near drowning. *Resuscitation*, **52**(3), 247–54.

Acute asthmatic attack

Present with a calm reassuring approach to both child/young person and family.

Assess ABC

- Is the child able to talk in single words or sentences?
- SpO_2
- Heart rate
- Respiratory rate
- Use of accessory muscles
- Level of consciousness/degree of agitation
- Peak flow

Assess and record above parameters every hour and before and after bronchodilator administration.

Administration of β_2-receptor agonist bronchodilators (salbutamol)

- In mild/moderate asthma: in aerosol form via a spacer (with or without a mask); spray in individual puffs, as inhalation is by tidal breathing.
- In severe/life-threatening asthma. In nebulized form, administered with O_2. May be given every 30 min.
- If no effective response:
  - administration of IV salbutamol as a loading dose, followed by continuous IV administration.
  - management should continue either within an HDU or an ICU.
  - cardiac monitoring is essential—salbutamol will produce sinus tachycardia and hypokalaemia (monitor serum potassium and supplement as necessary).

Aminophylline

- IV loading dose given over 20 min (cardiac monitoring—tachycardia and arrhythmias), followed by continuous infusion.
- Check theophylline levels at 1 hour following initial administration.

If child has had theophylline in the previous 12 hours, the loading dose should be omitted.

Administration of anticholinergic bronchodilator (ipratropium)

- In nebulized form, administered with O_2.
- May be repeated every 20–30 min in the first 2 hours.
- Maximum effect occurs after 30 min, but then lasts for 3–5 hours.

Corticosteroids

A single dose of prednisolone orally is effective if tolerated, otherwise IV administration of hydrocortisone.

Neil Bloxham, Plymouth Hospitals NHS Trust

Magnesium sulphate

Magnesium sulphate by slow infusion has shown some benefit when unresponsive to other therapies; ◆ however, there is inconclusive evidence as to its place in the routine management of asthma.

Observation and management

Moderate asthma

On a ward
• Find the position most comfortable for the child supported by parent, or lean forward with arms supported on a pillow on bed table.
• Observation frequency is determined by the response of the child/young person—initially observe hourly.
• O_2 by nasal prongs/humidified O_2 via face mask to maintain normal SpO_2.
• Bronchodilator: regularly. ▶ Ensure that there is medication prescribed to enable a prompt response to be made in the event of deterioration.
• Corticosteroid: orally, once daily.

Severe/life-threatening asthma

Within an HDU or an ICU.
• Find position most comfortable for child.
• Humidified O_2 via face mask to maintain SpO_2 above 95%.
• Continuous monitoring.
• Bronchodilators: frequent.
• Corticosteroid: IV.
• Manage IV therapy.
• Prepare equipment to enable intubation and subsequent ventilation.
• Prepare for transfer to an intensive care unit or retrieval to tertiary paediatric intensive care unit.

Discharge planning

• Ensure there is an asthma home management plan and explain it to child and parents.
• Provide sufficient medication.
• Inform asthma nurse/respiratory nurse within children's community nursing team.
• Discharge letter for GP.
• Appointment with GP or practice asthma nurse within 1 week of discharge.
• Appointment to see consultant respiratory paediatrician 4–6 weeks following discharge.

Further reading

Mackway-Jones, K., Molyneaux, E., Phillips, B., Wieteska, S. (ed.) (2005). *Advanced paediatric life support: the practical approach*, 4th edn. BMJ–Blackwell.
Rang, H.P., Dale, M.M., Ritter, J.M., Moore, P.K. (2003). *Pharmacology*, 5th edn. Churchill Livingstone.
Royal College of Paediatrics and Child Health and Neonatal and Paediatric Pharmacists Group (2003). *Medicines for children 2003*. RCPCH Publications.

The choking infant and child

Choking, i.e. obstruction of the airway by an aspirated foreign body, is a common problem in pre-school children.

Foreign bodies may consist of objects such as toys, marbles, coins, or, most commonly, food.

Infants and young children have:
• no or few teeth and narrow airways
• not fully developed the ability to chew and swallow, and the ability to time these with breathing.

As a consequence, objects placed in their mouths can be inhaled. Partial or total (rarely, if the object or piece of food is large enough) occlusion of the airway may result.

History

• Very important, because the diagnosis is rarely straightforward.
• Can help to establish whether the airway is obstructed by a foreign body or whether it results from underlying pathology, such as an allergic reaction or infection.

Ask:
• Were you or anyone else with the child at the time?
• What were they playing with?
• Did you see the child put anything in his/her mouth? If so, what?
• Have you brought a similar object with you?
• Has the child been ill with a recent respiratory illness?
• Has he/she had any recent difficulty in swallowing?
• Does he/she have any known allergies? If so, what?
• Was the child eating? Could he/she have eaten anything that he/she is are allergic to?

Signs and symptoms

Is the infant/child:
• talking?
• crying?
• coughing?
• wheezing?
• cyanosed (remember children do not go 'blue' but look pale with blue tinges to his/her lips, mucous membranes, and nails)?

▶ If the above are evident, the trachea is partially obstructed.

▶ The unresponsive child, with no spontaneous breathing, may have totally occluded his/her airway and should be managed as for choking.

Management

The management of choking in infants and children differs slightly. For the purposes of resuscitation and management of choking:
• infant: <1 year
• child: 1–8 years
• >8 years, adult methods apply.

Lesley Wayne, University of Plymouth

Physical methods of clearing the airway should be performed if:
   clear evidence of an inhaled foreign body and the infant/child has
   increasing dyspnoea or becomes apnoeic
   manoeuvres to open the airway of an apnoeic infant/child fail.

Keep calm. Do not increase the child's anxiety because this can cause
him/her to inhale the object and force it further down. Only if the foreign
body is easily visible and at the front of the mouth, should an attempt at
its removal be made by grasping the object firmly before removing.

Do not perform a blind finger sweep. This may push the foreign body
further down and/or cause trauma to the soft palate.

If the child is conscious, allow him/her to adopt the best position to
maintain his/her airway and encourage coughing. Administer high-flow O_2.

Management of airway obstruction

Management of the infant with airway obstruction

- Position infant in prone position with head down, along your thigh or knee for support.
- Support head by placing your hand under the chin, but take care not to obstruct airway further.
- Perform five firm back blows, between the shoulder blades, using palm of hand.
- Check mouth after each back blow.
- If still obstructed, turn the baby over to the supine position and perform five chest thrusts.
  - Use the same fingers and position as for chest compressions (one finger below nipple line using two fingers) in an upwards thrusting movement.
- Check mouth and remove any visible foreign body.
- If still obstructed, open airway using chin lift/jaw thrust.
- Assess breathing; if no spontaneous breathing is evident, perform rescue breaths, up to five attempts.
- Ensure that the infant exhales after each artificial ventilation.
- If two successful breaths in five are achieved, continue with rescue breathing until spontaneous breathing occurs or help arrives and baby is transported to emergency facility.
- If no successful breaths are achieved, continue with alternate 'back slaps', 'chest thrusts', and attempted rescue breathing.
- Transport infant to nearest medical facility via urgent ambulance.
▶ Abdominal thrusts are not recommended in infants because they may damage abdominal viscera.

Management of the child with airway obstruction

- Commence with five back blows, placing the child with the head lower than chest.
  - Either sit the child on your knee, leaning him/her forwards, or place the child over your knee, head down.
- Check mouth after each blow.
- If still obstructed, perform five chest thrusts.
- Stand the conscious child on a chair; if unconscious, place in the supine position on the floor. Use the same hand position adopted for cardiac compressions (one finger above xiphoid process). The technique used is the same as for compressions, but chest thrusts should be sharper and more vigorous.
- Check mouth and remove any visible foreign body.
- If still obstructed or if child is not breathing spontaneously, continue with rescue breathing (five attempted breaths).
- Ensure each ventilated breath is exhaled by the child.
- If two breaths in five are successful, continue with rescue breathing.
- If the child remains obstructed, perform five more back blows.
- Check mouth.

Lesley Wayne, University of Plymouth

- If the obstruction remains, continue by performing five abdominal thrusts.
  - To perform abdominal thrusts, place the child in the upright position, standing on a chair if conscious. Approach from behind and, using the heel of one hand positioned between umbilicus and xiphoid process, deliver five upwards thrusts towards the diaphragm.
  - If child is unconscious, place in a supine position and, using heel of one hand, deliver abdominal thrusts as described above.
- Continue with rescue breaths.
- The cycle of back blows, chest thrusts, rescue breaths, abdominal thrusts, and rescue breaths should be carried out until the obstruction is cleared or the child is transferred.

▶ Should the infant/child remain obstructed and subsequently become unconscious, remember to check for a pulse. If no pulse is detected or it is palpated at below 60 bpm, cardiac compressions should be commenced immediately and continued as for paediatric cardiopulmonary resuscitation.

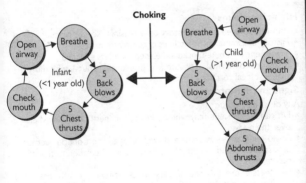

Further reading

BMJ (2001). *Advanced paediatric life support*, 3rd edn. BMJ, London.
Paediatric Life Support Working Party of the European Resuscitation Council (1994). Guidelines for paediatric life support. *British Medical Journal*, **308**, 1349–55.
Resuscitation Council (UK) (2000). Paediatric basic life support. Resuscitation Guidelines 🖥 www.resus.org.uk/pages/pbls.htm

Anaphylaxis

Severe, potentially fatal, hypersensitivity type 1 allergic reaction. An inappropriate and harmful response of the body's immune system to a normally harmless substance.

Aetiology

Activation/stimulation of sensitized mast cells by the allergic antibody immunoglobin E. This results in rapid degranulation and release of pharmacological mediators, e.g. histamine, causing local inflammation, urticaria, and angio-oedema. Any or all of the body's systems may be involved. Reaction usually starts within 15 min of exposure.

Triggers

Most commonly:
- foods—peanuts, milk, egg, tree nuts, seeds, fish, and shellfish
- medicines
- hymenoptera venom—wasps and bees
- animal hair
- latex.

High-risk groups

- Previous severe reaction/history of increasingly severe reactions
- History of asthma: most fatalities occur in asthmatics
- Treatment with beta-blockers—epinephrine less effective
- Reactions to minimal exposure (e.g. just touching nuts), with more than just local reactions

Signs and symptoms

Any or all may occur.
- Urticaria—transient itchy wheals, 'hives', and 'nettle rash' anywhere over the body.
- Angio-oedema—erythaema and swelling of any part of body because of vasodilation and release of mediators from circulation to tissues. If severe, may feel faint.
- Shortness of breath/wheeze/hoarse voice—airways go into spasm and produce lots of mucus, causing respiratory distress; child unable to speak in sentences.
- Distress—frightening experience, causing anxiety/confusion/ disorientation; feeling of doom.
- Pallor—clammy, cyanosis, and hypotension.
- Severe abdominal pain—leakage of mediators into bowel, causing nausea, vomiting, cramps, and diarrhoea.
- Collapse—cardiorespiratory arrest.

Assessment

- There can be great variations in the timing and nature of symptoms. Onset is usually within seconds or minutes but can be delayed more than an hour, and a late-phase reaction can occur (and continue for several hours), especially if allergen has been ingested and continued gastrointestinal absorption occurs.

Di Keeton, Southampton University Hospital NHS Trust

- Uniphasic or biphasic. If biphasic, patients seemingly recover from the initial reaction but have a second episode, often much more severe, a while later.
- Reactions occur along a continuum, and in combinations from mild to life threatening. ▶ If a single symptom of a severe reaction is present, the reaction should be treated as severe and epinephrine given.

Mild to moderate allergic reactions

- Urticaria and nettle rash: not life threatening; may be anywhere on body
- Rhinoconjunctivitis
- Angio-oedema: if mild and not affecting airways
- Abdominal pain: no cramps or diarrhoea
- Itchy/tingly mouth or throat: with normal voice, no stridor, wheeze, or respiratory compromise

Treatment

- Separate/remove allergen; ▶ Do not induce vomiting
- Oral liquid antihistamines (chlorphenamine)
- Mild wheeze; treat with nebulized β_2-receptor agonist (salbutamol)
- Observe for 2–4 hours for possible biphasic reaction

Severe anaphylactic allergic reactions

Assess ABC	Treatment
Airway: *blocked* • Hoarse, wheezy, swelling, itchy throat, lips, and eyelids • Stridor is sign of laryngeal oedema • May require urgent ENT and anaesthetic help	• IM ± nebulized epinephrine • IV chlorphenamine + IV hydrocortisone
Breathing: *changes* • Breathlessness: check noise, effort, efficiency, effect, and saturations • Unable to talk in sentences • Wheeze is a sign of bronchospasm • If necessary, follow guidelines for severe asthma (*asthma*) • May require ventilator support in very severe reactions	• IM ± nebulized epinephrine • IV chlorphenamine + IV hydrocortisone
Circulation: *not good* • Pale clammy circum-oral cyanosis, and severe abdominal pain • Tachycardia and hypotension • Ensure IV access; assess for shock	• IM epinephrine, treat shock with IV saline 10 mL/kg body weight • IV chlorphenamine + IV hydrocortisone

Further reading

Sicherer, S.H. *et al.* (2004). Advances in allergic skin disease, anaphylaxis and hypersentitivity reactions to foods, drugs and insect stings. *Journal of Allergy and Clinical Immunology*, **114**(1), 118–24.
Simons, F. (2004). First-aid treatment of anaphylaxis of food: focus on epinephrine. *Journal of Allergy and Clinical Immunology*, **113**(5), 838–44.
Anaphylaxis campaign. 🖳 www.anaphylaxis.org.uk

Management of hypothermia

A person is considered to be suffering from hypothermia if he/she has a core body temperature of 35°C or less.

Children and infants are more susceptible to developing hypothermia (i.e. the body loses its ability to keep warm) because of to their relatively large surface area for body mass and thinner layer of subcutaneous fat, so reducing their ability to conserve heat. Newborn babies are especially at risk because their temperature regulatory mechanisms are not well developed.

Resuscitation attempts and drug therapies are less effective in the hypothermic patient, and if steps are not taken to rectify the situation, the patient will die.

Hypothermia may occur for a variety of reasons, e.g. following near-drowning, burn victims, lengthy exposure of the sick or injured child or infant, metabolic disorders, sepsis, and drug overdose. Rarely, it has also been known to occur following the administration of antipyretic drugs, such as ibuprofen and paracetamol.

History
• What happened? When? How long? Environmental temperature?
• Known medications?
• Relevant past medical history?
• Known allergies?

Signs and symptoms of hypothermia
Mild (32–35°C):
• shivering
• slurred speech
• poor coordination/numb hands
• cool or cold skin/extremities.
Moderate (28–32°C):
• reduced level of consciousness/inability to make rational descisions
• pallor, mottling, and cyanosis
• muscle rigidity
• decreased respiration
• bradycardia/frostbite.
Severe (<28°C):
• loss of consciousness
• limbs rigid
• fixed dilated pupils
• cardiac arrhythmias
• respiratory arrest.

Management of mild to moderate hypothermia
• Warm patient gradually (move to a warm environment if possible).
• Remove wet clothing.
• Liquids by mouth if appropriate or consider use of warm IV fluids.

Lesley Wayne, University of Plymouth

- Monitor core temperature; consider use of thermal regulation equipment where appropriate.
- Monitor urinary output.

Management of severe hypothermia

- Airway management, high-flow/high-concentrated O_2, humidified and warmed to 40–42°C if possible.
- CPR as indicated.

▶ Avoid external re-warming of the whole body because this causes the blood vessels in the extremities to dilate, resulting in a secondary drop in the core temperature, hypovolaemia, and the possibility of fatal cardiac dysrhythmias.

Further reading

Desai P.R., Sriskandan S. (2003). Hypothermia in a child secondary to ibuprofen. *Archives of Disease in Childhood*, **88**, 87–88.

Kozole A. (1999). Hypothermia in a 7-year old boy: the Current Creek rescue. *Emergency Nursing*, **25**(1), 56–59.

Richardson J., Sills J. (2004). Hypothermia following fever. *Archives of Disease in Childhood*, **89**, 1177.

Multiple traumas

It is vital to assess/treat an injured child in a structured way, to ensure that nothing is missed and that you treat urgent life-threatening events first.

Structured approach:
- primary survey = AcBCDE
- secondary survey
- emergency treatment
- definitive care.

This approach has the same principles as basic life support/assessment of the seriously ill child (ABC); without the function of these, in that order, life is not sustainable.

Primary survey (AcBCDE)

- **A** = Assess/open airway:
  - use jaw lift technique (do not use head tilt/chin lift because these may cause worsening/death in children with cervical cord injury)
  - clear airway of any obstruction.
- **c** = Apply cervical collar:
  - only remove if neurological examination is normal
    ⚠ Normal cervical spine X-ray does not rule out spinal cord injury.
- **B** = Assess breathing once airway open:
  - give 100% O_2
  - if breathing, assist with bag–valve–mask/intubation
  - remember NG tube to ↓ gastric distension (oral route in cranio-facial trauma in case of basilar skull fracture).
- Treat life-threatening conditions now:
  - tension pneumothorax
  - simple/open pneumothorax
  - massive haemothorax
  - flail chest/cardiac tamponade.
- **C** = Cardiovascular status:
  - control blood loss
  - secure vascular access
  - if hypovolaemia present when external haemorrhage has been controlled, consider internal damage/haemorrhage
  - treat hypovolaemic shock using 20 mL/kg body weight of crystalloid/colloid; reassess regularly; second bolus/blood may be required
  - surgical involvement essential in all trauma cases
- **D** = Consciousness level: use AVPU
- **E** = Exposure: remove the child's clothes to assess for other injuries; keep room/child warm

Secondary survey

- Full examination, including log roll, X-rays, and history taking.
- Record vital signs regularly; if any deterioration, go back to start of primary survey.

Melanie Kelly, Royal Cornwall Hospital Trust

Emergency treatment

Treatments that need to start in the first hour to prevent the occurrence of life-threatening or limb-threatening events.

Definitive care

Appropriate referral to other professionals; may need retrieval to specialist care centre—vital to ensure optimum recovery.

This is a brief reference to multiple trauma only—further reading/training is vital.

Further reading

Advanced Life Support Group (2002). *Advanced paediatric life support: the practical approach*, 3rd edn. BMJ.

European Paediatric Life Support (2003). *European paediatric life support course: provider manual for use in the UK*, 1st edn. Resuscitation Council (UK).

Recovery position in children and young people

Although a number of recovery positions are currently advocated, no single one can be endorsed. However, the position adopted should:
- be stable
- maintain a patent airway
- maintain a stable cervical spine
- avoid application of pressure on the chest that restricts breathing
- minimize the risk of aspiration
- limit pressure on bony prominences and peripheral nerves
- enable visualization of the child's breathing and colour
- allow access to the child for interventions
- be easy and safe to achieve (including repositioning if required).

Unconscious infant (<1 year old)

Action	Considerations
Hold the child in your arms, *ideally face downwards*, with the head lower than the main part of child's body	To keep airway open
	To allow vomit and other fluids to drain from the mouth
	To keep neck and spine aligned

Child breathing but not responding

Action	Considerations
1. Straighten legs and position arm	If child is found on his/her side or front, not all these steps will be necessary to place them in the recovery position
Kneel beside child	
Remove any spectacles and bulky objects from his/her pockets	
Straighten the child's legs	
Place the nearest arm at right angles to the child's body, with the elbow bent and the palm facing upwards	
2. Move other arm and raise leg	
Bring the child's far arm across the chest, hold the hand, palm outwards, against the near cheek. With your other hand, grasp the far leg just above the knee and pull it up, keeping the foot flat on the ground	

Julie Black, Royal Aberdeen Children's Hospital

Contd.

3. Roll child towards you

With one hand, keep the child's hand pressed against the cheek to support the head	Tilt chin so that fluid can drain from the mouth
With the other hand, pull the far leg towards you, and roll the child towards you and onto his/her side	
Adjust the upper leg so that both the hip and knee are bent at right angles. Tilt the child's head back so that the airway remains open	The bent leg props up the body and prevents the child from rolling forwards. In an infant, this may require the support of a small pillow or rolled-up blanket placed behind the infant's back to maintain the position
If necessary, adjust the hand under the cheek to make sure that the head remains tilted and the airway stays open	

4. If child remains in the recovery position for longer than 30 min, roll child on to his/her back, then turn child on the opposite side—unless other injuries prevent you from doing this

Further reading

St John Ambulance, St Andrew's Ambulance Association, The British Red Cross Society (2002). *First Aid Manual*. Dorling Kindersley.

Resuscitation Council (UK) Paediatric Basic Life Support. ▣ www.resus.org.uk (accessed 13 May 2005).

Reasons why children arrest

The aetiology of cardiorespiratory arrest differs in children and adults. In children, physiology anatomical, and pathological differences more commonly lead to cardiorespiratory arrest—resulting from respiratory and/or circulatory failure—rather than cardiorespiratory arrest that results from cardiac disfunction/arrhythmia.

Primary cardiorespiratory arrest

- Cardiac arrhythmia, commonly ventricular fibrillation or pulseless caused by ventricular tachycardia.
- Onset abrupt and unpredictable, usually resulting from heart disease.
- Uncommon in children but can be seen with existing cardiac disease, after cardiac surgery, hypothermia, and poisoning.
- Immediate defibrillation is required. Delays reduce the chance of return to circulation by 10% per minute.

Secondary cardiorespiratory arrest

- Sequence more commonly seen in children: occurs because of the body's inability to cope with the underlying illness/injury.
- Pre-terminal rhythm is bradycardia → asystole or pulseless electrical activity.
- Can arise from respiratory failure → inadequate oxygenation → hypoxia + hypercapnia + acidosis → cell damage + death → cardiac arrest.
- Can arise from circulatory failure → organs deprived of essential nutrients/O_2 + unable to remove waste products → hypoxia + acidosis. Inadequate circulation → vital organs underperfused.
- Body will activate physiological responses → compensated respiratory/circulatory failure. If no medical interventions, → decompensated respiratory/circulatory failure. If still no medical interventions, → cardiac arrest.
- Respiratory and circulatory failure can occur separately or together; however, both will always unite as the body's condition worsens.
- Outcome of cardiorespiratory arrest is very poor. Early recognition of and intervention in the seriously ill child is vital.
- Knowledge of the underlying physiological and anatomical differences in children is important. These differences are often linked to the common illnesses/injuries that can lead to cardiorespiratory arrest.
- Always call for senior/specialist help as soon as possible.

Melanie Kelly, Royal Cornwall Hospital Trust

Common underlying causes in children

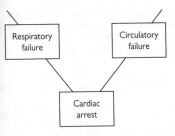

Respiratory		Circulatory	
Distress	**Depression**	**Fluid loss**	**Maldistributon**
Asthma	Convulsions	Blood loss	Septic shock
Croup	Head injury	Gastroenteritis	Anaphylaxis
Foreign body	Poisoning	Burns	Cardiac disease

Paediatric resuscitation trolleys

'The equipment used for cardiopulmonary resuscitation (including defibrillators) and the layout of equipment and drugs on resuscitation trolleys should be standardized throughout the institution'.[1]

It is essential that in all paediatric cardiac arrests, basic life support is carried out efficiently and effectively. No specific equipment is required for basic life support. As resuscitation equipment arrives, it should be used to enhance basic life support and initiate more advanced life support techniques.

Standardization of resuscitation equipment and trolley layout should reduce the likelihood of an equipment error occurring at arrest calls. A standardized layout will also enable ease of checking and formal regular audit.

A suggested equipment list that may be used as a template for the standardization of resuscitation trolleys follows. All areas where children are seen, from PICUs to out-patients, should have identical core resuscitation equipment in a standard format. Additional equipment may be permitted in specialist areas, relevant to the dependency of the children cared for. However, all additions should be discussed with, and approved by, the local resuscitation department/committee.

For ease of access, the trolley should be laid out following the ABCD approach. D relates to drugs and fluids, rather than disability.

Paediatric resuscitation equipment

Airway

- Oropharyngeal airways: 000, 00, 0, 1, 2, 3, 4
- Nasopharyngeal airways: child and adult
- ET tubes:
  - 2.0–6.0 (uncuffed; 1/2 size increments)
  - 6.0–8.0 (cuffed; 1/2 size increments)
- Laryngoscopes: × 2 + batteries
- Laryngoscope blades (fibre optic)
  - Miller 0
  - Miller 1
  - Robert Shaw 1
  - MacKintosh 2, 3, and 4
- ET CO_2 detectors
- Stethoscope
- Catheter mounts
- Ayres T-piece
- Tracheal stylet: small and medium
- Gum elastic bougie: 5 ch and 10 ch
- Magills forceps: paediatric and adult
- Tilly forceps: neonatal
- Lubricating gel
- Elastoplasts/cotton tape/duoderm
- Scissors: tough cuts

Pete Darley, Central Manchester and Manchester Children's University Hospitals NHS Trust

Breathing

- Bag–valve–masks: 1 × adult (1) and child (500 mL)
- Face masks: 00, 0/1, 2, 3, 4 (silicone clear)
- Oxygen masks: 1 × adult and child (Hudson non rebreath)
- Cricoid kit
- Pocket mask
- NG tubes: 6, 8, 10, 12
- Soft suction catheters: 6, 8, 10, 12
- Rigid-bore suction catheters: mini and adult
- Nebulizer kit: paediatric and adult

Circulation

- Alcohol skin wipes
- Cannulae: 14 g, 16 g, 18 g, 20 g, 22 g, 24 g
- Intra-osseous needle: 1 x size 14 and 1 x size 16
- Syringes: 1 mL, 2 mL, 5 mL, 10 mL, 20 mL, 50 mL
- Heparinized syringes
- Selection of needles
- Saline ampoules: 10 mL × 5
- Water ampoules: 10 mL × 5
- Extension sets: 10 cm and 50 cm
- T-piece extension sets
- Three-way taps × 3
- Bungs
- Gauze × 3
- Tape/cannula dressings
- IV administration sets: non-burette, free-flow set, and dedicated set

Drugs/fluids

- Drug trays × 2
- 0.9% sodium chloride: 500 mL bag × 2
- 10% dextrose: 500 mL bag × 2
- Haemaccel: 500 mL bag × 2
- 0.45% sodium chloride and 5% glucose: 500 mL bag × 1 (non-clinical areas)
- Mannitol 20%: 500 mL bag × 1

Outside of trolley

- Portable suction
- Defibrillator/ECG electrodes/gel pads
- Broselow tape/Oakley chart/profile charts
- Audit forms
- Cardiac arrest algorithms

1 Resuscitation Council (UK) (2004). *Cardiopulmonary Resuscitation: standards for clinical practice and training.*

Ward-based resuscitation

Resuscitation of children is often a stressful situation, requiring the nurse to concentrate extremely hard in a high-pressure moment in time. Even the most experienced children's nurse will find resuscitating children difficult and stressful. To reduce the stress and anxiety that children's nurses experience in paediatric resuscitation, training, teamwork, and preparation are key.

Each nurse has a responsibility to ensure he/she is adequately trained for the job he/she performs. Indeed, within the UK each NHS trust provides mandatory resuscitation training for their staff on a yearly basis. However, this is often not enough, because during a year resuscitation skills and knowledge are naturally lost. Therefore keeping basic resuscitation skills up to date is essential.

Regular scenario-based training should occur on each ward, with instruction from senior staff who are skilled in paediatric resuscitation and preferably hold advanced paediatric life support certificate or instructor status. These scenario-based sessions need not be difficult but should include the basics of ABC using a team approach.

Having a team approach is of great importance within the ward environment because you will be resuscitating with a resuscitation team and not on your own. Each member of the resuscitation team fulfils a specific role following the ABC approach, and each member of the team needs to be flexible enough to perform the roles of others. Again, it is the basics that are needed. The skill of opening the airway and using a bag–valve–mask is more important than being able to intubate.

Each team must have a leader who will follow the ABC approach and will ask what has happened prior to their arrival. If it is your patient, a brief explanation of the child's illness and what has happened is all that is needed, not a full hand-over!

Being prepared is equally important as training and teamwork. Knowing where the resuscitation equipment is and how to get it to the child is vitally important. In addition, knowing where the equipment is stored within the resuscitation trolley and how to access it is of great value in stressful situations. Most trolleys follow an ABC approach, but there is no national standard for resuscitation trolley layout, so you need to know your own trolley well.

Furthermore, it is vital that, as a paediatric nurse, you understand what each piece of equipment within the resuscitation trolley is and how it works. For example, a Miller laryngoscope blade is straight, while a Macintosh blade is curved. An introducer has a curved handle end, while a bougie is long and straight.

Bag–valve–masks come in different sizes, usually infant/child and adult sizes. However, the masks come in a wide range of sizes and two different shapes. Choosing a mask is easy, because it should cover the mouth and nose and not protrude into the eyes or past the chin.

Keith Bromwich, University of Coventry and Warwickshire

Part of preparation is to know the child you are looking after. This means being ready should the child become seriously ill. Make sure you know the basic and important information needed in an emergency. This would include the child's weight, which is the basis for working out vital medication doses in an emergency. The following table gives the vital basic calculations needed for any child if he/she were to become unwell.

	Calculation	Your dose/size
Weight	Age + 4 × 2	_____ kg body weight (age 1 year+)
Epinephrine	0.1 mL/kg body weight 1:10 000	_____ mL
Internal diameter of tube	Age/4 + 4	_____ internal diameter
Glucose	5 mL/kg body weight	_____ mL of 10%
How much direct current shock	1st and 2nd = 2 J/kg body weight	_____ J
	3rd = 4 J/kg body weight	_____ J
Tube length	Age/2 +12 (mouth)	_____ cm mouth
	Age/2 + 15 (nose)	_____ cm nose
Systolic blood pressure	Age x 2 +70	
Fluid challenge	20 mL/kg body weight	_____ mL (usually normal saline, 0.9%)

Know where to call for help. Shout for help; pull the emergency bell (it is not a cardiac arrest bell) and call 2222 (ensure that this is your hospital's emergency call number). If calling for help, be clear about exactly what you want. For example, 'Paediatric respiratory arrest ward 1'. Do use the term 'paediatric', otherwise you may end up with an adult resuscitation team!

Finally, the following table gives a brief overview of the basic roles in resuscitation of children. All resuscitation begins with the basics and advanced life support follows. Remember: these skills need practice on a regular basis to enable you to function effectively.

Basic roles in an emergency

Airway	Breathing	Circulation
Opening airway	Giving O_2	Chest compression
Suction	Bag–valve–mask	Drawing up medications
Inserting oral airway/nasal airway	Correct mask size	Recording observations

Basic life support

Basic life support for the child is not the same as for the adult. The general principles are the same, but specific techniques are required, depending on the age/size of the child.

Basic life support follows the ABC sequence.

- First ensure a safe environment for you and the child.
- Always stimulate the child first; if no response, start the basic life support sequence.

Airway
- Open airway:
  - infant—hand on forehead, tilt head = neutral position
  - child—same, but add chin lift = sniffing position
  ⚠ Suspected cervical injury, use jaw thrust
- Check airway for obvious foreign body—do not use a blind finger sweep

Breathing
- Look for chest movements, listen for breath sounds, and feel for expired breaths (take no more than 10 s).
- If nothing, give five rescue breaths (ensure two effective breaths). Each breath should last 1–1.5 s; take a breath between each breath delivered.
- Ensure chest rises/falls each time (reassess airway if it does not or follow foreign body algorithm if there is no effect on repositioning airway).
- Only move to 'circulation' when effective breaths have been given.

Circulation
- Feel for pulse:
  - infant—brachial/femoral
  - child—carotid.
  - if unsure, check for signs of life.
- If no pulse or <60 bpm or no signs of life, start external chest compressions.

External chest compression
Compression of chest up to half/one-third of the chest depth:
- rate 100 times min
- rhythmical movements
- compression to ventilation ratio:
  - 5:1 infant/child
  - 15:2 older child.

Landmarks for external chest compression
- Infants:
  - two-fingers on the lower/centre sternum and one finger below inter-nipple line
  - two rescuers: both thumbs in the same position, hands circling chest/supporting back.

Melanie Kelly, Royal Cornwall Hospital Trust

- Child:
  - heel of hand on sternum, with one finger above xiphoid process, shoulders straight
  - body weight used to compress.
- Older child (8 years):
  - two-handed adult technique: two fingers above xiphisternum.

Regularly assess ABC, keeping to that sequence until help arrives or breathing/circulation returns.

This is a brief reference guide only; further reading and regular training are recommended.

Further reading

Advanced Life Support Group. (2002). *Advanced paediatric life support: the practical approach*, 3rd edn. BMJ.

European Paediatric Life Support. (2003). *European paediatric life support course: provider manual for use in the UK*, 1st edn. Resuscitation Council (UK).

Airway adjuncts, uses, sizing, and potential hazards

An airway adjunct is used to maintain airway patency and avoid significant hypoxia-related complications.

There are two main devices: the oropharyngeal (Guedel) and nasopharyngeal airways. Both are simple and safe if used appropriately by trained and competent professionals and in conjunction with the correct airway-opening manoeuvres.

The oropharyngeal (Guedel) airway
- Prevents the tongue from occluding the oropharynx and supports an open canal from the teeth to the posterior pharyngeal wall.
- Commonly used in the unconscious patient and during the recovery period following tracheal extubation.
- It may not be tolerated if the patient has an intact gag reflex, because it may stimulate choking, vomiting, and laryngospasm.

The nasopharyngeal airway
- Passes from the nostril to the posterior pharyngeal wall and is tolerated well, even by the conscious patient.
- Do not use if a fractured base of the skull is suspected.
- The nasal mucosa is highly vascular and friable and there is a risk of haemorrhage on passing the airway, so it is not recommended if the patient has coagulopathy.
- Caution must also be noted if adenotonsillar hypertrophy is evident.
- It has been very successful in the management of Pierre Robin syndrome.
- If a small nasopharyngeal tube is required a cut-down ET tube can be used.

Airway insertion
- As with all procedures, explain the procedure carefully using understandable terminology and reassure the patient and his/her parents/carers prior to airway insertion.
- Once the device is *in situ* re-evaluation of the airway is vital to ensure patency has been achieved.
- Always ensure O_2 and suction are to hand.
- Any patient with a potential airway obstruction/difficulty must be monitored and never left unattended.

⚠ If a patient has a GCS score of 8 or less, their ability to protect their own airway will be compromised.

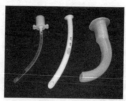

Lisa Marie Wilkie, Royal Devon and Exeter NHS Foundation Trust

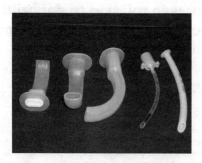

	Guedel airway	Nasopharyngeal airway
Sizing	Mid-incisor to the angle of the jaw against the face, concave side up	Tip of the nose to the tragus of the ear. The diameter of the tube must pass easily into the nostril, without causing sustained blanching to the alae nasi
Caution	Too short and it is ineffective; too long and laryngospasm, airway obstruction, and vomiting may occur	Too short and it is ineffective; too long and the oesophagus may be intubated
Insertion	In a child <8 years, use a tongue depressor and slide the Guedel, convex side up, over the tongue and into position. In a patient ≥8 years, insert the airway, concave side upwards, until the tip reaches the soft palate, then rotate it through 180° and slide it back over the tongue	Place a large safety pin through the flange of the tube prior to insertion or reconnect ET connector if cutdown ET tube is used. Direct the tube into the nostril and feed it in a posterior direction along the floor of the nose and rotate slightly as it passes the turbinates. Continue until the safety pin/connector is resting at the nostril
Caution	Risk of soft palate trauma in infants/small children if the Guedel is rotated, which could obstruct airway. Care must be taken not to damage the teeth or delicate mucosal tissue	Try other nostril or smaller size if insertion is difficult. Risk of inhaling the tube if not secured at the nostril end with safety pin or connector
	Reassess ABC	Reassess ABC

Further reading

Advanced Life Support Group. (2001). Advanced paediatric life support: the practical approach. BMJ.

ECG traces in relation to defibrillation use in children/automated external defibrillators in children

The aetiology of cardiorespiratory arrest in children is normally associated with respiratory insufficiency when the heart stops because of ischaemia or hypoxia secondary to another condition. The arrest rhythm is usually bradycardia, progressing to asystole, and successful outcome depends on prevention or prompt resuscitation.

In comparison, the aetiology of cardiorespiratory arrest in adults is normally associated with an arrhythmia (more commonly ventricular defibrillation or pulseless ventricular tachycardia). Hypoxia and acidosis are not initially present and successful outcome depends on early defibrillation.

The incidence of ventricular defibrillation in the paediatric population in the past has been reported as extremely rare; however, more recent evidence suggests that ventricular fibrillation as the primary arrhythmia occurs more frequently with increasing age.

In the paediatric casualty, basic life support with airway adjuncts is normally established before placement of a cardiac monitor to determine the rhythm, which may account for primary ventricular fibrillation not being identified.

If early recognition and defibrillation in adult victims improves outcome, one could assume that early defibrillation in paediatric patients presenting in ventricular fibrillation has potential to improve outcome.

Defibrillators

- To use manual defibrillators requires comprehensive training and knowledge to analyse the rhythm strip to inform diagnosis. The skills of ECG analysis and interpretation require practice, confidence, and competence, which limits the use of manual defibrillators to specialist practitioners.
- Automated external defibrillators and semi-automatic external defibrillators provide a series of spoken and visual prompts for the operator, interpret the patient's heart rhythm, and, if required, complete the process of defibrillation automatically.
- The main advantage of the automated external defibrillator is that the user does not require the skills of ECG analysis and interpretation.
- Automated external defibrillators may be used for children aged 1–8 years who have no signs of circulation. The device should deliver a paediatric dose.
- The paediatric automated external defibrillator has the ability to identify paediatric arrhythmias and achieves optimum specificity and sensitivity. Defibrillators for use in children are currently being developed that will deliver a fixed shock of 50 J via specific paediatric pads.

Further reading

Samson, R., Berg, B., Bingham, R. (2003). Use of automated external defibrillators in children: an update. An advisory statement from the Paediatric Advanced Life Support Task Force, International Liaison Committee on Resuscitation. *Resuscitation*, **57**, 237–43.

Marie Elen, Napier University Edinburgh

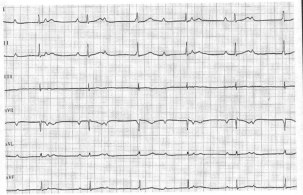

Complete heart block

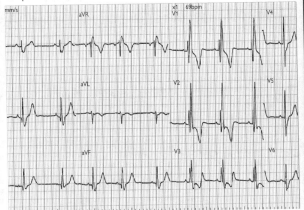

rbbb

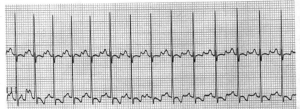

Sinus tachycardia

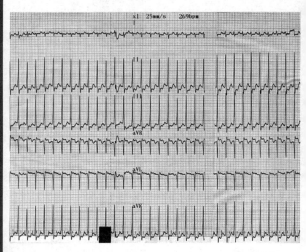

Supraventricular tachycardia

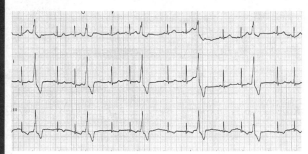

Ventricular ectopics

First-line drug and fluid resuscitation in paediatric arrests

In all paediatric cardiac arrests, it is imperative that the following actions are undertaken as a matter of priority before commencing any drug or fluid intervention:

• commence basic life support
• secure the airway
• deliver high-flow O_2
• assess cardiac arrest rhythm.

Attention should now move on to drug and fluid interventions.

Drugs

Epinephrine (adrenaline)

This is a powerful inotrope and vasoconstrictor, which is given to increase coronary perfusion pressures and improve oxygenation of the myocardium. This is vital for a successful resuscitation.

• Indication: absent pulse/low output state.
• Dose: first and subsequent doses:* 10 μg/kg body weight (0.1 mL/kg body weight 1:10 000 epinephrine).
• Frequency: Every 3 min until the return of spontaneous circulation or resuscitation abandoned.
• Route: IV/intra-osseous. Can be given via ET tube at a 10-fold dose (100 μg/kg body weight) via a suction catheter or NG tube passed to the tip of the ET tube.
• Notes:*An increase in the dose of epinephrine for second and subsequent doses is no longer recommended as routine. However, increasing the second dose to 100 μg/kg body weight (0.1 mL 1:1000 epinephrine) should be considered in an arrest associated with a vasodilatory pathology (septic shock).

Amiodarone

Amiodarone should be administered to patients with rhythms resistant to cardioversion or whose rhythms repeatedly revert to ventricular fibrillation/pulseless ventricular tachycardia following successful cardioversion. In all other circumstances, management should be discussed with a paediatric cardiologist or paediatric intensivist before administering therapy.

• Indication: refractory ventricular fibrillation or pulseless ventricular tachycardia. (Also used to treat supraventricular tachycardia or low output ventricular tachycardia to prevent progression to cardiac arrest.)
• Dose: 5 mg/kg body weight (maximum 300 mg).
• Frequency: single dose.
• Route:IV/intra-osseous.
• Notes: should also be *considered* for use in supraventricular tachycardia and ventricular tachycardia (with output) after discussion with cardiac specialist.

Pete Darley, Central Manchester and Manchester Children's University Hospitals NHS Trust

Sodium bicarbonate

Cardiac contractility is reduced in response to acidosis. Administration of bicarbonate will reduce the acidosis and improve the response to exogenously administered inotropes (epinephrine).

• Indication: prolonged cardiac arrest or cardiac arrest associated with documented severe metabolic acidosis.
• Dose: 1 mL/kg body weight of 8.4% solution.
• Frequency: every 5 min.
• Route: IV/intra-osseous.
• Notes: if possible give via a separate IV line to epinephrine because residual bicarbonate will inactivate subsequent epinephrine doses. If only single access is available, always use large flush of saline after each drug to purge the line.

Atropine

• Indication: atropine should only be used in the face of bradycardia causing a low-output state, with a strong suspicion of vagal overstimulation.

Calcium

A calcium bolus used to be included in cardiac arrest protocols. However, concerns that it may be harmful at a cellular level, together with an absence of evidence for its efficacy, has led to its removal from protocols. It should still be administered to patients with hypocalcaemia and hyperkalaemia.

• Indication: treatment in definitive cases of hypocalcaemia and hyperkalaemia.

Fluids

Crystalloid/colloid/blood

• Dose: 20 mL/kg body weight immediately as bolus
• Notes: each bolus should be administered rapidly followed by a re-evaluation of clinical signs before repartition

The ideal type of fluid to be administered remains a subject of debate. However, current recommendations support the use of human albumin solution for patients with meningococcal sepsis.

Recent trials have also suggested that crystalloids should be used as first-line therapy following trauma. It is also advised that the aliquots of fluid be reduced to 10 mL/kg body weight where intracranial injury is suspected.

The use of blood should always be considered after 2–3 boluses of fluid (40–60 mL/kg body weight).

10% dextrose

• Dose: 5 mL/kg body weight
• Notes: for the correction of hypoglycaemia. Dextrose solutions should not be used for fluid replacement because they will cause a precipitous drop in plasma sodium. In the presence of shock and hypoglycaemia, the dextrose volume should be given in addition to the fluid boluses.

Parents witnessing arrest procedures

Despite parents' right to stay with their child in hospital, it is particularly during cardiac arrest and resuscitation attempts that they are often denied this right. Despite growing evidence that supports parental presence, and the 2000 International Liaison Committee on Resuscitation's explicit guidelines stating that the opportunity to stay must be offered, allowing parental presence during resuscitation remains dependent on the views of the individual staff attending the arrest.

When parents are not present during resuscitation, they experience:
• greater uncertainty
• greater feelings of helplessness and loss of parental role
• poor understanding of the resuscitation event, including lack of understanding of the terminology used
• little opportunity to say goodbye when necessary
• greater feelings of guilt and of letting their child down
• feelings of mistrust in staff and subsequent greater vigilance if the child survives, creating reluctance to leave again.

Benefits to parents who are present:
• comforted by seeing everything has been done in the attempt to save their child
• the opportunity to prepare for possible death of their child and say goodbye
• a greater understanding of the resuscitation, with fewer unanswered questions
• feeling a part of the team and having the opportunity to contribute to the decision to stop a futile attempt
• regaining a parental role
• recognition that the reality of the resuscitation scene is less traumatic than that imagined
• no long-lasting traumatic memories of the event experienced, whether the child survived or died.

Parent responses and needs

• Parents exhibit a variety of behavioural responses. Crying is not an indication of not coping; stoic parents may be in crisis and unable to cope.
• Consider *individual* parents' responses and do not make judgements on perceived coping abilities.
• Witnessing resuscitation does not always imply parents will understand terminology used.
• Repetitive, easy to understand explanations are required. Try not to use terms such as 'resuscitation' or 'cardiac arrest' without clarifying understanding.
• The opportunity to make the decision to stay or leave the scene must be offered to parents. This must be repeated at regular intervals, because their decisions may alter during the event. The ability to leave and return frequently must be supported.

Fiona Maxton, Napier University Edinburgh

- Parents welcome the chance to touch their child's hand or foot. This should be encouraged wherever possible.
- A support person, preferably an expert nurse, rather than social workers or clergy, is recommended to keep parents informed and supported during the resuscitation.
- Silent support is often sufficient. It is difficult for parents to assimilate too much information.
- Remember to offer/provide support for those parents who choose not to witness the resuscitation.
- Parents are not concerned with assessing staff performances or detecting mistakes. Fears of litigation are unsubstantiated, despite this factor being cited as a reason to deny parental access.

▶ Parents experience great distress when their child requires resuscitation. This distress is not exacerbated if they choose to be present and, indeed, may be eased. *Not* being present does not reduce anguish and distress and can intensify these feelings.

Family and staff support following resuscitation

Following an unsuccessful resuscitation, parents need:
- Clarification and explanations, particularly if parents had not been present. This should be carried out through a multidisciplinary approach with appropriate personnel, including medical staff, nursing staff, social workers, and members of religious groups if relevant.
- Facilitation of parents' progression back into their lives without prolonged over-dependence on hospital staff.
- Ongoing and appropriate follow-up. This may be initially through the hospital social work department or liaison nurse practitioner, to address any unanswered questions and facilitate the grieving process.
- Referral/contact information on national community supportive groups such as Cruse.[1]

Following a successful resuscitation:
- Parents still require clarification of events with the use of simple, easy to understand terminology. Continually confirm parents' understanding of explanations, because they will often be uneasy about asking questions for fear of being considered foolish.
- Need support in gaining confidence to leave the bedside again without excessive fear of further cardiac arrests.

Staff needs:
- Informal and formal debriefing sessions are necessary to manage more emotive feelings that exist when parents have been present during a resuscitation attempt.
- Effective mentoring of inexperienced staff by expert nurses or medical personnel who are experienced in performing resuscitation, while at the same time caring for and supporting parents.

Summary points
- Parents have an inherent need to be with their child during periods of crisis that must be recognized and supported.
- Being present comforts parents by being able to provide comfort and love for their child, irrespective of their own anguish.
- Consider importance of family-centred care philosophy.
- Assess the individual families' needs appropriately.
- Never prevent parents from being present during resuscitation attempts.
- Provide appropriate support.
- Not every parent will wish to be present. Their wishes must also be respected without pressure to stay.

Fiona Maxton, Napier University Edinburgh

Further reading

American Heart Association in collaboration with the International Liaison Committee on Resuscitation (AHA/ILCR) (2000). Guidelines 2000 for cardiopulmonary resuscitation and emergency cardiovascular care. *Circulation*, **102** (Suppl. 8), I-1–I-139.

Eichhorn D.J., Meyers T.A., Guzzetta C.E., Clark A.P., Klein J.D., Taliaferro E., Calvin A.O. (2001). Family presence during invasive procedures and resuscitation: hearing the voice of the patient. *American Journal of Nursing*, **101**(5), 48–55.

Maxton, F.J.C. (2005). Sharing and surviving the resuscitation. Parental presence during resuscitation of a child in PICU: the experiences of parents and nurses. Unpublished PhD thesis, University of Western Sydney, Australia.

Tucker T.L. (2002). Family presence during resuscitation. *Critical Care Nursing Clinics of North America*, **14**, 177–85.

Basic life support teaching tool for parents/carers

Introduction

Basic life support consists of simple, yet life-saving, actions that can keep someone alive until help arrives. It is a useful skill for all to learn, particularly parents/carers of children who are at risk of respiratory/cardio-respiratory arrest.

Nurses may be asked to teach basic life support to parents/carers. The following framework may assist nurses in teaching and assessing, and can be used as an aide-memoire for parents.

Instructions should be kept simple and concise so that they are easily remembered. Arrange for an interpreter to be present as required.

The SAFE approach and ABC algorithm (APLS) are simple and easy to remember.

Teaching may be split into stages.
- Demonstrate basic life support, using resuscitation teaching dolls. Explain each stage: what, how, and why.
- Observe the parent/carer practising the procedure on the doll. Prompt him/her as necessary, being clear and calm in your instructions. He/she may feel anxious and will need support and encouragement. Enable parents to practise as many times as they wish.
- Ask the parent to recite the steps in the SAFE approach and ABC algorithm.
- Document details of the training in the child's medical records, nursing care plan, and teaching package if available.
- Arrange a date to reassess his/her knowledge and skills, and document competence/learning needs.
- Discuss arrangements for regular reassessment: 'use it or lose it'!

What to do	How to do it	Why it is necessary
Call for help — **SAFE** approach	**S**hout for help. Phone 999. **A**pproach with care. **F**ree from danger. **E**valuate **ABC**	Can save your child's life
Check responsiveness	Call your child's name. Gently shake or pinch a limb. Do not shake child's head because this can be dangerous	May cause your child to breathe. If no response, quickly move on to the next step
A Open the airway	Tilt your child's head back to the 'neutral' position for an infant/ 'sniffing' position for a child	So air can be blown into the lungs

Andrea Macarthur, Central Manchester and Manchester Children's University Hospitals NHS Trust.

Contd.

B	Check breathing	**Look**	—is the chest moving?	If your child is not breathing quickly, move on to the next step
		Listen	— can you hear any breathing?	
		Feel	— can you feel any breath on your cheek?	
	Breathe		Breathe in, then place your mouth over your child's mouth, or mouth and nose. If using mouth alone, pinch closed your child's nose. Give **5** quick breaths. Check that the chest rises and falls each time	Puts O_2 into your child's lungs. It might stimulate your child to breathe
C	Check the pulse		Feel for a pulse for **10** s in your child's neck or arm at the front of the elbow	To assess if heart is pumping. If no signs of life, quickly move onto next step
	Compress your child's chest		*<1 year* — put two fingers on the sternum (breast-bone) just below the nipple line and quickly press five times, moving the sternum one-third of the chest depth	To pump O_2 around body
			>1 year — put heel of your hand on the sternum one finger up from the bottom of the breast bone and quickly press five times, moving the chest one-third of chest depth	
	Continue basic life support		**One breath: five compressions.** Continue giving one breath to five compressions for 1 min or 20 times. After 1 min, call the emergency services if not already called	Pumps O_2 round your child's body until help arrives

Minor injuries

Minor injuries: overview

Within the UK, every year approximately 2.3 million children attend the accident and emergency department as a result of sustaining an injury, the majority of which are minor. However, it should be remembered that 'accidents' are the most common cause of death in children under 15 years of age.

Types of minor injuries
- Wounds
- Burns/scalds
- Soft tissue injuries
- Injuries to upper and lower limbs
- Pulled elbow
- Fractures
- Finger injuries
- Hand injuries
- Minor head injuries
- Bites and stings
- Foreign bodies
- Ingestions

Pain assessment
Nearly all children attending the accident and emergency department with an injury will be experiencing pain; therefore accurate pain assessment is vital. Various tools are available for measuring pain and these can be used quickly and effectively. Adequate analgesia should always be given prior to examination of any child attending with an injury.

History taking
Accurate history taking is vital, because obtaining a detailed history will alert the practitioner to potential problems of any underlying significant injuries.

Essential skills:
- knowledge of childhood milestones, growth, and development
- ability to take good history, remember the child may be unable to give reliable history
- build up a good rapport with the child.

Essential information:
- time, date, and place of injury
- was the injury witnessed?
- mechanism of injury
- previous medical history, including previous injury
- allergies
- immunization status
- consider non-accidental injury.

Melanie Hutton, Royal Hospital for Sick Children Glasgow

Examination

Prior to examining any child, always prepare the environment, ensure that all toys and equipment are developmentally appropriate and, where possible, there is child-friendly décor and a separate children's area.

How to examine.
- Always allow parents/carers to be present.
- Examine on parent's knee or where child is comfortable.
- Give a good explanation of procedure.
- Observe the child through play: distraction and other cognitive techniques may be useful.
- Use information obtained during history taking.
- Head-to-toe assessment.
- *Do not* focus only on the obvious injury.

Management

The correct management will depend on the type of injury sustained. However, in the case of all minor injuries, remember that there is always the potential for a more serious underlying condition to be present.

Discharge advice

- Arrange follow-up care if appropriate.
- Give appropriate written/verbal instructions.
- Give pain-relief advice.
- Advise on accident prevention/health education.

Further reading

Barnes, K. (2003). *Paediatrics: a clinical guide for nurse practitioners*. Butterworth-Heinemann.
Beattie, T.F., Hendry, G.M., Duguid, K.P. (1997). *Paediatric emergencies*. Mosby-Wolfe.
Davies, F.C.W. (2003). *Minor trauma in children*. Arnold.

First aid for burns

Commonly, burns can be attributed to several causes, and while each has distinct characteristics, they all require similar responses, with the notable exception of chemical burns.

First aid for burns is given according to the following simple steps. ▶ The person attempting to provide first aid must also ensure that their safety is not compromised, because the source of the burn may still pose a threat.

Stop the burning

Remove the source of the burn, thus reducing the child's exposure to heat energy. This may be achieved, for example, by putting out flames in the case of flame burns. Chemical burns should be irrigated liberally with running water to help dilute and/or wash away the chemical agent responsible for the burn. People suffering from electrical burns should be disconnected from the source of electricity in the first instance, taking care to avoid contact.

Cool the burn

Running cold water over the affected part for *at least* 10 min, and preferably up to 20 min, will dissipate heat energy to slow up and stop the destructive burning processes taking place. It is important that this is done promptly. Care must be taken not to induce hypothermia in children, and running water should be applied to the burn and not the whole child.

Relieve pain

The amount of pain that a child is suffering is not to be underestimated, and the best pain relief available should be administered while maintaining safety.

Cover the wound

While the wound should be uncovered to remove any clothing that could still be retaining heat, if anything is stuck to the wound it should be left until later. Forcibly removing material from the burn could potentially cause more damage. When providing a dressing for a burn in the field, nothing more than clingfilm should be used, so that the injury is not obscured. It is important to remember the formation of oedema and be sure not to wrap the clingfilm around limbs because it could act in a similar fashion to a circumferential burn. Blisters should be kept intact until the child has been admitted to the burns unit. However, if the blister is big enough to be painful and in danger of shearing off, then aspiration of the fluid may be indicated. In any event, the blister skin should again be left on until seen by a burns surgeon.

If it is suspected that the burn is in excess of 10% of the surface area of the childs body, an advanced life-support algorithm should be adopted that involves a primary survey of ABC, such as that supplied by the emergency management of severe burns course.[1]

Brian McGowan, University of Ulster

- **A**: airway maintenance with cervical spine control
- **B**: breathing and circulation
- **C**: circulation with haemorrhage control
- **D**: disability—neurological status
- **E**: exposure and environmental control
- **F**: fluid resuscitation proportional to burn size

1 Hudspith, J., Rayatt, S. (2004). ABC of burns: First aid and treatment of minor burns. *British Medical Journal*, **328**, 1487–9.

Poisoning management

With the array of colourful medications and attractively packaged household products, it is not surprising that childhood is the most common period of development in which accidental poisoning occurs.

Emergency measures

Whereas most children who overdose on drugs show few signs or symptoms, those who are severely poisoned require rapid and effective intervention. The assessment of the child should follow the basic principles of primary assessment and resuscitation, as required.

▶ In all cases of serious poisoning, early consultation with a poisons centre is essential.

Lethality assessment

At the end of the primary assessment, it is important to assess the potential lethality of the overdose. This requires knowledge of the substance taken, the time it was taken, and the dose. This information may be unattainable in the unwitnessed poisoning episode of a toddler or that of an unconscious or uncooperative adolescent. Some clues about the drug ingested may be available from physical signs noted during the primary assessment.

Tablets and capsules bought in with the patient should be examined for size, shape, colour, and markings, and a poisons information centre or drug information pharmacist should be contacted to undertake identification.

If the drug overdose is assessed as having a potentially high lethality or its exact nature is unknown, measures to minimize the blood concentration of the drug should be undertaken.

Activated charcoal

Activated charcoal, by virtue of its large surface area, absorbs many drugs and toxins without being systemically absorbed. It is used orally to limit drug or toxin absorption and is now widely used in cases of poisoning. As with most medications, giving activated charcoal to children can often be difficult. Great care should be taken if altering the taste of the preparation because some additives can reduce the charcoal's activity.

To aid administration, the activated charcoal can be given via a NG tube. It is important to note that aspirated charcoal causes severe lung damage, so airway protection is especially important in the child who is not fully conscious.

Gastric lavage

This can be indicated in children who have ingested significant amounts of drugs at high lethality, but is only likely to be effective if performed within 1 hour of ingestion. Its use also carries dangers, including aspiration, induction of hypoxia and tachycardia, and rarely, perforation of the oesophagus.

Stefan Cash, University of Central England Birmingham

Emesis

Attempting to empty the stomach by inducing emesis is no longer considered useful, regardless of the age of the patient or the method used.

The National Poisons Information Service (NPIS) enquiry number is 0870 600 6266

Poisons information can also be accessed via the NPIS web site TOXBASE 🖳 www.spib.axl.co.uk/

Further reading

Advanced Life Support Group (2001). The poisoned child. In *Advanced paediatric life support*, pp. 149–58. BMJ.
Olson, K. (2004). *Poisoning and drug overdose*, 4th edn. Lange Medical Books.

Reference section

Types of communication

- Communication is a transfer of information, and the flow of communication will be hindered if the non-verbal cues and the spoken message are incongruous.
- Effective communication requires good active-listening skills.
- In verbal communication, 7% of what we pick up relates to the content, 38% is vocal cues, such as voice, style, and volume, and body language, including facial expression, makes up 55%.

Verbal communication

- Voice and tone convey different messages, including pleasure, anger, frustration, and understanding.
- Using an interpreter, if the recipient does not have English as a first language, aids understanding.
- Accent, dialect, jargon, and language can detract from the message.
- Tone and intonation of voice can reflect one's emotion or attitude.

Non-verbal types of communication

- Physical aspects:
  - facial expressions, such as raised eyebrows, frowning, smiling, staring, and yawning, convey information
  - eye contact, such as staring, direct focus, or blinking, may indicate emotion and listening, but be aware of cultural differences
  - gestures—hand movements are most commonly used when expressing a message and tactile information demonstrates emotional expression; remember to be sensitive towards personal space.
- Creative communication, also known as aesthetic communication, includes creative expression, such as play and music.
- Symbolic communication makes use of religious, cultural, and cult symbols, which may include clothing, jewellery, and behaviour.
- Environment and smell, including furniture arrangement and the use of space and décor, enhance or detract from the communication process.
- Movement, such as rushing past a patient, can suggest a message or children may communicate their emotions through movement, such as rocking. Silence can convey comfort, tension, confusion, lack of understanding, fear, and reflection.

Communication systems

- Makaton, sign language, and Braille are universally recognized as formal types of communication.
- Picture books, photographs, drawings, shapes, and models are used successfully to convey messages.
- Written information, including email, internet, text, poetry, and prose, are examples of communication that are used widely nowadays.

Hermione Montgomery and Janet Hetherington, Birmingham Children's Hospital NHS Trust

- Storytelling, including the patient's stories, can share experiences, feelings, and feedback.
- Multimedia, electronic voices, and audio devices can offer alternative approaches to communication.

Action for Sick Children

Action for Sick Children is a registered charity, which was founded over 40 years ago, at a time when parents were actively discouraged from staying with their child and visiting hours were very restricted. The charity's mission is to ensure that healthcare in the UK meets the unique needs of all children, young people, and their families.

Action for Sick Children campaigns on all aspects of healthcare, whether in hospital or at home, and from national policies to individual family cases. The charity believes that family-focused environments, in addition to excellent medical services, are important to aiding recovery. At both local and national levels the charity harnesses the experience and expertise of children, young people, and their families, as well as experience and expertise of healthcare professionals. Action for Sick Children develops standards in child healthcare and lobby to implement them.

The charity is unique because it champions *family*-orientated health care. Action for Sick Children advocates a coordinated perspective that incorporates the views of families, children, young people, and healthcare professionals regarding the needs of *all* children and young people who access health services.

Today, the charity focuses on national issues together with its network of branches, who also work locally to improve health services for children and young people. The charity acts as a consumer information base via free leaflet guides for parents and a freephone helpline number (0800 074 4519), funds hospital facilities, such as play programmes and parents' accommodation, and sets up services to facilitate family visiting.

Major improvements in children's health services have taken place, and the charity continues to have an influential consultative role with key policy makers and government in the development of healthcare policies for children. Action for Sick Children has an established presence in the field of health education. The charity organizes and participates in training courses on health issues affecting children, young people, and their families, which are aimed at providers and commissioners of health services. The continuing changes in health service organization make education an important area in securing high standards in service delivery. The charity's long-standing expertise of consulting children, young people, and their families, together with experience in delivering training, makes them unique for this area of education.

Fiona Moore, Action for Sick Children London

The role of the Citizen's Advice Bureau (CAB)

Socio-economic influences on the health of children are well documented, and inequalities in health result in higher rates of admission for certain groups of children. Many of the families of these sick children may have personal, legal, and financial problems, which can negatively impact on their abilities to cope when a child becomes ill and is in need of hospital admission. The CAB service is a registered charity, which has been helping people to resolve issues such as these since 1939. Additionally, children and young people themselves may need the impartial advice that this service can offer. This is especially true of young people, who may themselves be parents and have credit card and other types of debt. The Office of Fair Trading has launched a campaign to help young people make sound choices when they are buying, for example, from internet companies using credit cards.

The CAB can help vulnerable families, in person, by phone, or email, or through outreach sessions in places such as family health centres. During the events at Alder Hey Children's Hospital and after the Redfern Inquiry, the CAB set up a centre within the hospital's patient and advocacy liaison unit to help the distressed families deal with the aftermath of the organ-retention scandal. Families can also access CAB information online, including frequently asked questions in a variety of ethnic languages, and download pertinent fact sheets.

The CAB is:
- Independent: CAB advisers always act in the interests of their clients.
- Impartial: they do not make judgements or assumptions about their clients. Importantly, the service is open to everyone.
- Confidential: the anonymity of their clients is respected and CAB will not pass on anything a client reports to them without their permission.
- Free—for all.

CAB advisers are able to:
- interview clients face to face and by phone to problem solve
- access the regularly updated electronic information database for current information
- help families to negotiate with people, such as creditors, or to appeal against decisions, e.g. social security benefit claims
- write letters or phone individuals on behalf of clients
- help clients to prioritize their problems, e.g. to sort out which debts are most important
- help clients with form filling, e.g. to claim for social security and other benefits (this is an especially useful function for families who may have literacy or other problems which inhibit them from accessing services or potential benefits)
- represent clients in court and at tribunals
- refer clients to CAB specialist caseworkers for complex problems or other agencies, as appropriate.

James E. Glasper, Citizens Advice Bureau Lymington Hampshire

The ongoing mission of the CAB is to ensure that social policy at local and national levels is responsive to the needs of all citizens.

Further reading

📖 www.oft.gov.uk/consumer/credit
📖 www.citizensadvice.org.uk/macnn

Common investigations

Barium meal/barium swallow/barium enema

Barium (Ba) is a radiopaque substance that can be swallowed as a porridge-like mixture. Moving X-ray images, called fluoroscopy, capture images of the gastrointestinal system as barium is swallowed and passed from the stomach to the small bowel. This can aid diagnosis of swallowing and digestion problems. A barium enema is passed up into the rectum and colon to aid diagnosis of large bowel disorders.

Bloods

Blood can be taken from a vein, an artery, or from the capillary bed (heel prick or finger prick). The blood may be sent for a full blood count (FBC), biochemical analysis (U&Es, TFTs, bone, etc.), microbiological studies (blood culture, antibiotic assay), blood gas analysis, cytogenetic studies, or numerous other tests. The type of test required dictates where the blood comes from, which blood bottle it is put into, and where it is sent to.

Bone marrow aspirate and trephine

Bone marrow may be drawn from the iliac crest under local or general anaesthetic and sent to haematology for in-depth study. This may aid the diagnosis and staging of leukaemias and other blood disorders. A trephine takes a small core of the bone marrow tissue for similar reasons but can give more information than an aspirate.

Bone scan (scintigraphy)

A bone scan involves injecting a low-risk radioactive isotope into the bloodstream. Following this, a few hours later, the patient lies on a scanning table. The scanner detects where the isotope is collecting in the bones by picking up the radiation emissions from the body. The detection of 'hot spots' aids diagnosis of conditions such as osteomyelitis and healing fractures of the bone. Particular care is required when handling the patient's bodily fluids (e.g. nappies) for 24 h after the injection.

CT scan

CT stands for computed tomography and was previously known as a CAT scan (computed axial tomography). A CT scan involves the patient lying on a scanner table which moves into a scanner shaped like a large polo mint. The scanner emits X-ray radiation through the selected part of the body in 'slices'. The computer displays the slices in order and allows the radiologist to diagnose hard and soft tissue disorders inside the body. More modern scanners, known as spiral CT, can produce better images more rapidly by spinning at speed around the patient in a spiral. CT is commonly used in cases of head trauma or abdominal and pelvis trauma, as well as many other conditions.

Andrew J.S. Brown, Derriford Hospital, Plymouth

Chlamydia swab

A chlamydia swab involves swabbing between the lower eyelid and the surface of the eye to remove some cells. These cells are then prepared and sent to the lab to diagnose the presence of chlamydia, a common sexually transmitted infection. A baby can contract the infection at birth from an infected mother.

DMSA (2,3-dimercaptosuccinic acid) scan

A DMSA scan is used to visualize renal scars and differential renal function, commonly after pyelonephritis or urinary tract infections. The scan involves intravenous injection of a radioactive isotope and then studying its passage through the kidney. It is conducted in the Nuclear Medicine department. As with the bone scan, particular care is required when handling the patient's bodily fluids (e.g. nappies) for 24 h after the injection.

EEG

EEG, or electroencephalography, is a study of the patterns of electrical activity within the brain. It forms part of a range of studies known as neurophysiology. An EEG involves the application of many electrodes to the scalp with glue and tape. These are then attached to a computer which traces the activity in various leads and produces a graph. The neurophysiologist can then decode the patterns and aid diagnosis of disorders such as epilepsy. The EEG study can be a one-off snapshot of a few minutes' duration, a continuously recorded study of several hours, or continuous EEG video telemetry, whereby a video camera records the patient's activity simultaneously with EEG tracing.

ECG

ECG stands for electrocardiography, and is the process of recording the electrical activity of the heart muscle. It involves the application of either three or ten electrodes to the chest wall and limbs. The computer records the activity between any two electrodes and produces a graph for interpretation by the doctor or nurse. This procedure aids diagnosis of heart conditions. The ECG can, like the EEG, be conducted intermittently or continuously. ECG monitoring can be used at the patient's bedside where there may be actual or potential concern about heart rhythms.

Echocardiogram

Echocardiography may be conducted to study the structure and function of the heart and its valves. It uses a probe on the skin to emit high frequency sound waves, ultrasound, which passes harmlessly through body tissue and reflects back off structures to provide an image of the echoes on a monitor. The operator can examine blood flow rates and pressures through the heart chambers and valves, as well as detect abnormalities such as atrial or ventricular septal defects, patent ductus arteriosus, and arterial stenosis.

Faecal occult blood

Faecal occult blood, or FOBs, is an investigation of the patient's stool for traces of altered blood. This might indicate a problem higher up the G tract or one involving swallowing blood. Pea-sized quantities are spread onto special collecting cards on three consecutive days and then sent to the laboratory for examination.

Immunofluorescence

This is the laboratory study of a specimen for the presence of particular viruses. It is commonly performed on a nasopharyngeal aspirate to screen for the presence of RSV (respiratory synctial virus).

IVU/IVP

IVU, or intravenous uretogram, and IVP, or intravenous pyelogram, are X-ray studies of the kidneys and ureters. They involve the rapid injection of a radiopaque dye into a vein and subsequent plain X-ray films at timed intervals thereafter. This shows the dye travelling from the bloodstream, through the kidneys and down the ureters into the bladder. It may demonstrate obstruction of the kidney or ureter due to stenosis, renal stones, etc.

Linogram/tubogram

This is simply the X-ray study of a line or tube, such as a Hickman line or nasojejunal tube. It is performed by administering a radiopaque dye into the line or tube and observing what happens to it. It can be used to confirm the placement and function of the line or tube if there is otherwise any doubt.

Lumbar puncture

A lumbar puncture is performed to obtain a specimen of cerebrospinal fluid (CSF) for lab analysis, or to measure the pressure of the fluid surrounding the brain and spinal cord. The LP may be performed on the ward and involves the child being held and supported curled up in a ball on their left side while a doctor passes a spinal needle between the vertebrae of the lumbar spine. Several drops of CSF can be collected from the needle or a manometer attached. The procedure is usually carried out to confirm the diagnosis of diseases such as meningitis, Guillain–Barré, etc.

MAG$_3$ (mercaptoacetyltriglycine) scan

A MAG$_3$ scan, like a DMSA scan, is used to determine kidney function and evaluation of upper urinary tract obstruction, particularly after serious or repeated urinary tract infections. The scan involves intravenous injection of a radioactive isotope and then studying its passage through the kidney. It is conducted in the Nuclear Medicine department. Particular care is required when handling the patient's bodily fluids (e.g. nappies) for 24 h after the injection.

MRI

An MRI, or magnetic resonance imaging, scanner produces detailed images of slices through the body in a similar way to a CT scanner. It has the advantages over CT of not using X-ray radiation with its associated risks. In addition, MRI produces clearer images of soft tissues. The patient lies on a table which moves deep inside a magnetic coil. This can be quite claustrophobic and noisy. The coil produces a strong magnetic field and the scanner detects the magnetic echoes generated within the water molecules in the body. The computer generates images of slices in any of the three dimensions and can even build a 3D model on screen. The images can be T_1 or T_2 weighted to show different structures in different ways. The magnetic field can be strong enough to remove metal from the body, so patients who have metal implants, pacemakers, etc. cannot be scanned.

Micturating cystogram

A micturating cystogram is an X-ray investigation of the lower urinary tract. It involves instilling a radiopaque dye into the bladder via a urinary catheter and observing what happens to it on X-ray fluoroscopy while the bladder fills and when it is subsequently voided. It can detect problems such as ureteric reflux and other problems of the bladder and urethra, particularly following a serious urinary tract infection.

M, C & S

This stands for microscopy, culture and sensitivity, which is the laboratory study conducted on many types of specimen to detect and identify bacteria and ascertain their sensitivity to antibiotics. The specimen is first examined under a microscope for bacteria or their indicators such as pus cells, white blood cells, etc. Then the specimen is smeared on an agar plate and placed in conditions conducive to bacterial growth. This is the culture phase. When bacteria have been grown they are subjected to a number of antibiotics and the effects noted. In this way their sensitivity or resistance to antibiotics can be ascertained. A full report on the specimen will not be available for 5 to 7 days, although a positive result may come back in a day or two.

NPA

An NPA is a nasopharyngeal aspirate and is obtained using a fine suction catheter and a sputum trap. The aspirate is sent to the lab for microbiological examination. The most common investigation is immunofluorescence for RSV, although other investigations can be performed. The result can be obtained within an hour or so upon request, and may be important in terms of the nursing management of the patient.

Pernasal swab

A pernasal swab is a specimen collected from deep within the nasal passages using a fine, flexible wire swab. It is usually collected to ascertain whether the patient is colonized with the bacteria that causes pertussis (whooping cough).

Swab

A swab is a sterile cotton bud used to collect any bacteria or viruses from a number of sites on the body, including wounds, nose, throat, eyes, etc. The swab is placed into the relevant transport medium and sent to the lab for processing. A result will normally be available in a few days.

Ultrasound scan

Ultrasound uses harmless high-frequency sound waves to provide a non-invasive means of visualizing structures inside the body. The ultrasound signal is generated in a probe and sent through the body tissues, using a gel on the skin surface to improve the signal quality. The sound waves echo off body structures and fluids and are detected by the probe. The computer generates a visual picture of these echoes which the operator can interpret. It has very many uses and is widely used in children as it is non-invasive and generally painless. Ultrasound may be used to guide a needle for biopsy of a tissue or aspiration of a cyst. In addition, when used in Doppler mode, ultrasound may demonstrate and measure the flow of blood through vessels and structures.

Urine

Urine can be collected as a mid-stream sample, from a catheter, from a nappy pad, or directly from the bladder using a syringe and needle (suprapubic aspirate). Many investigations can be performed on urine, including simple dipstick urinalysis, MC&S, toxicology, and other bio-chemical studies. The particular study required will dictate how the urine is stored for transport to the lab. A 24-hour urine involves collecting each urine passed in a 24-hour period, storing it in a large container and sending the whole lot to the lab.

X-ray

X-rays are a form of radiation generated in a controlled manner, which are able to pass through body tissues. The extent to which X-rays penetrate the various tissues depends upon their density. Air in the lungs, for example, will appear black on an X-ray film whereas the much denser bone appears white. When the X-rays exit the body they then strike a plate behind. This will either be a traditional film plate or, in the case of modern digital imaging, an electronic receiver. The films are developed and a translucent film can be viewed on a screen. Digital images can be viewed on a monitor or hardcopy prints produced on film. X-rays can use moving image technology, known as a fluoroscope or image intensi-fier, to view real-time moving images which can be stored. X-rays are not without their potential hazards, like any form of radiation, so their use is strictly controlled and due consideration given to the necessity of repeated studies.

Index